Soft Tissue and Esthetic Considerations in Implant Therapy

Soft Tissue and Esthetic Considerations in Implant Therapy

ANTHONY G. SCLAR, DMD
PRIVATE PRACTICE
MIAMI, FLORIDA

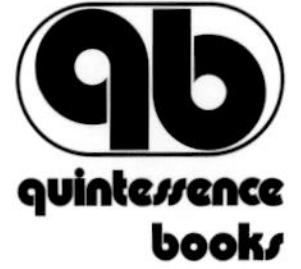

QUINTESSENCE PUBLISHING CO, INC
Chicago, Berlin, Tokyo, Copenhagen, London, Paris, Milan, Barcelona, Istanbul, São Paulo, New Delhi, Moscow, Prague, and Warsaw

Library of Congress Cataloging-in-Publication Data

Sclar, Anthony.
Soft tissue and esthetic considerations in implant dentistry / Anthony G. Sclar.
p. ; cm.
Includes bibliographical references and index.
ISBN 0-86715-354-7 (hbk.)
1. Dental implants. 2. Dental implants--Aesthetic aspects.
[DNLM: 1. Dental Implantation--methods. 2. Esthetics, Dental. WU 640 S419s 2003] I. Title.
RK667.I45 S385 2003
617.6'9--dc21

2002154463

Quintessence Publishing Co, Inc
551 Kimberly Drive
Carol Stream, IL 60188
www.quintpub.com

Editor: Lisa C. Bywaters
Design and Production: Dawn Hartman
Cover Design: Eric O'Malley

Printed in Japan

Table of Contents

Dedication

To my father, Seymour Sclar, for teaching me the virtues of choosing a profession that I love, achieving my personal best, helping others, and maintaining a sense of humor even in the toughest of times.

To my mother, Susan Sclar, for teaching me the values of discipline, a healthy work ethic, and a large dose of persistence in the pursuit of my dreams.

To my wife, Susan Ynclan Sclar, soul mate, love of my life, and the most solid person I have ever known, for unwavering love and support without which I could not have completed this book or enjoyed the limitless pursuit of excellence within my profession.

To my children, Samantha and Matthew, unknowing contributors to this project, giving of their precious time with Papa. I love you both fifty times around the moon!

Preface

Since Brånemark et al's elucidation of the scientific basis for osseointegration and the methodology for achieving long-term clinical success with implant-supported restorations, the dental literature has been replete with scientific and clinical information emphasizing refinements in implant hardware and detailing the surgical techniques to achieve regeneration of alveolar bone. As a result, the clinical applications of osseointegration have gradually been expanded to include the treatment of edentulous maxillary arches, various degrees of alveolar atrophy, and partial edentulism.

Although the immobility of the bone-implant interface was initially credited as the breakthrough for overcoming the biologic soft tissue problems that plagued predecessor implants anchored via fibrous encapsulation, the mechanism by which a stable soft tissue environment developed around the osseointegrated implant was far from understood. Furthermore, the detrimental effect of mobility of peri-implant soft tissues on the long-term prognosis of an osseointegrated implant was either ignored or greatly underestimated. As information concerning the anatomic similarities and important differences between periodontal soft tissues and peri-implant soft tissues became available, the profession made great strides in understanding the biologic processes involved in the formation and maturation of the structural relationship between the soft tissues and an emerging implant. Through experience, clinicians were also gaining a greater appreciation for the importance of establishing a stable peri-implant soft tissue environment. In particular, when osseointegrated implants were first used for esthetic tooth replacements, the lack of predictability and the unacceptable rate of compromised outcomes underscored the importance of proper surgical and prosthetic soft tissue management. While the profession focused on "magical incisions and flap designs" that would ensure pleasing esthetic results, many factors now known to play an important role, such as the history leading to tooth loss and the periodontal phenotype, went largely unrecognized. Although there was an evident lack of consensus in the implant literature regarding the need for attached tissues around implant restorations, experienced clinicians correlated the presence of attached (nonmobile) tissues with a decrease in soft tissue–related complications, facilitation of prosthetic procedures for the restorative dentist, and greater satisfaction by their patients.

Despite these developments, the need for practical guidelines and detailed information concerning the surgical management of peri-implant soft tissues in individual case situations and patient types has largely gone unanswered. This book was written to fill that void. It combines original concepts and techniques with information extrapolated from the specialties of oral and maxillofacial surgery, plastic and reconstructive surgery, and periodontology. Although the majority of the material covered is clinical in nature, the scientific basis and pertinent surgical anatomy for the successful use of the techniques and treatment protocols are introduced early on and reinforced throughout wherever applicable.

The reader is led through a systematic evaluation of the esthetic implant patient, including consideration of the various conditions and anatomic limitations that adversely affect or limit treatment outcomes. From there, a new classification system for alveolar ridge defects specific to esthetic implant therapy is presented; each of these defects is subsequently correlated with appropriate treatment options later in the book. Surgical instrumentation, criteria for optimal flap designs, general soft tissue management considerations, guidelines for the use of surgical maneuvers, and surgical techniques for management of peri-implant soft tissues in specific case types are all presented in detail. In addition, the rationale and indications for use of periodontal soft tissue grafting techniques are provided, with details of surgical technique as well as guidelines for peri-operative patient care.

Two innovative techniques are presented in separate sections. The impetus for the development of the Bio-Col alveolar ridge preservation technique is explained, along with expanded clinical applications and long-term clinical results. The vascularized periosteal-connective tissue flap (VIP-CT flap), which enables predictable hard and soft tissue site development of anterior maxillary implant sites, also is presented, including the rationale, anatomic considerations, and a summary of my clinical experience in using it.

The final section of this book presents a comprehensive approach to esthetic implant therapy and depends to some degree on the reader's understanding of the sections preceding it. Following a philosophy of care for the esthetic implant patient, hard and soft tissue implant site-development techniques are presented in correlation with the classification system for alveolar ridge defects introduced earlier. Prosthetic and surgical considerations for enhancing outcomes in esthetic implant therapy, such as the use of custom healing abutments, laser soft tissue sculpting and resurfacing, and platelet-rich plasma, are then described. Finally, a conceptual framework for esthetic implant site development is presented to give the implant surgeon an understanding of the sequence and timing of procedures. The treatment algorithms included in the Appendix help the reader navigate the challenges of treatment planning esthetic implant therapy in an abbreviated and easy to follow format.

The many clinical cases presented throughout the book demonstrate surgical detail in specific scenarios and can be used as a reference for the implant surgeon treating cases with similar history, anatomic presentation, and patient types. It is my sincere hope that the information in this book will help clinicians master new esthetic techniques that will ultimately benefit their patients.

Acknowledgments

Much credit is owing to the many individuals who helped shape my career and contributed to this project. First and foremost, the comprehensive training that I received in reconstructive maxillofacial surgery provided the foundation for my current treatment philosophy and led to the development of the new surgical techniques and approaches presented in this book. For this I thank Robert E. Marx, who provided an optimal learning experience during each resident surgery and always emphasized that it was a sound knowledge of anatomy and basic sciences that distinguished a true surgeon from a technician. A special acknowledgement goes to Stuart N. Kline, whose wisdom, discipline, and respect instilled in me a compassionate approach to patient care and the understanding that documentation and critical review of surgical outcomes play an important role in the professional development of a surgeon. I would also like to acknowledge Steven M. Holmes, who has played many roles—teacher, partner, and friend—during my surgical career. Thank you for providing a unique private practice environment that allowed me to focus on continued education, professional development, and quality patient care. Special mention goes to Matthew B. Hall, my mentor during dental school, with whom I shared many brainstorming sessions and published and presented my first research paper in oral and maxillofacial surgery, the profession that I love. Special mention also goes to Stephen E. Feinberg, who helped me organize and host the first implant soft tissue management course at the University of Michigan and then encouraged me to share my clinical experience by writing a book on the subject.

I would also like to acknowledge the many participants and colleagues who initially asked the questions addressed in this book during the lectures, conferences, and symposium presentations that I have given over the past decade. Special acknowledgment also must be made of the many restorative dentists who contributed to the results published in this book and of our local dental laboratory technicians: Peter Kuch, Klaus Lampman, Heike Alvarez, and Dale Cornelius. Thanks to each of the patients whose cooperation enabled us to continually refine our techniques and approaches, to the benefit of future patients and everyone reading this book.

I would like to thank my publisher, Tomoko Tsuchiya, for giving me the opportunity to write this book and for her patience, guidance, and encouragement throughout the process. A most deserved acknowledgement goes to Lisa Bywaters, the principle editor of this book, for her patience with my hectic schedule, her sacrifice of family time to work unusual hours and weekends, her continued encouragement, and her extraordinary skill and professionalism. I would like to thank François Fache for the many hours spent together working on the illustrations initially used in lectures and eventually included in this book. A very special thank you to Carmen Carnero, a highly skilled and talented surgical assistant, for her excellence in clinical photography, for managing the clinical images and compiling the statistical data presented in this book, and most of all for her enthusiastic oversight of procedural details that enable us to provide the highest level of care for our patients. A special mention goes to Elizabeth Suarez, our patient educator and treatment coordinator, for her professionalism and skill in educating patients about the quality-of-life benefits that implant therapy can provide and for closely coordinating their care with the restorative dentists and other implant team members. Recognition also goes to my clinical team—Tiffany Lutz, Fernando Venegas, Nan Boyle, and the entire staff at South Florida OMS—for their understanding and support during this project and during the related teaching activities that directly or indirectly impact their work environment.

Finally, I would like to acknowledge and thank my family and friends for all the support and encouragement they gave me during this project, despite the sacrifice and burden that it often imposed upon them.

CHAPTER 1

Beyond Osseointegration

Echoing the relationship between the periodontal tissues and a natural tooth, the supporting tissues of an osseointegrated implant must be organized not only to anchor the implant in the bone, but also to form a protective soft tissue seal around the implant as it emerges into the oral cavity. This so-called biologic soft tissue seal protects the implant by resisting the challenges presented by bacterial irritants as well as the mechanical trauma resulting from restorative procedures, masticatory forces, and oral hygiene maintenance. It has long been recognized that to be clinically successful, a titanium dental implant must form and maintain integration not only with bone but also with connective tissue and epithelium.[1] The term *soft tissue integration* describes the biologic processes that occur during the formation and maturation of the structural relationship between the soft tissues (connective tissue and epithelium) and the transmucosal portion of the implant. Although experimental and clinical research have only recently begun to focus on improving our understanding of the factors that can affect this soft tissue environment, our current knowledge indicates that the maintenance of a healthy soft tissue barrier is as important as osseointegration itself for the long-term success of an implant-supported prosthesis. The information in this chapter correlates the theory of soft tissue integration with the clinical practice of implant therapy.

Anatomy and Biology of Peri-implant Soft Tissues

An understanding of both periodontal and peri-implant anatomy and biology is necessary for successfully managing the soft tissues during implant therapy. Similarities between the periodontal and peri-implant soft tissues provide the anatomic and biologic bases for applying basic periodontal flap techniques and reconstructive periodontal surgery in implant therapy, while differences reveal the limitations that can be expected when various periodontal surgical techniques are used during implant therapy. Understanding these similarities and important differences, the surgeon can modify standard periodontal techniques to make them more suitable for use in implant therapy. Armed with this knowledge, the surgeon can formulate a soft tissue treatment plan that includes the appropriate selection and timing of soft tissue management procedures to ensure a healthy peri-implant soft tissue environment and the successful reconstruction of natural-looking soft tissues from which an esthetic implant restoration can emerge.

Comparative anatomy of periodontal and peri-implant soft tissues

If it is true that form follows function, as nature often demonstrates, then it should come as no surprise that peri-implant and periodontal soft tissues are remarkably similar. Various studies have demonstrated histologic, histochemical, and ultrastructural similarities in the architecture of periodontal and peri-implant soft tissues in animals and humans.[1–7] Studies such as these confirm the body's ability to organize soft tissues based on the functional need for transmucosal seal and stability shared by both a natural tooth and a dental implant (Fig 1-1).

Periodontal soft tissue anatomy

The macroscopic, microscopic, and ultrastructural characteristics of periodontal soft tissues have been described in detail.[8–12] The tooth is secured in the alveolar bone by a combination of connective tissue and epithelial attachments. Connective tissue attaches to a tooth in two distinct areas: (*1*) below the alveolar crest, the periodontal ligament secures the tooth root in the alveolar socket; and (*2*) Sharpey's connective tissue fiber bundles extend from the socket walls and are embedded in the acellular root cementum. Above the alveolar crest, gingival fiber bundles provide additional attachments to secure the tooth in the alveolus, but they also serve to immobilize the gingival tissues in relation to the supra-alveolar portion of the root cementum. Each gingival fiber bundle has a functional orientation and is identified according to its insertion and the distinct path it follows through the tissue. For example, the *transseptal* fibers anchor each tooth to its neighboring dentition. Running directly over the interdental septum and embedding in the supra-alveolar cementum of adjacent teeth, these fiber bundles contribute significant stability to each tooth in the arch. The *dentoperiosteal* and *dentogingival* fibers also are embedded in the supra-alveolar cementum and extend inferiorly and superiorly into the attached and free gingiva, respectively. The *circular* fibers run circumferentially through the free gingiva, splicing the fiber bundles running vertically to encircle the tooth. In addition to securing the tooth in the alveolus, the dentoperiosteal, dentogingival, and circular fibers play an important role in immobilizing the gingival tissues that surround the tooth. This tissue immobility, along with resistance to bacterial and mechanical challenges, contributes to the maintenance of a permucosal seal.

The epithelial tissues of the periodontium are divided into three types according to their form and function. The *junctional* epithelium attaches to the tooth and occupies the area between the most coronal attachment of supra-alveolar connective tissue and the base of the gingival crevice. The cells of this specialized epithelium are larger and have wider intercellular spaces and fewer desmosomes compared with those found in the sulcular epithelium. The junctional epithelial cells secrete a basal lamina on the surface of the tooth, and their attachment to the tooth is mediated through hemidesmosomes. Together with the underlying connective tissue attachments described above, the junctional epithelium forms a permucosal seal for the emerging tooth. The thin, nonkeratinized *sulcular* epithelium lines the entire gingival sulcus and provides the first line of defense against bacterial ingress or toxin penetration into the underlying connective tissue. The *oral* epithelium lines the external gingival surface from the crest of the free gingiva to the mucogingival junction. This relatively thick, keratinized epithelium, which is firmly attached to the underlying connective tissue via a network of rete pegs, provides resistance to the forces of mastication and oral hygiene.

An understanding of the vascular supply to the periodontal soft tissues provides the basis for successful soft tissue management during periodontal surgery, as well as the application of reconstructive periodontal techniques. The blood supply to the periodontium is derived from three main sources: the supraperiosteal

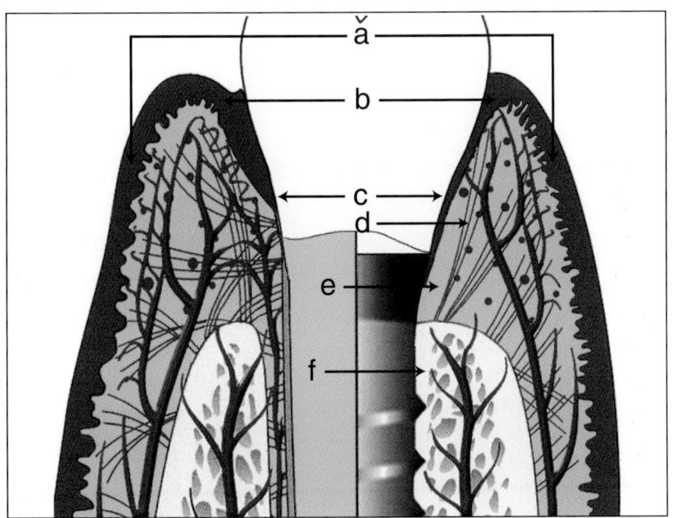

Fig 1-1 Comparative anatomy of periodontal and peri-implant soft tissues. The similarities between periodontal and peri-implant soft tissues are limited to the structure and function of analogous epithelial tissues: *(a)* Oral epithelium; *(b)* sulcular epithelium; *(c)* junctional epithelium. Important differences in peri-implant soft tissues include: *(d)* lack of connective tissue attachment; *(e)* hypovascular-hypocellular connective tissue zone adjacent to the implant; and *(f)* absence of periodontal ligament blood supply.

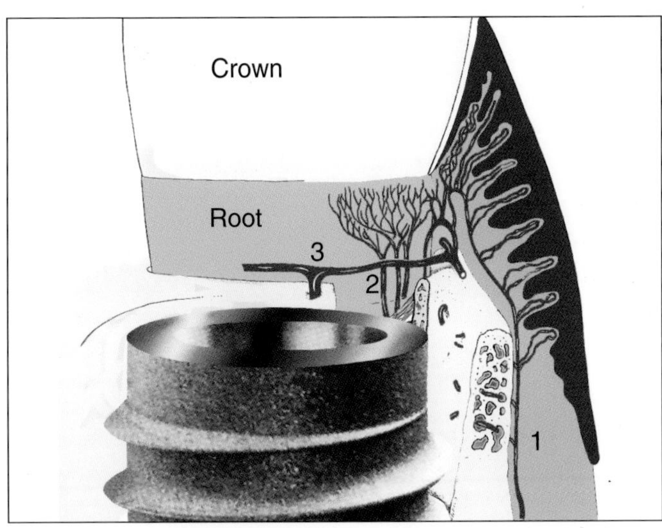

Fig 1-2 The three main sources of blood supply to the periodontium: (*1*) supraperiosteal vessels supply the free and attached gingiva; (*2*) blood vessels of the periodontal ligament form a vast network around the root of the tooth and extend beyond the alveolar crest to contribute to the circulation of the free gingiva, including the col; and (*3*) blood vessels of the alveolar bone send perforating branches, which form anastomotic connections with supraperiosteal and periodontal ligament vessels before extending beyond the alveolar crest to contribute additional blood supply to the free gingiva. (Adapted from Carranza[13] with permission from WB Saunders.)

blood vessels, the blood vessels of the periodontal ligament, and the blood vessels of the alveolar bone (Fig 1-2). While each of these vascular sources is primarily responsible for circulation to a defined area, several existing and potential anastomotic connections are also available between the main vessels. For example, although the main blood supply to the free gingiva is derived from the supraperiosteal blood vessels, a significant portion of the circulation to this area is derived from anastomosis with blood vessels from the periodontal ligament and the alveolar bone. The number of anastomotic connections increases in response to periodontal inflammation such as that typically associated with early postsurgical wound healing and active periodontal disease. The clinical relevance of this becomes clear when one considers that the interdental papilla and the col also derive a significant portion of their circulation from these anastomotic connections and that certain surgical approaches may needlessly sever these anastomotic connections, resulting in unwanted loss of interdental tissue volume. Furthermore, the successful application of periodontal plastic surgical techniques often requires the exploitation of these potential anastomotic connections to provide sufficient peripheral vascular supplies to sustain free tissue grafts secured over partially avascular recipient sites.

Peri-implant soft tissue anatomy

In general, the similarities between periodontal and peri-implant soft tissues are limited to the form and function of the analogous epithelial structures.[1–7,14–17] The oral, sulcular, and junctional epithelia in peri-implant soft tissues are nearly identical in form and function to their periodontal counterparts. A junctional epithelium forms and attaches to a titanium dental implant in a manner analogous to the epithelial attachment that forms to a natural tooth (ie, a hemidesmosomal attachment). In both cases, the junctional epithelial attachment is an important component of the protective permucosal soft tissue seal. Similarly, the sulcular epithelium that forms adjacent to a dental implant provides cellular immunologic protection analogous to that found in the periodontium, and when present, the thick, keratinized oral epithelium also provides protection from the mechanical forces of mastication, restorative procedures, and oral hygiene. However, although periodontal and peri-implant oral and sulcular epithelia are supplied by a rich vascular plexus,

Table 1-1 Internal and external factors that affect the health of the peri-implant soft tissues

Internal factors
Age of patient
General health
Periodontal status of remaining dentition
Host resistance
Systemic disease
Periodontal phenotype
Pre-existing bony dehiscence
Vestibular depth
Aberrant frenum
Thickness of attached tissue
Apicocoronal dimension of attached tissue, if present
External factors
Tobacco use
Use of medications
Oral hygiene
Implant design and surface characteristics
Submerged vs nonsubmerged technique
Surgical approach
Location of implant
Depth of implant placement
Prominence of implant position in the alveolus
Restorative technique
Restorative materials
Restorative margin vis-à-vis biologic width

the epithelia surrounding a dental implant do not enjoy the potential vascular anastomotic connections derived from the vessels of the periodontal ligament.

There are also important differences between periodontal and peri-implant soft tissues about which the implant surgeon should be familiar. Obviously, the tissues that anchor the implant in the alveolus lack both cementum and a periodontal ligament; instead, the implant is directly connected to bone below the alveolar crest. In addition, there are no gingival fiber bundles analogous to the dentoperiosteal and dentogingival fiber bundles that are attached to the natural tooth, although there is a zone of supra-alveolar connective tissue surrounding the emerging implant. Immobility of attached peri-implant soft tissues is derived not from a connective tissue attachment to the implant but rather from the splicing of connective tissue fiber bundles running from the alveolar crest to the free gingiva and from the circular connective tissue fiber bundles running circumferentially around the implant.[1-7,18] Finally, the connective tissue immediately adjacent to the implant is relatively acellular and avascular compared with analogous periodontal tissues, which enjoy a rich vascular plexus derived from periodontal ligament vessels. In general, the dense connective tissue found immediately adjacent to a dental implant is histologically similar to scar tissue—that is, rich in collagen and poor in cellular elements—in contrast to the connective tissue found further away from the implant, which is typically rich in fibroblasts and circulatory elements. These differences in the peri-implant connective tissue render the implant more susceptible than the natural tooth to mechanical and bacterial challenges. When esthetics must be considered, differences in the orientation, composition, and circulation of the peri-implant connective tissue zone may limit opportunities to influence surrounding soft tissue architecture with prosthetic-guided soft tissue healing techniques (see chapter 7).

Need for attached peri-implant soft tissues

While it is generally recognized that a stable peri-implant soft tissue environment is one that provides a transmucosal seal against bacterial irritants and sufficient structural stability to withstand the mechanical trauma commonly encountered in the oral cavity, there is a lack of consensus in the literature concerning the need for attached tissues surrounding implant restorations and whether they provide any long-term biologic advantage over alveolar mucosa.

Although many investigators have concluded that so-called attached peri-implant soft tissues provide no long-term advantage over alveolar mucosa,[19-21] a growing number of investigators correlate the presence of attached tissues with improved soft tissue health, greater patient satisfaction, and fewer complications.[1,17,22,23] The latter group believes that attached, nonmobile soft tissues resist disruption of the junctional epithelial seal to the implant and may even limit the apical spread of marginal inflammatory lesions that can lead to bone loss and eventually to implant failure. The lack of consensus in the literature regarding this issue should not be surprising when one considers how many different factors may affect the health of the peri-implant soft tissues (Table 1-1).

Because so many factors can influence the health of the peri-implant soft tissues and the long-term success of an osseointegrated implant, it is difficult to design a study isolating the effects that attached tissues may have on the health or longevity of an implant restoration. Therefore, for the present time the conclusion as to whether attached tissues are necessary must be based on clinical observations rather than on scientific studies.

Clinical rationale for attached peri-implant soft tissues

Several authors have presented sound rationales for the presence of attached tissues around implant restorations.[22–26] In general, these rationales are based on an understanding of the vulnerability of the peri-implant soft tissue seal and oral hygiene's critical role in ensuring long-term success in implant therapy. Attached peri-implant soft tissues provide the restorative practitioner with a "prosthetic-friendly" environment, which facilitates not only the precise prosthetic procedures but also the oral hygiene maintenance required for long-term success. Attached tissues resist recession, maintain predictable levels over time, and enhance esthetic blending. In addition, those with appropriate contours create a self-cleansing environment for the implant restoration by minimizing food accumulation. This fulfills the patient's expectation of a replacement tooth that functions in the same fashion as the lost tooth, greatly increasing patient satisfaction.

In addition to the challenges presented by oral hygiene procedures and the forces of mastication, the peri-implant soft tissues are routinely threatened by numerous additional mechanical challenges. Abutment connection procedures, removal and replacement of provisional abutments, implant-level impression procedures, preparation and delivery of subgingival restorations, framework try-ins, and the movements allowed by resilient attachments securing removable implant prosthetics all represent challenges that could result in disruption of the junctional epithelial seal and underlying connective tissue zone, potentially jeopardizing the long-term success of the implant.

In summary, most experienced clinicians agree that an adequate zone of attached soft tissues with intimate adaptation to the emerging implant structures is critical for the long-term success of an implant restoration in the partially edentulous patient. Moreover, there is a higher incidence of soft tissue complications related to implant therapy performed in atrophic edentulous arches with minimal attached tissues. Therefore, a strong clinical rationale exists for attached tissues and adequate vestibular depth in partially and completely edentulous patients when tissue mobility and inadequate access for oral hygiene will predictably increase soft tissue complications and thereby decrease patient satisfaction with the implant restoration.

Concept of biologic width

To understand the significance of biologic width in implant therapy, it is useful to review the definition of this concept as it relates to the natural dentition and contemporary restorative dentistry.

Biologic width represents the clinical application of histometric measurements of the dimensions of the human dentogingival junction obtained from preserved cadaver specimens at different phases of passive eruption of the teeth. In 1924, Orban and Kohler[27] first reported the results of a histometric study of the human dentogingival junction following Gottlieb's[28] initial discovery and description of the epithelial attachment of the gingiva in 1921. In addition to the dimensions of the newly discovered epithelial attachment, Orban and Kohler also reported on the dimensions of the connective tissue attachment and the relationship of the base of the gingival sulcus, the alveolar crest, and the most apical portion of the epithelial attachment to the position of the cementoenamel junction during the then-accepted four phases of passive eruption. During the 30 years that followed, many questioned the existence of an epithelial attachment, as well as its mechanism and strength.[29,30] Eventually, the exact nature of the epithelial attachment to enamel and cementum was elucidated, and a consensus on the modes of periodontal soft tissue attachment was reached.[31–34]

It soon was accepted as fact that the epithelial attachment of the gingiva was mediated by the secretion from the epithelium of a cementing substance and that this epithelial attachment did not provide the mechanical strength of a physical union of ameloblasts to the forming and maturing enamel rods, as originally envisioned by Gottlieb. It was Sicher[31] who first proposed a physiologic division of labor for the supporting tissues making up the dentogingival junction, emphasizing the physiologic importance of the tenuous epithelial attachment. In his simplified model, the functional dentogingival junction had two separate components that together provided for the integrity and maintenance of the periodontal soft tissue attachments: The epithelial attachment provided for the "biologic protection" of the dentogingival junction, while the connective tissue attachment provided the mechanical "firmness" of the gingival attachment.

In 1961, Gargiulo, Wentz, and Orban[35] conducted a landmark study of the dimensions of the dentogingival junction in humans in order to understand the effects that periodontal surgery and disease might have on these dimensions. These investigators re-evaluated and added to the original data by Orban and Kohler. They measured 30 additional human cadaver arches and reported the range and mean values for the six individual measurements as performed in the original study. Their results confirmed the validity of the dentogingival junction and the duality of its functional components (epithelial and fibrous connective tissue). The greatest variability was found in the dimensions of the epithelial attachment and the least variability in the dimensions of the connective tissue attachment, while the depth of the gingival sulcus remained relatively constant during the phases of passive eruption. The measurements obtained from this study served to define the dimensions of the *physiologic dentogingival junction* in humans and established a basis for those who subsequently formulated the clinical application of this information with the concepts associated with the term *biologic width*.

Whereas the descriptions of the physiologic dentogingival junction and the clinical concept of biologic width originally included only the combined dimensions of the supra-alveolar connective tissue and the epithelial attachments to a natural tooth, some authors include the dimensions of the gingival sulcus in their discussions of biologic width. This discrepancy seems to be related to a confusion of terminology regarding the *functional* dentogingival junction (sulcus depth plus length of epithelial attachment plus length of connective tissue attachment) and the *physiologic* dentogingival junction (length of epithelial attachment plus length of connective tissue attachment), which has become synonymous with modern concepts of biologic width.

For this discussion, biologic width will be defined as the combined dimensions of the supra-alveolar connective tissue attachment and the junctional epithelial attachment to a natural tooth or emerging implant. The currently accepted combined mean value of biologic width is 2.04 mm, based on the study by Gargiulo et al[35]; it represents a mean dimension of 1.07 mm for connective tissue attachment and 0.97 mm for epithelial attachment. While the total dimension of 2.04 mm is a useful reference, it is important to remember that it was derived from individual measurements taken on the mesial, distal, vestibular, and oral surfaces of the dentition of preserved cadaver specimens during the different phases of passive eruption. The standard techniques used for preservation and decalcification of the specimens measured in the studies introduced significant dimensional changes, and no consideration was given to the effect that tooth location (maxillary vs mandibular, anterior vs posterior), periodontal phenotype, or root morphology might have had on the dimensions of the dentogingival junction. Furthermore, it is important to realize that although the mean measurements varied little, the individual measurements varied greatly. Furthermore, in clinical situations the biologic width will vary on different tooth surfaces and in different areas within the same individual.

A more recent study by Vacek et al[36] confirmed these concepts and added to our understanding of biologic width. These investigators examined the natural dimensions of the dentogingival junction in 10 adult human cadaver arches. Mean measurements for sulcus depth (1.34 mm), epithelial attachment (1.14 mm), connective tissue attachment (0.77 mm), and loss of attachment (ie, distance from the cementoenamel junction to the coronalmost aspect of connective tissue attachment) (2.92 mm) were measured histomorphometrically for 171 individual tooth surfaces. The range of biologic width reported in this study was 0.75 to 4.33 mm, reinforcing the clinical concept of a variable supracrestal attachment area to allow for a range of epithelial and connective tissue attachments. Although individual measurements varied greatly, these investigators again observed no significant differences in the mean dimensions of the dentogingival tissues measured on different tooth surfaces (buccal, lingual, mesial, and distal). No correlation was found between loss of attachment and the dimensions of connective tissue attachment or the biologic width (epithelial attachment plus connective tissue attachment). These investigators observed that of all the tissue dimensions measured, the length of connective tissue attachment varied the least. Of particular significance, the epithelial attachment was significantly greater on tooth surfaces adjacent to subgingival restorations, and both the epithelial and connective tissue attachments (biologic width) were significantly greater in posterior sextants when compared with the dimensions measured on the anterior dentition.

Clinical significance of biologic width in restorative and implant dentistry

Many clinicians have recognized and described the clinical significance of biologic width in restorative and periodontal therapy.[37–42] In addition, the anatomy of the peri-implant soft tissues has been described and the histometric dimensions of the implantogingival junction have been reported.[1–7] However, despite the many validations of the biologic width phenomenon as it applies both to periodontal and to peri-implant soft tissues, the clinician should realize that the minimum morphologic dimensions compatible with gingival and peri-implant soft tissue health in humans have yet to be established. Nevertheless, although the ideal dimensions of biologic width for a particular clinical situation cannot be determined by the results of any study to date, the concepts derived from these studies can serve as important guidelines in the clinical practice of restorative and implant dentistry.

In restorative dentistry, the concept of biologic width becomes clinically significant only when intracrevicular restorative margins are necessary for functional or esthetic reasons. In these situations, the clinician must recognize that a minimum dimension of sound tooth structure between the restorative margin and the alveolar crest is necessary to accommodate connective tissue and epithelial attachment and to provide a safe distance from the base of the crevice. In clinical practice, a distance of 0.5 to 1.0 mm between the restorative margin and the base of the crevice is generally considered to be safe. When the depth of the crevice is less than 1.5 mm, it becomes more difficult to prepare the tooth without damage to the soft tissue attachments. As a consequence, soft tissue recession may occur, possibly exposing the restorative margin. This is the challenge that the restorative clinician faces when preparing intracrevicular restorations in esthetic areas. *Invasion of the biologic width* is the terminology commonly used to describe a restorative margin that encroaches upon this safe distance. Injuries to the gingival attachment as a result of tooth preparation and impression procedures are also considered violations of biologic width. They have a detrimental effect on the stability of the gingival attachment apparatus and can result in pocket formation or apical migration of the periodontal attachment apparatus.

To assist the restorative clinician in maintaining the health and stability of the periodontium when intracrevicular restorative margins are indicated, Maynard and Wilson[40] described the physiologic dimensions of the area of the periodontium relevant to the restorative clinician. They divided the dentogingival unit into three conceptual components: superficial physiologic dimension, crevicular physiologic dimension, and subcrevicular physiologic dimension. The superficial physiologic dimension comprises the attached and free gingiva. The authors suggested that approximately 5 mm of keratinized tissue, composed of 2 mm of free gingiva and 3 mm of attached gingiva, is necessary to maintain the health of the periodontium when the margins of the restorations are extended into the sulcus. Although they conceded that intracrevicular restorations could be successfully placed in the presence of a smaller amount of keratinized tissue, they emphasized that predictability was far greater when these minimum dimensions were present prior to the initiation of the restorative procedures. In addition, the authors recognized and discussed the importance of the thickness of the gingival tissues in tolerating intracrevicular restorative procedures. They presented a rationale for increasing both the width and the thickness of keratinized tissue around dentition requiring intracrevicular restorations prior to initiation of the restorative procedures.

The authors' description of the crevicular physiologic dimension included both the depth and breadth of the sulcus. To ensure an esthetic and physiologic intracrevicular restoration, they suggested a minimum depth of 1.5 to 2.0 mm from the free gingival margin to the base of the crevice prior to intracrevicular margin preparation. The authors pointed out that when restorative therapy is planned following periodontal surgery, the customary 6-week waiting period often is inadequate for the development of a new gingival crevice of a depth sufficient to tolerate the procedures necessary to produce an esthetic and physiologic intracrevicular restoration. Their description of the breadth of the sulcus included both the circumferential extension and volume capacity of the gingival crevice. They stressed the importance of avoiding injury to the crevicular epithelium during tooth preparation, impression procedures, and cementation of the final prosthesis. They also differentiated between quantitative violations (overcontoured restorations) and qualitative violations (maladapted restorations) of the gingival crevice and explained how these can contribute to chronic inflammation of the marginal tissues, leading to pocket formation or apical migration of the periodontal attachment.

The authors defined the subcrevicular physiologic dimension as the distance from the base of the gingival crevice to the alveolar crest. Their definition included the junctional epithelium and supra-alveolar connective tissue fiber, which is equivalent to our current concept of biologic width. They recognized that the restorative procedures required for intracrevicular restorations (tooth preparation, retraction procedures, impression techniques, and placement of a provisional restoration) can disrupt the periodontal soft tissue attachments, potentially causing a progressive inflammatory process. Furthermore, they understood that cementation of a final restoration under these conditions would only maintain the injury and eventually lead to pocket formation or apical migration of soft tissue attachment and loss of alveolar bone. Most important, these authors recognized the need for a variable supracrestal attachment area to allow for the dimensional range of epithelial and connective tissue attachments. The information presented by these authors provides a conceptual framework for our current understanding of the periodontal restorative interrelationships and the significance of biologic width in restorative dentistry.

Although similarities in the structure of periodontal and peri-implant soft tissues make it tempting to extrapolate our understanding of the significance of biologic width directly to implant therapy, our lack of knowledge concerning the functional significance of the differences in the composition of connective tissue, the orientation of collagen fiber bundles, and the distribution of vascular elements adjacent to the permucosal portion of a titanium implant do not allow us to do so. Our current understanding of the possible significance of biologic width in implant therapy has primarily been derived from animal research. Berglundh et al[43] and Buser et al[4] performed studies on canine models demonstrating that peri-implant soft tissues around both unloaded two-piece submerged and one-piece nonsubmerged implants share many features with the gingival tissues around teeth. Both studies demonstrated that epithelial downgrowth did not extend to the alveolar crest. Instead, these investigators demonstrated the existence of a zone of dense connective tissue interposed between the junctional epithelium and the alveolar bone crest at implant sites in the dog model. They demonstrated that this connective tissue zone had consistent dimensions and that its histologic characteristics were similar to those of scar tissue. Abrahamsson et al[7] documented similar peri-implant soft tissue attachment characteristics using both a one-piece nonsubmerged and different two-piece submerged implant systems.

Despite the similarity of these findings, controversy still exists over the significance of slight differences observed in the dimensions of the implantogingival junction around submerged and nonsubmerged implants. Some investigators, such as Weber et al[44] and Hürzeler et al,[45] have demonstrated that the epithelial attachment is more apical and always located below the microgap in submerged compared with nonsubmerged titanium implants; other investigators, such as Chehroudi et al,[46] have demonstrated greater connective tissue height and less epithelial downgrowth around submerged two-piece titanium implants. The relevance of these observed differences is not known. In addition, although many agree that direct attachment of connective tissue to titanium implants does not occur, some evidence suggests that the presence of a connective tissue zone in contact with the implant may inhibit apical epithelial migration and is an important factor in maintaining stability of the peri-implant soft tissues.[46]

Berglundh and Lindhe[6] conducted a study that added to our understanding of the significance of biologic width in implant therapy and the importance of the supra-alveolar connective tissue zone to the stability of the peri-implant soft tissue. In this unique animal study, submerged two-piece titanium implants were placed bilaterally 3 months after the removal of all premolars, following standard protocol. At abutment connection, the tissue thickness (about 4.0 mm) was maintained on one side and surgically reduced via excision of connective tissue to 2.0 mm or less on the contralateral side. After a 6-month period of plaque control, the dimensions of the peri-implant soft tissues were compared. The investigators found that although the tissue thickness at abutment connection was significantly different, the combined dimensions of the junctional epithelium and the supra-alveolar connective tissue (ie, biologic width) around the implants at test and control sites were similar 6 months later. Furthermore, they observed that wound healing at the sites where the tissue had been thinned consistently showed bone resorption. It was apparent that the bone resorbed to accommodate a minimum biologic width of approximately 3.0 mm at these particular implant sites. The authors suggested that the soft tissue attachments (biologic width), once established, were nature's mechanism for protecting the zone of osseointegration from the bacterial and mechanical challenges of the oral cavity. This study validates the clinical rationale for augmenting soft tissue prior to abutment connection or nonsubmerged implant placement when thin mucosal tissues are present.

Abrahamsson et al[47] performed a study to evaluate the effect of different abutment materials on the health and stability of the peri-implant soft tissues in the beagle dog model. They reported that gold alloy and dental porcelain abutments were inferior to titanium- and aluminum-based sintered ceramic abutments and that their use resulted in bone resorption, apical migration of the soft tissue, and formation of the protective barrier (biologic width) on the surface of the implant body. Another animal study, performed by Cochran et al,[48] not only demonstrated the existence of biologic width around one-piece nonsubmerged implants but also added to our understanding of the stability of peri-implant soft tissues following different periods of loading. In this study, nonsubmerged implants were placed 3 months after removal of all four premolars and first molars on six American foxhounds. The dimension of the biologic width was evaluated at 3 months in the unloaded group, at 6 months in the group loaded for 3 months, and at 15 months in the group loaded for 12 months following implant placement. They compared their findings with those of previous histometric studies of the human dentogingival junction on preserved cadaver specimens.[36] Their data suggested that a biologic width exists around nonsubmerged one-piece titanium implants and that this physiologically formed and stable structure is similar to that found on the human natural dentition. As in previous studies, the dimensions of the supra-alveolar connective tissue, once formed, remained relatively stable, while the dimensions of the junctional epithelium and sulcus depth demonstrated more variability.

Guidelines based on principles of biologic width

Although our current understanding of the factors that influence biologic width in implant therapy is incomplete, the information that we have can be used to guide clinicians, just as the original histometric data of the dimensions of the human dentogingival junction guided restorative clinicians in the management of important periodontal relationships. Based on the results of animal research and on the author's experience, it is reasonable to conclude that the delivery of implant restorations with intracrevicular margins presents significant challenges to the peri-implant soft tissues and can cause progressive inflammatory lesions (peri-implantitis). Furthermore, since the results of animal studies have suggested that peri-implantitis lesions eventually involve bone and may lead to implant failure,[42] the author believes it is prudent to embrace a rationale that requires adequate width and thickness of keratinized tissue around implant restorations when intracrevicular restorative margins are planned. The author suggests applying this rationale whenever an implant will emerge through thin or mobile mucosal tissues. In these situations, oral soft tissue grafting procedures should be performed to improve the ability of the peri-implant soft tissues to withstand the trauma of abutment connection and intracrevicular restorative procedures as well as the subsequent mechanical challenges of masticatory forces, hygiene maintenance, and the repeated mechanical stresses that removable restorations secured with resilient prosthetic attachments present.

Whenever an implant is placed in an area of esthetic concern, a certain amount of biologic risk will be encountered. An understanding of the concepts encompassed by the term *biologic width* allows the clinician to calculate the risk for a particular situation. In esthetic implant dentistry, the goal is to provide excellent esthetics and peri-implant soft tissue health and stability with little or no crestal bone loss or remodeling. This can occur only when the biologic width requirement for a particular site is matched exactly with an implant of the appropriate diameter placed at the ideal depth and angulation to maintain the three-dimensional scalloped osseous anatomy and the thickness of the overlying soft tissue drape. Since the dimensions of the biologic width vary on different teeth and different surfaces in the same individual, it is nearly impossible for any single type of prefabricated, cylindrical, titanium, root-form implant system to satisfy the circumferential biologic width requirements of every implant site. Although the introduction of multiple implant diameters, collar heights, and customizable abutments of appropriate materials has moved us closer to our goal for esthetic implant dentistry, in many instances biologic compromises are necessary.

With this in mind, the clinician must seek a balance between esthetics, peri-implant soft tissue stability, and preservation of alveolar bone levels. The surgical dimensions and topography of a particular site, the proximity of adjacent dentition or implants, the periodontal phenotype, and knowledge of ideal crown-to-implant ratios should guide the surgeon in placing an implant of the appropriate diameter at an ideal depth for each particular site. Experienced clinicians know that deeper implant placements make it easier to fabricate an esthetic restoration with natural emergence. Because deeper implant placements are associated with apical migration of the peri-implant soft tissues to accommodate the circumferential biologic width requirements of the site, the author routinely performs soft tissue augmentation when working in areas of esthetic concern in order to strike a balance between depth of implant placement, maintenance of esthetic restorative emergence, and soft tissue stability.

It is important to point out that because of the multitude of factors that can potentially influence the biologic width requirements for a particular implant restoration, variability in the soft tissue dimensions from one site to another should be anticipated. Further research is needed to determine the influence that the following factors have on the dimensions and long-term stability of the peri-implant soft tissues: implant design and surface characteristics, location and depth of implant placement, type of approach (submerged vs nonsubmerged), abutment materials, implant-abutment microgap, cemented restorations with intracrevicular margins, periodontal phenotype, and reconstructive hard and soft tissue procedures.

Choosing Between a Submerged and Nonsubmerged Approach

The decision to use a submerged or nonsubmerged approach in implant therapy cannot be made on the basis of results from any of the studies performed to date. Instead, the clinician should consider the clinical and "theoretical" biologic advantage or disadvantage that each approach might provide for a patient in a particular situation.

The evolution of implant design from a two-piece system with separate interosseous and permucosal components to a one-piece system in which interosseous and permucosal components comprise a single unit is the factor that initiated interest in the application of nonsubmerged techniques. The most significant advantage of a nonsubmerged implant approach is that it provides sufficient time for mature soft tissue integration prior to initiation of the restorative process. This allows for stabilization of the junctional epithelium and sulcus depth dimensions during

One-piece nonsubmerged approach

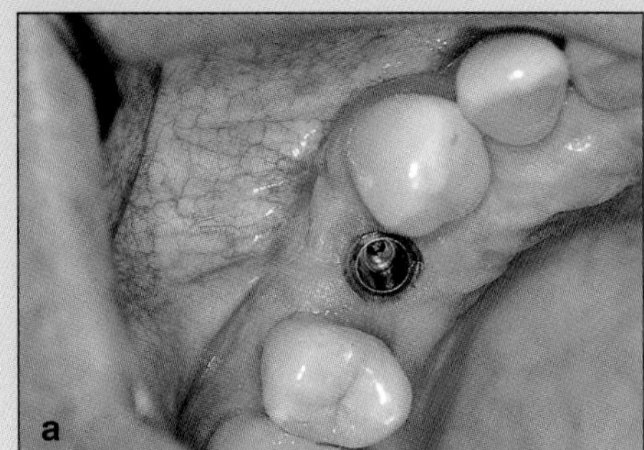
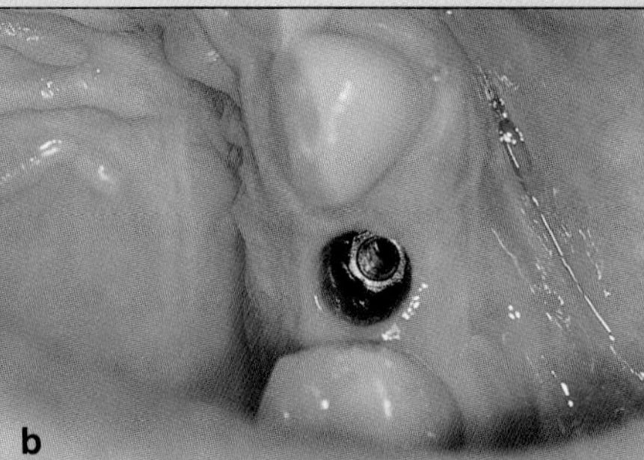

Fig 1-3a Despite the highly scalloped osseous anatomy and thick soft tissue drape at this maxillary premolar implant site, the use of a one-piece nonsubmerged implant with a standard collar height provides a "prosthetic-friendly" environment. The soft tissue seal is not disrupted by removal of the healing abutment, and subsequent prosthetic procedures are facilitated.

Fig 1-3b In a similar situation, the use of a two-piece implant system via a nonsubmerged approach with a provisional titanium healing abutment has several disadvantages. Removal of the provisional abutment severs the junctional epithelial attachment and disrupts the peri-implant connective tissue zone. Subsequent prosthetic procedures are difficult to perform and damage the peri-implant soft tissues, potentially causing apical migration at the expense of underlying alveolar bone.

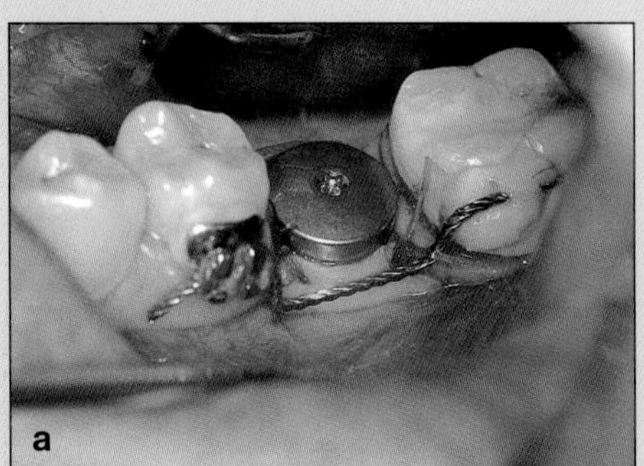
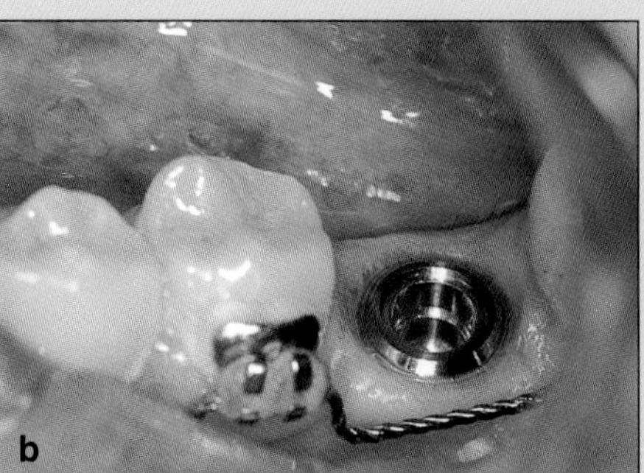

Fig 1-4a A one-piece nonsubmerged implant placed at a deeply scalloped molar site provided for mature soft tissue integration and soft tissue stability prior to the fabrication of the molar restoration.

Fig 1-4b After 3 months of healing, removal of the closure screw did not disrupt the tenuous junctional epithelial seal. The support provided by the healing abutment during the soft tissue integration period has maintained soft tissue architecture and papillary volume, thus preventing unwanted food impaction. The wide-diameter prosthetic connection ensures a natural restorative emergence.

Two-piece nonsubmerged approach

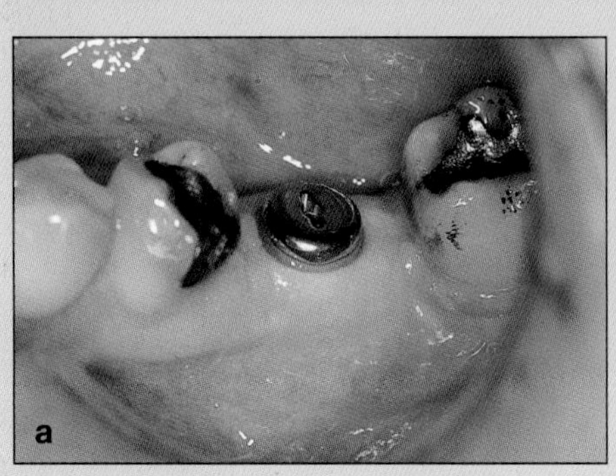
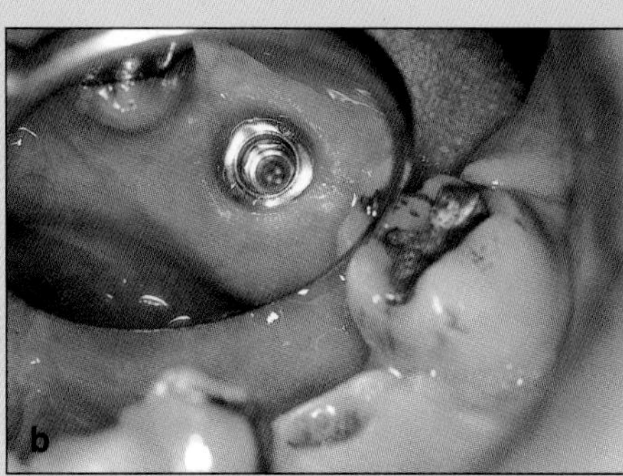

Fig 1-5a An implant restoration with flat osseous anatomy, minimal bone height above the inferior alveolar nerve, and reduced interarch dimension was desired at this mandibular molar site. A two-piece nonsubmerged implant with provisional healing abutment provided an ideal solution for this clinical situation.

Fig 1-5b Removal of the provisional healing abutment reveals mature soft tissue healing without collapse of the soft tissues over the abutment-connection surface.

the hard and soft tissue integration periods. Furthermore, the nonsubmerged approach eliminates the need to disrupt mature peri-implant soft tissues with abutment connection procedures or occasional surgical soft tissue refinements, thus providing a prosthetic-friendly environment and improving the long-term predictability of the restoration (Figs 1-3a and 1-4 to 1-8). Because a nonsubmerged approach requires fewer surgical procedures, circulation to the area is preserved, treatment time and patient discomfort are reduced, and patient acceptance is improved.

A theoretical biologic advantage unique to a one-piece implant placed in a nonsubmerged fashion is that it is closed to the ingress of bacterial contami-

One-piece nonsubmerged approach

Figs 1-6a and 1-6b Nonsubmerged placement of a one-piece implant with shortened collar height and Esthetic-Plus (Straumann USA, Waltham, MA) healing abutment preserves the volume of the facial gingival tissues, thus simplifying the subsequent fabrication of an esthetic intracrevicular implant restoration.

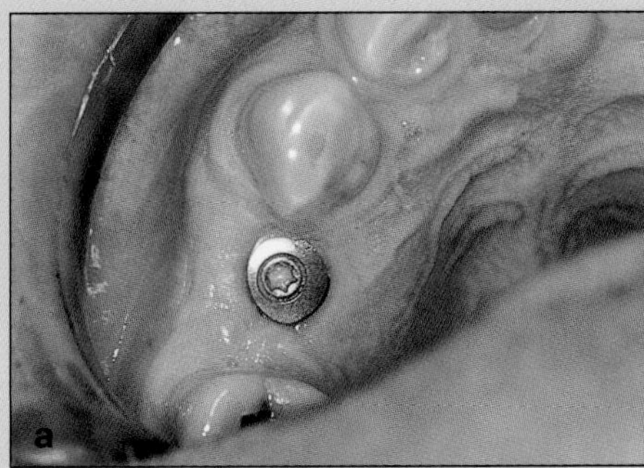

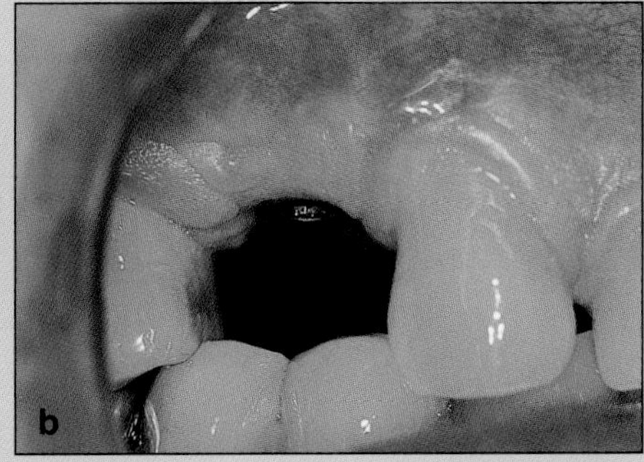

Fig 1-7a A one-piece nonsubmerged implant with Esthetic-Plus healing abutment was placed in a semi-submerged fashion, providing support for adjacent papillae while avoiding recession of facial soft tissues by allowing them to collapse over the facial bevel of the anatomic healing abutment.

Fig 1-7b The final restoration can now be delivered without the need for implant exposure. Mature soft tissue integration improves the predictability of the restoration, eliminating the need for prolonged use of a provisional restoration.

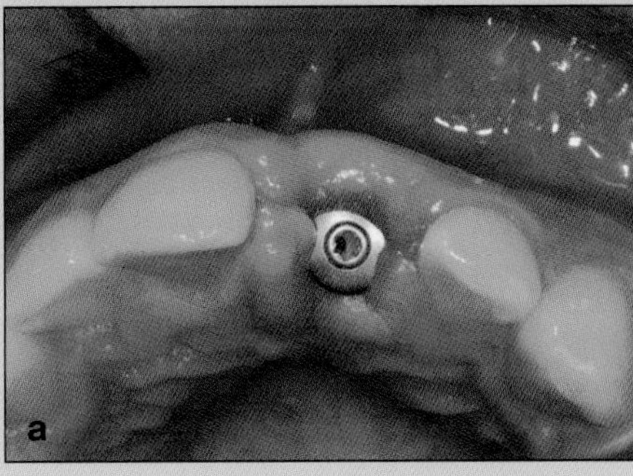

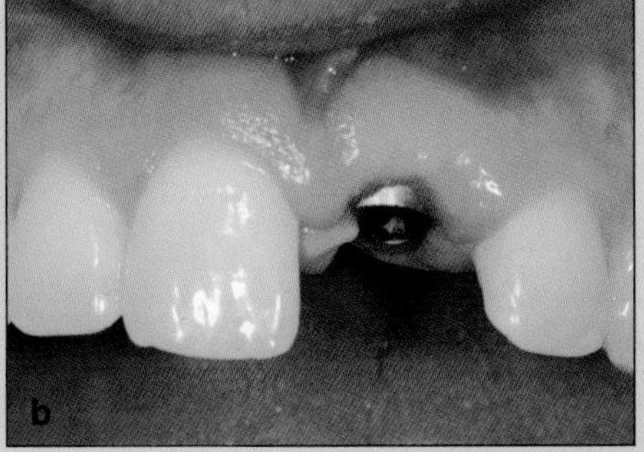

Fig 1-8a Eight-week postoperative view of four one-piece nonsubmerged implants used for replacement of maxillary incisors. The delivery of custom tooth-form healing abutments at the time of nonsubmerged implant placement provides immediate support for peri-implant soft tissues, thereby ensuring positive gingival architecture.

Fig 1-8b Four months after nonsubmerged implant placement, custom tooth-form healing abutments were removed and prosthetic abutments delivered. Note the health and stability of the peri-implant soft tissues. Prosthetic procedures are limited to the intracrevicular area, thereby enhancing esthetic predictability.

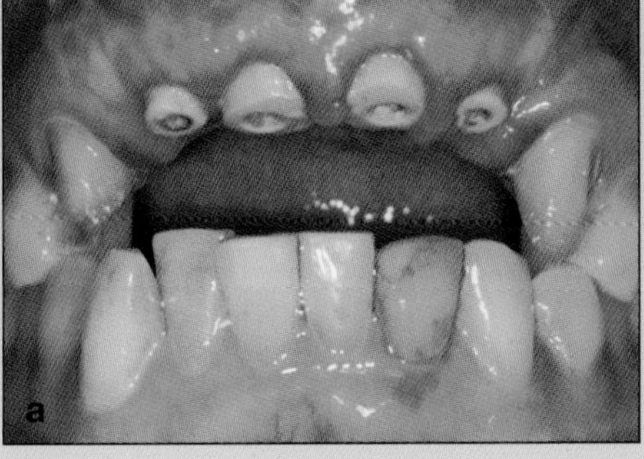

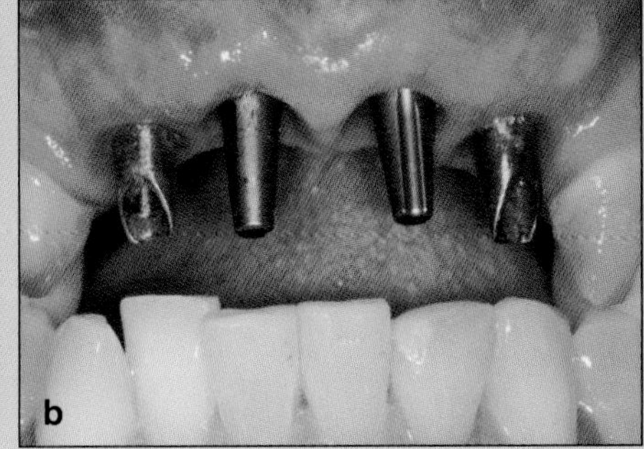

nants, the full clinical significance of which is still not understood. While two-piece implants placed in a nonsubmerged fashion with simultaneous delivery of the permanent abutment provide advantages similar to those of one-piece implants, use of provisional healing abutments may not provide the same clinical and theoretical biologic advantages. This is particularly true when the underlying osseous anatomy dictates that the level of abutment connection be deep within the tissue. Subsequent replacement of the provisional abutment with a permanent abutment or implant-level restorative procedures will by definition sever the junctional epithelium and disrupt the zone of connective tissue adaptation adjacent to the implant, potentially causing apical migration of the soft tissue attachments with resorption of underlying alveolar bone. Moreover, in these instances the restorative clinician is faced with a less-than-desirable environment for the completion of the precision prosthetic procedures (Fig 1-3b).

When the underlying osseous contours at the implant site are flat, use of a two-piece nonsubmerged implant provides clinical advantages similar to those of a one-piece implant and, in situations where interocclusal space is limited, may offer additional prosthetic flexibility (see Fig 1-5).

While most clinicians generally prefer a submerged approach for esthetic implant therapy, use of a nonsubmerged approach (see Figs 1-6 to 1-8) offers significant advantages for everyone involved. By using prefabricated anatomic or custom tooth-form healing abutments to support the existing or reconstructed soft tissues immediately at the time of implant placement, the surgeon enjoys the benefit of increasing the likelihood of maintaining or developing positive soft tissue architecture at the site. This early employment of prosthetic-guided soft tissue healing also prevents soft tissue shrinkage and eliminates the need for a second surgical procedure for implant exposure. In addition, this affords the surgeon the opportunity to monitor the soft tissue volume and architecture and to perform soft tissue refinements as needed without significant inconvenience to the patient. The restorative dentist also enjoys the benefit of working in a stable (intracrevicular) soft tissue environment following the osseointegration and soft tissue integration period, further enhancing prosthetic predictability. The laboratory technician enjoys the advantage of fabricating provisional and definitive restorations on a master cast that represents mature soft tissue profiles, thus facilitating abutment selection. Finally, the patient benefits from the reduced treatment time and the need for fewer surgical procedures to obtain a stable soft tissue environment with pleasing peri-implant soft tissue esthetics.

When combined and appropriately sequenced with indicated site-preservation and site-development techniques, the use of the nonsubmerged approach simplifies implant therapy and provides unsurpassed esthetic predictability as well.

CHAPTER 2

Systematic Evaluation of the Esthetic Implant Patient

This chapter presents information necessary for the implant surgeon to perform a systematic evaluation of the esthetic implant patient. Although a complete review of dentofacial and dentoperiodontal esthetics is beyond the scope of this book, surgeons involved in esthetic implant therapy should have a working knowledge of smile esthetics and smile design. In essence, smile esthetics includes an understanding of how facial features, muscular activity, and the relationships between the visible dentition and gingival tissues combine to create the unique appearance of an individual's smile. Although everyone's smile is unique, there are common elements that combine to form a smile that is esthetically pleasing. Similarly, there are identifiable elements that detract from the esthetic appearance of a smile. The implant surgeon should be familiar with both the elements that enhance and those that detract from smile esthetics. The practitioner's smile design process, then, involves the systematic quantification of these positive and negative elements. The next step is to visualize an ideal final esthetic result and identify any anatomic limitations that might preclude achieving it. Subsequently, a treatment plan is formulated that takes into consideration the patient's individual needs and desires as well as the expected response to surgical procedures indicated by the patient's periodontal phenotype. To simplify this process, this chapter introduces a new classification of alveolar ridge defects specific to esthetic implant sites that is correlated with the selection and sequencing of surgical procedures required for predictable esthetic outcomes in implant therapy and, more importantly, emphasizes the clinical conditions that preclude achieving ideal esthetics.

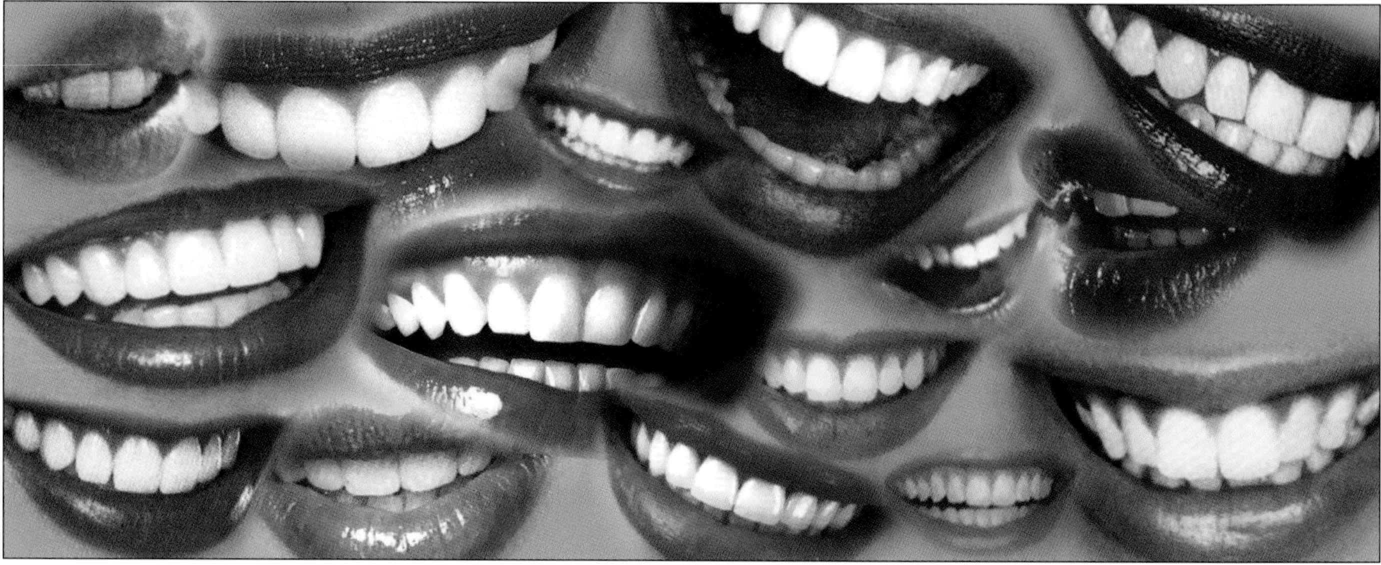

Fig 2-1 Evolving trends in dental esthetics are evident in today's print media. The implant surgeon can study these examples to develop a sense of what elements combine to create an esthetically pleasing smile.

A Simplified Approach to Patient Evaluation

Smile design, in its simplest form, involves eliminating or minimizing those elements that detract from the esthetic appearance of a smile and creating or emphasizing those elements that can enhance the smile within the limitations of the patient's facial features, muscular activity, clinical crown dimensions, root length, three-dimensional position and axial inclination of individual dentition, and quantity and health of periodontal soft tissues. Patients seeking esthetic implant replacements can often greatly benefit from the smile-design process and, if educated about the possibilities, are often eager to undergo a complete smile transformation. This process may involve orthodontic therapy, cosmetic and reconstructive periodontal surgery, cosmetic dentistry, or even orthognathic surgery, all properly sequenced with implant-site development, implant placement, provisional restoration, and delivery of the final esthetic implant restoration. This multidisciplinary approach to esthetic implant therapy is the topic of chapter 7.

When implant therapy is contemplated for an area of esthetic concern, the pretreatment evaluation performed by the surgeon must include a complete functional and esthetic periodontal evaluation. Focusing attention solely on the area of planned implant restoration often results in esthetic compromises that could have been avoided. While it is important for the surgeon to be able to quantify dentoperiodontal esthetics, it is critical that any existing or potential dental and periodontal deficiencies be identified prior to implant therapy.

This chapter provides the surgeon with the information needed to perform a presurgical esthetic dentofacial and dentoperiodontal evaluation of patients undergoing esthetic implant therapy. In addition, it discusses the identification of existing or potential periodontal defects and anatomic limitations that may compromise the final esthetic results. Although this evaluation is not comprehensive, it provides the basic information required for the surgeon participating in the diagnostic and treatment-planning process described above. For the reader seeking more detail, Chiche and Pinault[1,2] and Levin[3] each provides a comprehensive review and discussion of facial, dental, and periodontal esthetics.

The author recommends that the implant surgeon practice the following simplified approach to functional and esthetic dentofacial and dentoperiodontal evaluation on a daily basis when examining patients. It is also helpful to study the many examples of ideal dentofacial esthetics found in today's print media (Fig 2-1). This will give the surgeon a good understanding of what is considered an esthetically pleasing smile in today's culture. The surgeon will become familiar with evolving trends in dental esthetics, such as the increasing acceptance of the diversity inherent in a natural smile as opposed to the artificially uniform appearance once demanded from dental restorations. Although the surgeon must be able to systematically quantify the individual elements that come together to create a pleasing smile, with practice, esthetic dentofacial and dentoperiodontal evaluation becomes second nature, and clinical measurements merely confirm what the experienced eye is immediately able to discern.

Facial and Dental Symmetry

The functional and esthetic dentofacial and dentoperiodontal examination begins with an evaluation of facial symmetry. Chiche and Pinault[1] point out that although dentofacial features do not need to be completely symmetrical to impart beauty, significant asymmetry near the facial or dental midline always detracts from esthetics. Conversely, lateral asymmetries are acceptable and can actually be pleasing to the eye.

The surgeon should begin the evaluation of facial and dental symmetry by determining the position of the facial midline. In most cases, this determination is made relative to a level interpupillary line. The facial midline then forms a perpendicular to the interpupillary line and is located at the midpoint between the patient's pupils in a forward gaze. Sitting directly in front of the patient, the author uses a McCoy Facial Tri-Square (Padget Instruments, Kansas City, MO) to determine the facial midline. When this tool is aligned with a level interpupillary line, the clinician can easily visualize the perpendicular center at the midpoint between the pupils relative to prominent facial and dental anatomy. Facial symmetry is easily evaluated by determining whether the nasal midline, upper lip philtrum, and chin midline are coincident with the facial midline (Fig 2-2a). Dental symmetry is also evaluated relative to the facial midline (Fig 2-2b). The position of the papilla between the maxillary central incisors, as well as the location and axis of the maxillary and mandibular dental midlines, is evaluated relative to the facial midline. Although the location of the maxillary and mandibular dental midlines need not coincide with the facial midline, their axes should be close to parallel to the facial midline.[1] A canted dental midline forms an angle to the facial midline, detracting far more from esthetics than does noncoincidence of facial and dental midlines. In addition, the clinician should evaluate the incisal, occlusal, and gingival planes for their orientation relative to the level interpupillary line. A parallel orientation is considered esthetically pleasing.

Upper lip line

The form of the upper lip and its relationship to the underlying dentoperiodontal structures are the most important considerations when evaluating dental esthetics. The ideal relationship of the maxillary teeth to the upper lip is the starting point for esthetic dental reconstruction. This relationship determines what therapeutic modalities will be needed to obtain an esthetic result. It also determines the esthetic importance of reconstructing harmonious dentoperiodontal structures and, as in the treatment planning for surgical correction of dentofacial deformities, is often the limiting factor in the smile-design process.

The position of the lip should be evaluated at rest, during conversation, during a relaxed moderate smile, and when the patient is highly animated. The clinician should first evaluate the amount of dentogingival exposure when the patient is completely relaxed and the lips are naturally positioned (Fig 2-3a). This can be achieved by having the patient lick the upper and lower lips, gently rub them together, and allow them to part naturally. Alternatively, the clinician can establish the tooth-to-lip relationship in the relaxed lip position by having the patient pronounce the letter *m* several times and then allow the lips to gently part. Both methods allow the clinician a quick glimpse of dentogingival exposure with the lips in a truly relaxed position, which can be photographically recorded for future reference.

Clinical measurements of tooth and gingival exposure taken during examination of a patient's smile often are inaccurate because the patient postures the lips rather than allowing them to assume a natural position. Therefore, to determine natural lip positions, it is useful to observe the patient interacting with office personnel or other patients (Figs 2-3b and 2-3c). Phonetics can aid in the observation and recording of maximum dentogingival exposure. The patient's pronunciation of the letter *e* in an exaggerated way will approximate the maximum dentogingival exposure, even though it results in an unnatural lip position and posture (Fig 2-3d).

A working knowledge of the average maxillary incisor display with the lips at rest is useful, because it is the most accurate of the clinical lip measurements. The average maxillary incisor display with the lips in a rest position is 1.91 mm in men and 3.40 mm in women.[1] In addition, younger patients tend to display more maxillary tooth structure than do older patients, and patients with longer upper lips display less maxillary tooth structure than do those with shorter lips.

As previously mentioned, it is important to evaluate the amount of gingiva displayed with the lips in various positions. While a display of more than 3.0 mm of gingival tissue during a moderate smile has been described as a "gummy" smile, there is a wide range of acceptability for gingival exposure during smiling.[1] The evolving trend toward a full-volume smile has been accompanied by increased acceptance of greater gingival exposure in the esthetically pleasing smile (see Fig 2-1). It is important for the clinician to evaluate the display of the dentition and gingival tissues not only in the anterior maxillary area but also in the buccal corridor or vestibular space. Significant exposure of posterior dentition and gingival tissues is considered esthetically desirable today. From a diagnostic standpoint, this issue becomes important when reconstruction of posterior maxillary areas is contemplated with implant therapy. In these instances, esthetics may dictate arch expansion or alveolar ridge augmentation to create harmony with the anterior dentition and the posterior esthetic implant reconstruction.

Lower lip line

The relationship of the lower lip to the maxillary anterior dentition helps the clinician evaluate the curvature and orientation of the incisal plane and the oral-facial–incisal edge positions of the maxillary incisors.[1] In general, the incisal plane should follow the gentle curvature of the lower lip when the patient is relaxed and smiling moderately (Fig 2-4). Furthermore, when the patient pronounces the letter *f* or *v*, the incisal edges should make a definite contact at the inner vermilion border or wet-dry line of the lower lip. Incisal edge contact facial or lingual to the inner vermilion border may indicate inappropriate contouring of existing dental restorations or malposition of incisor dentition.

Incisal plane

As previously mentioned, the incisal plane should be parallel to the level interpupillary line and follow the gentle curvature of the lower lip when the patient is smiling. A mild canting of the incisal plane relative to the interpupillary line can be esthetically acceptable. When the interpupillary line is canted, the incisal plane should be perpendicular to the facial midline as determined using alternate landmarks such as the midpoint between the pupils and the center of the upper lip philtrum.

The surgeon should understand that esthetic incisal plane morphology involves more than orientation. An esthetically pleasing incisal plane follows either a mild convexity from central incisor to canine or a "gull wing" pattern, where the edge length of the lateral incisors is slightly shorter than the neighboring central incisor and canine[2] (Fig 2-5a). Either of these incisal plane morphologies can exist bilaterally or in combination with the other to create an esthetically pleasing incisal plane.

The morphology and relationship of the incisal embrasures of the maxillary anterior teeth also can enhance or detract from smile esthetics. The incisal embrasures are formed by the edges and separations between the maxillary anterior teeth and should progressively widen from the central incisors to the canines to enhance smile esthetics (Fig 2-5b).

Although flat incisal plane morphology is considered acceptable only for older patients, the author finds that many older patients, when educated about esthetic options, select a convex incisal plane morphology associated with a youthful smile. This is consistent with today's culture, where reversal of the visible signs of aging has become the focus of plastic surgery, cosmetic dentistry, and the health and nutrition industries. Finally, a concave incisal plane (commonly known as a *reverse smile line*) or an excessively convex incisal plane always detracts from dentofacial esthetics and should be avoided (Fig 2-5c).[2]

The surgeon evaluating incisal plane orientation and morphology should be aware that any alterations observed during examination may have resulted from altered eruption of individual teeth, uneven incisal edge wear, or inappropriate restorations. In addition, the restoration of an esthetic incisal plane may be subject to functional occlusal limitations and must be planned to be in harmony with the lips and face. When implant therapy is planned in the maxillary anterior area with pre-existing aberrations in the incisal plane, shortening or lengthening the incisal edge positions of the maxillary anterior dentition may require orthodontic therapy, corrective jaw surgery, and esthetic crown lengthening or root coverage procedures to obtain or maintain harmonious tooth proportions.

Occlusal plane

The incisal and occlusal surfaces of the teeth determine the occlusal plane. The occlusal plane, which should parallel the level interpupillary line, is best evaluated from a sagittal perspective relative to the Frankfort horizontal plane. This relationship is commonly evaluated by correlating cephalometric tracing and three-dimensional analysis of study casts mounted on a semi-adjustable articulator using a facebow transfer. The occlusal plane can also be evaluated clinically from a sagittal perspective relative to the Camper plane, which extends from the inferior border of the ala of the nose to the superior border of the tragus of the ear. When the occlusal plane does not correspond to the incisal plane, the clinician must determine whether the occlusal plane appears to have the expected relationship to the above-mentioned references. If it does, this indicates a discrepancy in the

Evaluation of facial and dental symmetry

Fig 2-2a McCoy Facial Tri-Square is used to evaluate facial symmetry. The facial tri-square is superimposed over the patient's face. The tri-square is aligned with a level interpupillary line and centered at the midpoint between pupils. Nasal midline, upper lip philtrum, and chin midline are evaluated for coincidence with facial midline. The surgeon should be positioned directly in front of and at eye level with the patient.

Fig 2-2b After evaluation of facial symmetry, dental symmetry is evaluated by determining whether the position of the papilla between the maxillary central incisors as well as maxillary and mandibular dental midlines are coincident with or parallel to the facial midline. Incisal, occlusal, and gingival planes are evaluated for parallel orientation relative to a level interpupillary line.

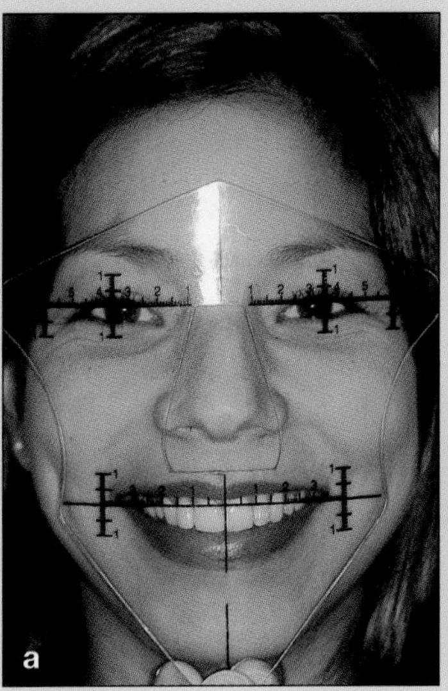

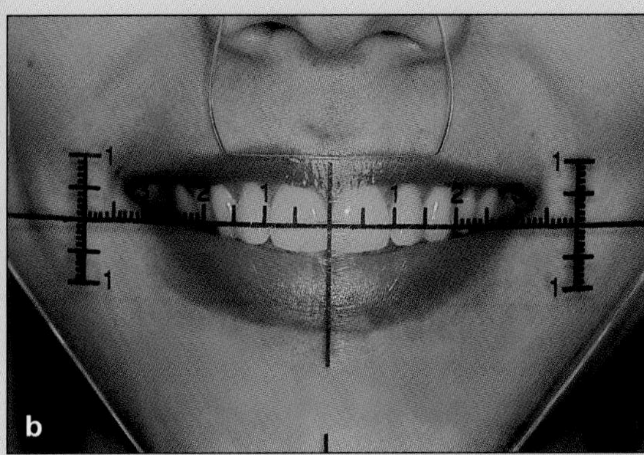

Upper and lower lip lines

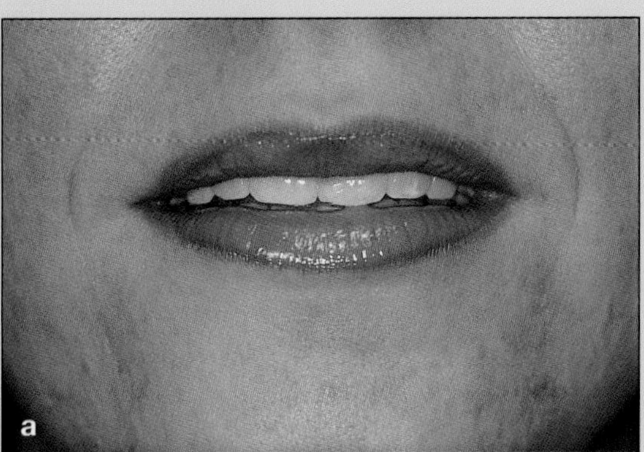

Fig 2-3a Evaluation of dentogingival exposure when the upper lip is relaxed and naturally positioned can be achieved by having the patient lick their lips, rub them together, and gently allow them to part. Alternatively, the patient is asked to pronounce the letter *m* several times, after which the upper lip assumes a relaxed position.

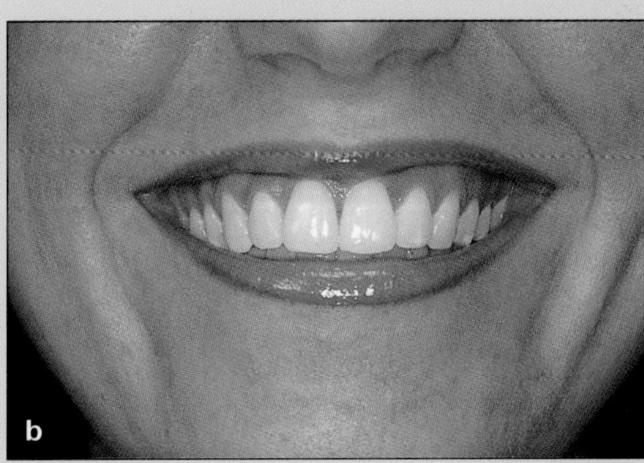

Fig 2-3b Maximum dentogingival exposure captured when the patient was fully animated during conversation. Although increased activity of peri-oral and associated facial musculature is evident when compared to the phonetic method demonstrated in Fig 2-3d, dentogingival exposure is only slightly greater.

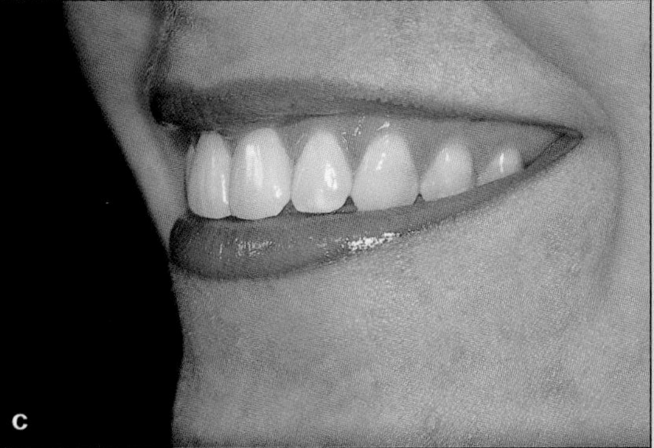

Fig 2-3c When the patient says the letter *f* or *v*, the incisal edge contact at the inner vermilion border or wet-dry line of the lower lip indicates esthetically pleasing oral-facial positions of the maxillary incisors.

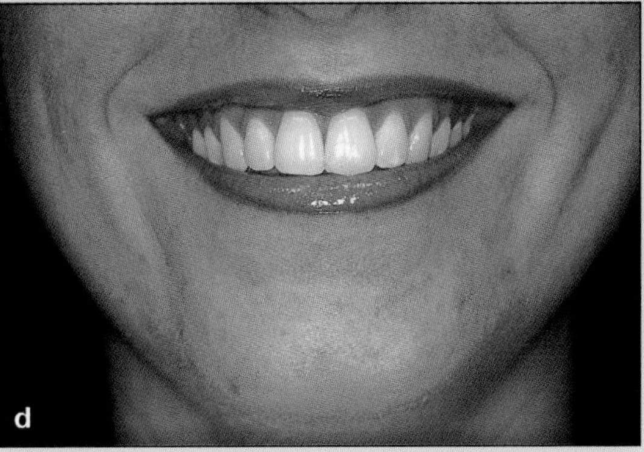

Fig 2-3d Phonetic method for approximating maximum dentogingival exposure. The patient is asked to pronounce the letter *e* in an exaggerated way, allowing the surgeon to repeatedly evaluate dentogingival exposure in a clinical setting.

incisal plane, which may be corrected with orthodontics, orthognathic surgery, cosmetic periodontal surgery, or restorative modalities, as previously mentioned. When the occlusal plane is canted in reference to the level interpupillary line or does not have the expected relationship to the Frankfort horizontal plane or the Camper plane, the patient may have a skeletal problem requiring surgical correction.

Prior to implant therapy, the occlusal plane should be evaluated as described above. Partially edentulous patients with removable partial dentures require special considerations. Because of frequent discrepancies between the occlusal and incisal planes secondary to altered eruption of the dentition, it may be difficult to restore the edentulous spans without significant functional and esthetic compromises. Again, diagnostic templates will indicate the need for orthodontic, periodontal, restorative, or surgical therapy on the remaining natural dentition and prevent unforeseen compromises.

Tooth proportions and relationships

Many formulas, rules, and concepts can help the clinician determine pleasing intrinsic proportions for individual anterior teeth, as well as the optimum relationships among the central incisors, lateral incisors, and canines. In addition to these useful guidelines for establishing esthetic dental proportions, the restorative clinician must also consider the framework of the patient's lips and face. Even the most pleasing dentogingival proportions can lack esthetic appeal if the amount of dentogingival exposure does not complement the patient's face. Nevertheless, these guidelines are useful for the implant surgeon who desires to systematically evaluate dental and periodontal esthetics before commencing implant therapy in esthetic areas.

For the proportions of a maxillary central incisor, an intrinsic width-to-length ratio of 75% to 80% is considered esthetically pleasing.[2] Various pleasing tooth outlines can be produced within this width-to-length ratio to establish the appropriate shape in relation to the patient's face. The so-called golden proportion can be used as a guide for establishing harmonious tooth-to-tooth proportions.[3] In applying the golden proportion to the anterior maxillary dentition, the clinician should keep in mind that harmony is based on what is visualized from the front rather than on an actual mesiodistal measurement of each anterior tooth. According to the golden proportion, a harmonious recurring proportion is established when the central incisor appears 60% wider than the lateral incisor and the lateral incisor appears 60% wider than the mesial aspect of the canine, as observed from the front (Fig 2-6a). Recurring proportional relationships of teeth that appear to decrease in size away from the midline are pleasing.

The axial inclinations and rotational positions of the maxillary anterior dentition contribute significantly to a harmonious visual impact. In general, smile esthetics are enhanced when the clinical crowns of the maxillary anterior teeth are tipped medially, or toward the midline. Furthermore, if the medial tipping increases progressively from central incisor to lateral incisor and from lateral incisor to canine, the visual impact of pleasing recurring proportions that progressively decrease in size away from the midline is reinforced (Fig 2-6b). This is an important consideration during orthodontic detailing of patients prior to esthetic implant therapy (Figs 2-7 and 2-8).

Another important esthetic visual relationship in the anterior dentition involves the area or zone in which the adjacent teeth appear to touch. The connector zones should be distinguished from the actual points of contact between the dentition, which are much smaller.[4] The height of the interdental papillae, the depth of the incisal embrasures, and the axial inclinations of the approximating dentition determine the size of each individual connector zone (Fig 2-9). Here again, the goal is to establish a pleasing recurring proportional relationship between the connector zones progressing away from the midline. Morley[4] suggests that the ideal connecter zones for optimal smile esthetics are as follows: 50% of the length of the maxillary central incisors for the connector zone between these teeth, 40% of the length of the central incisor for the connector zone between the maxillary central and lateral incisors, and 30% of the length of the central incisor for the connector zone between the lateral incisor and the canine when observed from a lateral view. This relationship between connector zones also reinforces the general concept of using pleasing proportions for the maxillary anterior teeth, that is, making the dentition appear to decrease progressively in size away from the midline.

In short, implant surgeons and restorative clinicians who can evaluate intrinsic dental proportions and tooth-to-tooth proportional relationships of the maxillary anterior dentition (including incisal embrasure morphology, axial inclinations, and size of connector zones) have powerful tools. They can then determine whether presurgical orthodontic therapy, cosmetic periodontal surgery, or cosmetic dentistry will be indicated to obtain the best possible esthetic results or to establish or maintain harmony between the implant reconstruction and the natural dentition within the confines of the facial and lip musculature.

Although specific ratios have been discussed, Chiche and Pinault[2] prefer to emphasize general concepts and establish relative priorities in smile design. According to these authors, the maxillary central inci-

Incisal plane morphology

Fig 2-4 In addition to paralleling a level interpupillary line, an esthetically pleasing incisal plane follows the curvature of the lower lip when the patient is relaxed and smiling moderately. When the incisal edges follow a mild convexity from central incisor to canine, esthetic appearance is enhanced.

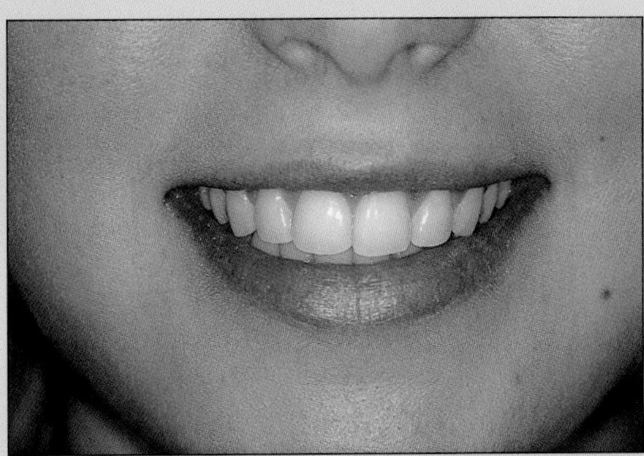

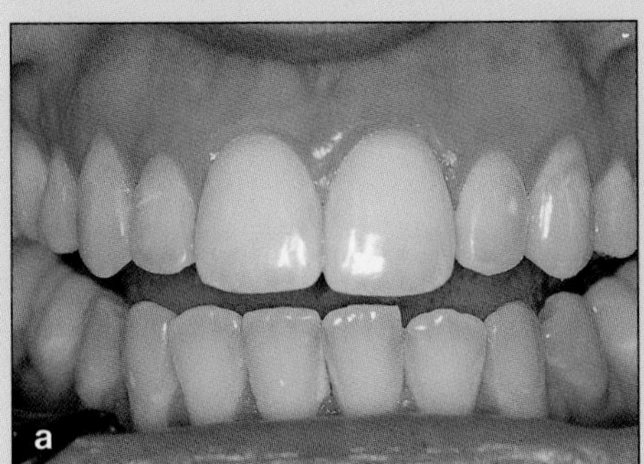

Fig 2-5a An incisal plane with "gull wing" morphology is also considered esthetically pleasing. Note that the incisal edge of the lateral incisor is slightly shorter than the neighboring central incisors and canines.

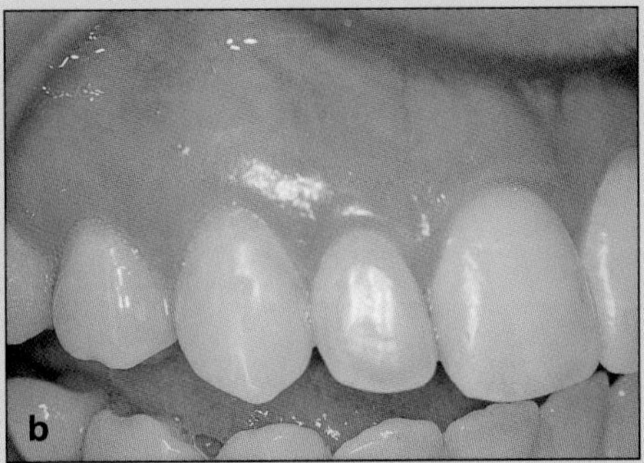

Fig 2-5b Incisal embrasures that progressively widen from central incisors to canines enhance esthetics by contributing to the harmonious visual impact of a decrease in the size of the maxillary anterior dentition as one moves away from the midline.

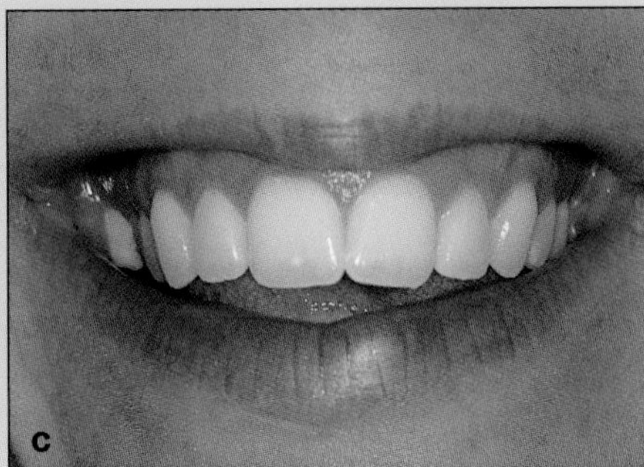

Fig 2-5c Concave incisal plane morphology, commonly known as a reverse smile line, detracts from dentofacial esthetics. Note that the incisal plane diverges from the lower lip line when the patient is relaxed and smiling moderately.

Tooth proportions and relationships

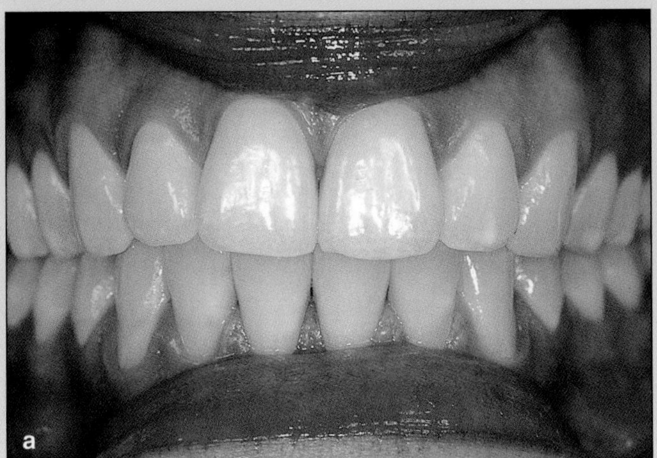

Fig 2-6a Esthetically pleasing dental proportions. The central incisors dominate the smile and have intrinsic width-to-length ratios approximating 75% to 80%. There is a pleasing recurring tooth-to-tooth relationship with the central incisors appearing to be wider than the lateral incisors and the lateral incisors appearing to be wider than the canines from a frontal view.

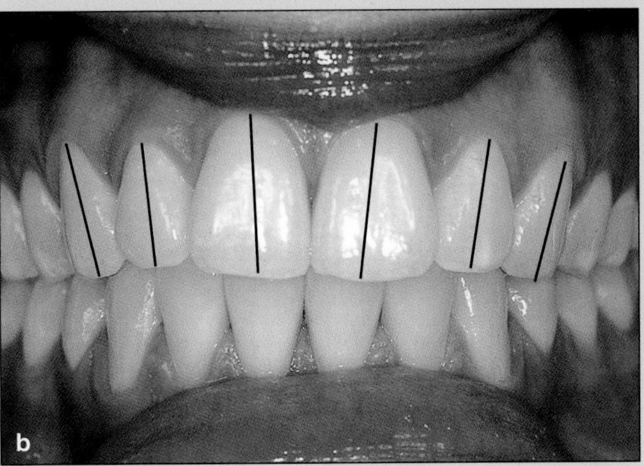

Fig 2-6b Axial inclination of maxillary incisors can contribute to or detract from dental esthetics. A progressive increase in medial tipping from the central incisor to the canine greatly enhances the esthetics of this dentition by reinforcing the visual impact of pleasing dental proportions that decrease in size away from the midline.

Tooth proportions and relationships

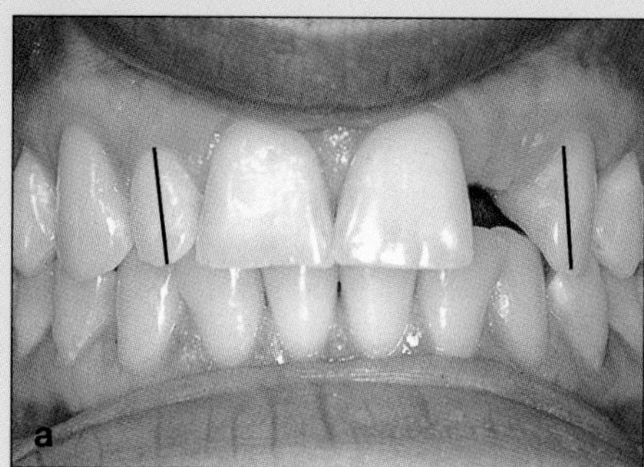

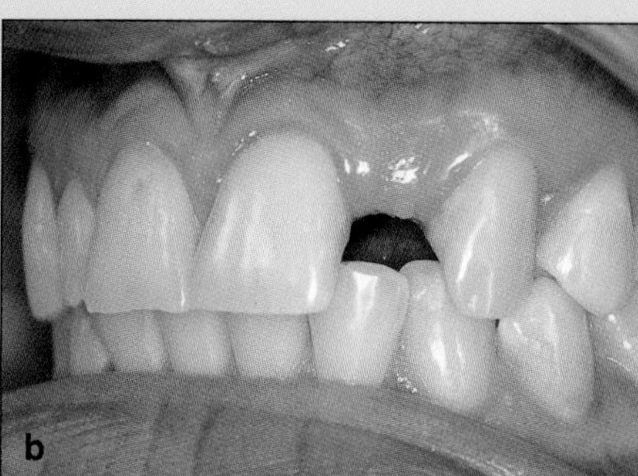

Fig 2-7a Evaluation of this lateral incisor implant site for an esthetic restoration involves an assessment of the axial inclination and rotational positions of the neighboring dentition. In this case, orthodontic intervention to accomplish further medial tipping and counterclockwise rotation of the canine will establish an ideal functional canine relationship and greatly enhance the final esthetic result obtainable by the restorative dentist.

Fig 2-7b Rotational correction and medial tipping have provided functional coupling of canines, ensuring a canine-protected occlusion. Progressive medial tipping from the central incisor to the canine provide the ideal environment for a harmonious implant restoration. (Orthodontics by Dr Richard Mariani Jr, Miami, FL.)

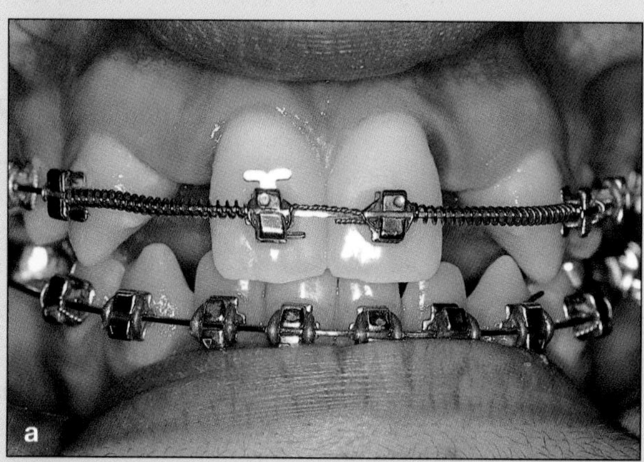

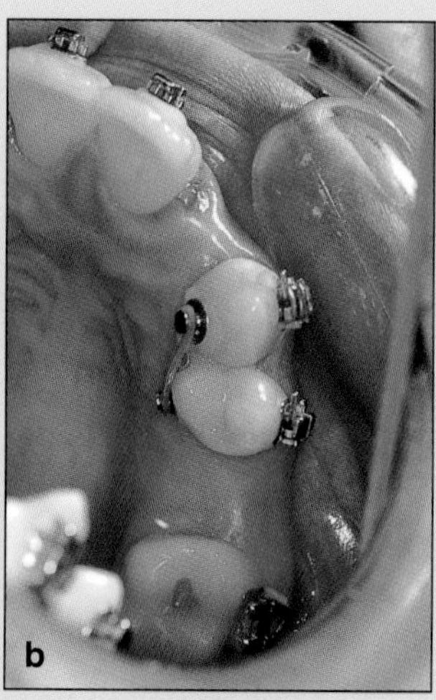

Fig 2-8a Although sufficient mesiodistal space has been obtained presurgically through orthodontic movement, rotational position and axial inclination of incisors and canines would detract from smile esthetics if implants were placed at this time. Instead, rotational corrections and medial tipping will provide the visual impact of pleasing recurring proportions that progressively decrease in size away from the midline.

Fig 2-8b After initial alignment and equalization of lateral incisor spaces has been achieved, additional orthodontic appliances are subsequently placed to accomplish subtle rotational corrections required prior to implant placement. (Orthodontics by Dr Richard Mariani Jr, Miami, FL.)

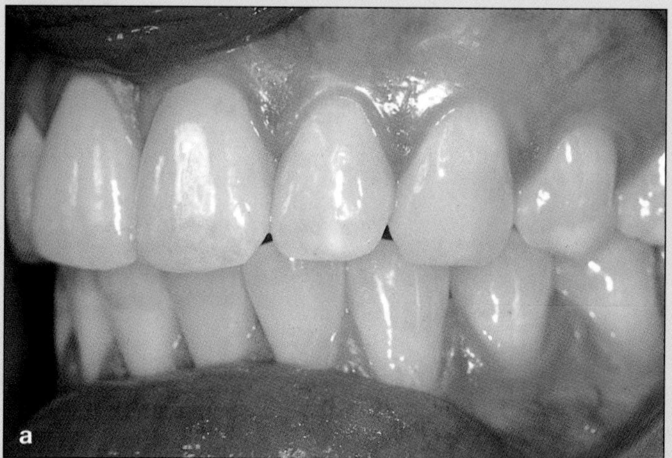

Fig 2-9a Connector zones represent the area or zone where adjacent maxillary teeth appear to touch. The height of the interdental papillae, depth of the incisal embrasures, and axial inclinations of the teeth define them. The proportional relationship between the connector zones forms an important esthetic visual relationship that contributes to the appearance of pleasing recurring proportions that appear to decrease in size as they progress away from the midline. Note the progressive decrease in size of the connector zones between the central incisors compared to those between the central and lateral incisors and between the lateral incisor and the canine.

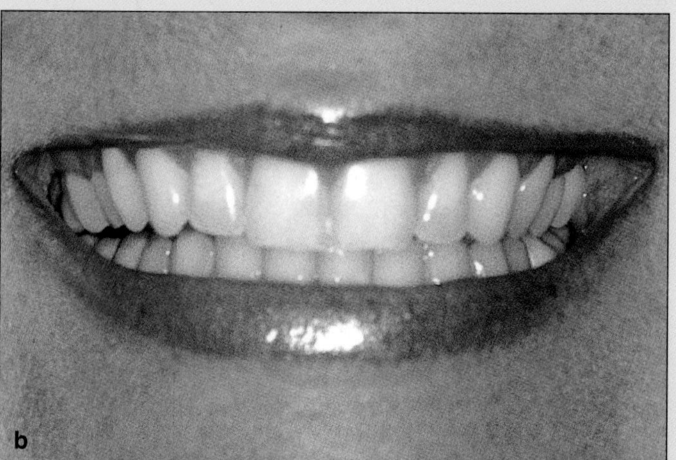

Fig 2-9b Dental elements that combine and contribute to this beautiful smile include pleasing intrinsic dental proportions, recurring tooth-to-tooth proportional relationships, harmonious incisal plane and incisal embrasure morphology, progressive medial tipping, and pleasing proportional relationship of connector zones that decrease in size away from the midline.

sors should have pleasing intrinsic proportions and should dominate the smile. This is consistent with the concept of establishing a focal point for the smile that is symmetrical, dominant in size, and located in the center of the face. Chiche and Pinault also suggest that a pleasing proportional relationship be established between the central and lateral incisors. They suggest that establishing pleasing proportions between the lateral incisor and the canine, as well as recurring proportions between all the maxillary anterior teeth, although ideal, is only a relative priority. Again, this is consistent with the general concept of maintaining symmetry close to the facial and dental midlines and incorporating or accepting mild asymmetry or irregularity away from the midlines. Excessive asymmetry or irregularity away from the midlines, however, will detract from the esthetics of a smile.

Gingival plane and gingival outline

The gingival plane should be parallel to the level interpupillary line or, when the interpupillary line is canted, perpendicular to the facial midline. In addition, the gingival plane should parallel the incisal plane. Mild canting of the gingival plane relative to the level interpupillary line or incisal plane is acceptable. Correction of significant canting of the gingival plane may require orthodontics, periodontal surgery, restorative dentistry, or orthognathic surgery. Chiche and Pinault[2] identify two esthetically pleasing patterns or morphologies for the gingival outline. The first is a sinuous pattern that occurs when the lateral incisor gingival margin is just coronal to the neighboring central incisor and canine unilaterally (Fig 2-10a). The second is a straight pattern that occurs when the gingival margins of the central incisor, lateral incisor, and canine are all at the same level unilaterally (Fig 2-10b). Both patterns can exist bilaterally or in combination on either side of the midline (Fig 2-10c).

When the sinuous pattern is exaggerated, the gingival outline becomes displeasing (Figs 2-11a to 2-11c). It is important to recognize that an exaggerated form of the sinuous pattern results in an unesthetic gingival appearance. Another displeasing gingival outline results when the gingival margin of the lateral incisor is apical to the neighboring central incisor and canine, forming an arch (Figs 2-12b and 2-12c). The displeasing arch pattern is common when full clinical crown exposure of the central incisors, canines, or both is not present or when the lateral incisors are congenitally missing and the residual alveolar ridge has atrophied (Figs 2-12a to 2-12c).

Predicting the gingival pattern that will result after implant placement is important when replacement of any of the maxillary anterior dentition is contemplated. Again, if the patient displays the gingival tissues, symmetry between the gingival margins of the central incisors is mandatory, while mild asymmetry between the gingival margins of the lateral incisors and canines may be acceptable. Obtaining a harmonious gingival appearance in these situations may involve augmentation of the edentulous area with hard or soft tissue and esthetic crown lengthening of the adjacent dentition (Figs 2-12d and 2-12e).

The implant surgeon should select and properly sequence the surgical procedures required to eliminate the functional and esthetic periodontal defects identified at the presurgical evaluation. These soft tissue defects may exist at the implant site or may involve the adjacent dentition. Most often, cosmetic periodontal surgery is indicated for the correction of displeasing gingival outlines and the improvement of tooth proportions by relocation of gingival margins (Figs 2-13 and 2-14). In addition, augmentation of soft tissue and/or hard tissue volume at implant and pontic sites, orthodontic therapy, and/or cosmetic dentistry may be required in certain cases to obtain an optimal esthetic result (see Fig 2-12). When a single maxillary central incisor is to be replaced with an implant restoration, the surgeon must ensure that the final position of the marginal tissues will match those of the adjacent central incisor to avoid an unacceptable midline asymmetry. If this cannot be achieved, even with the aid of soft tissue augmentation, then the surgeon should consider alteration of the soft tissue level on the adjacent central incisor. When both maxillary central incisors are to be replaced with implants, the surgeon's first priority is to ensure that the final soft tissue levels are the same. In addition, the relationship of the gingival levels predicted for the central incisor implant restorations relative to the adjacent lateral incisors and canines must be evaluated. In some instances an ideal esthetic result can be obtained only with significant modification of the gingival levels of the adjacent dentition through orthodontic, periodontal, and restorative intervention. This explains why successful implant restoration of maxillary central incisors in a patient with a high smile line can challenge the implant team and require comprehensive treatment planning and a multidisciplinary approach. The replacement of maxillary lateral incisors and canines often presents less of a challenge because mild lateral asymmetries are often esthetically acceptable.

Gingival plane and gingival outline

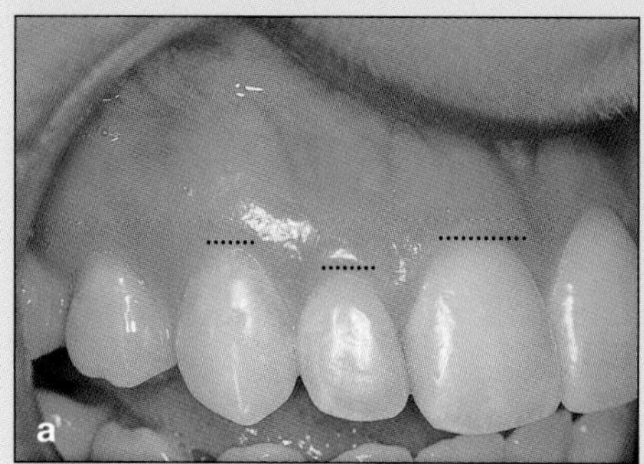

Fig 2-10a A gingival outline that forms a slightly sinuous pattern contributes to an esthetically pleasing smile. Note that the lateral incisor gingival margin is located just coronal (2 mm or less) to a tangent drawn between the neighboring central incisor and canine gingival margins.

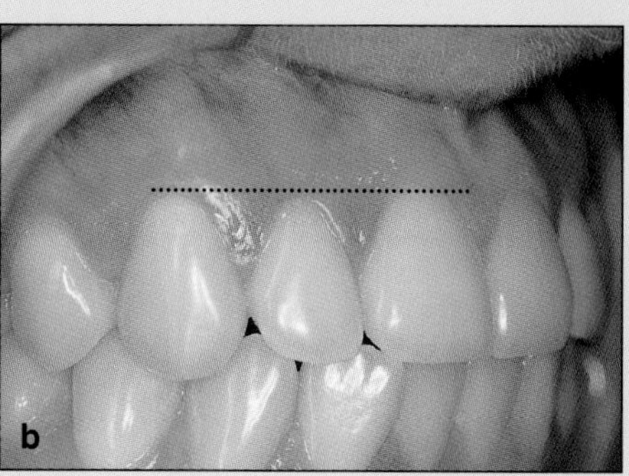

Fig 2-10b A gingival outline that forms a straight pattern also contributes to an esthetically pleasing smile. Note that the lateral incisor gingival margin falls on the tangent drawn between the neighboring central incisor and canine gingival margins.

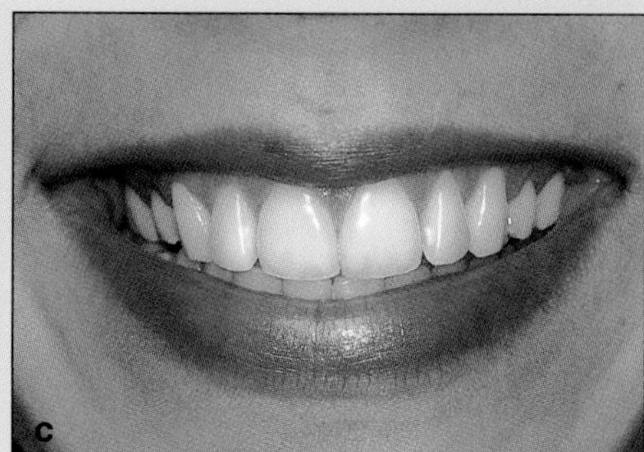

Fig 2-10c A combination of the sinuous and straight gingival patterns contributes to the esthetic appearance of this smile.

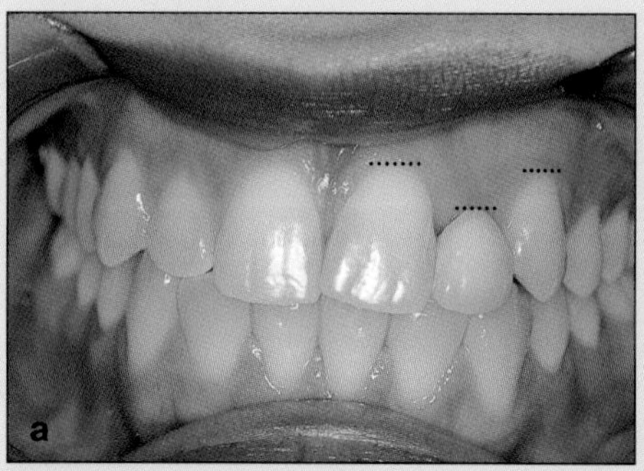

Fig 2-11a Displeasing gingival outline with exaggerated sinuous pattern bilaterally. The locations of the lateral incisor gingival margins are greater than 2 mm below a tangent drawn between the neighboring central incisor and canine gingival margins. The left lateral incisor is an unesthetic pontic of a failing resin-bonded restoration to be replaced by an implant restoration. The gingival margin of the pontic appears to be 4 mm below the gingival margins of the adjacent dentition.

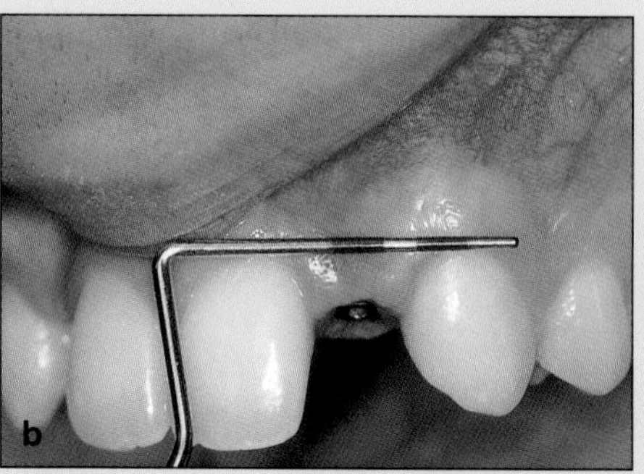

Fig 2-11b The implant was placed at a depth to improve but not to fully correct the gingival outline. To eliminate the displeasing gingival outline, deeper fixture placement and esthetic crown lengthening of the right lateral incisor were recommended.

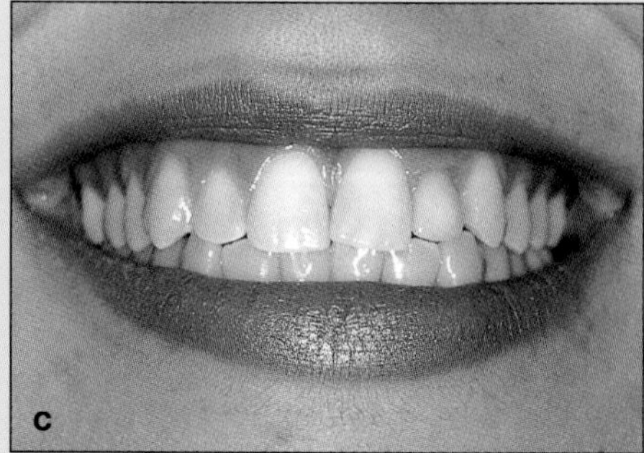

Fig 2-11c Although the implant restoration was an improvement over the resin-bonded restoration, the persistence of an exaggerated sinuous pattern bilaterally and the resultant disproportional relationships between the maxillary anterior dentition detract from the esthetic appearance of the smile.

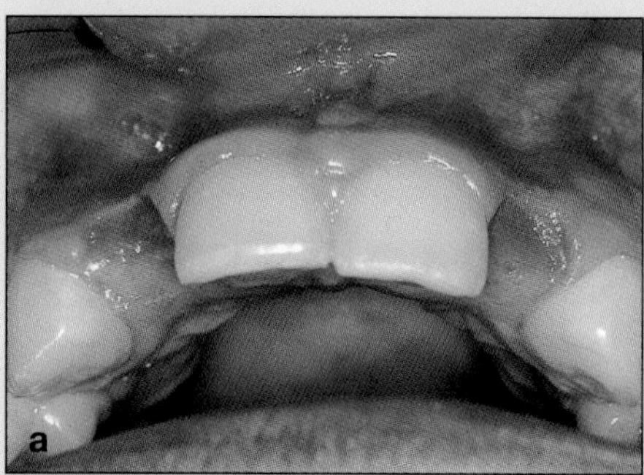

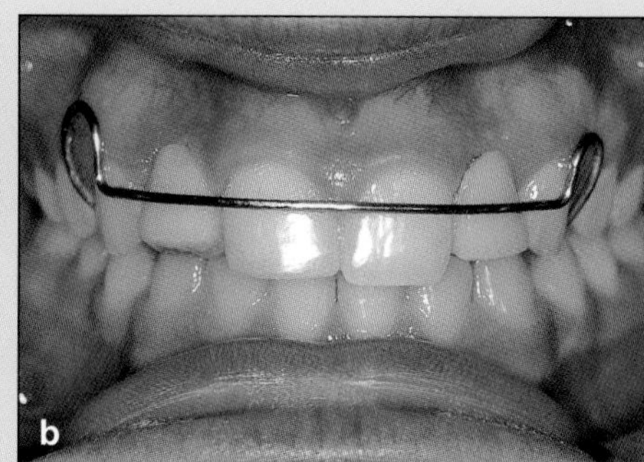

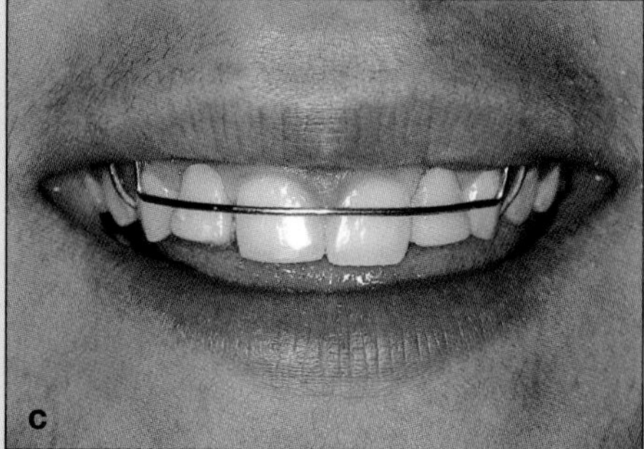

Figs 2-12a to 2-12c Displeasing gingival outline with arch pattern. Pretreatment view of patient with congenitally missing lateral incisors to be replaced by implant restorations. Subepithelial connective tissue grafts performed at the time of implant placement will correct small-volume soft tissue ridge defects present at the implant sites. The absence of full clinical crown exposure of the central incisors and canines, if uncorrected, will limit the esthetic appearance of the implant restorations.

Figs 2-12d and 2-12e Posttreatment views demonstrate establishment of pleasing gingival outlines and harmonious implant restorations. Visualization of the desired gingival margin positions for the implant restorations and adjacent natural dentition was required before commencing with implant therapy. Harmony was achieved through crown lengthening performed after stable soft tissue levels were obtained at the lateral incisor implant sites. Note the tremendous improvement in smile esthetics compared to the pretreatment condition shown in Figs 2-12b and 2-12c.

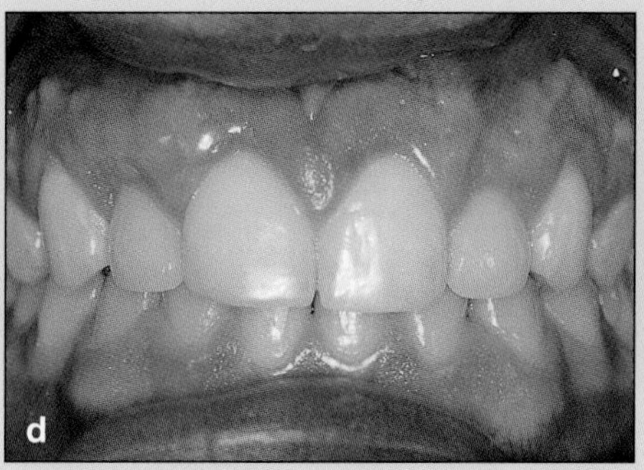

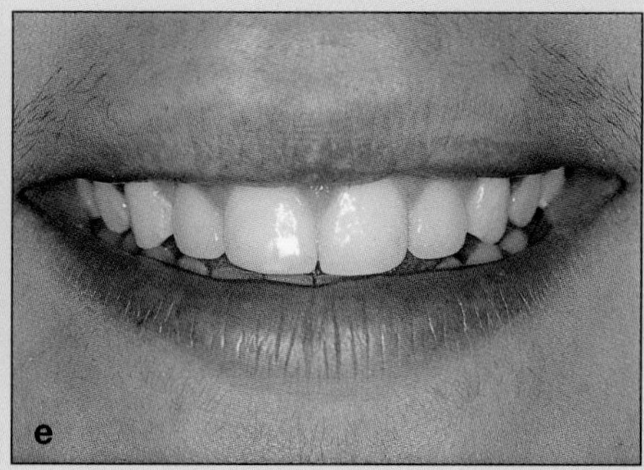

Figs 2-13a and 2-13b Displeasing gingival outline evident with discrepancy of central incisor gingival margin positions. This unacceptable midline asymmetry greatly detracts from the esthetic appearance of the patient's smile.

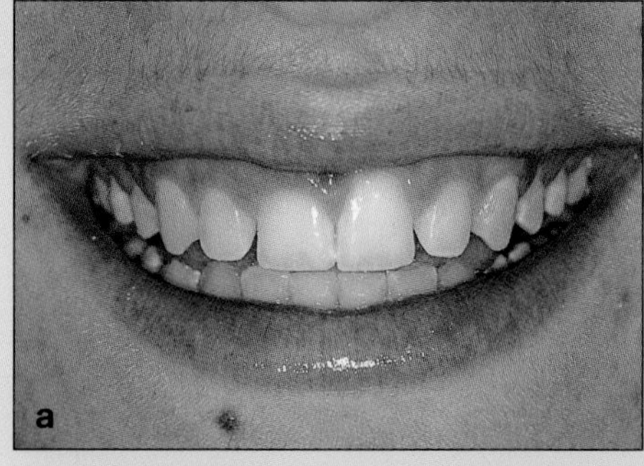

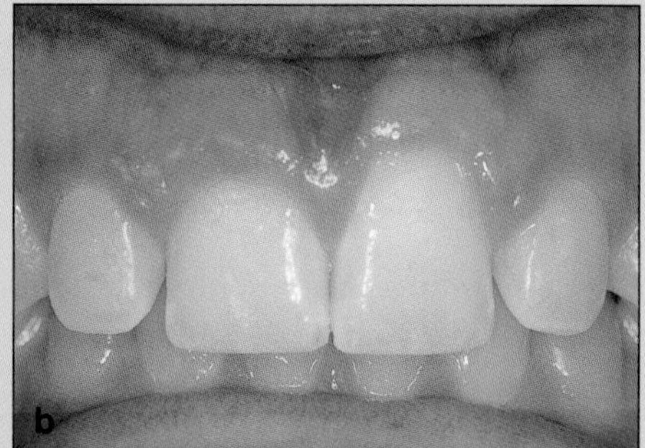

Figs 2-13c and 2-13d Following esthetic hard and soft tissue crown lengthening performed via a papilla-sparing approach, midline symmetry is obtained and smile esthetics are greatly enhanced.

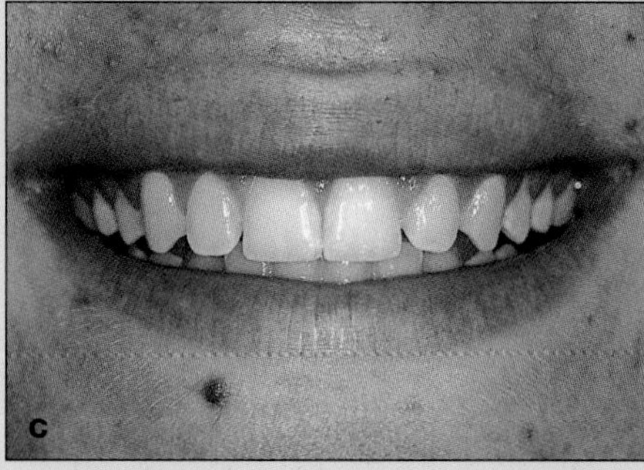

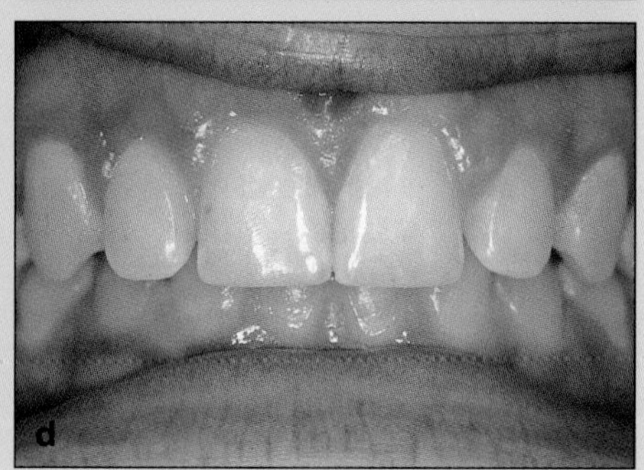

Figs 2-14a and 2-14b Excessive gingival display and displeasing dental proportions detract from smile esthetics.

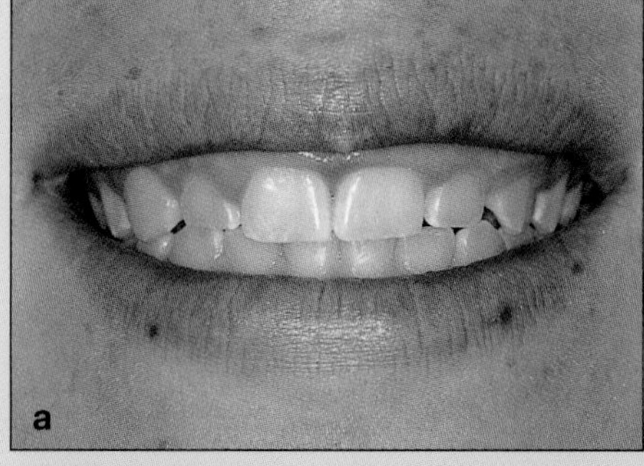

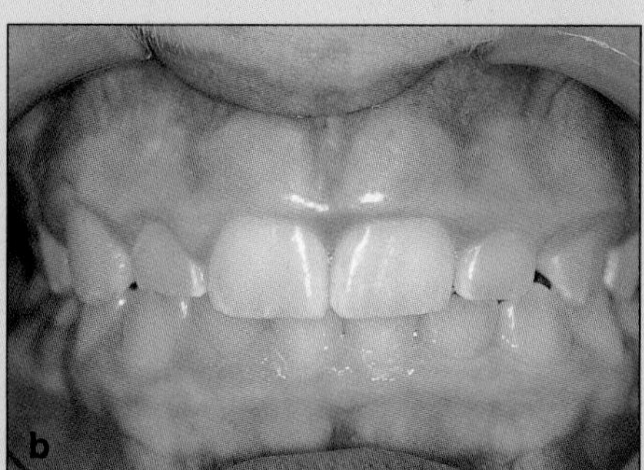

Fig 2-14c Initially following CO_2 laser–assisted soft tissue esthetic crown lengthening, gingival display is greatly improved and dental proportions are harmonious.

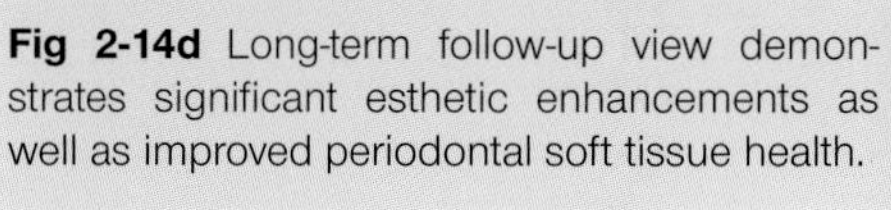

Fig 2-14d Long-term follow-up view demonstrates significant esthetic enhancements as well as improved periodontal soft tissue health.

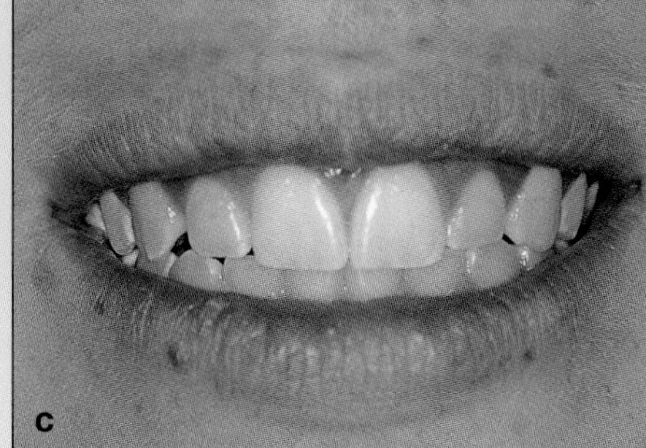

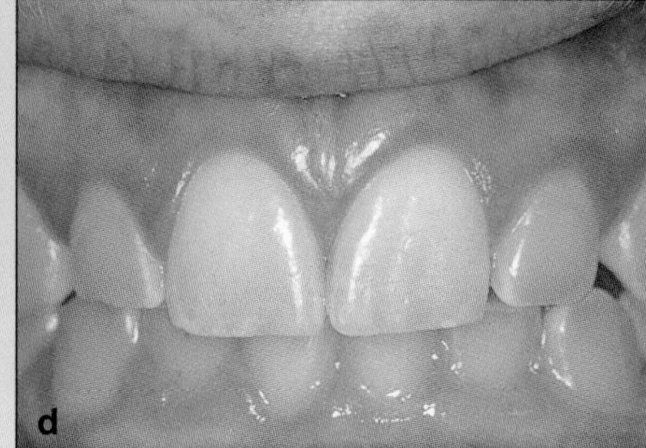

Periodontal Biotype

The patient's periodontal biotype is one of the most important factors in determining the outcome in esthetic implant therapy. The surgeon who understands how the different periodontal biotypes respond to the many surgical and restorative interventions involved in implant therapy can customize the treatment plan, properly sequence necessary adjunctive procedures, and select the surgical approaches that consistently lead to desirable esthetic outcomes. This is analogous to the facial cosmetic surgeon who evaluates a patient's skin type, cartilage support, and nasal morphology before functional and esthetic rhinoplasty. By determining the patient's periodontal biotype, the implant surgeon can establish realistic expectations for the esthetic outcomes and plan surgical approaches that optimize the results.

Two distinct periodontal biotypes have been described by Olsson and Lindhe.[5] Each periodontal biotype responds to surgical and restorative interventions in a predictable fashion, which either detracts from or favors ideal esthetic implant outcomes. The following is a brief description of the periodontal biotypes and their significance in the surgical and prosthetic phases of esthetic implant therapy.

Thin, scalloped periodontium

The thin, scalloped periodontium has a pronounced positive periodontal architecture with a delicate, friable soft tissue curtain. Attached soft tissue is minimal, and bony dehiscence and fenestration defects characterize the underlying osseous structure. This periodontal type has been associated with a specific tooth morphology characterized by triangular anatomic crowns with small interdental contacts at the incisal third. The clinical crowns either are flat in the cervical area or emerge with subtle convexities. The thin, scalloped periodontium reacts to surgical or prosthetic interventions with soft tissue recession, apical migration of attachment, and loss of underlying alveolar volume (Figs 2-15a and 2-15b).

In a patient with a thin, scalloped periodontium, the surgical and restorative interventions involved in esthetic implant therapy will result in some degree of soft tissue recession. In addition, the thin maxillary buccal plate underlying the friable soft tissue curtain is predisposed to defect formation secondary to remodeling and resorption of bone following tooth removal or osteotomy preparation and implant placement. Therefore, the implant team must make every effort to preserve the existing hard and soft tissue anatomy at the implant sites by employing minimally traumatic surgical and restorative techniques. The alveolar ridge preservation techniques that are described in chapter 4 should be performed following tooth removal in preparation for delayed implant placement or in conjunction with immediate implant placement. When immediate implant placement follows the removal of a maxillary anterior tooth, primary stability should be obtained without jeopardizing the integrity of the buccal wall of the socket. The author recommends maintaining a void between the implant body and the buccal wall of the socket, which is grafted with deproteinized bovine bone mineral (Bio-Oss; Osteohealth, Shirley, NY), as described in detail in chapter 4. Prosthetic soft tissue support with anatomically correct provisional restorations or prosthetic components is mandatory in the thin, scalloped periodontium; this is because peri-implant soft tissues, particularly the interdental papillae, collapse almost instantly following tooth removal, and subsequent re-creation of the papillae in the thin, scalloped periodontium is extremely difficult.

The author recommends the use of so-called flapless surgery whenever possible for immediate implant placement and the use of a U-shaped peninsula flap or tissue punch approach (see chapter 3) when site development is not indicated or desired in conjunction with delayed implant placements (see Figs 3-34 to 3-36). The U-shaped peninsula flap preserves the circulation to the area and allows direct visualization of the buccal, interproximal, and palatal alveolar crest levels, thus providing much-needed information to guide accurate three-dimensional implant placement. When combined with prosthetic soft tissue support, flapless surgery preserves the soft tissue volume and architecture at the implant site. Thus, the author prefers the U-shaped peninsula flap for implant placement for the reasons stated above but prefers the tissue punch approach to expose submerged or semi-submerged implants.

When soft tissue augmentation is performed in conjunction with implant placement, a pouch dissection or a flap design that preserves the circulation to the implant site and avoids elevation of the papillary or col tissue (as described in chapters 3 and 5) should be used. When hard tissue grafting is indicated to reconstruct missing bone volume, an exaggerated curvilinear-beveled flap design is preferred.

Restorative procedures in esthetic implant therapy also can cause a loss of soft tissue volume or blunted soft tissue architecture in the thin, scalloped periodontium, especially when a submerged approach with a two-piece implant system is used. In most esthetic

Clinical relevance of periodontal biotype in implant therapy: Thin, scalloped periodontium

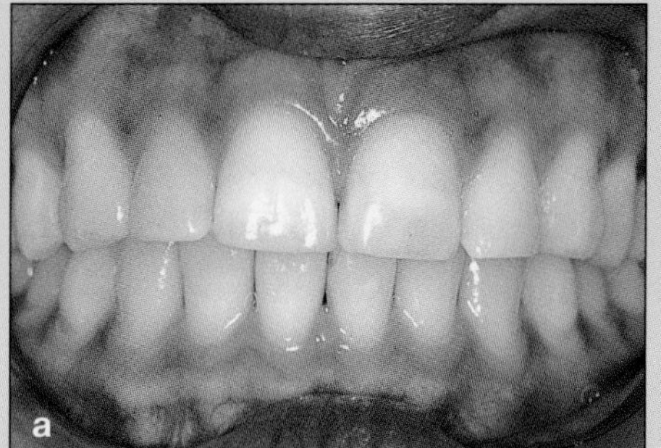

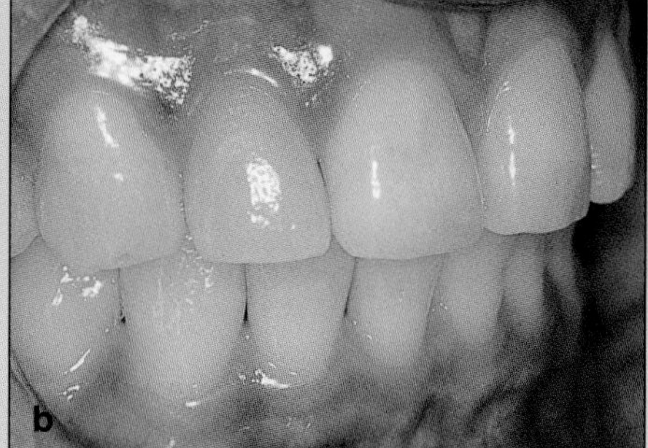

Figs 2-15a and 2-15b Thin, scalloped periodontal biotype. Note the pronounced positive gingival architecture with delicate, friable soft tissues. There is a minimal amount of attached tissue, and the interdental papillae adjacent to the failing right lateral incisor are already blunted. The incisors are flat in the cervical area and emerge with subtle, if any, convexity. The clinical crowns are triangular with small interdental contacts located at the incisal third.

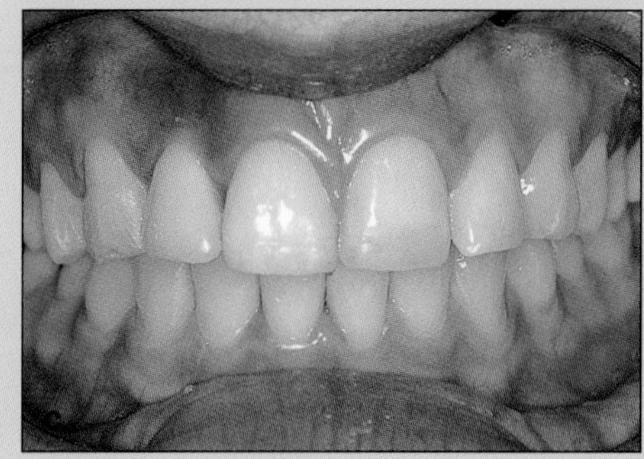

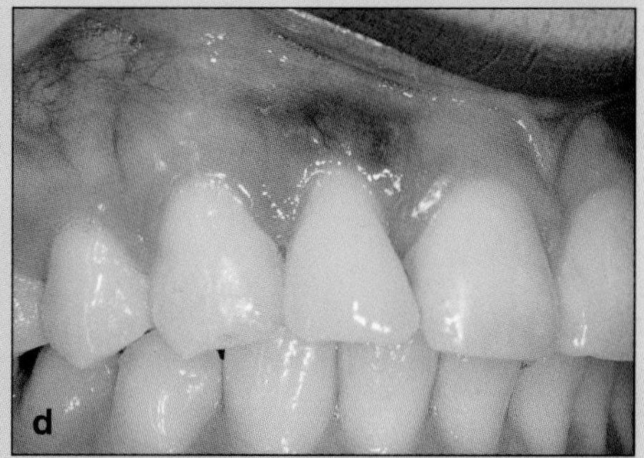

Figs 2-15c and 2-15d One-year posttreatment. The right lateral incisor was removed with a minimally traumatic technique, and an immediate submerged implant was placed with the Bio-Col ridge-preservation technique. Soft tissues were immediately supported by modifying the clinical crown of the lateral incisor into an ovate pontic and securing it to the adjacent dentition via resin-bonding. Despite "flapless" surgery and application of ridge preservation, peri-implant soft tissue recession and persistent soft tissue inflammation and sensitivity developed, preventing normal oral hygiene and jeopardizing the long-term prognosis of the implant restoration.

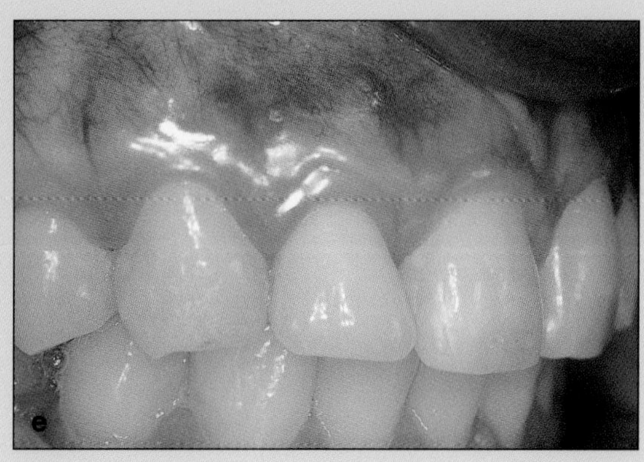

Fig 2-15e A subepithelial graft was performed via a closed pouch recipient site dissection 2 years earlier. Note the dramatic increase in the width of attached tissue surrounding the lateral incisor implant restoration when compared to the pretreatment photographs. Excellent esthetic blending of the grafted tissue was obtained, which is typical with the thin, scalloped periodontium. (Restoration by Dr Ricardo Gonzales, Miami, FL.)

cases, the 4- to 6-week period allowed for soft tissue healing following the placement of titanium healing abutments is insufficient for the soft tissue integration process. Consequently, the soft tissue stability required for delivery of a predictable permanent esthetic restoration is not achieved, and esthetic compromises become apparent after the inevitable recession of soft tissue, resulting in tissue discoloration or exposure of the restorative margin. In addition, when nonanatomic healing abutments are used, the dense connective tissue scar that forms immediately adjacent to the provisional abutment usually keeps the clinician from taking advantage of prosthetic-guided soft tissue healing. In essence, the tissues have been guided to heal in a nonanatomic, unesthetic fashion. Although there is evidence that the peri-implant soft tissues can eventually regain an esthetic morphology following the delivery of restorations with proper contours, the author finds this approach to be less predictable and practical because of the 12- to 18-month period often required. In most cases, prosthetic compensations (closure of gingival embrasures) are built into the restorations, which prevents full papillary return even when anatomically favored by appropriate interdental bone support. Furthermore, the removal and replacement of the healing abutments and implant-level prosthetics (impression procedures or delivery of permanent abutments) can cause apical migration of the peri-implant soft tissues in the thin, scalloped periodontium.

Whenever possible, at second-stage surgery, custom abutments and provisional restorations should be delivered by the surgeon in a minimally traumatic fashion to provide anatomic support and prosthetic-guided soft tissue healing. Registering implant position at the time of implant placement facilitates this process. An indirect technique is then used to fabricate a customized abutment and provisional restoration. Alternatively, an implant-supported provisional restoration can be fabricated directly to a prefabricated permanent abutment delivered by the surgeon at implant uncovering, but this approach may be more traumatic to the surrounding tissues and may cause soft tissue recession. Although the use of a two-piece implant system with a nonsubmerged approach allows more time for soft tissue integration, implant-level prosthetics may still result in apical migration of soft tissues in the thin, scalloped periodontium.

When a nonsubmerged or semi-submerged approach is used with a one-piece implant, anatomic support of the surrounding soft tissues is immediately obtained from the transmucosal portion of the implant and through the use of prefabricated anatomic abutments or customized "tooth-form" provisional abutments fabricated directly or indirectly. Because the permucosal portion of the implant provides an area for connective tissue adaptation and junctional epithelial attachment formation, the delivery of anatomically correct provisional abutments at the time of implant placement supports and guides the soft tissue healing only in the superficial areas that are eventually critical for prosthetic emergence. Following the osseointegration–soft tissue integration period, removal of these custom tooth-form components generally is atraumatic, as the connective tissue zone and junctional epithelial attachment are not disrupted and sufficient time has been allowed for the development of an adequate peri-implant sulcus.

In addition to heeding the surgical and prosthetic considerations described above, the restorative clinician, laboratory technician, and implant surgeon working with a thin, scalloped periodontium must ensure that healing abutments and provisional restorations have contours identical to the teeth they are meant to replace. Specifically, the buccal contour must be flat or emerge with a subtle convexity, and the interproximal contours must properly support the interdental papillae. Overcontouring of the facial aspect of the restoration results in soft tissue recession and an unesthetic implant restoration that is longer than the neighboring dentition in the apicocoronal dimension. Undercontoured proximal surfaces result in loss of papillary height and morphology. Accordingly, the surgeon must ensure that prefabricated or customized tooth-form healing abutments match the mesiodistal dimensions and proximal contours of the teeth that are being replaced and are slightly undercontoured or beveled to prevent the recession that predictably occurs when the facial restorative contours are excessive. Similarly, the laboratory technician and restorative clinician must be aware of the importance of proper emergence contours of provisional and permanent restorations in the thin, scalloped periodontium.

Despite the previously described efforts to preserve the existing soft tissue volume and architecture at the site, soft tissue grafting is almost always indicated to counteract the loss of soft tissue volume that predictably occurs when implant therapy is performed on a patient with a thin, scalloped periodontium. In the author's experience, the need for soft tissue grafting is constant and is not influenced by implant type or by the use of a submerged vs nonsubmerged approach. The ease with which the tissues of this periodontal type are managed makes these patients excellent candidates for soft tissue grafting procedures. Esthetic blending after soft tissue grafting procedures are performed on these patients is generally excellent. In addition, incision lines are easily camouflaged and often inconspicuous (Figs 2-15c to 2-15e) when compared with those that generally result from grafting procedures in the thick, flat periodontium. Accordingly, the surgeon should tell the patient about the expected loss of soft tissue volume at the implant site during therapy and plan for one or more soft tissue augmentation procedures to obtain the desired functional and esthetic result. The surgeon also should anticipate the possible need for guided bone regeneration to treat bony dehiscence and fenestration defects that may develop or be exacerbated after implant placement. The surgeon should consider performing guided bone-regeneration procedures whenever thin areas are observed in the buccal plate during tooth removal or implant placement. This will avoid late, unexpected esthetic complications related to remodeling and resorption of crestal alveolar bone with exposure of a portion of the titanium implant.

Thick, flat periodontium

A relatively flat soft tissue and bony architecture characterizes the thick, flat periodontium. There is significantly less disparity between the buccal marginal and interproximal soft tissue levels when compared with the thin, scalloped periodontium. The soft tissue curtain is dense and fibrotic, and there is an abundance of attached soft tissue. The underlying osseous form is composed of thick, dense bone. Square anatomic crowns that have bulbous convexities in the cervical third characterize the associated tooth form. The contact points and connector zones between the clinical crowns are large and often extend into the cervical one-third area. As a consequence, the interdental papillae are short compared with those found in the thin, scalloped peri-

Clinical relevance of periodontal biotype in implant therapy: Thick, flat periodontium

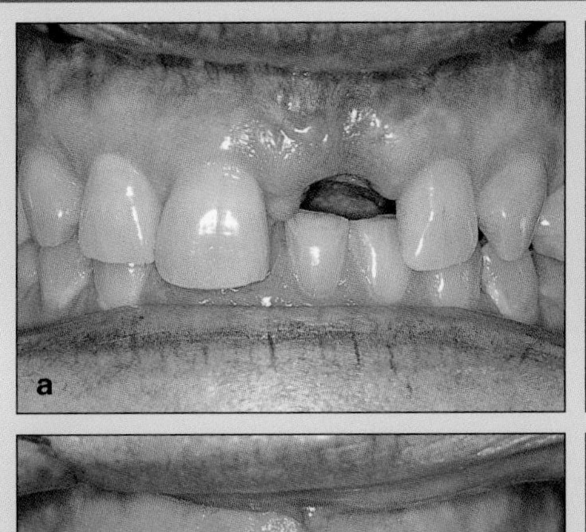
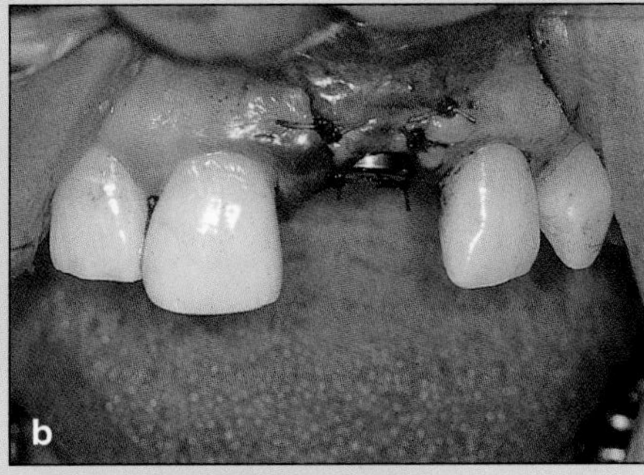

Fig 2-16a Thick, flat periodontal biotype. Patient had a midline diastema prior to loss of the left central incisor. Note that the soft tissue curtain is dense and fibrotic and there is an abundance of attached soft tissue at the implant site and around the adjacent dentition. The clinical crowns of the anterior teeth are square and have bulbous convexities in the cervical one third. The contact points and connector zones are large, extending into the cervical one third of the teeth. The interdental papillae are short.

Fig 2-16b A nonsubmerged implant was placed using an exaggerated curvilinear flap design with beveled incisions. Meticulous alignment of wound margins was accomplished during closure.

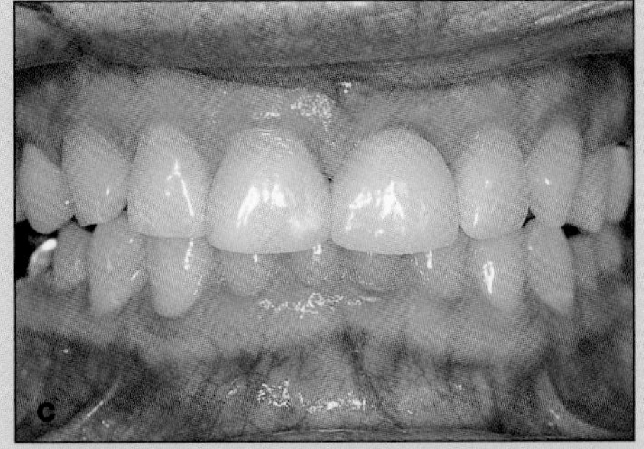
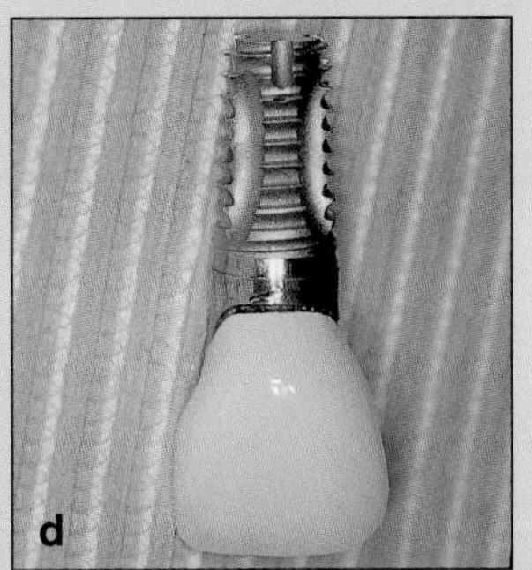

Fig 2-16c View of final implant restoration, which failed when the implant lost osseointegration 6 months later. The implant was removed, and the Bio-Col ridge preservation technique was performed. No osseous defect was noted after removal of the implant.

Fig 2-16d Failed implant demonstrated little evidence of osseointegration, perhaps secondary to decreased circulation to the site as a result of previous trauma and multiple endodontic procedures.

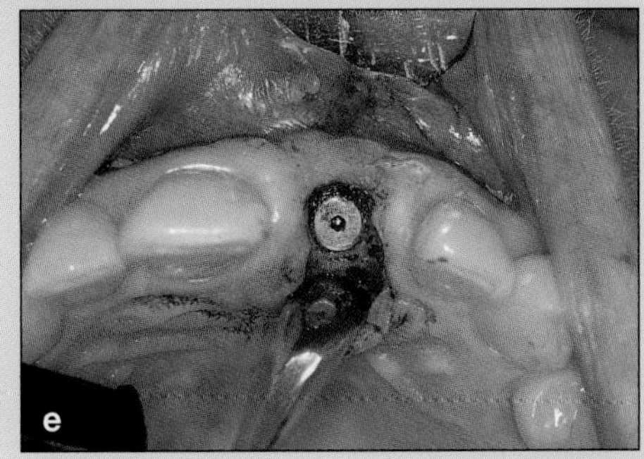
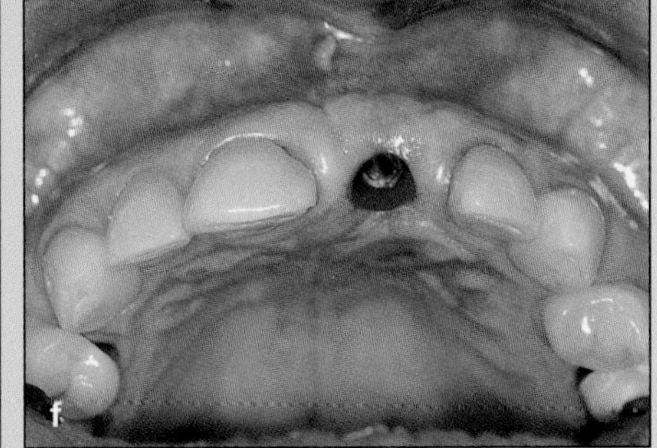

Fig 2-16e U-shaped peninsula flap used for implant replacement. Note that the initial incision lines, while not unesthetic, are noticeable. The use of this conservative approach avoided additional scarring that characteristically occurs with the thick, flat periodontium.

Fig 2-16f Tissue punch approach used for implant exposure and abutment connection.

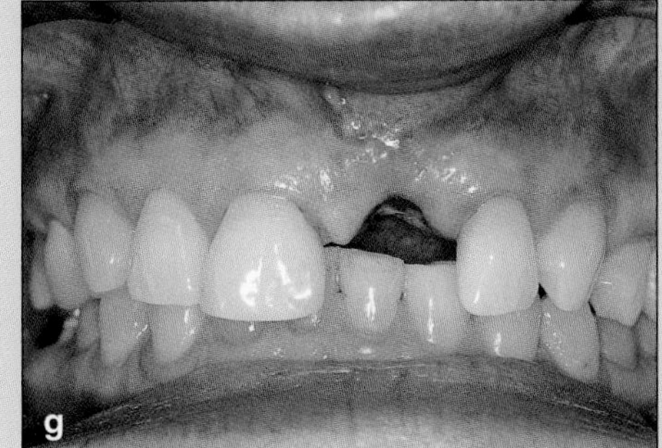
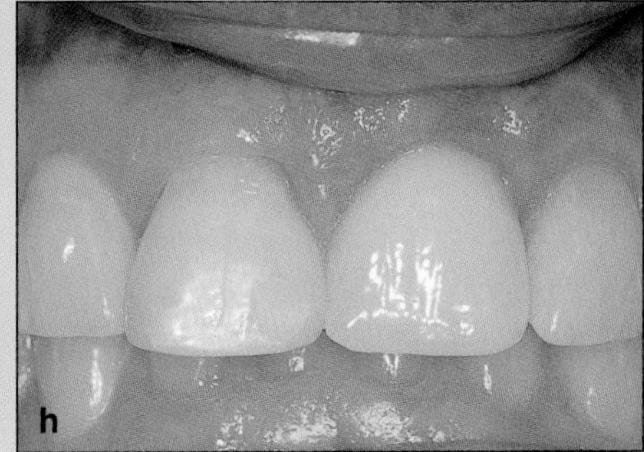

Fig 2-16g Frontal view immediately prior to final impression. Despite compromised dental history and subsequent failure and replacement of the implant, minimal alveolar ridge shrinkage has occurred. Specifically, there is no evidence of loss of soft tissue volume or architecture. The interdental papillae have maintained their pretreatment size and shape.

Fig 2-16h Three years after delivery of the final implant restoration, the peri-implant soft tissue volume and architecture are unchanged. No soft tissue recession has occurred despite multiple procedures performed; this is characteristic of the thick, flat periodontium. (Restoration by Dr Richard Mariani Sr, Miami, FL.)

odontium. The thick, flat periodontium resists recession and reacts to surgical and restorative insults with pocket formation (Fig 2-16).

The surgeon planning implant therapy for a patient with a thick, flat periodontium must be aware that while the thick fibrotic soft tissues resist recession, they are predisposed to forming unsightly notches and scars that can jeopardize the final esthetic and functional results. In addition, when soft tissue plastic surgery is performed to correct these conditions, the results are not always as desired, and multiple revisions are often needed. The fibrotic nature of the soft tissues makes them difficult to manage and can limit the esthetic success of soft tissue grafting procedures.

Therefore, whenever possible, the surgeon should avoid incisions through the buccal tissues during implant placement. Instead, the U-shaped peninsula flap described in chapter 3 should be used. When site-development procedures requiring elevation of a buccal flap are indicated, the use of an exaggerated curvilinear flap design with beveled incisions, as described in chapter 3, will allow for less conspicuous incisions after healing. The surgeon should make every effort to properly align the marginal soft tissues during wound closure and eliminate tension at the wound closure site. Failure to do so will result in a wide, uneven scar that is esthetically unacceptable. Notching of the marginal tissues results in both a functional and an esthetic compromise that is difficult to eliminate with soft tissue plastic surgery. In most cases, the only possible improvement is through soft tissue augmentation procedures performed using a closed pouch approach and subsequent laser soft tissue resurfacing and sculpting procedures, as presented in chapter 7. Finally, in patients with a thick, flat periodontium, immediate implant placement following tooth removal through a flapless approach, combined with prosthetic support for the surrounding soft tissues, results in a high degree of functional and esthetic success with good long-term stability.

Performing a systematic evaluation

This esthetic-conscious patient is unhappy with her smile and would like to improve it. She cannot identify what is wrong, but would like to know what treatment options are available to improve her smile. Can you help her?

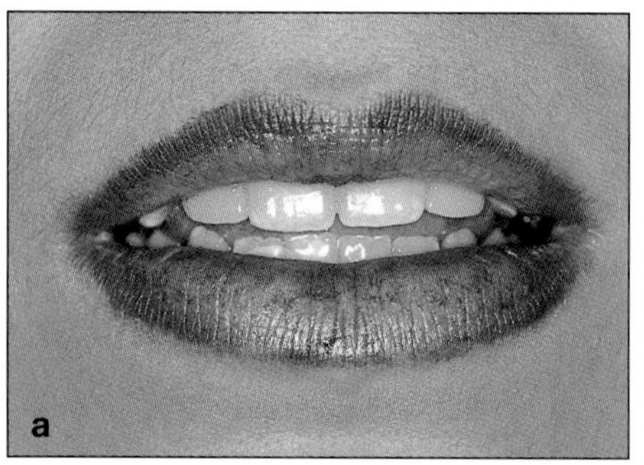

Fig 2-17a Resting lip position

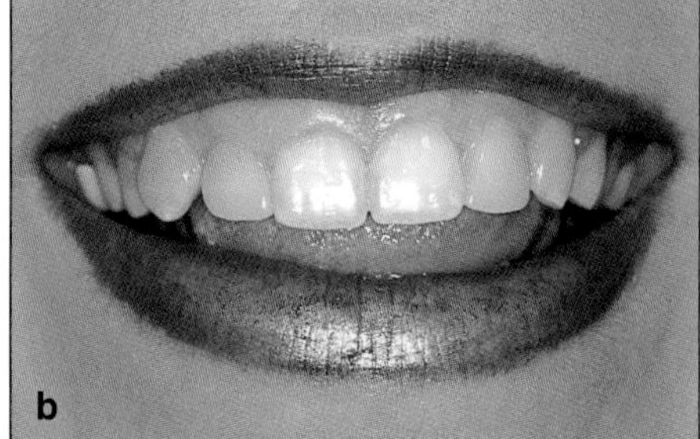

Fig 2-17b Relaxed smile

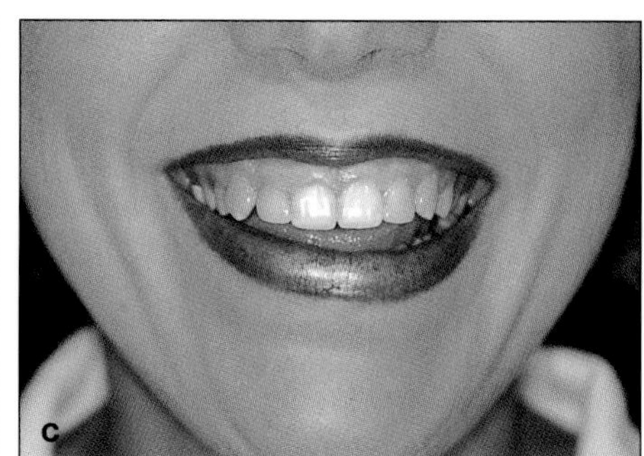

Fig 2-17c Fully animated smile

This 30-year-old female has a negative dental history and no dental or periodontal problems. Cephalometric analysis indicates vertical maxillary excess resulting in an anterior open bite. Based on the limited visual information available in Figs 2-17a to 2-17c, perform a systematic evaluation of this patient's smile. Make the assumption that although the patient has mild facial asymmetry, the facial and dental midlines are coincident and the dental midline is slightly canted to the right when compared to the facial midline. Make a list of those elements that detract from the esthetic appearance of her smile and compare your list to the list below. Rank the esthetic importance of each negative element listed below based on the priority of establishing a focal point for her smile that is symmetrical in shape, dominant in size, and located in the center of the face, as well as on the relative priority of establishing symmetry away from the midline. Formulate priority-based treatment options with the assumption that the existing dentition has a good long-term prognosis with more than ideal crown-to-root ratios and adequate width of attached tissues.

Systematic evaluation of smile esthetics

1. Discrepancy between central incisors creates an unacceptable midline asymmetry (Figs 2-17b and 2-17c).
2. The central incisors fail to dominate the smile (Figs 2-17b and 2-17c).
3. Intrinsic dental proportions of the central incisors are displeasing. The lateral incisors and canines also appear short and wide (Figs 2-17b and 2-17c).
4. The proportional relationship of the anterior maxillary dentition is displeasing (Figs 2-17b and 2-17c).
5. Axial inclination of anterior dentition detracts from esthetics. Progressive medial tipping is absent.
6. Connector zones appear to be disproportionately long when compared to the recommended 50%–40%–30% rule suggested by Morley.[4] The connector zone appears to be approximately 80% between central incisors, 70% between the central and lateral incisors, and 60% between the lateral incisors and the canines.
7. Rotational position and excessive buccal axial inclination of the right maxillary canine greatly detract from esthetics.
8. Flat incisal plane does not follow the gentle curvature of the lower lip (Figs 2-17a, 2-17b, and 2-17c).
9. Excessive gingival display is evident when the patient is animated. There is mild inferior canting of the gingival plane and more gingival display on the right (Fig 2-17c).
10. A discrepancy is evident between the incisal plane and the occlusal plane bilaterally. The entire maxilla is slightly canted inferiorly on the right (Fig 2-17b). An anterior open bite exists as a result of posterior occlusal prematurities. Transverse discrepancy of the maxilla and tooth malposition detract from esthetics in the buccal corridor.

Visualizing the final esthetic results

Option 1 Minor orthodontics/cosmetic periodontal surgery/conservative cosmetic dentistry

a. **Minor orthodontics:** Parallel dental and facial midlines, correct rotational discrepancy of the right maxillary canine, improve axial inclination with progressive medial tipping, and introduce slight incisal plane convexity.

b. **Cosmetic periodontal surgery:** Esthetic crown lengthening of anterior dentition to improve intrinsic and tooth-to-tooth proportional relationships, minimize gingival exposure, and create an esthetically pleasing gingival plane and outline. Esthetic crown lengthening of maxillary premolars harmonizes anterior and posterior gingival outlines.

c. **Conservative cosmetic dentistry:** Enameloplasty to idealize incisal embrasures and fine tune incisal plane morphology and tooth shapes and proportions. Possible need for esthetic bonding or veneer restorations.

Option 2 Cosmetic periodontal surgery/endodontic therapy/restorative dentistry

a. **Cosmetic periodontal surgery:** Esthetic crown lengthening of anterior dentition to improve intrinsic and tooth-to-tooth proportional relationships, minimize gingival exposure, and create an esthetically pleasing gingival plane and outline. Esthetic crown lengthening of maxillary premolars harmonizes anterior and posterior gingival outlines.

b. **Endodontic therapy:** Right maxillary canine in preparation for full-coverage restoration.

c. **Restorative dentistry:** Partial or full-coverage restorations as needed to parallel dental and facial midlines, correct rotational discrepancy of the right maxillary canine, improve axial inclination of the anterior dentition with progressive medial tipping, introduce slight incisal plane convexity, and idealize functional anterior guidance.

Figs 2-18a to 2-18c Predicted enhancement of smile esthetics obtainable with either Option 1 or Option 2

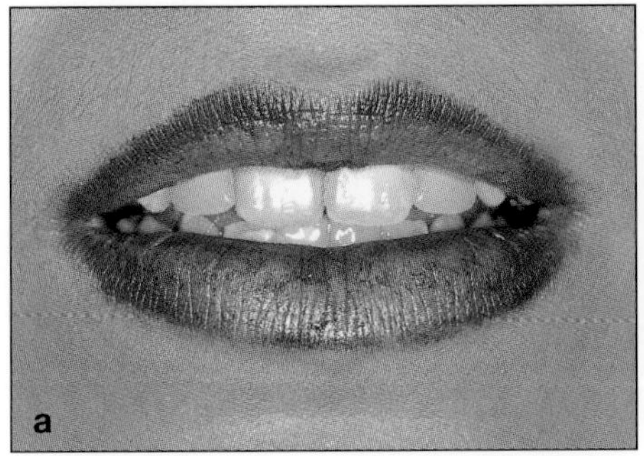
a

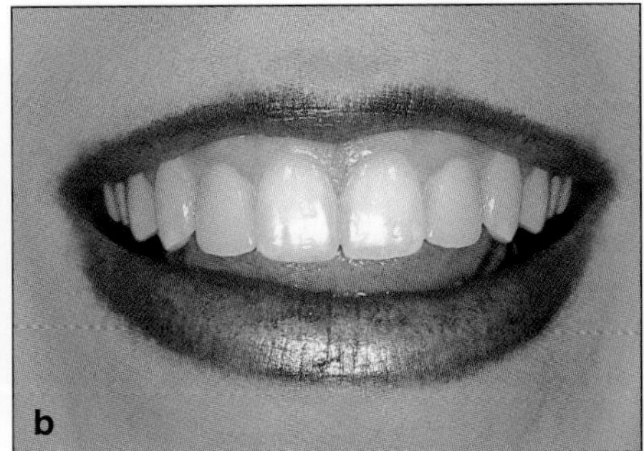
b

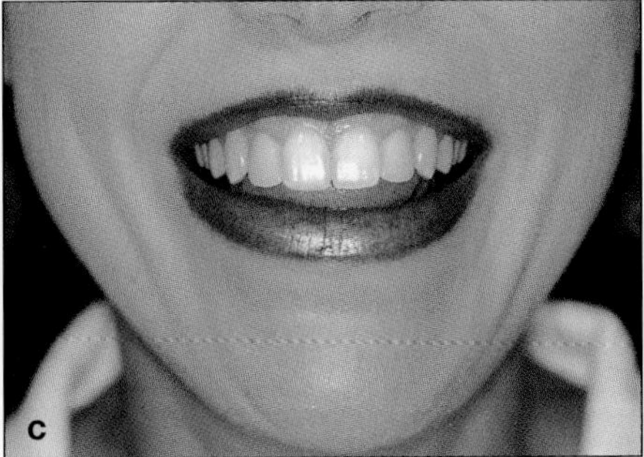
c

Option 3 Orthognathic surgery/cosmetic periodontal surgery/conservative cosmetic dentistry

a. **Combined orthodontic-surgical approach for correction of maxillary asymmetry and vertical maxillary excess:** After leveling, alignment, and coordination of maxillary and mandibular arches, orthognathic surgery performed to level canted maxillary occlusal and incisal planes and parallel and align dental and facial midlines. Superior repositioning of the maxilla is planned with knowledge of gingival margin positions following esthetic crown-lengthening procedures. Expansion of the maxilla will result in a full-volume smile that fills the buccal corridors. Axial inclinations will be improved with introduction of progressive medial tipping. A convex incisal plane that corresponds with a level occlusal plane, both of which parallel a level interpupillary line, will be achieved to enhance dentofacial esthetics. Autorotation of mandible results in a reduction of lower face height, relaxation of perioral musculature, and establishment of functional guidance.

b. **Cosmetic periodontal surgery:** Esthetic crown lengthening of anterior dentition to improve intrinsic and tooth-to-tooth proportional relationships and create an esthetically pleasing gingival plane and outline. Esthetic crown lengthening of maxillary premolars harmonizes anterior and posterior gingival outlines.

c. **Conservative cosmetic dentistry:** Enameloplasty to idealize incisal embrasures and fine tune incisal plane morphology and tooth shapes and proportions. Possible need for esthetic bonding or veneer restorations.

Figs 2-19a to 2-19c Predicted enhancement of smile esthetics obtainable with Option 3

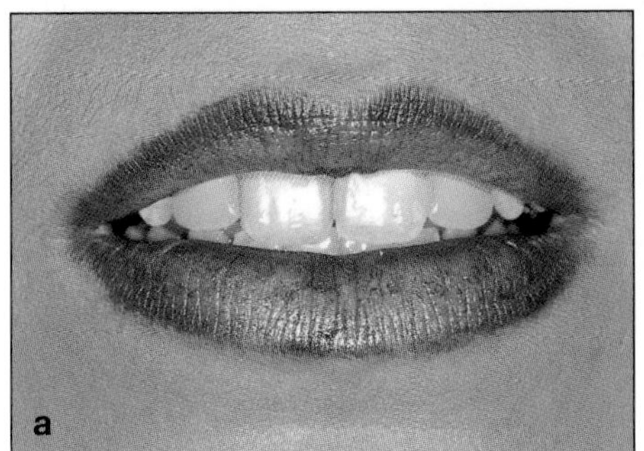
a

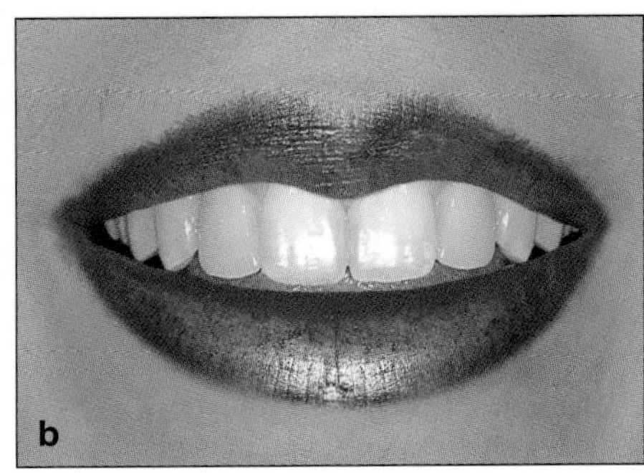
b

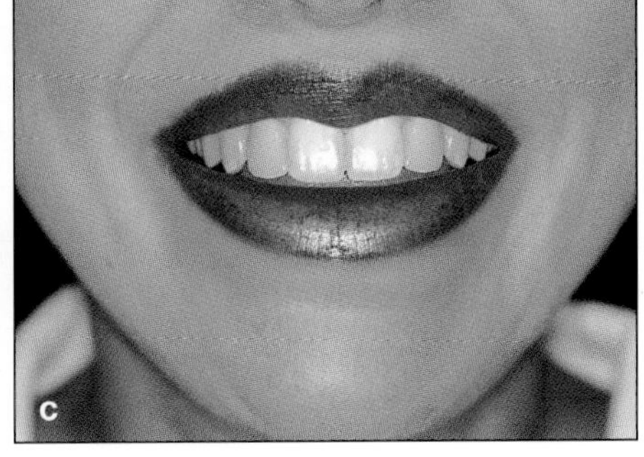
c

Anatomic limitations: Vertical maxillary deficiency and compromised bone height or width on adjacent dentition

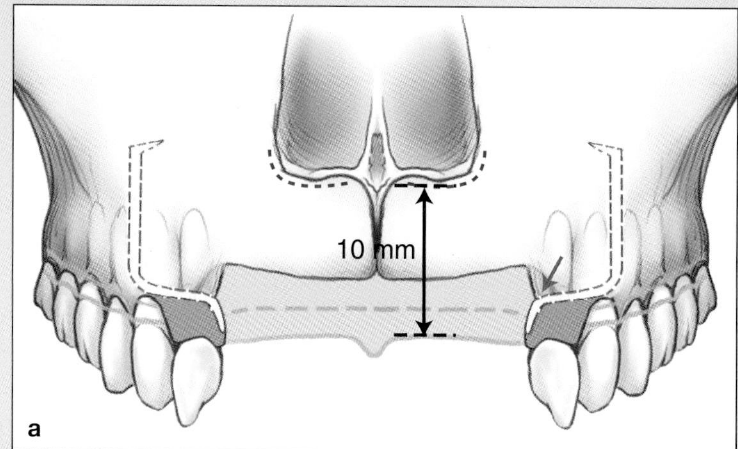

Fig 2-20a Vertical deficiency in the anterior maxillary area presents an anatomic limitation that may compromise functional and esthetic results in implant therapy. Apical migration of soft tissues following implant exposure is common. In addition, the proximity of the anterior nasal spine and piriform apertures of the nose limit the mobilization and coronal advancement of the soft tissues necessary for successful hard and soft tissue site development. Note outline of proposed flap design for surgical access. Compromised bone height or width on adjacent dentition *(blue arrow)* is an anatomic limitation that limits both vertical hard and soft tissue site development. Esthetic outcomes are limited when interdental bone height or width at the crest is insufficient to support a papilla and thereby ensure a harmonious connector zone between the implant restoration and adjacent natural tooth.

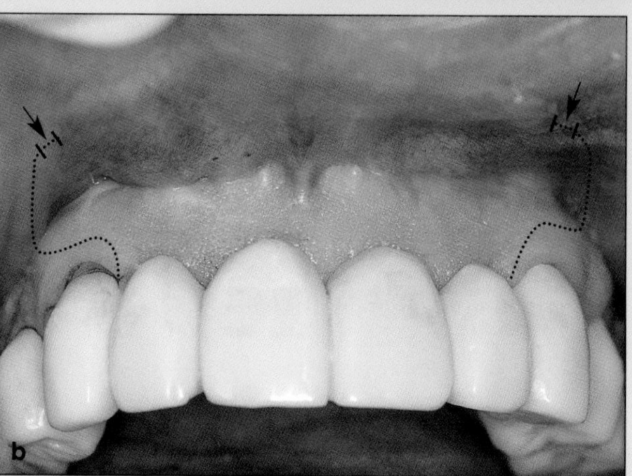

Fig 2-20b Presurgical view of maxillary central and lateral implant sites with large-volume hard tissue defect. Vertical deficiency in the anterior maxillary area, a short upper lip, and a concavity in the anterior maxillary alveolus are noted on palpation. The distance between the palpable anterior nasal spine and the coronal peak of the central incisor interdental papilla is 9 mm.

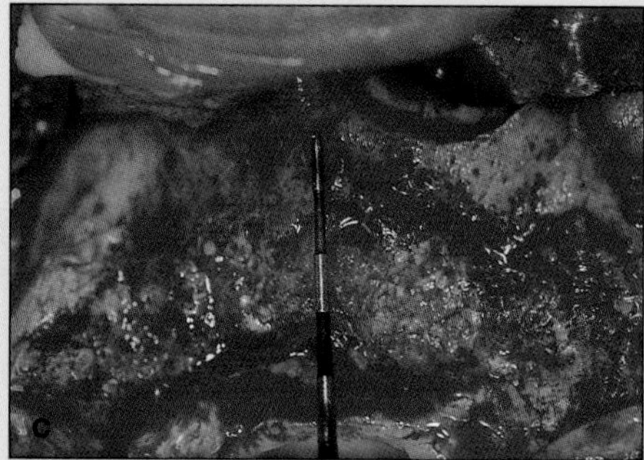

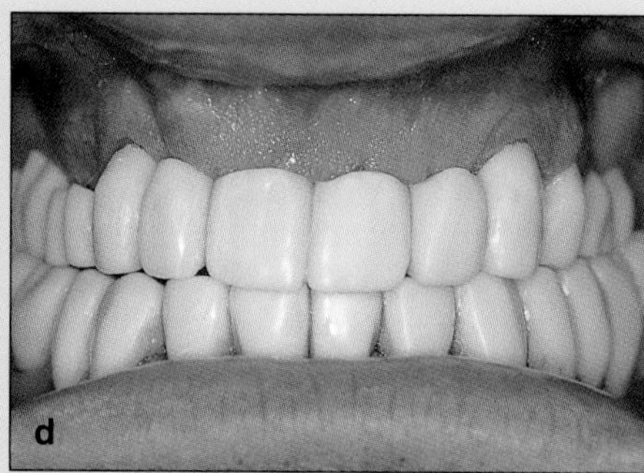

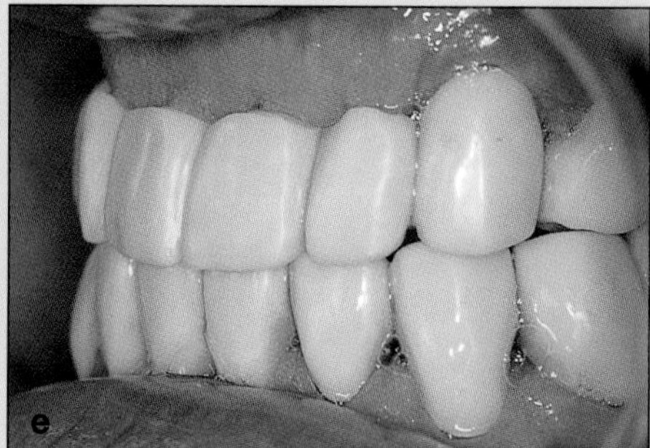

Fig 2-20c An exaggerated curvilinear-beveled flap design with tension-releasing cutback incisions was used to gain wide exposure of the area for site-development procedures. This approach incorporates more elastic mucosal tissues within the flap, thereby improving the ability to obtain tension-free closure over the necessary large-volume hard and soft tissue grafts. Note that the distance between the anterior nasal spine and the central papilla measures less than 10 mm. Osseous reduction of the anterior nasal spine will be performed. Periosteal releasing incisions have been made at the confluence of the alveolar ridge and nasal floor periosteum (see Fig 2-20a, *dotted red line*). Perinasal lip elevator musculature has been reflected.

Figs 2-20d and 2-20e Despite anatomic limitations, successful vertical and buccal augmentation was achieved through modification of flap design, osseous reduction of anterior nasal spine, and the use of periosteal releasing incisions to allow tension-free closure of the buccal flap over large-volume corticocancellous block grafts and bilateral VIP-CT flaps, which were performed simultaneously.

Anatomic Limitations

Vertical maxillary deficiency

The surgeon planning esthetic implant therapy for a patient with vertical deficiency of the anterior maxillary region should be aware of anatomic limitations that can compromise functional and esthetic outcomes. Typically, these patients have a short upper lip length as measured clinically or cephalometrically from subnasale to stomion. The clinical norm for upper lip length in males is 22 mm ± 2 mm and in females, 20 mm ± 2 mm. Therefore, male patients are considered to have a short upper lip when the length is less than 20 mm and female patients when the length is less than 18 mm. Intraoral palpation reveals deficient vestibular depth in the anterior maxillary region with a shortened distance (< 10.0 mm) measured from the coronalmost aspect of the interdental papilla between the central incisors and the palpable anterior nasal spine (Fig 2-20a). In addition, the nasal floor and piriform apertures are closely approximated to the roots of the lateral incisor and canine teeth as determined on radiography or direct visualization after exposing the area at the time of surgery. On occasion, patients with vertical maxillary deficiency also have a concave alveolar ridge and perinasal anatomy, making surgical management of soft tissues and site-development procedures even more difficult to perform due to further reduction of the reconstructive soft tissue envelope.

In patients with these anatomic characteristics, the author has identified a predisposition for apical migration of soft tissues following implant placement, exposure, or site-development procedures. The proximity of the anterior nasal spine and the nasal floor significantly limits the surgeon's ability to obtain passive flap adaptation during hard and soft tissue augmentation because of decreased ability to gain coronal flap advancement over these grafts (Fig 2-20b). Consequently, flap elevation for implant placement usually extends beyond the mucogingival junction, resulting in a tendency for apical soft tissue migration. When planning esthetic implant therapy for patients with these anatomic limitations, the author recommends discussing with them the increased need for hard or soft tissue augmentation to overcome the anatomic limitations and to offset predictable soft tissue retraction and associated loss of hard tissue.

Surgical management includes an exaggerated wide-base curvilinear flap design with beveled incisions, as described in chapter 3. It is also necessary to carefully elevate the periosteum from the piriform aperture just entering the nasal floor. Periosteal releasing incisions are sometimes made at the confluence of the alveolar ridge and nasal floor periosteum to obtain tension-free adaptation of flaps upon wound closure. Elevation of periosteum in these areas improves the overall elasticity of the flap and detaches the levator labii superioris and zygomaticus minor muscles, thereby reducing upper lip activity in the immediate postoperative period. In addition, exposure of the anterior nasal spine and, on occasion, reduction osteoplasty are performed as part of recipient-site preparation for bone-grafting procedures or prior to wound closure (Figs 2-20c to 2-20e). Subsequently, localized vestibuloplasty is often indicated to re-establish adequate vestibular depth after site-development procedures.

Compromised bone height or width on adjacent dentition

Loss of height or width of the interdental bone between a tooth and an implant site presents another anatomic limitation that can limit vertical hard and soft tissue site development or esthetic results obtainable from adjacent implant restorations. This anatomic limitation results in blunting or absence of the interdental papilla, thus detracting from the establishment of a harmonious gingival appearance around the implant restoration. In addition, air escape between the maxillary anterior dentition can interfere with phonetics and is rarely acceptable to patients. In most of these instances, prosthetic compensation via closure of the gingival embrasure is necessary; however, doing so results in compromised oral hygiene maintenance of the area, which can further propagate bone loss and ultimately may jeopardize osseointegration of the implant and the long-term prognosis of the adjacent tooth.

Tarnow and coworkers[6] correlated the loss of interdental soft tissues with the distance in height between the base of the contact or connector zone and the interdental bone crest. They found that when this dimension was 5.0 mm or less, the interdental papilla would fill the gingival embrasure 100% of the time. When this distance increased to 6 mm or even 7 mm or greater, the interdental papilla could be expected to fill the gingival embrasure 56% and 27% of the time, respectively. While these guidelines are helpful for evaluating esthetic implant sites in partially edentulous patients prior or subsequent to tooth loss, the implant surgeon must also take into account such factors as periodontal biotype, tooth malposition when present, and whether prosthetic support for the interdental tissues was maintained at edentulous sites following tooth removal.

In addition, the width of interdental bone on adjacent teeth appears to be as critical as the height in determining the final esthetic outcome (see Fig 2-20a). When the interdental bone crest between a natural tooth and an implant site is less than 2 mm in width, an esthetic risk exists. If immediate implant placement is to follow tooth removal, care should be taken to maintain a minimum distance of 1.5 to 2.0 mm between the implant body and the adjacent tooth root. This will ensure optimal bone volume to support the overlying papilla. When the implant body encroaches on this minimum distance, interdental bone height is lost, jeopardizing osseointegration of the implant and the periodontal prognosis of the adjacent tooth.

Whenever the implant surgeon has the opportunity to evaluate a compromised tooth prior to its removal, careful attention should be given to the height and width of the interdental bone between the adjacent teeth. Loss of interdental hard and soft tissues is often camouflaged by edema from chronic inflammation of the periodontal soft tissues secondary to mobility of the tooth, violations of biologic width or leakage from existing restorations, and noninfectious resorption of the tooth. In these situations, it is best to avoid immediate implant placement in favor of an alveolar ridge preservation technique, even if all other parameters of the examination are ideal. Re-evaluation several months later

Miller class I recession:
Marginal tissue recession does not extend to the mucogingival junction, and there is no loss of interdental bone or soft tissue. Root coverage of 100% can be anticipated.

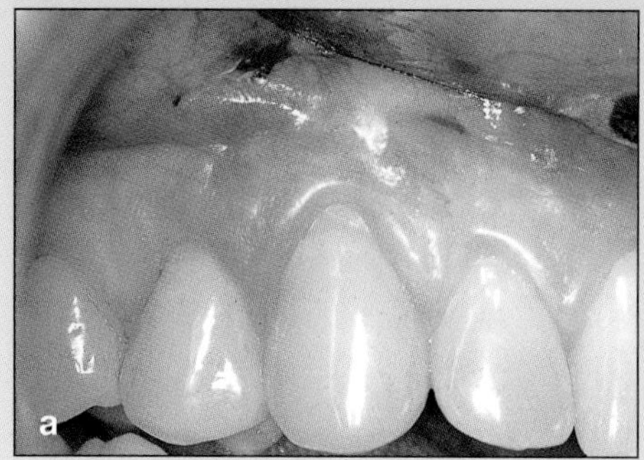

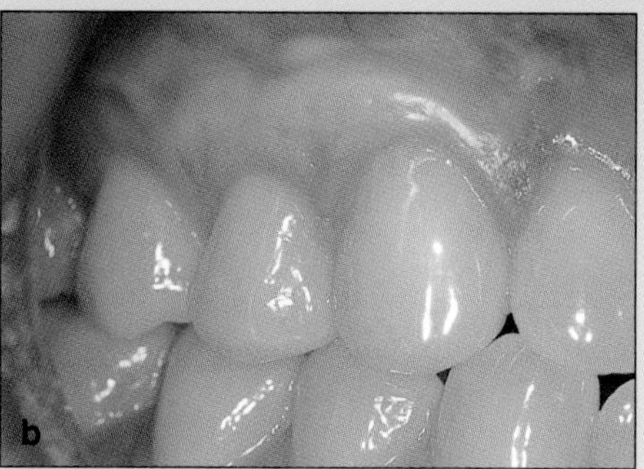

Fig 2-21a Miller class I recession defect on the maxillary canine.

Fig 2-21b Root coverage of 100% obtained with subepithelial connective tissue grafting via a closed recipient site pouch.

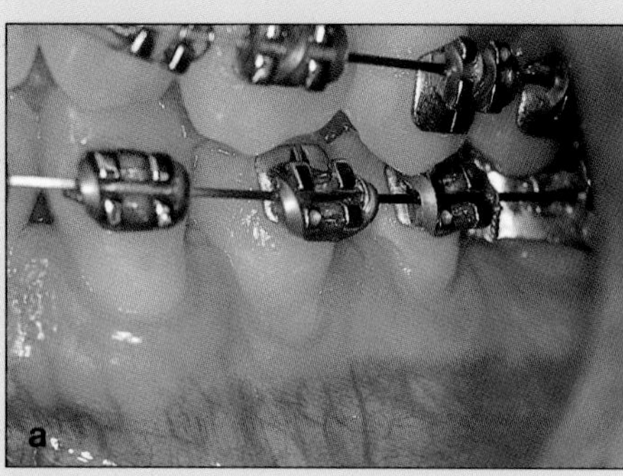

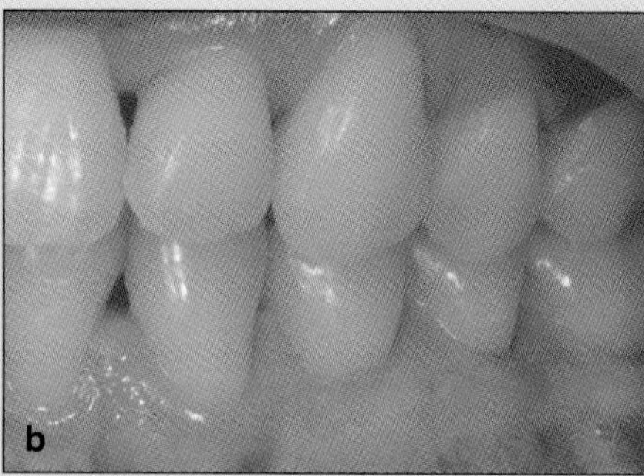

Fig 2-22a Miller class I recession defect involving mandibular premolars noted during orthodontic therapy.

Fig 2-22b Root coverage of 100% obtained with subepithelial connective tissue grafting via an open recipient site flap.

will allow an accurate appraisal of remaining hard and soft tissue volume and architecture at the site and ensure proper selection and sequencing of site-development procedures if indicated.

When evaluating a partially edentulous site for hard and soft tissue site development, the height and width of crestal bone on the natural teeth adjacent to the site are the major criteria to consider. Here too, the remaining bone height and width appear to be of equal importance. In the author's experience, the volume outcomes from hard tissue site development immediately adjacent to a natural tooth are most predictable when the width of bone on the adjacent natural tooth is 2.0 mm or greater. This provides a solid base for graft adaptation and subsequent integration of the graft via the bridging phenomenon. When there is compromised height or width of the crestal bone on a natural tooth adjacent to an implant site, forced orthodontic eruption is one option for overcoming or diminishing the severity of this anatomic limitation. Alternatively, the tooth can be removed and the area of site development extended, or the patient can accept an esthetic compromise, and esthetic crown lengthening of neighboring dentition can be used to camouflage the esthetic defect (see chapter 7 and Appendix).

Marginal Tissue Recession

The evaluation and classification of marginal tissue recession is an important part of the pretreatment evaluation of partially edentulous patients undergoing esthetic implant therapy. Root-coverage procedures on adjacent dentition may be indicated to establish an esthetic gingival appearance. The surgeon must determine the cause of localized recession defects, and when recession is determined to be progressive, measures to correct the situation should be included in the patient's therapeutic plan. In addition, a predisposition for tissue recession (thin, scalloped periodontium) signals the need for soft tissue grafting in conjunction with implant therapy.

Sullivan and Atkins[7] proposed a classification for marginal tissue recession that described four types of defects: shallow-narrow, shallow-wide, deep-narrow, and deep-wide. Miller[8] subsequently proposed an expanded classification of marginal tissue recession that not only described the morphology of recession defects but also correlated the morphology with the ability to achieve complete or partial root coverage. Miller's classification also takes into account the relationship of the recession defect to the mucogingival junction, the degree of interdental hard and soft tissue loss, and the prominence of the tooth in the arch. In essence, Miller

Miller class II recession:
Marginal tissue recession extends to or beyond the mucogingival junction, and there is no loss of interdental bone or soft tissue. Root coverage of 100% can be anticipated.

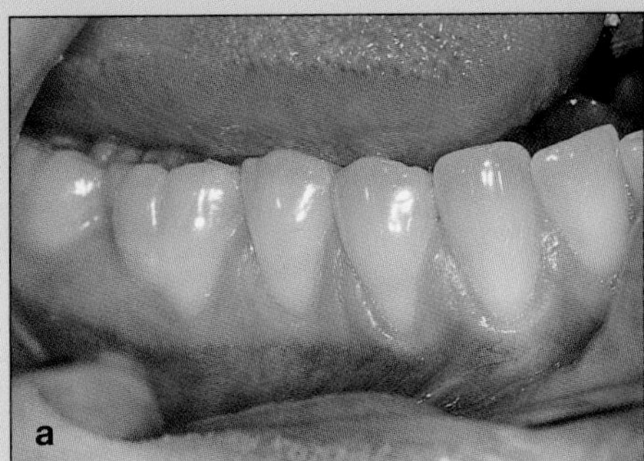

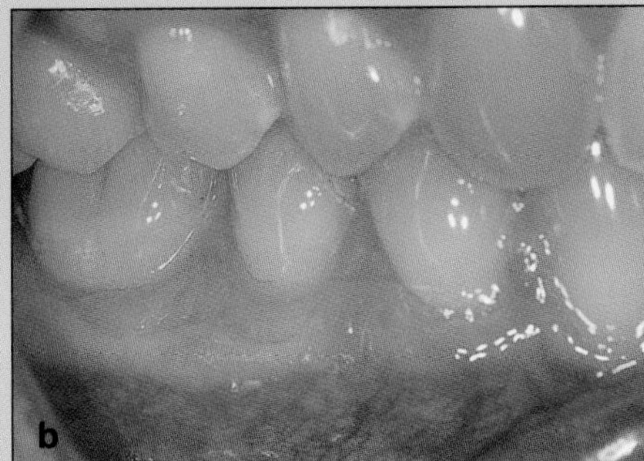

Fig 2-23a Miller class II recession defect on the mandibular second premolar and first molar. Recession progressed to the mucogingival junction prior to surgical correction.

Fig 2-23b Root coverage of 100% obtained with a subepithelial connective tissue graft via an open recipient site flap.

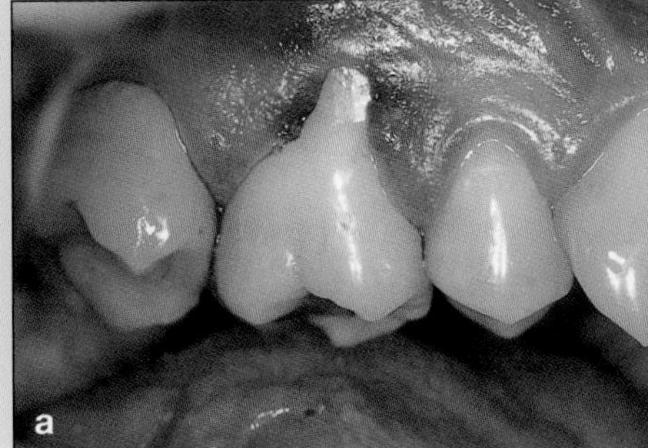

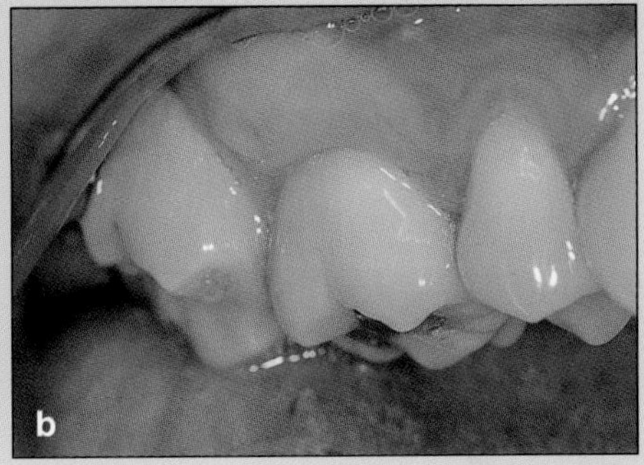

Fig 2-24a Miller class II recession on maxillary first molar extended beyond the mucogingival junction.

Fig 2-24b Root coverage of 100% obtained with subepithelial connective tissue graft via a double papilla flap.

expanded upon the descriptive classification proposed by Sullivan and Atkins by correlating the type of defect with the surgeon's ability to use the peripheral vascular supply (interdental tissues) to nourish and sustain free soft tissue grafts placed over avascular root surfaces. In addition, he emphasized the relationship between buccal-lingual tooth position, the prominence (convexity) of the exposed root surface, and the size of the avascular root surface to be covered with the amount of peripheral vascular supply available to support soft tissue reconstruction. Most important, he described the anatomic circumstances that limit or preclude attempts at root coverage by the surgeon (Figs 2-21 to 2-28).

Because Miller's classification of marginal tissue recession provided the anatomic basis for consistent prediction of the outcome of root-coverage procedures, its publication was a breakthrough for the periodontal plastic surgeon. In addition, this classification is a useful communication tool for educating patients and restorative dentists about the possibilities and limitations of root coverage, thereby ensuring realistic expectations for surgical outcomes. If the tooth is positioned within the alveolar housing or can be mechanically reduced to eliminate excessive prominence, the surgeon can show the patient or restorative dentist the level of root coverage attainable. To do so, the surgeon places a periodontal probe horizontally across the recession at the coronal level of the interdental soft tissue on either side of the defect. The relationship of the probe to the cementoenamel junction determines the level of root coverage attainable.

Miller's classification of marginal tissue recession:

- Class I. Marginal tissue recession does not extend to the mucogingival junction, and there is no loss of interdental bone or soft tissue. Root coverage of 100% can be anticipated (Figs 2-21 and 2-22).
- Class II. Marginal tissue recession extends to or beyond the mucogingival junction, and there is no loss of interdental bone or soft tissue. Root coverage of 100% can be anticipated (Figs 2-23 and 2-24).
- Class III. Marginal tissue recession extends to or beyond the mucogingival junction, and loss of interdental bone, loss of soft tissue, or tooth malposition prevents 100% root coverage. Partial root coverage can be anticipated (Figs 2-25 and 2-26).
- Class IV. Marginal tissue recession extends to or beyond the mucogingival junction, and loss of interdental bone, loss of soft tissue, or tooth malposition is severe enough to preclude attempts at root coverage (Figs 2-27 and 2-28).

Miller class III recession:
Marginal tissue recession extends to or beyond the mucogingival junction, and loss of interdental bone, loss of soft tissue, or tooth malposition prevents 100% root coverage. Partial root coverage can be anticipated.

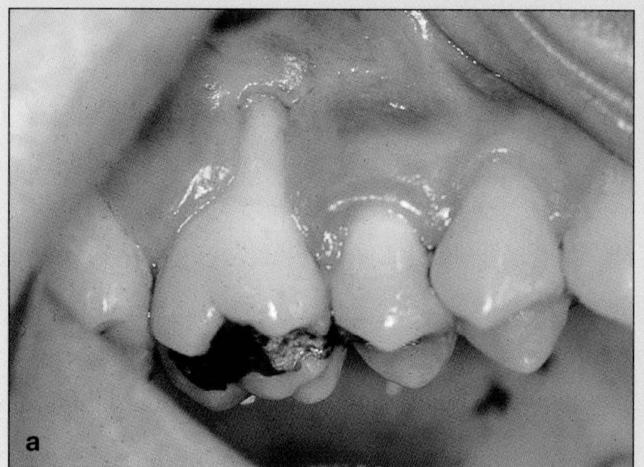

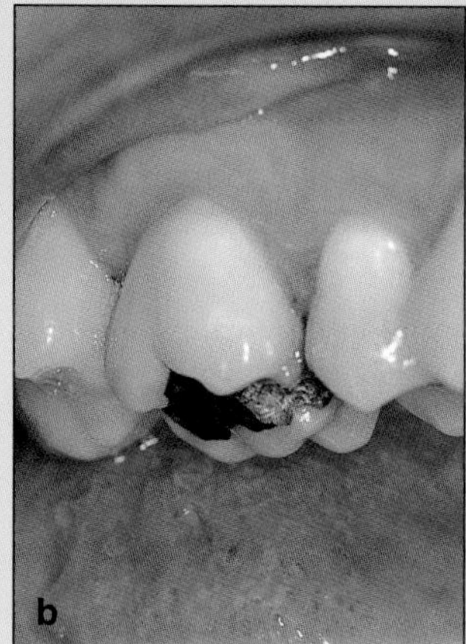

Fig 2-25a Miller class III recession defect on the maxillary molar extends beyond the mucogingival junction. While there is no loss of interdental bone or soft tissue, the prominence of the root could preclude complete root coverage.

Fig 2-25b Root coverage of 100% obtained after root prominence was mechanically reduced with hand instrumentation, thereby converting it to a Miller class II defect.

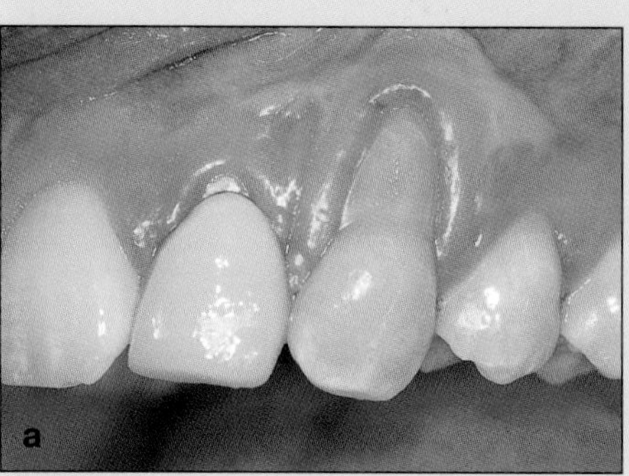

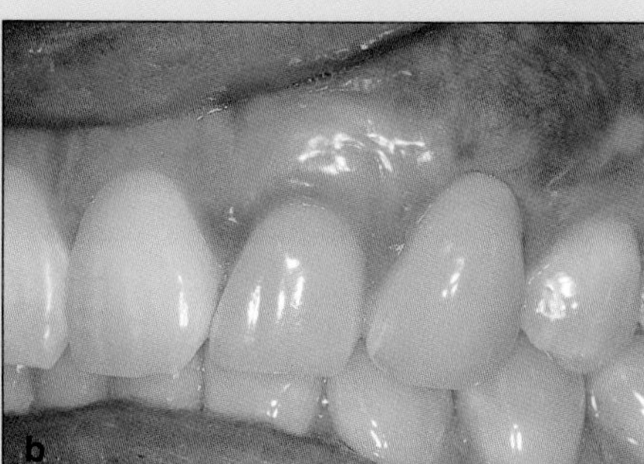

Fig 2-26a Miller class III recession on the canine and Miller class II recession on the lateral incisor. Two previous attempts at root coverage using epithelialized palatal grafts without mechanical reduction of root prominence failed. The portion of the previous grafts that survived can be seen above the canine. The canine was previously treated with endodontic therapy.

Fig 2-26b Root coverage of 100% obtained via two subepithelial grafts. Mechanical reduction of root prominence was performed during the first grafting procedure. This effectively converted the Miller class III defect into a Miller class II defect. The second procedure involved coronal advancement of the cover flap over an additional subepithelial graft. (Restoration by Dr Larry Grillo, Aventura, FL.)

Recession of peri-implant soft tissues

In the author's experience, with certain exceptions, Miller's classification is equally useful for evaluating marginal tissue recession and predicting the outcomes of oral soft tissue grafting procedures performed around dental implants. When marginal tissue recession occurs around a single-tooth implant, the surgeon can use the peripheral circulation provided by the neighboring dentition to support and nourish the graft. However, uncorrectable implant or abutment malposition can preclude a successful outcome.

Miller's classification system can be used to predict outcomes for abutment coverage. When marginal tissue recession occurs in a patient with multiple implants, and soft tissue coverage of an abutment or abutments is desired, lack of contribution from the periodontal ligament circulation to the peri-implant soft tissues should be considered. Whenever possible, the recipient site and graft should be enlarged to take advantage of all available peripheral circulation to compensate for the decreased circulation available to the peri-implant soft tissues. Although the surgeon can compensate by adjusting the size of the recipient site, the volume of inter-implant hard and soft tissue available or the degree of implant malposition may limit the amount of abutment coverage possible with multiple implants. Thus, the clinician must recognize the limitations imposed by diminished circulation of peri-implant soft tissues or by implant or abutment malposition.

Other limitations are due to the fact that the nature of the soft tissue attachment to an exposed natural tooth root may differ from that found on an implant abutment following oral soft tissue grafting for correc-

Miller class IV recession:
Marginal tissue recession extends to or beyond the mucogingival junction, and loss of interdental bone, loss of soft tissue, or tooth malposition is severe enough to preclude attempts at root coverage.

Figs 2-27a and 2-27b Loss of bone and soft tissue on the mesial aspect of the mandibular premolar precludes attempts at root coverage because there is an absence of vascularity to nourish a soft tissue graft at the mesial aspect of the site, thereby eliminating the bridging phenomenon.

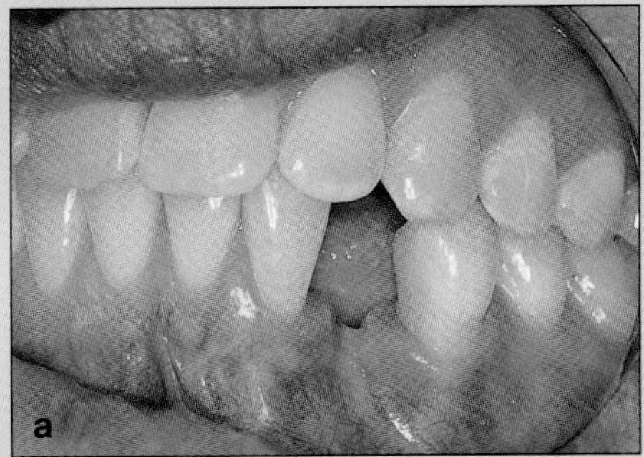

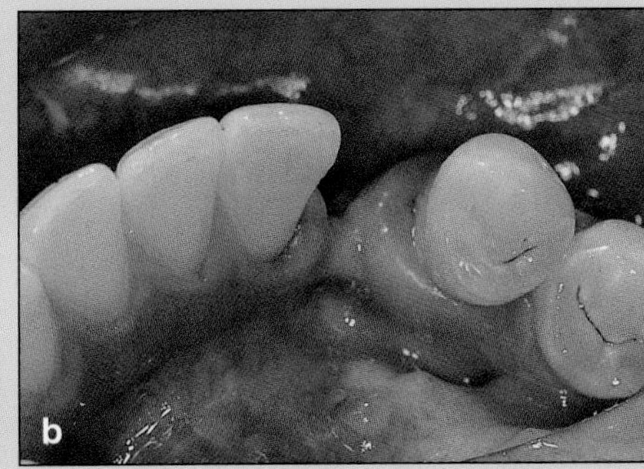

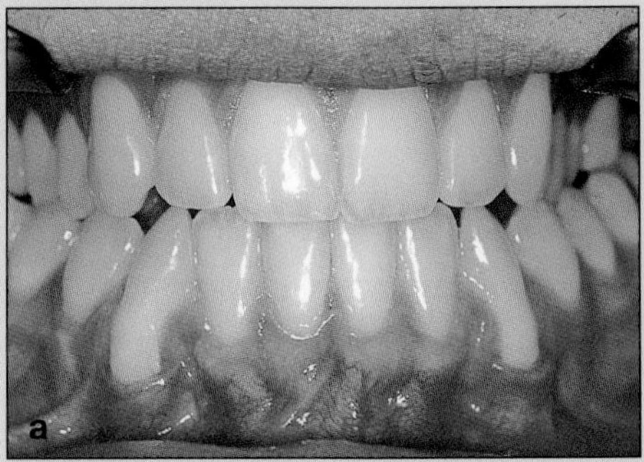

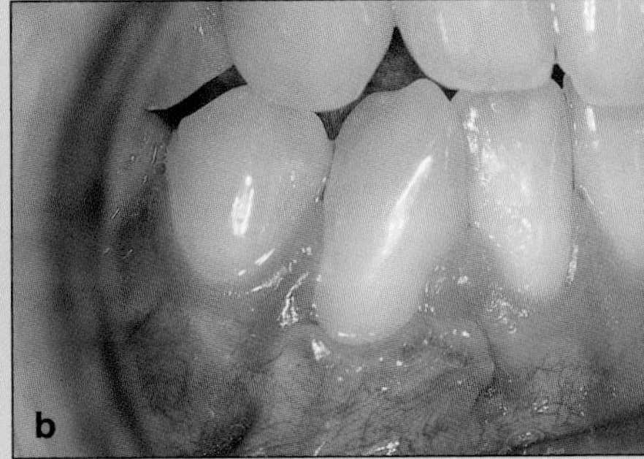

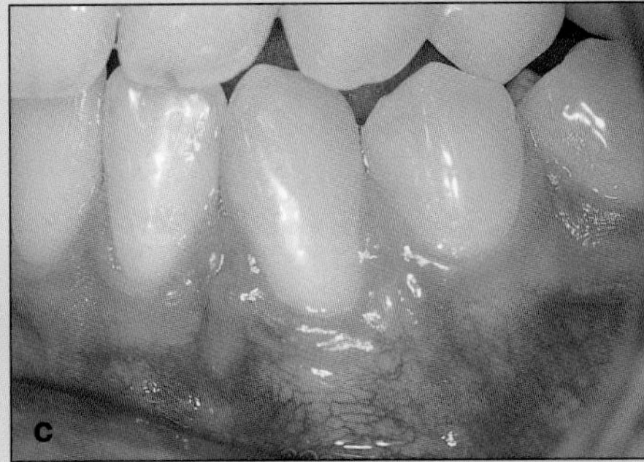

Fig 2-28a Miller class IV recession on both mandibular canines. Although tooth malposition is severe enough to preclude root coverage, the abundant volume of adjacent interdental papillae makes partial root coverage feasible if substantial mechanical reduction of the prominent roots is possible. Endodontic therapy should be considered if pulp exposure is anticipated.

Figs 2-28b and 2-28c Partial root coverage obtained with a subepithelial connective tissue graft after significant mechanical reduction of exposed roots effectively reduced the severity of these defects to Miller class III.

tion of recession. While an exposed root surface can be mechanically and chemically modified to promote attachment of collagen fibrils to cementum, there is histologic evidence that following root-coverage procedures in humans, collagen fibril attachment may occur only at the periphery of the prepared root surface, with junctional epithelial attachment predominating in the central portions of the root.[9] Nevertheless, the natural tooth will maintain connective tissue attachment to root cementum apical to the grafted recession defect, and a stable attachment mediated by junctional epithelium and connective tissue adaptation or attachment results in long-term functional and esthetic success following root-coverage procedures. In contrast, collagen fibril attachment to titanium implants is currently not possible. Therefore, when oral soft tissue grafting is performed to augment peri-implant soft tissues, actual attachment to a titanium implant or abutment is mediated solely by the junctional epithelium. Nevertheless, the collagen fibrils contained within the graft run parallel to the implant abutment surface and anchor the marginal tissues to the crest of the alveolus; this arrangement provides the tissue immobility needed to maintain soft tissue integration and a biologic soft tissue seal. Therefore, despite a lack of connective tissue attachment to the implant surface following soft tissue grafting, the grafting does restore a duality of function between existing epithelial structures and grafted connective tissue elements, similar to that found around a natural tooth. The result is enhanced esthetic contours and a stable peri-implant soft tissue environment that can withstand the bacterial and mechanical challenges present in the oral cavity (see Figs 2-15c to 2-15e).

Classification of Alveolar Ridge Defects in Esthetic Implant Therapy

Evaluating alveolar ridge defects and determining whether to reconstruct them in a staged fashion before or at the same time as implant placement is one of the most important clinical decisions facing the implant surgeon. When site-development procedures are indicated, the implant surgeon must be able to select and appropriately sequence procedures according to the specific type of alveolar ridge defect encountered and the esthetic importance of the site. Doing so not only improves the long-term functional results achieved with implant therapy but also allows the surgeon to realistically predict esthetic outcomes. Because of the increased complexity and biologic requirements of reconstructing alveolar ridge defects at esthetic implant sites, the author distinguishes the classification and reconstruction of these defects from defects found in nonesthetic areas or from alveolar ridge defects associated with conventional fixed restorations.

The existing classification systems for alveolar ridge defects focus on morphologic descriptions of pontic site defects, with correlations to surgical management limited to camouflaging the defect with soft tissue grafting or the use of nonresorbable bone graft substitutes in preparation for conventional fixed partial dentures.[10] Although useful, these classifications provide little guidance for the implant surgeon when reconstruction of missing hard and soft tissue volume is required at an esthetic implant site. They do not provide guidance in selecting and sequencing site-development procedures or in determining advantageous surgical approaches, predicted outcomes, or potential limitations. Esthetic implant therapy often necessitates biologic reconstruction of missing hard tissue anatomy in conjunction with soft tissue reconstruction to allow accurate three-dimensional implant placement, predictable osseointegration, and the development of a healthy peri-implant soft tissue environment with harmonious soft tissue contours and pleasing soft tissue color. These requirements cannot be fulfilled by the camouflaging procedures required for the development of a pontic site for conventional fixed restorations or by the same reconstructive sequence used for site development in nonesthetic areas.

To simplify the evaluation and surgical management of alveolar ridge defects in esthetic implant therapy, the author developed a new classification system that not only describes the defect but also correlates specific types of ridge defects with the selection and sequencing of procedures recommended for successful reconstruction. In addition to providing a conceptual framework for surgical management of alveolar ridge defects at esthetic implant sites, the classification system identifies the limitations to complete reconstruction in specific defect types.

When evaluating alveolar ridge defects for esthetic dental implant reconstruction, the author primarily uses visual inspection, palpation, radiographic evaluation, and bone sounding under local anesthesia with a surgical template to determine if the defect is primarily due to loss of hard tissue, loss of soft tissue, or a combination of both. In some cases, a radiographic template may be used in conjunction with computerized tomography to gain additional information about the nature of an existing alveolar ridge defect. A diagnostic waxup of the final restoration evaluated on articulated study casts or directly in the patient's mouth provides additional information about the volume and nature of the defect relative to the planned final restoration.

Based upon the presurgical evaluation, the author classifies alveolar ridge defects according to volume (large or small) and nature (hard tissue, soft tissue, or combination hard and soft tissue). When specific types of alveolar ridge defects pre-exist, emphasizing the volume and nature of the defect rather than the defect's morphology (vertical or horizontal) allows the formation of useful algorithms to guide the implant surgeon in the selection and sequencing of reconstructive procedures required for successful site development (see Appendix). The surgeon must keep in mind that the recommended treatment algorithms take into consideration the effect that hard tissue reconstructive procedures or surgical access for placement or exposure of an implant will have on the volume, architecture, and topography of the overlying soft tissues at the site according to the periodontal phenotype of the patient. Consequently, in esthetic implant site development, many hard tissue alveolar ridge defects are ultimately treated in the same fashion as combination hard and soft tissue defects. Similarly, because the resorption and remodeling of alveolar bone that predictably occurs following the loss of an anterior maxillary tooth usually involves loss of ridge height and width, most esthetic implant site defects are truly combination vertical and horizontal defects in morphology and rarely are exclusively vertical or horizontal defects. Therefore, reconstructive efforts at esthetic implant sites usually involve more than replacing missing hard and soft tissue volume and architecture to allow ideal implant placement and esthetic restorative emergence. These efforts usually also involve compensating for soft tissue shrinkage or less-than-ideal volume yields from hard tissue grafting, with prophylactic soft tissue augmentation

Large-volume hard tissue defect

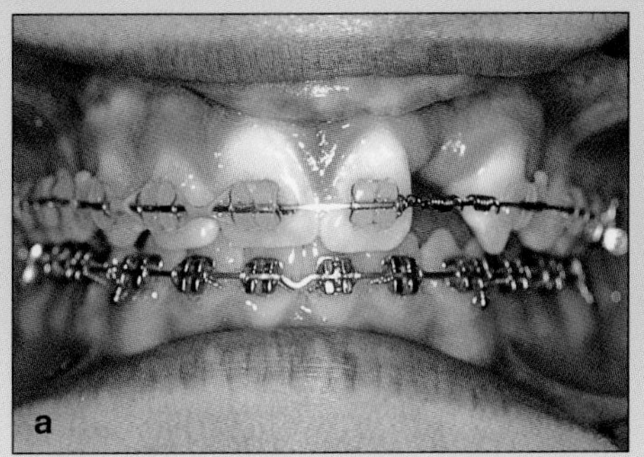

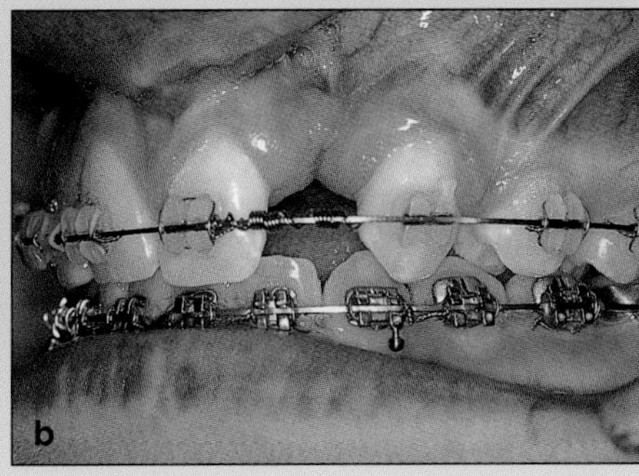

Figs 2-29a and 2-29b A large-volume hard tissue defect is evident at this lateral incisor implant site with pre-existing alveolar cleft. Staged reconstruction of these defects is always indicated. Although hard tissue reconstruction will enable proper three-dimensional implant placement, soft tissue grafting is often required to offset the loss of soft tissue volume that occurs as a consequence of the bone-grafting procedures. (See chapter 3 for treatment details.)

performed to offset expected soft tissue loss or to camouflage a slight deficiency in hard tissue contours.

Six individual types of alveolar ridge defects are distinguished, based upon the volume and nature of the defect: large-volume hard tissue defect, small-volume hard tissue defect, large-volume soft tissue defect, small-volume soft tissue defect, and large- and small-volume combination defects. Once the defect is classified, the morphology of the defect can then be described as vertical; horizontal; or most commonly, a combination of vertical and horizontal at maxillary sites. Bone loss involving periodontal support of the adjacent dentition, which presents an anatomic limitation (as previously discussed), is emphasized. Each defect classification is correlated with the appropriate selection and sequencing of various hard and soft tissue grafting procedures required for predictable esthetic outcomes, as described below. The differences in reconstructive requirements for the same types of alveolar ridge defects found at nonesthetic implant sites are also discussed to emphasize the additional requirements for surgical management of ridge defects in areas of esthetic importance.

Large-volume hard tissue defect

A large-volume hard tissue defect (Fig 2-29) prevents ideal three-dimensional implant placement and in both esthetic and nonesthetic areas is most appropriately reconstructed in a staged fashion prior to implant placement. For reconstruction of these types of defects, the author uses autogenous corticocancellous block grafts in combination with particulate grafts, as described in chapter 7. When the defect is entirely horizontal, with no loss of vertical bone height, the surgeon can anticipate complete restoration of hard tissue volume at the site. When the defect includes loss of vertical bone height, complete reconstruction may be limited.

The limiting factor in reconstruction of large-volume bone defects with loss of vertical bone height in edentulous patients is the ability to expand and suspend the soft tissue drape to accommodate sufficient vertical bone graft volume and minimize subsequent graft resorption caused by contraction of the soft tissue envelope or early postsurgical loading. In addition to the soft tissue considerations outlined above, the coronal level, thickness, and volume of interdental bone remaining on the adjacent natural dentition determine the limit of vertical bone augmentation possible at partially edentulous sites. When there is no loss of bone height or volume on the adjacent dentition in a single-tooth gap, complete reconstruction is possible. As the width of vertical bone defect increases, complete vertical bone reconstruction becomes less likely. Additional limitations to vertical bone regeneration should be expected when bone loss extends to the root surfaces of adjacent natural dentition, since the root surface is avascular and cannot contribute to the survival of the graft by the bridging phenomenon. Vertical bone regeneration becomes totally dependent upon the blood supply that may emanate from the periodontal ligament circulation, as well as the overlying soft tissue drape and the acceptance of the graft to the exposed root surface. In these instances, vertical bone regeneration is currently not predictable. Future success will depend on a greater understanding of the complex process involved in regeneration of the periodontal structures, which include cementum, the periodontal ligament, and epithelial structures, in addition to bone.

When a vertical bone defect is present, staged reconstruction is always indicated. Distraction osteogenesis, though difficult to apply in esthetic areas, should be considered in conjunction with bone grafting. Orthodontic eruption with subsequent restoration or removal of compromised dentition adjacent to an esthetic ridge defect is another strategy for improving hard and soft tissue volume prior to surgical site-development efforts. In most esthetic areas, large-volume hard tissue defects

Small-volume hard tissue defect

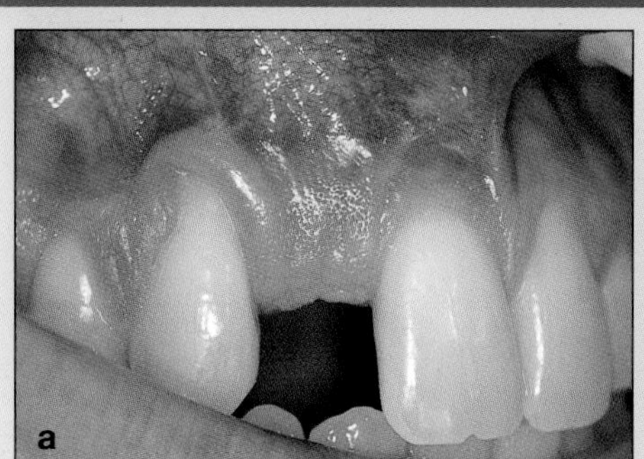

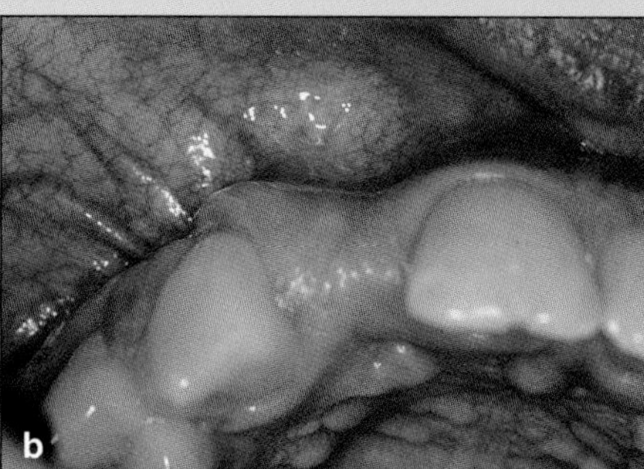

Fig 2-30a A small-volume hard tissue defect is present at this lateral incisor implant site. Palpation and bone sounding demonstrate that the defect does not involve the alveolar crest, allowing simultaneous reconstruction at the time of implant placement. The Miller class I recession defect on the adjacent canine will be corrected after bone graft maturation and implant integration have occurred.

Fig 2-30b Occlusal view demonstrates more than adequate width at the crest of the ridge for ideal implant placement. (See chapter 7 for treatment details.)

require both hard and soft tissue to compensate for the loss of soft tissue volume that occurs as a result of the bone grafting and implant procedures.

Small-volume hard tissue defect

A small-volume hard tissue defect (Fig 2-30) does not affect three-dimensional implant placement or primary implant stability and thus allows simultaneous reconstruction at the time of implant placement. Although small-volume fenestration defects are usually managed with a guided bone regeneration procedure performed at the time of implant placement, reconstruction of small-volume hard tissue defects involving or jeopardizing the alveolar crest (the area critical for prosthetic emergence) is most predictably managed with a staged approach, as described in chapter 7. The correction of a small-volume hard tissue defect in conjunction with esthetic implant therapy may require subsequent soft tissue grafting to offset the soft tissue shrinkage that occurs as a result of the initial guided bone-regeneration procedure. While patients with a thin, scalloped periodontium are at greatest risk, surgeons should discuss with all patients the possibility of the need for subsequent soft tissue grafting procedures to obtain the desired esthetic outcome.

Large-volume soft tissue defect

A large-volume soft tissue defect (Figs 2-31 and 2-32) prevents the development of a stable peri-implant environment or provides inadequate soft tissue coverage for successful hard tissue site-development procedures. In addition, in esthetic areas, a large-volume soft tissue defect prevents the emergence of an implant restoration that is in harmony with the adjacent dentition.

In nonesthetic areas, large-volume soft tissue defects are most often corrected at the time of implant exposure or nonsubmerged implant placement using epithelialized palatal mucosal grafts, as described in chapter 5. Although poor color matching limits the use of palatal mucosal grafts in esthetic areas, these grafts can be used to successfully reconstruct large-volume soft tissue alveolar ridge defects in a staged fashion with horizontal augmentation preceding and providing the foundation for subsequent vertical soft tissue augmentation. One or more subepithelial connective tissue grafts also are usually required to reconstruct large-volume soft tissue defects in conjunction with esthetic implant therapy. These subepithelial connective tissue grafts are performed prior to implant placement, at the time of implant placement, during the osseointegration period, or at the time of implant exposure, depending on the quality of the soft tissues that pre-exist at the site and whether a submerged or nonsubmerged implant approach is planned, as described in chapter 5. Alternatively, the vascularized interpositional periosteal–connective tissue (VIP-CT) flap may be used to reconstruct large-volume soft tissue defects in conjunction with esthetic implant therapy in the maxillary anterior area. A single procedure is performed prior to implant placement, at the time of implant placement, or during the osseointegration period, as described in chapter 6.

Small-volume soft tissue defect

A small-volume soft tissue defect (Figs 2-33 and 2-34) results in a volume of attached tissue surrounding an implant restoration that is less than ideal for predictable long-term stability or esthetic emergence. In nonesthetic areas, small-volume soft tissue defects are managed with one of the surgical maneuvers described in chapter 3. In esthetic areas, small-volume soft tissue defects are most often managed at the time of submerged or nonsubmerged implant placement with subepithelial connective tissue grafts secured in closed pouch recipient sites (horizontal defects) or in con-

Large-volume soft tissue defects

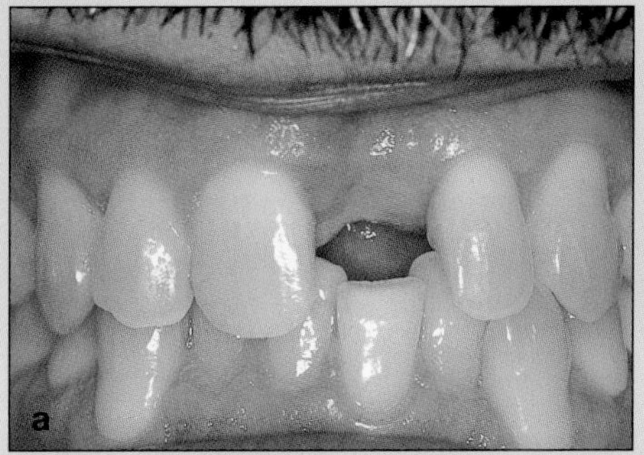
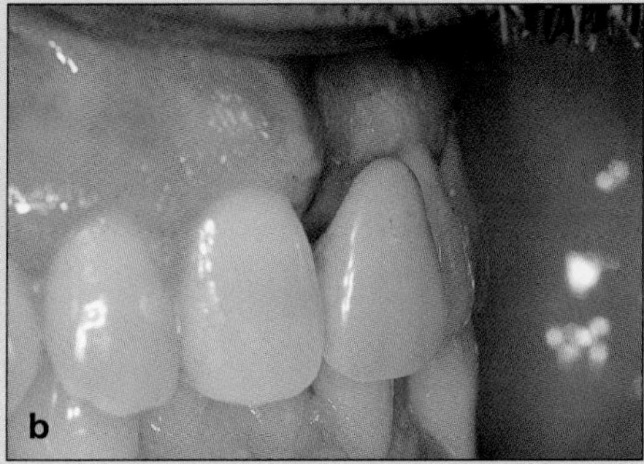

Figs 2-31a and 2-31b This large-volume soft tissue defect located at a central incisor site must be corrected in order to establish a healthy peri-implant soft tissue environment and ensure an acceptable esthetic result from future implant restoration. Because of the magnitude of the defect, several subepithelial connective tissue grafts or a VIP-CT flap is indicated for reconstruction. (See chapter 7 for treatment details.)

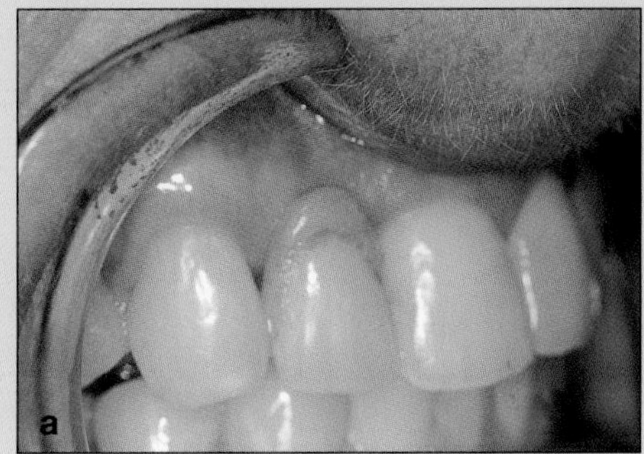
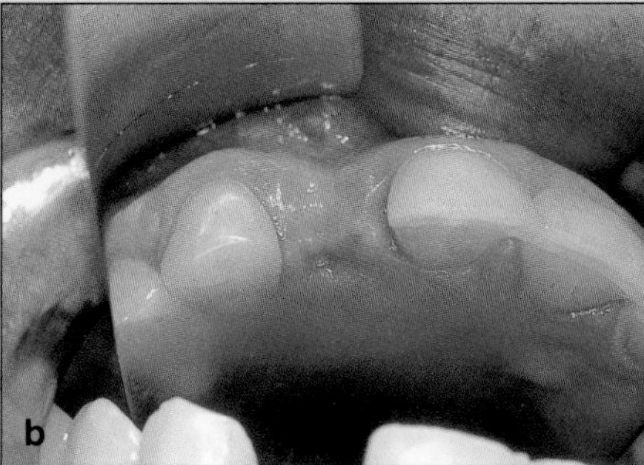

Figs 2-32a and 2-32b Large-volume soft tissue defect present in the area critical for prosthetic emergence. A significant vertical soft tissue deficiency is evident as indicated by the removable interim provisional restoration. Several subepithelial connective tissue grafts or a VIP-CT flap is indicated for reconstruction. (See chapter 6 for treatment details.)

Small-volume soft tissue defects

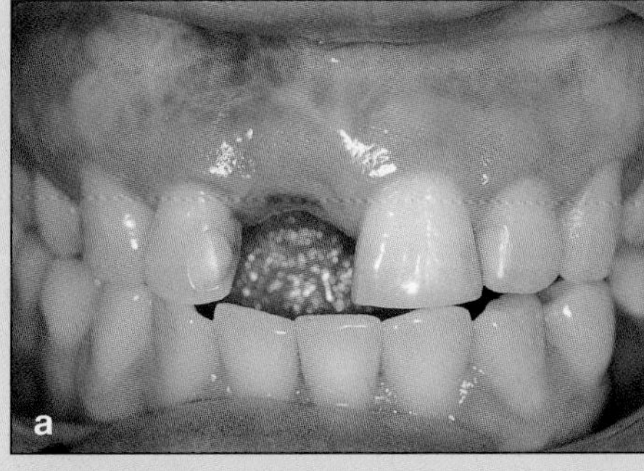
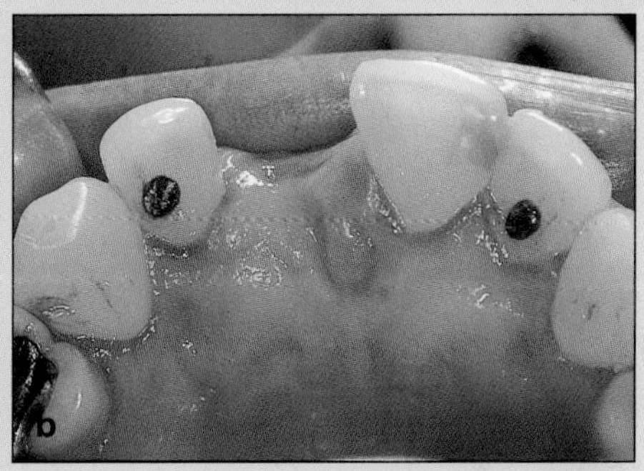

Figs 2-33a and 2-33b A small-volume soft tissue defect exists in the area critical for prosthetic emergence. Reconstruction with a subepithelial connective tissue graft prior to or synchronous with implant placement is indicated. (See chapter 7 for treatment details.)

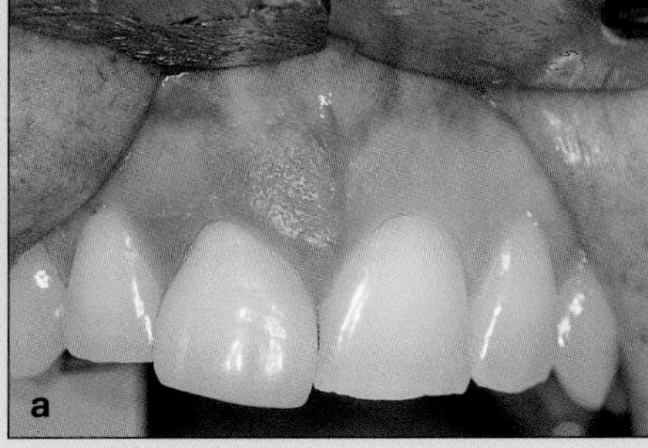
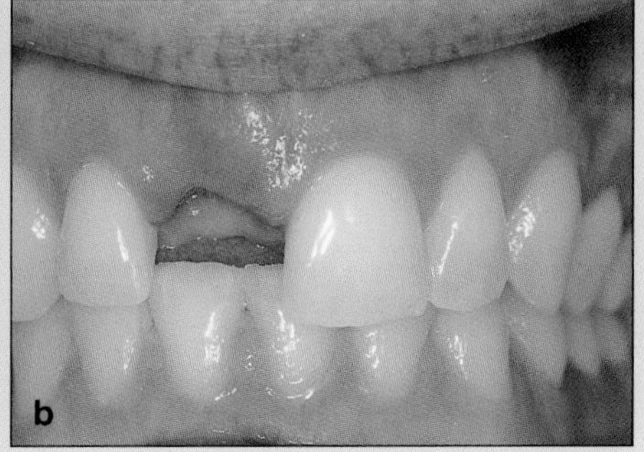

Fig 2-34a Significant edema is evident around this failing central incisor, giving the false impression that there is more than enough soft tissue present for successful esthetic implant restoration.

Fig 2-34b Small-volume soft tissue defect becomes evident following tooth removal despite minimally traumatic tooth removal and use of the Bio-Col technique. Simultaneous reconstruction of the soft tissue defect at the time of implant placement is predictable. (See chapter 7 for treatment details.)

junction with coronally repositioned flaps (vertical defects), as described in chapters 5 and 7.

The surgeon must understand that although small-volume soft tissue defects are detected prior to initiating implant therapy, many result from soft tissue shrinkage following surgical and restorative procedures commonly performed in esthetic implant therapy. Therefore, the surgeon should discuss the possible need for so-called soft tissue touch-up procedures with patients contemplating esthetic implant therapy.

Combination hard and soft tissue defects

Combination hard and soft tissue defects (Figs 2-35 to 2-40) are the most common types of defects en-

Combination hard and soft tissue defects

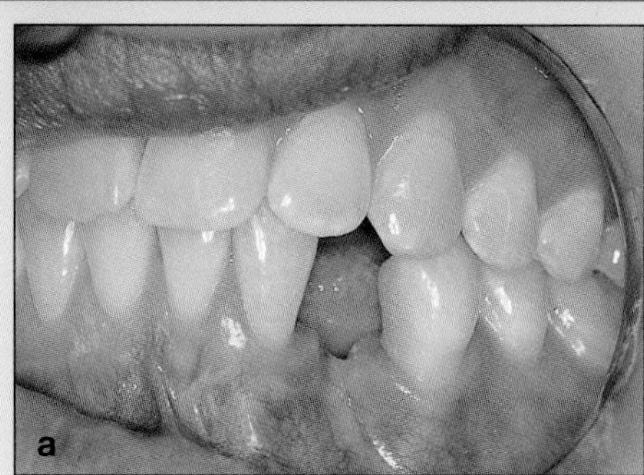

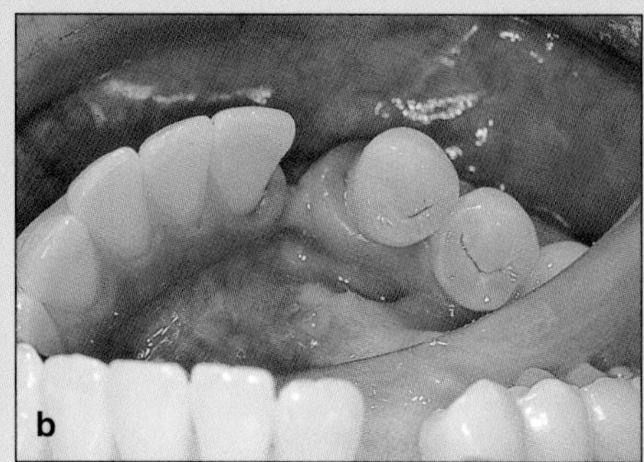

Figs 2-35a and 2-35b A large-volume combination hard and soft tissue defect exists at this mandibular canine implant site following failure of an intentional reimplantation procedure. Thin mucosal tissues at the site provide an inadequate soft tissue cover to support indicated bone grafting. An epithelialized palatal graft is indicated to improve soft tissue quantity and to provide thick keratinized tissue at the site in preparation for bone-graft reconstruction.

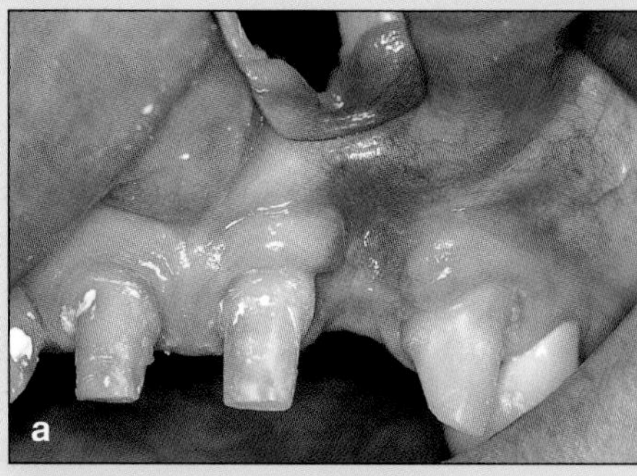

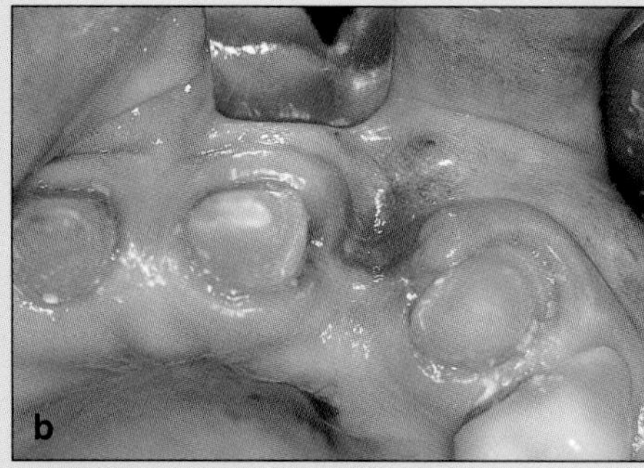

Figs 2-36a and 2-36b A large-volume combination hard and soft tissue defect exists at this lateral incisor site following failure of previous bone-graft procedure. The soft tissues at the site are extremely thin and scarred and of inadequate quality to support the needed bone-graft reconstruction. Therefore, soft tissue reconstruction with a VIP-CT flap is indicated prior to hard tissue grafting. (See chapter 6 for treatment details.)

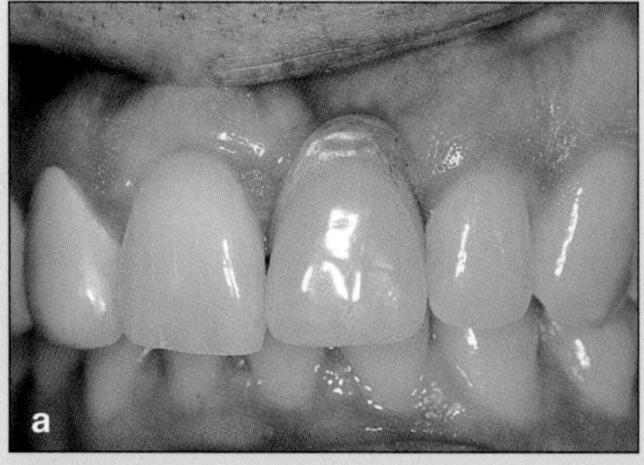

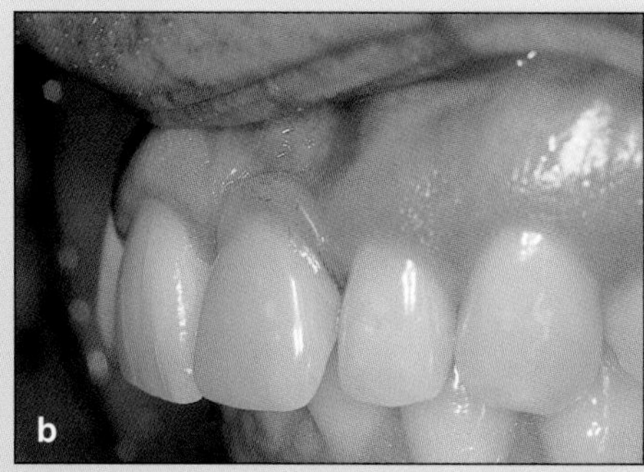

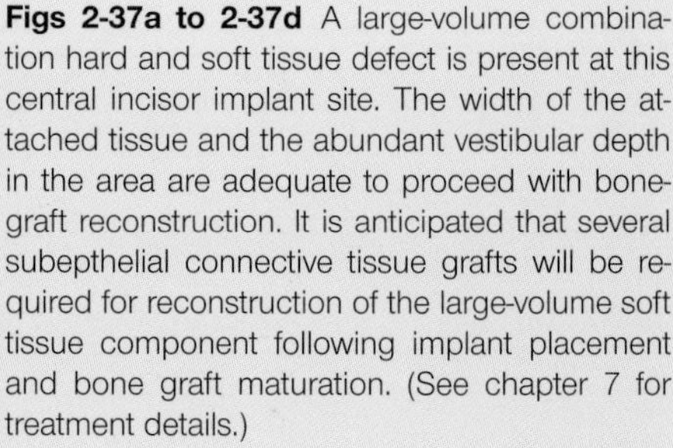

Figs 2-37a to 2-37d A large-volume combination hard and soft tissue defect is present at this central incisor implant site. The width of the attached tissue and the abundant vestibular depth in the area are adequate to proceed with bone-graft reconstruction. It is anticipated that several subepthelial connective tissue grafts will be required for reconstruction of the large-volume soft tissue component following implant placement and bone graft maturation. (See chapter 7 for treatment details.)

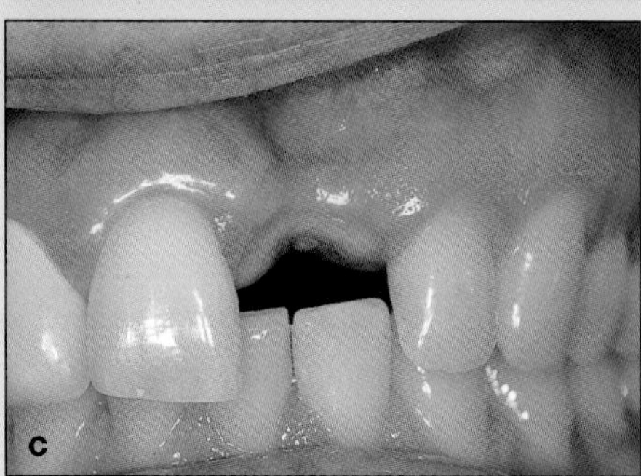

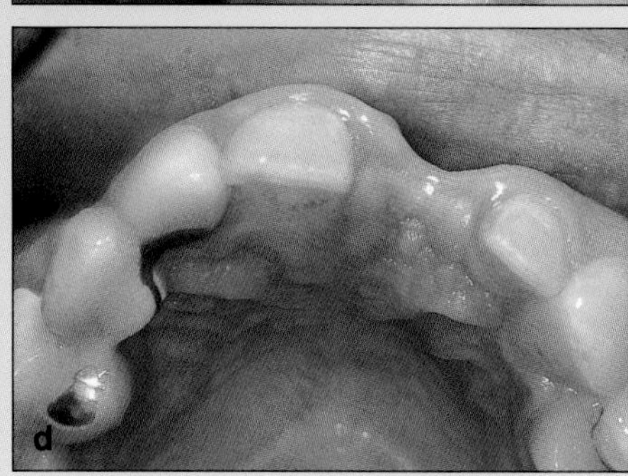

countered at esthetic implant sites. For the implant surgeon, managing large-volume combination defects can be challenging not only because they prevent ideal implant positioning but because they also compromise the surgeon's ability to establish a stable peri-implant soft tissue environment. Furthermore, although large-volume combination defects are always reconstructed in stages prior to implant placement regardless of location, they present the additional challenge of restoring positive esthetic soft tissue architecture when encountered at esthetic sites.

When evaluating a large-volume combination defect, the surgeon must first determine whether the quality of the existing soft tissues is adequate to accommodate the bone augmentation. An assessment of the width of attached tissue as well as the vestibular depth in the area is needed to determine whether soft tissue grafting will be necessary prior to the bony reconstruction (see Fig 2-37). In addition, if the soft tissues are extremely thin or inelastic or are characterized by scar tissue, then soft tissue grafting prior to bone grafting is strongly recommended. This scenario is common when the site has a history of trauma, infection, or multiple surgical interventions preceding tooth loss. In these instances, performing a soft tissue graft as a first step improves both the volume of soft

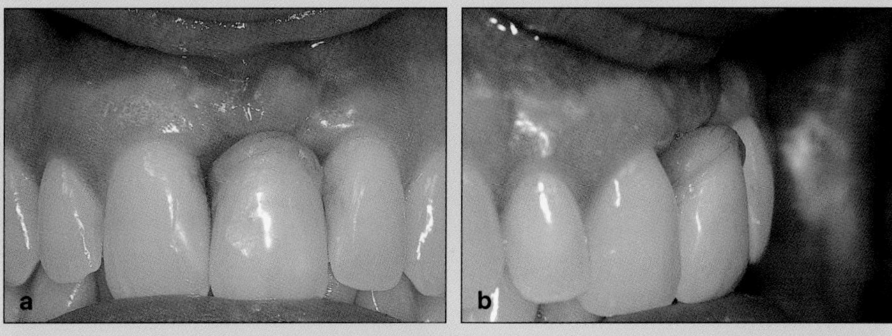

Figs 2-38a and 2-38b A large-volume combination hard and soft tissue defect is evident at this central incisor implant site. Simultaneous hard and soft tissue grafting with block bone graft and VIP-CT flap is indicated in preparation for implant placement. (See chapter 6 for treatment details.)

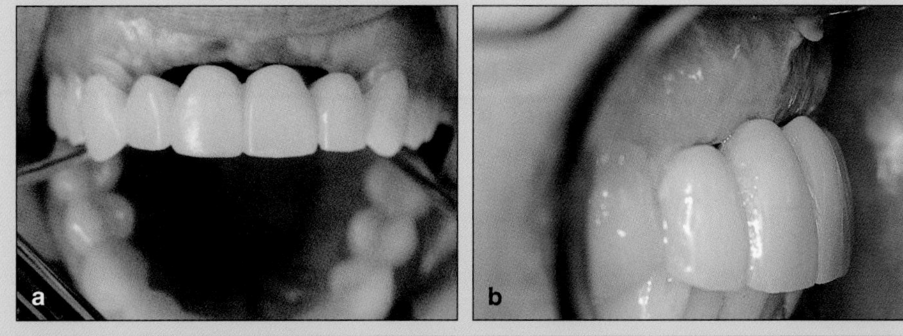

Figs 2-39a and 2-39b A large-volume combination hard and soft tissue defect exists following removal of all four incisors and the subsequent failed attempt at bone-graft reconstruction. Both hard and soft tissue components are large in volume. Previous surgical procedures have diminished the circulation at the sites. Simultaneous hard and soft tissue reconstruction is indicated with autogenous block bone grafts and VIP-CT flaps. (See chapter 7 for treatment details.)

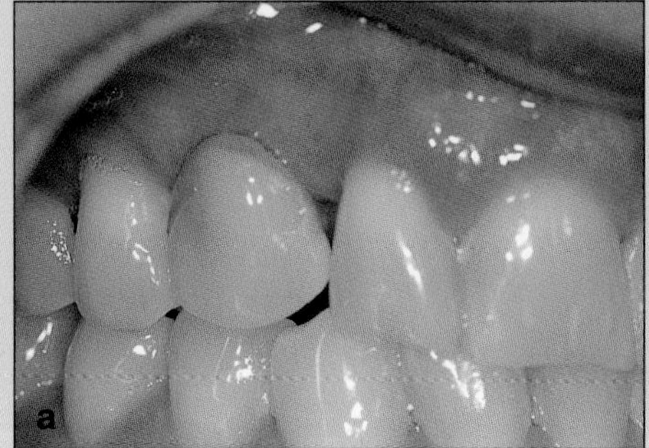

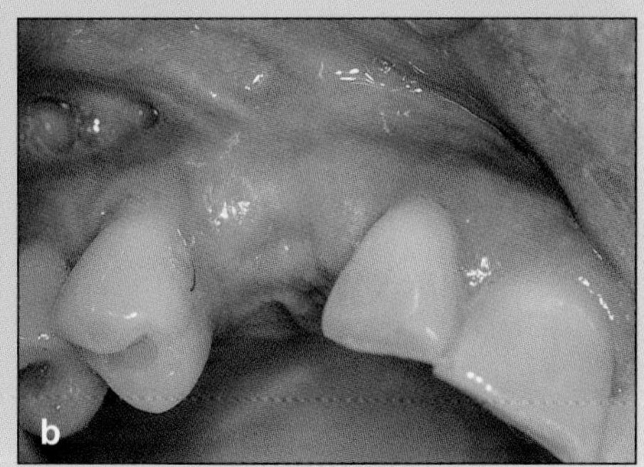

Figs 2-40a and 2-40b A small-volume combination hard and soft tissue ridge defect exists at this maxillary canine site. Prior to tooth removal, soft tissue recession with underlying root dehiscence existed. The loss of osseous ridge contour was not sufficient to affect ideal implant placement. Therefore this type of defect is usually camouflaged with a soft tissue graft or synthetic bone graft material if soft tissue cover is thick enough to mask the underlying graft. (See chapter 7 for treatment details.)

tissue cover available for the bone graft and the quality of the mesenchymal tissue available to support phase-two healing of the subsequent bone graft. The result is a reduction in exposure-related bone graft complications and improved incorporation and remodeling of the bone graft at the recipient site. Either a subepithelial connective tissue graft or an epithelialized palatal mucosal graft will provide adequate soft tissue quality and volume at the site prior to bone grafting (see Fig 2-35). Alternatively, VIP-CT flap will provide a large volume of soft tissue as well as significant improvement in the amount of circulation available at maxillary anterior sites prior to bone grafting (see Fig 2-36).

When both the width of keratinized tissue and the vestibular depth are adequate, bone grafting can be performed first followed by soft tissue grafting performed simultaneously with implant placement or during the osseointegration period (see Fig 2-37). Alternatively, simultaneous hard and soft tissue reconstruction with corticocancellous block grafts and VIP-CT flaps offer predictable results when large-volume combination esthetic ridge defects are present (see Figs 2-38 and 2-39). Finally, epithelialized palatal mucosal grafts are preferred as a first step in managing large-volume combination defects resulting from traumatic avulsion injuries because they provide keratinized tissue cover in a relatively short period, thus facilitating subsequent simultaneous hard and soft tissue reconstruction with corticocancellous bone grafts and VIP-CT flaps.

Small-volume combination hard and soft tissue esthetic ridge defects, in contrast, do not compromise ideal implant positioning or the opportunity to establish a stable peri-implant soft tissue, but they do result in subtle ridge contour defects that compromise esthetics. Such defects are usually camouflaged either with a subepithelial connective tissue graft or with a VIP-CT flap performed simultaneously with implant placement to camouflage missing hard and soft tissue contours (see Fig 2-40). Alternatively, alloplast graft materials can be used to camouflage these defects provided the existing soft tissue cover is adequate to mask the underlying graft.

CHAPTER 3

Surgical Techniques for Management of Peri-implant Soft Tissues

This chapter presents practical and effective methods for the surgical management of peri-implant soft tissues in a wide variety of case types and situations. An understanding of the suggested flap designs and guidelines for the use of specific surgical maneuvers will enable the implant surgeon to manage the peri-implant soft tissues with a high degree of predictability and success in most clinical situations. Coupled with knowledge of the peri-implant soft tissue anatomy and biology provided in chapter 1 and the basics of patient evaluation presented in chapter 2, the information in this chapter will serve as the basis for a flexible surgical technique that can be adapted for successful management of peri-implant soft tissues in individual case scenarios.

Instrumentation for Soft Tissue Management in Implant Therapy

Before discussing the specifics of surgical philosophy or technique, it is useful to review the basic instruments used in managing the soft tissues during implant-related surgery. Successful management of peri-implant soft tissues requires the ability to perform precise incisions that are often beveled and follow a curvilinear path. The surgeon must also be able to carefully elevate, retract, and meticulously readapt delicate mucoperiosteal tissues. Appropriate instrumentation is needed for performing osseous surgery or soft tissue grafting procedures at the implant site and, on occasion, cosmetic periodontal procedures on adjacent dentition to create harmony with the implant restorations. Although individual preference should dictate the contents of the surgical implant tray, the following instruments will enable a surgeon to perform the most common soft tissue surgical maneuvers required in implant therapy.

A no. 5 round scalpel handle (Fig 3-1a) provides superior dexterity and control for performing precise curvilinear-beveled incisions. The no. 5A scalpel handle (Fig 3-1b), which has an offset design, provides an advantage for incisions made in posterior quadrants and in palatal areas when mouth opening is limited. A no. 15C disposable scalpel blade (Fig 3-1c) has a low profile that is ideally suited for performing beveled incisions adjacent to other dentition. The no. 15C blade is also useful for resective contouring of mucoperiosteal flaps, which facilitates circumferential soft tissue readaptation around permucosal implant structures.

The no. 3/9A periosteal (Fig 3-1d) is a multipurpose instrument. The sharp perforated paddle is used for elevating mucoperiosteal flaps as well as stabilizing soft tissues during suturing procedures. The flat end serves as a retractor for delicate mucoperiosteal flaps and for soft tissue grafting and guided tissue regeneration procedures. The Buser elevator (Fig 3-1e) is a delicate periosteal elevator that facilitates gentle elevation of mucoperiosteal tissue flaps. The spear-shaped end is especially suited to initiating flap elevation and releasing adherent fibrous tissues from residual osseous defects underlying the flap. The small paddle-shaped end is used to continue flap reflection. The paddle can also be used during the harvest of subepithelial connective tissue grafts. The Lucas surgical curette (Fig 3-1f) is a useful instrument for initiating flap elevation in areas where access is limited and for removal of granulomatous tissue from osseous defects or extraction sites.

The Corn suture pliers (Fig 3-1g) are helpful for passing sutures through delicate soft tissue flaps or grafts. The unique design allows the surgeon to pass the suture through the tissue while the pliers gently stabilize the tissue. Additionally, the off-axis design makes these tissue pliers useful when access is limited. The Adson and Micro-Adson tissue pliers (Fig 3-1h) are used for gentle manipulation of mucoperiosteal tissues during flap elevation and readaptation. The Micro-Adson is particularly useful when working with delicate periodontal tissues and for handling donor and recipient tissues during oral soft tissue grafting procedures.

The curved Iris scissors (Fig 3-2a) are used for precision trimming of mucoperiosteal flaps as well as donor and recipient tissues during oral soft tissue grafting procedures. The Dean scissors (Fig 3-2b) are primarily used for cutting sutures. The long handle and off-axis orientation of the cutting surfaces of these scissors facilitate accurate cutting even when access is compromised.

The general-purpose Crile Wood needle holder (Fig 3-2c) accommodates suture sizes from 3-0 to 6-0, and its firm beak is suited for working with medium-sized suture needles such as the FS2. The Mini Ryder needle holder (Fig 3-2d) has a fine beak that accommodates suture sizes as small as 10-0 and is suitable for working with smaller suture needles such as the P3. It is reserved for the delicate suturing required during soft tissue grafting procedures, as well as the precise reapproximation of soft tissue flaps required to successfully camouflage the incisions made in esthetic areas. The narrow tapered beak is especially useful for suturing in interproximal and papillary areas.

Tissue nippers (Fig 3-2e) aid in the removal of loose tissue tags from the periosteum during the preparation of a uniform recipient site during soft tissue grafting procedures. The membrane placement instrument (Fig 3-2f) is another combination instrument that is useful during implant surgery and for both membrane and soft tissue grafting procedures. The spiked end can be used to stabilize a membrane or a soft tissue graft while it is adapted and secured at the recipient site. The long, thin paddle is designed to aid in membrane placement and adaptation. The paddle also functions as a fine periosteal elevator during the harvest of subepithelial connective tissue grafts from the palate and as a blunt probe for evaluation of blind dissections in envelope or pouch recipient sites prior to securing subepithelial connective tissue grafts.

In addition to these instruments, periodontal chisels and files should be included as part of the implant soft tissue armamentarium, since osseous modifications are often indicated around implants or adjacent dentition to create a positive osseous architecture in support of an esthetic soft tissue drape (Fig 3-3). Rotary instru-

Instrumentation for soft tissue management in implant therapy

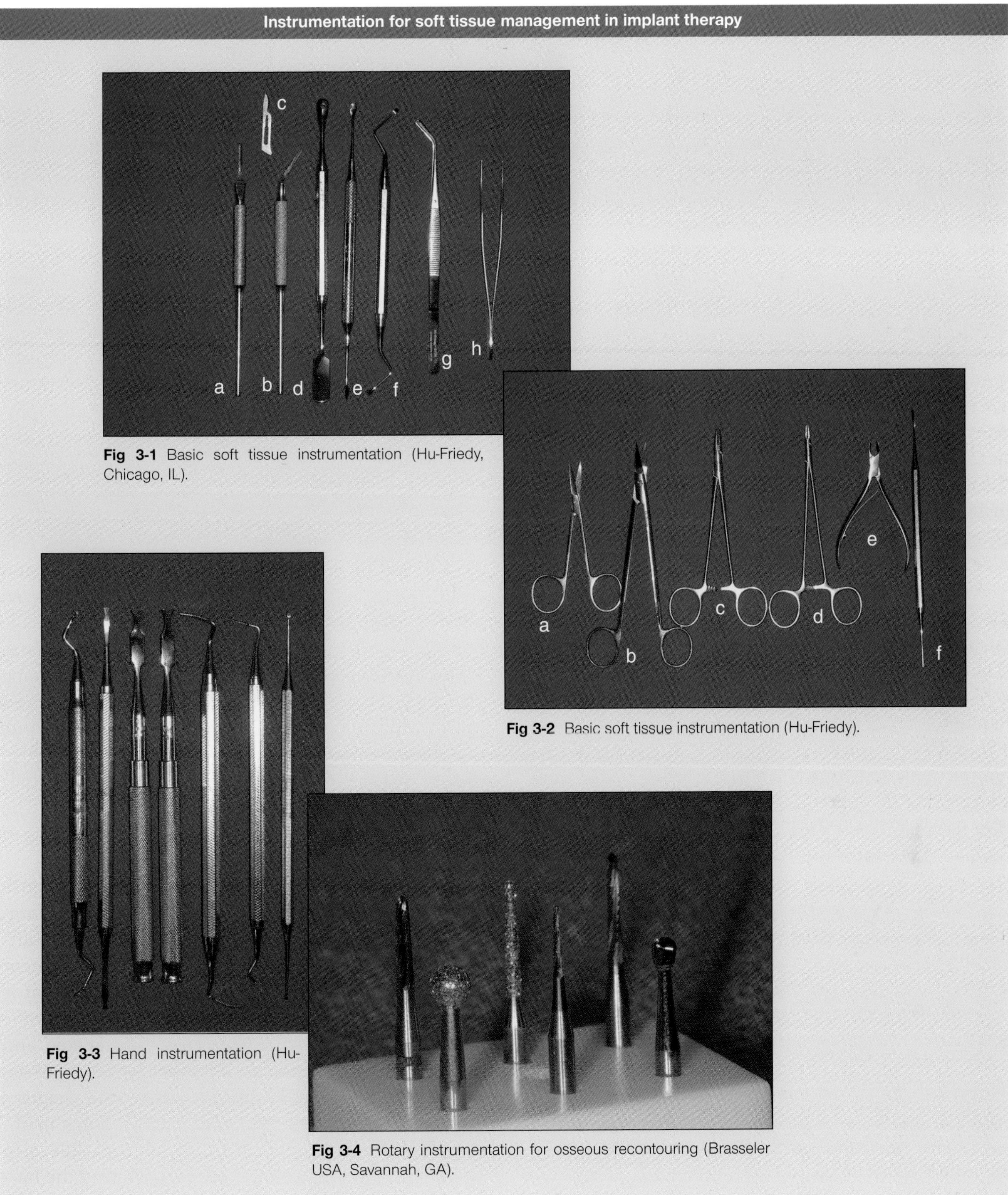

Fig 3-1 Basic soft tissue instrumentation (Hu-Friedy, Chicago, IL).

Fig 3-2 Basic soft tissue instrumentation (Hu-Friedy).

Fig 3-3 Hand instrumentation (Hu-Friedy).

Fig 3-4 Rotary instrumentation for osseous recontouring (Brasseler USA, Savannah, GA).

ments are also useful for this purpose, and a variety of burs are recommended for osseous recontouring (Fig 3-4). The author prefers to use absorbable suture material on atraumatic needles. For general wound closure after placement of submerged implants or during certain site-preparation procedures, 3-0 and 4-0 chromic gut suture is used on FS2 needles. During oral soft tissue grafting procedures and for readapting mucoperiosteal tissues around permucosal implant structures at abutment connection or nonsubmerged implant placement, 4-0, 5-0, and 6-0 chromic gut suture is used on a smaller P3 needle.

Criteria for Optimal Flap Design in Implant Therapy

When designing mucoperiosteal flaps for use in implant therapy, certain important criteria must be kept in mind. The flap should be designed to preserve both the vascular supply to the implant site and the surrounding topography of the alveolar ridge and mucobuccal fold. Failure to do so will result in increased wound dehiscence due to compromised circulation to flap margins, in addition to the damage created by ill-fitting removable provisional restorations. The flap design should facilitate the identification of important anatomy (such as bony concavities), the position and angulation of adjacent tooth roots, and the location of the maxillary sinus and the mental neurovascular bundle, while providing access for implant instrumentation and the use of surgical guides. Whenever possible, the flap should be designed to provide access for local bone harvest. This will avoid the need for a separate surgical site in the event that autogenous bone is needed for grafting unexpected osseous defects encountered during implant placement. Additionally, to minimize bacterial contamination, the flap design should provide for closure away from augmentation sites. When performing abutment connection to a submerged implant or when placing a nonsubmerged implant, the flap should be designed to facilitate circumferential adaptation of attached soft tissues around the permucosal implant structures. This will provide the anatomic components (epithelium and connective tissue) needed for the formation of a stable peri-implant soft tissue environment during the soft tissue integration period, thereby protecting the underlying alveolar bone levels. For practical purposes, a flap for use in implant therapy should always be designed to facilitate elevation, retraction, repositioning, and tension-free closure of the soft tissues at the surgical site.

The two basic flap designs traditionally advocated for use in implant therapy are distinguished by the location (vestibular or crestal) of the horizontal access incision. Brånemark et al[1] originally recommended a vestibular incision for implant placement in the edentulous mandible. Buser et al[2] also advocate a variation of the vestibular flap for localized bone augmentation in the mandible. Although a high degree of success is obtained when a vestibular flap design is used in localized ridge augmentation procedures performed in the mandible, the vestibular flap can be difficult to execute and often requires a large amount of periosteal stripping to provide adequate access for implant instrumentation. In addition, the vestibular flap design interferes with the use of surgical templates, alters the topography of the alveolar ridge and mucobuccal fold, and seldom fulfills the criteria for optimal flap design for implant surgery.

Guidelines for designing mucoperiosteal flaps used in implant therapy:

- Preserve blood supply
- Preserve the topography of the alveolar ridge and mucobuccal fold
- Facilitate identification of important anatomic structures
- Provide ample access for implant instrumentation and use of surgical guides
- Provide access for harvesting of local bone
- Provide for closure away from implant placement or tissue augmentation sites
- Minimize bacterial contamination
- Facilitate circumferential closure around permucosal implant structures

In contrast, a buccal flap initiated with a pericrestal incision provides the surgeon with a practical and effective approach for the management of soft tissues in most dental implant surgeries. This flap design is easily modified to bring about the desired surgical objectives in a wide variety of clinical situations. The buccal flap for implant surgery is outlined by a pericrestal incision and one or more curvilinear-beveled vertical releasing incisions made mesial and distal to the site of implantation. By changing the position and bevel of the pericrestal incisions, the buccal flap becomes suitable for both submerged and nonsubmerged implant surgeries (Fig 3-5). An identical flap design is used for abutment connection to submerged implants and placement of nonsubmerged implants. The flap used for submerged implant placement differs only in the position and bevel of the pericrestal incision and the degree of lingual or palatal flap elevation.

Use of beveled pericrestal incisions in implant therapy

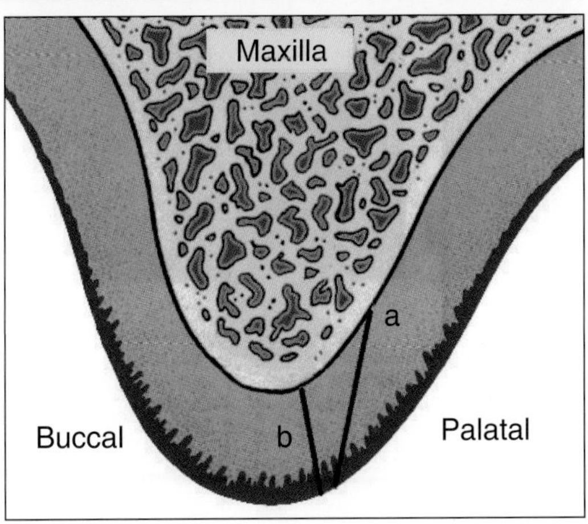

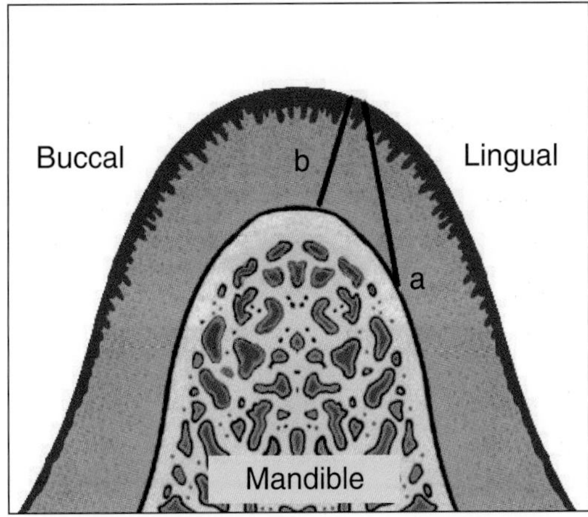

Fig 3-5 *(a)* Line representing the path of the palatal and lingual beveled incisions made for submerged implant placement. Note that the incisions are initiated on the palatal or lingual aspect of the ridge. *(b)* Line representing the path of incisions made for abutment connection and nonsubmerged implant placement. The buccal bevel maximizes the tissue that remains on the buccal flap for readaptation around the permucosal implant structures. Note that the incisions are initiated in a position that ensures adequate apicocoronal dimension of attached palatal and lingual tissues.

Application of Plastic Surgery Principles in Implant Therapy

In its simplest form, implant therapy requires a surgical procedure that is properly classified as plastic and reconstructive. The placement of an osseointegrated implant is a reconstructive procedure that forms the foundation for subsequent functional and esthetic dental rehabilitation.

One of the most significant advances in implant therapy is the adoption of the "plastic and reconstructive surgery mindset," which embraces the need for a sequence of surgical procedures performed to achieve the desired result. The selection and sequencing of each procedure is based on the regenerative potential of the individual site and the total volume of tissue to be reconstructed.

Recent biotechnologic advances have greatly enhanced the possibilities for hard and soft tissue site development. Coupled with the application of plastic surgery principles and mindset, we are now able to provide functional and esthetic implant restorations with impressive predictability. Of greater significance is our understanding and awareness of the factors that will limit the volume yields from various reconstructive procedures. This insight guides us in the formulation of treatment-planning options and surgical approaches that have anatomic and biologic bases for success. As such, the application of plastic surgery principles and the anatomic and biologic bases for the flap designs and soft tissue surgical maneuvers presented below are emphasized.

Curvilinear-beveled incisions

The application of plastic surgery principles in implant therapy dictates the use of flap designs that incorporate inconspicuous incisions and facilitate reconstructive procedures by allowing tension-free closure while preserving circulation to the flap margins. The use of curvilinear releasing incisions is a basic plastic surgery technique that provides significant advantages when compared with the linear vertical releasing incisions traditionally incorporated in trapezoidal flap designs. An incision that follows a curvilinear path is, by definition, longer than a straight incision. When curvilinear incisions are used, a greater volume of mucosal tissue can be incorporated in the flap, improving its overall elasticity. This facilitates passive flap coaptation and, when necessary, coronal advancement without embarrassment of circulation to the flap margin. The curvilinear design facilitates precise wound closure by providing a visual guide for the surgeon. In addition, the increased length of the curvilinear incision provides the opportunity for the placement of additional sutures, if needed, to accurately secure the flap during wound closure. By passing the incision through or parallel to existing anatomic landmarks such as interdental grooves and the mucogingival junction, the curvilinear incision is easily camouflaged and becomes less conspicuous when compared with a linear incision.

Application of plastic surgery principles in flap design

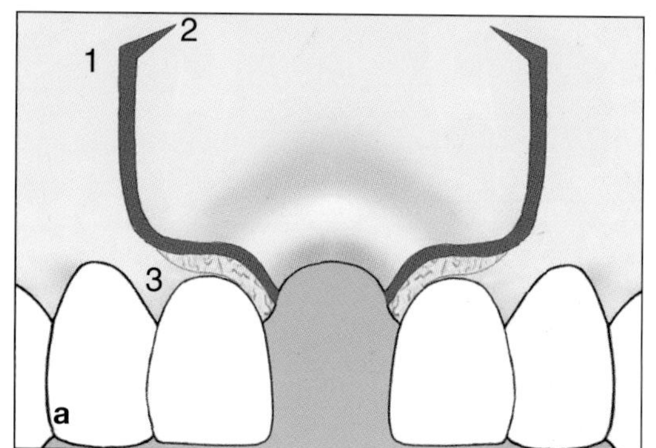

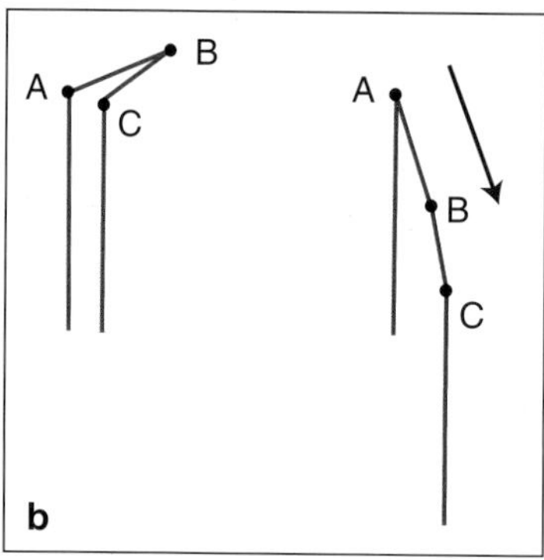

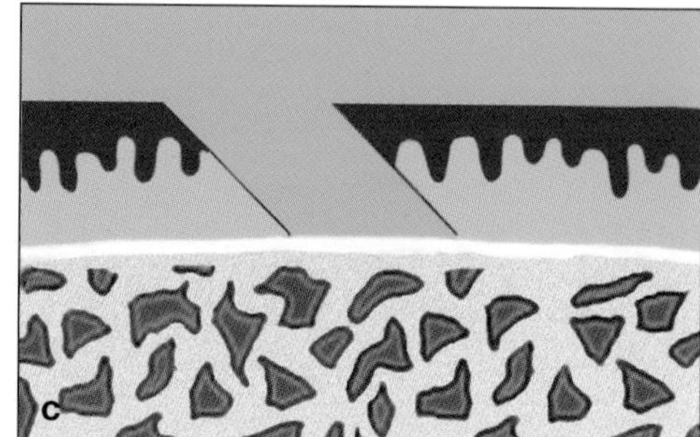

Fig 3-6 Curvilinear-beveled incisions. *(a)* The incision is initiated at the height of the vestibule in the mucosal tissues overlying the nearest interdental area (1). A cutback incision is made while the mucosal tissues are still held under tension (2). De-epithelialization of the adjacent papilla (3) provides a connective tissue base for coaptation of the coronally advanced flap and avoids entrapment of epithelium at the incision line. *(b)* The tension-releasing cutback incision facilitates coronal advancement of the flap. The amount is demonstrated by the movement of points B and C. *(c)* Beveled incision extends area of flap coaptation. Tangential orientation results in an inconspicuous incision line after healing.

The curvilinear incision is initiated under tension in the alveolar mucosa at the depth of the vestibule apical to the interdental papilla of the teeth adjacent to the site. The incision continues coronally passing through the interdental groove, a landmark identified in the mucosa, and follows a gentle curve as it approaches and then continues in the mucogingival junction toward the implant site. The path of the incision completes a sinuous pattern as it extends over the ridge crest through the attached tissues, terminating on the palatal or lingual aspect of the ridge (Figs 3-6a and 3-7a). Generally, use of this incision allows for inconspicuous correction of small-volume hard and soft tissue defects simultaneous with implant placement (Fig 3-7b).

When large-volume site-development procedures are performed, the author recommends increasing the width of the flap base by initiating the incision further away from the implant site or sites (second or third interdental area mesial and distal to the site). This will result in an exaggerated curvilinear flap design. In these situations, the incision will parallel the mucogingival junction for a greater distance before changing direction. This modification will facilitate passive wound closure by ensuring passive accommodation of the flap over large-volume hard and soft tissue grafts (see Fig 3-31). In addition, the use of tension-releasing "cutback incisions" will preserve circulation to the flap margin by allowing for additional coronal flap advancement without exceeding the elastic limit of the flap (Fig 3-6b). These full-thickness incisions are directed into the base of the flap at a 45- to 60-degree angle and are executed initially while the mucosal tissues are still under tension. Doing so ensures precise placement and angulation of these tension-releasing incisions and avoids unnecessary trauma from retraction during site-development procedures (Figs 3-7c and 3-7d). Traditional use of periosteal releasing incisions, which extend across the base of the flap and thereby reduce circulation to the flap margin, are seldom necessary when a curvilinear flap design with tension-releasing cutback incisions is used during site-development procedures. This is an important consideration, because marginal flap necrosis or wound dehiscence can result in graft exposure and decreased volume yields from the hard or soft tissue augmentation procedures.

The use of beveled incisions in implant surgery and site-development procedures is another plastic surgery technique that offers significant advantages over conventional techniques (Fig 3-6c). Beveling an incision extends the wound margin area and increases the surface area available for flap coaptation, enhancing the stability of the wound complex during early healing. Flap retraction is minimized, as are the unsightly notches and scars that can diminish esthetic results. Additionally, a properly beveled incision will camouflage the resulting scar, making it less conspicuous when compared with an incision made at 90 degrees to the tissue surface. This camouflaging effect occurs because the thickness of the flap margin gradually increases from partial to full thickness and is coapted to the recipient site, which also is beveled. The result is a tangential orientation of the incision and resulting scar with improved light transmission when compared with incisions that are not beveled (Figs 3-8 to 3-10; see also Fig 3-6). When used in implant therapy, the beveling technique decreases dehiscence of wound margins and dramatically improves incision line esthetics.

Advantages of using curvilinear incisions

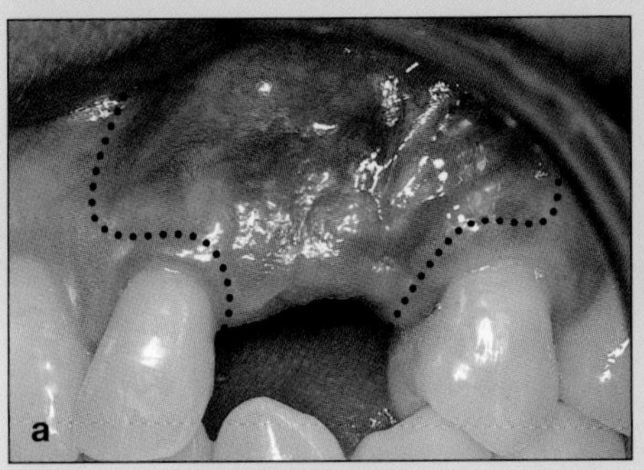

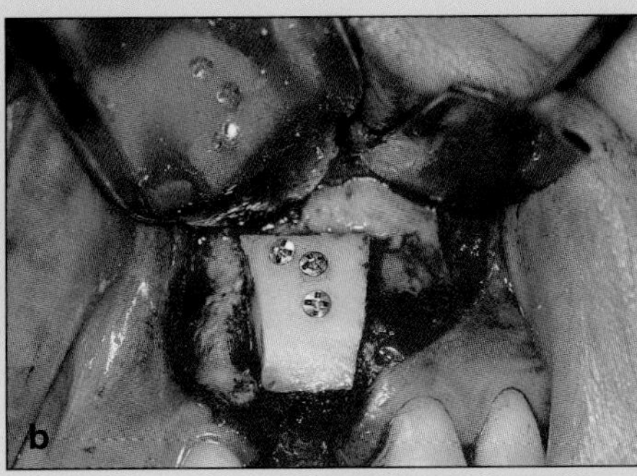

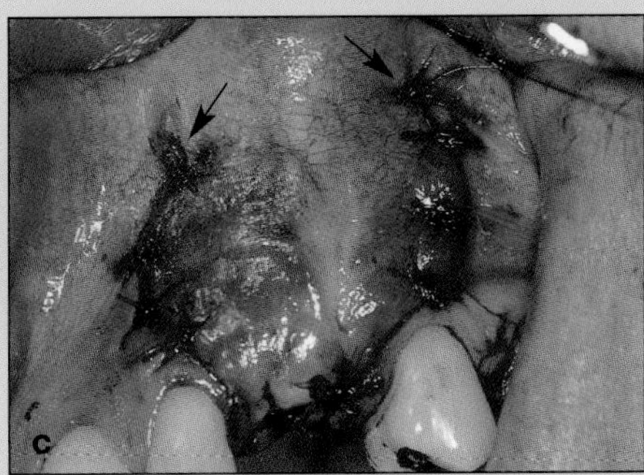

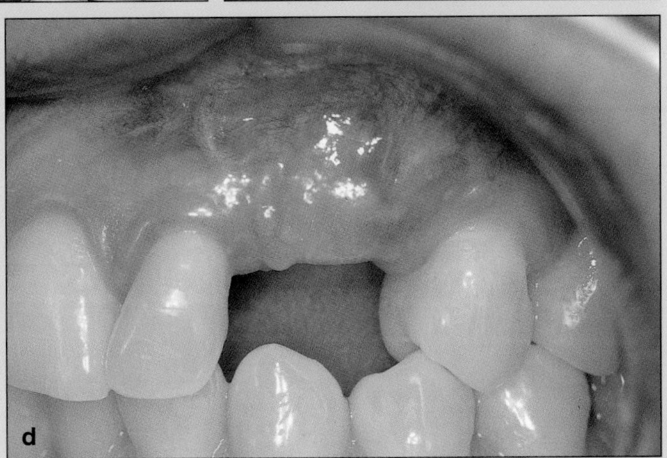

Fig 3-7a Compromised site following previous bone graft and implant failure. Significant scarring and chronic inflammation exist. Note position and path of curvilinear-beveled incisions that outline access flap for hard tissue graft procedure.

Fig 3-7b Tension-releasing cutback incisions facilitate access to apical portions of bone graft, fixation screw placement, subsequent particulate bone graft, and barrier membrane adaptation.

Fig 3-7c Coronal flap advancement and tension-free closure over corticocancellous block graft obtained without periosteal releasing incisions. Circulation to flap margin remains intact after closure. Note position of tension-releasing cutback incisions *(arrows)*. Coronal advancement of the flap provides for straight-line closure.

Fig 3-7d Inconspicuous incision line esthetics and minimal soft tissue shrinkage are apparent 4 months after procedure. Note improvement of soft tissue health and osseous volume at the site.

Advantages of using beveled incisions

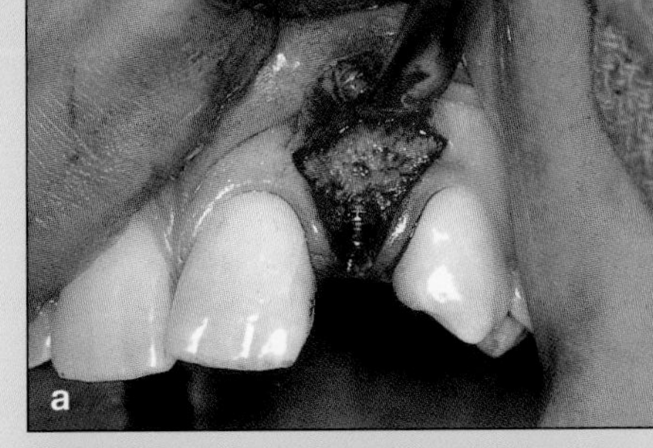

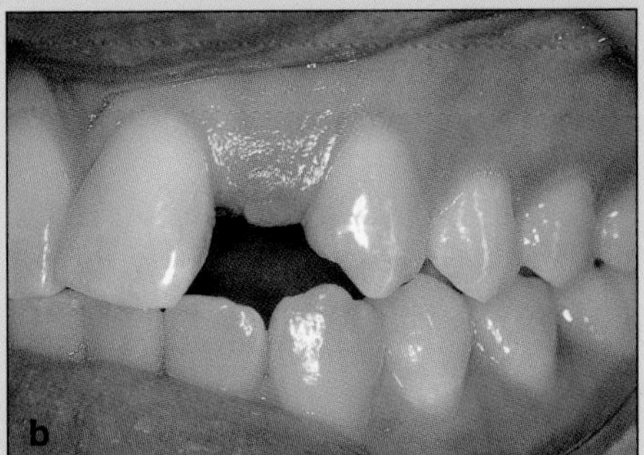

Fig 3-8a Abbreviated beveled incisions outline a conservative approach for implant placement and surgical indexing. Soft tissue recession is limited by avoiding extension of the incisions beyond the mucogingival junction.

Fig 3-8b Excellent incision line esthetics noted 6 weeks postoperatively. Soft tissue volume has been maintained.

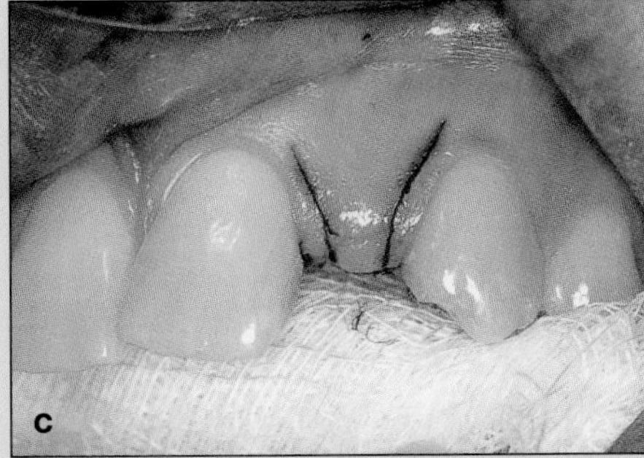

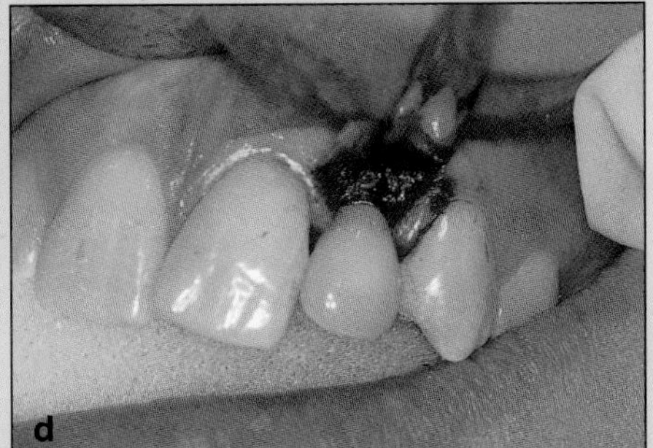

Figs 3-8c and 3-8d To preserve soft tissue volume, abbreviated beveled incisions were used for implant exposure and delivery of custom abutment and provisional restoration.

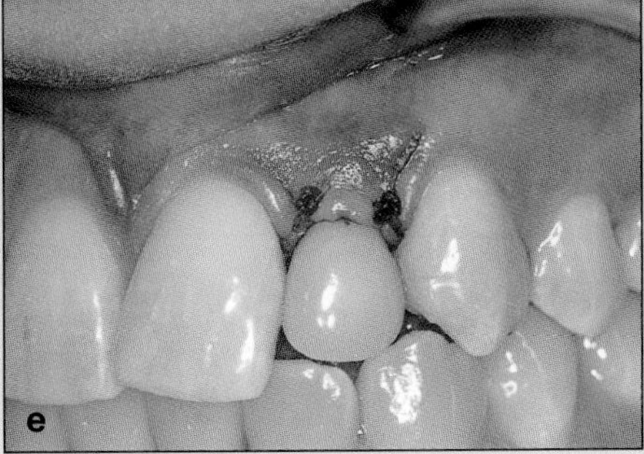

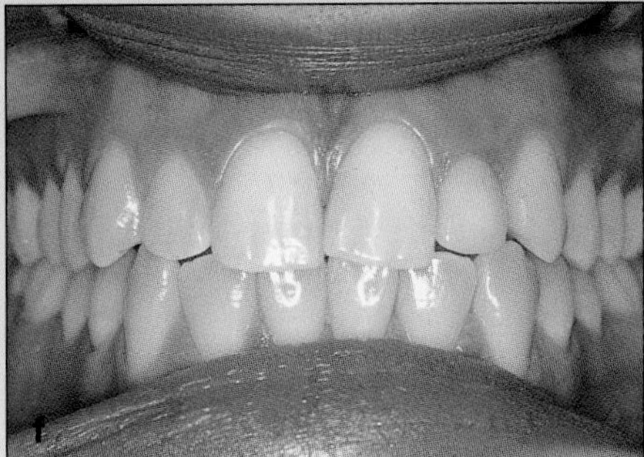

Fig 3-8e Wound closure obtained with 4-0 chromic gut suture on a P3 needle.

Fig 3-8f Excellent incision line esthetics noted after delivery of final restoration. (Restoration by Dr Faustino Garcia, Coral Gables, FL.)

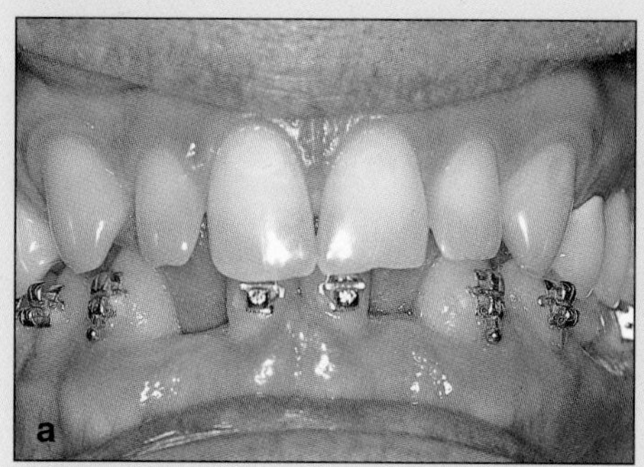

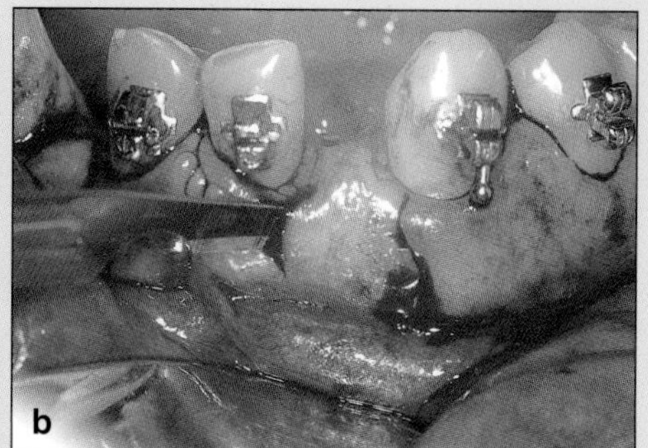

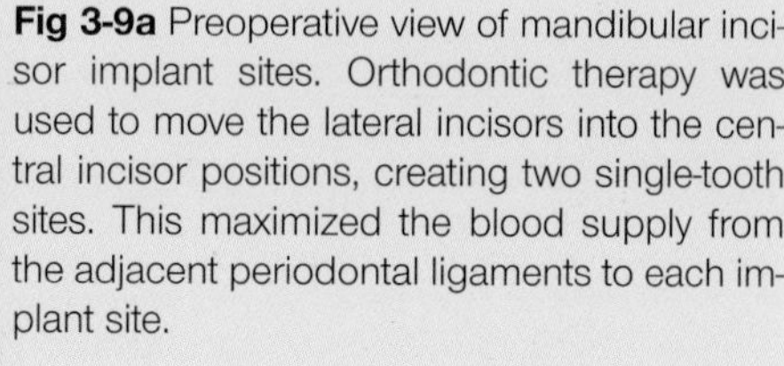

Fig 3-9a Preoperative view of mandibular incisor implant sites. Orthodontic therapy was used to move the lateral incisors into the central incisor positions, creating two single-tooth sites. This maximized the blood supply from the adjacent periodontal ligaments to each implant site.

Fig 3-9b Limited access necessitated reorientation of the scalpel to obtain appropriate beveling of the incision through attached tissues at the ridge crest.

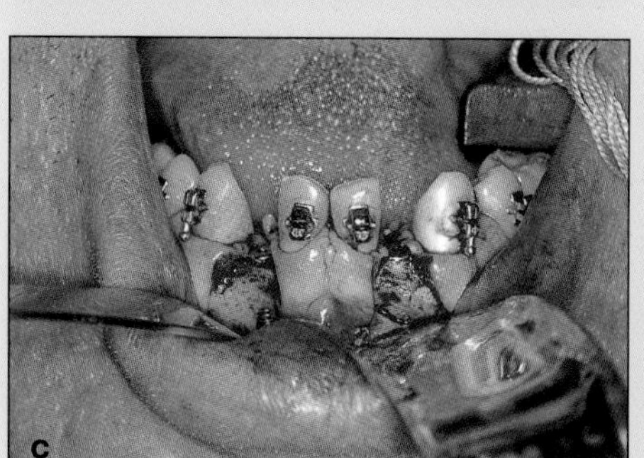

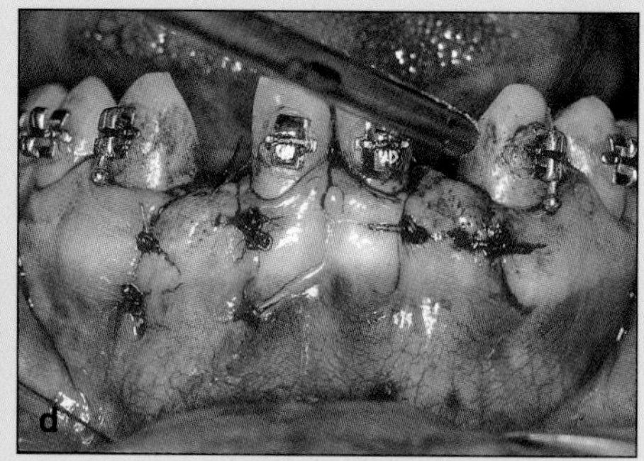

Fig 3-9c Despite reduced access, elevation of papillary and col tissues was avoided during implant placement. Access for grafting of apical fenestration defects was enhanced by the flap design.

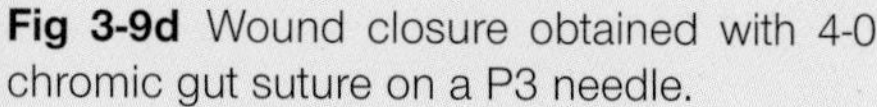

Fig 3-9d Wound closure obtained with 4-0 chromic gut suture on a P3 needle.

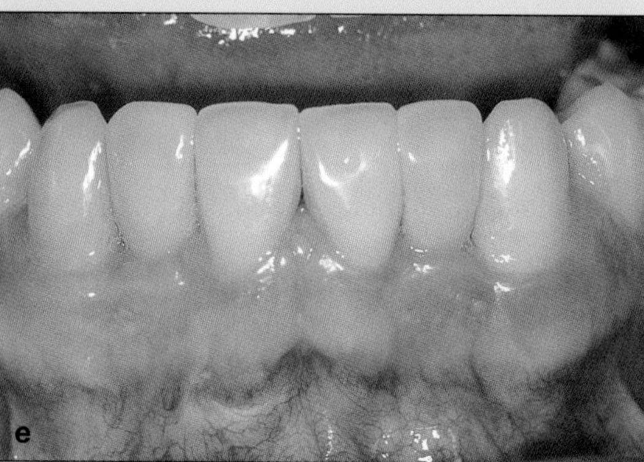

Fig 3-9e Flap design with beveled incisions resulted in inconspicuous incision line esthetics and negligible flap retraction. Maintenance of natural soft tissue architecture ensured natural- appearing emergence of the restorations. (Orthodontics by Dr Richard Mariani Jr, Miami FL; restoration by Dr Cecil Abraham, Miami, FL.)

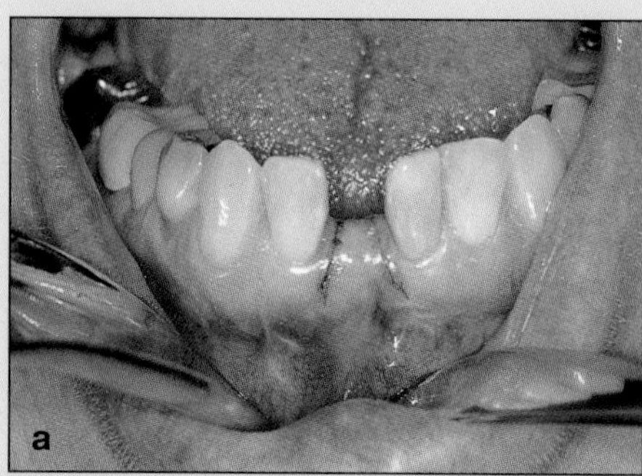

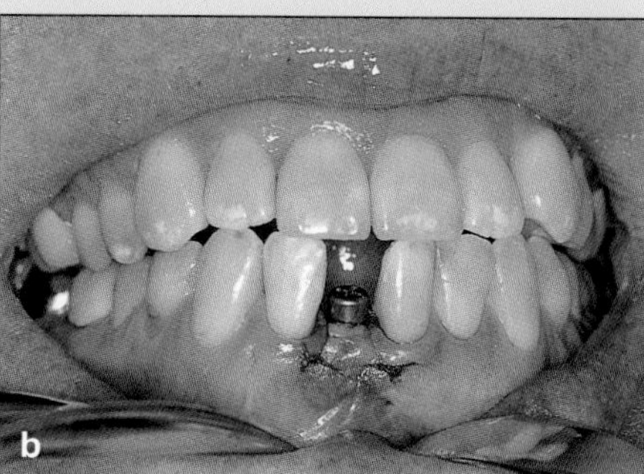

Fig 3-10a Beveled incisions outline the access flap for nonsubmerged implant replacement of mandibular central incisor. Note that the col and papillary tissues are not included in the flap even though the incisor site is small.

Fig 3-10b Closure around nonsubmerged implant abutment obtained with 4-0 chromic gut suture on a P3 needle.

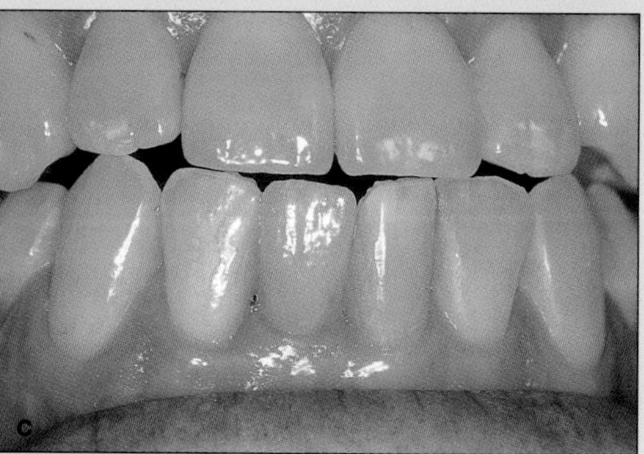

Fig 3-10c Flap design with beveled incisions resulted in inconspicuous incision line esthetics and maintenance of natural soft tissue architecture at the site. Final restoration has a natural appearance. (Restoration by Dr Ernie Rillman, Miami, FL.)

When beveling a curvilinear incision in implant therapy, the scalpel blade is oriented toward the center of the flap at approximately a 45-degree angle to the tissue surface. The orientation of the scalpel blade is maintained as the incision is continued through the attached tissue over the alveolar ridge crest (see Fig 3-6). A scalpel blade with a narrow profile will facilitate maintenance of proper angulation as the incision continues over the crest of the alveolar ridge. When a flap incorporating beveled incisions is coapted, the incision lines immediately become inconspicuous.

Flap Management Considerations

The primary goal of implant soft tissue management is to establish a healthy peri-implant soft tissue environment. This goal is accomplished by obtaining circumferential adaptation of attached tissues around the permucosal implant structures, thereby providing the connective tissue and epithelium needed for the formation of a protective soft tissue seal. In addition, when implant therapy is performed in esthetic areas, the recreation of natural-appearing soft tissue architecture and topography at the prosthetic recipient site becomes necessary. To achieve these goals, the surgeon must carefully preserve and manipulate existing soft tissues at the implant site and, when indicated, perform soft tissue augmentation. The quantity, quality, and position of the existing attached tissues relative to the planned implant emergence should be evaluated prior to implant surgery. The flap should be designed to ensure that an adequate band of attached, good-quality tissue always remains lingual or palatal to the planned implant emergence. Designing the flap in such a fashion is practical because subsequent correction of soft tissue problems occurring in lingual and palatal areas is difficult. Preoperative evaluation with the aid of a surgical template will help the surgeon visualize whether adequate tissue quality and volume are available in the area critical for prosthetic emergence. The surgeon can then decide where the incisions will have to be made or how the existing soft tissues must be manipulated with specific surgical maneuvers to establish a stable peri-implant soft tissue environment in each individual case as per the guidelines presented below.

Submerged implant placement

When placing a submerged implant, the buccal flap must be designed to preserve both the blood supply to the implant site and the topography of the alveolar ridge and mucobuccal fold. The pericrestal incision is beveled to the lingual or palatal (see Fig 3-5).The incision is initiated over the lingual or palatal aspect of the ridge crest, and the scalpel blade is angled to make contact with the underlying bone. Reflection of the buccal flap exposes the entire ridge crest and provides ample access for implant instrumentation. This is accomplished with minimal lingual or palatal flap elevation, thus preserving periosteal circulation and providing attached tissue to anchor the buccal flap during subsequent wound closure. The stability of the postoperative wound complex is improved, and the topography of the alveolar ridge and mucobuccal fold is preserved. As a result, wound dehiscence is decreased, and the use of a provisional prosthesis during the osseointegration period is facilitated.

Abutment connection and nonsubmerged implant placement

An identical flap design is used for abutment connection to submerged implants and for nonsubmerged implant placement (see Fig 3-5). The pericrestal incision is initiated in a position that ensures the maintenance of approximately a 3-mm apicocoronal dimension of attached lingual tissue or good-quality palatal mucosa (free of rugae) for re-adaptation around the emerging implant structures. The quantity and position of the existing soft tissues will guide the location of the incision. In general, this incision will be located closer to the midcrestal position than the incision made for submerged implant placement. The scalpel blade is held so as to create a buccal bevel. The buccal bevel facilitates abutment connection and implant placement while preserving periosteal blood supply by minimizing the need for lingual or palatal flap reflection. Additionally, the buccal bevel maximizes the amount of attached tissue reflected with the buccal flap (see Fig 3-10).

Surgical Maneuvers for Management of Peri-implant Soft Tissues

Once the flap has been outlined in a manner that ensures an optimal lingual and palatal soft tissue environment, the surgical maneuvers that will be used for managing the resulting buccal flap during abutment connection and nonsubmerged implant placement can be determined, for the most part, by the apicocoronal dimension of the attached tissue remaining on the buccal flap margin. Using this dimension as a guideline, other factors should be taken under consideration, including the thickness and health of the attached tissue remaining on the buccal flap and whether the margin of the planned restoration will be supragingival or intracrevicular. It is important to understand that whenever an intracrevicular restoration is planned, the peri-implant soft tissues must initially be able to withstand the trauma of the multiple procedures required to fabricate and deliver the final prosthesis. Subsequently, the tissues will have to tolerate the stringent hygiene maintenance required for long-term success and patient comfort. These considerations are of paramount importance for the partially edentulous implant patient, but they are also of significance for edentulous implant patients with atrophic alveolar ridges, where a lack of attached tissue is often accompanied by inadequate vestibular depth for proper oral hygiene maintenance. To establish sufficient vestibular depth in these patients, vestibular extension with or without soft tissue grafting is often indicated. Similarly, clinical observations of soft tissue recession, soft tissue mobility, or peri-implant soft tissue inflammation may indicate the need for subsequent soft tissue augmentation in both partially edentulous and edentulous patients, despite initial surgical judgment indicating adequate soft tissue volume at the time of wound closure according to the guidelines presented below.

The author commonly uses three distinct soft tissue surgical maneuvers to achieve the desired outcome of obtaining primary closure with circumferential adaptation of attached tissues around emerging implant structures: resective contouring, papilla regeneration, and lateral flap advancement. Although the minimum width of attached tissue necessary to establish a stable peri-implant soft tissue environment has not been established, the following guidelines for using each of the soft tissue maneuvers will provide consistent results in most clinical situations. These surgical maneuvers may be used for abutment connection to submerged implants and for placement of nonsubmerged implants. The author would like to emphasize that the use of a specific maneuver is based primarily on the apicocoronal dimension of attached tissue remaining along the buccal flap margin at each implant site. A combination of these surgical maneuvers is often indicated because the width of attached tissue remaining on the buccal flap varies as a result of necessary adjustments made in the path of the crestal incision to maintain an adequate width of attached tissue on the lingual or palatal flap.

Resective contouring

When the width of the gingival tissues remaining on the buccal flap is 5 to 6 mm, the author performs resective contouring to facilitate circumferential adaptation of the soft tissues around the emerging implant structures. A fine scalpel blade held in a round handle is used to perform a gingivectomy on the buccal flap corresponding in shape and position to the anteriormost abutment or nonsubmerged implant neck (Fig 3-11a). After resective contouring, the tissue is adapted around the emerging implant structure, and this process is repeated sequentially around each implant, moving in a distal direction (Fig 3-11b). The contoured flap is then apically repositioned and secured around the abutments with a suture passing through each inter-implant area, resulting in circumferential adaptation of attached tissues around emerging implant structures. Sutures are then placed to close the curvilinear releasing incisions that define the buccal flap outline (Fig 3-11c).

Papilla regeneration

When the width of the gingival tissues remaining on the buccal flap is 4 to 5 mm, the author recommends the use of the papilla regeneration maneuver advocated by Palacci.[3] This maneuver facilitates primary closure and circumferential adaptation around the permucosal implant structures while maintaining an adequate band of attached tissue around the emerging implant structures. The papilla regeneration maneuver is especially useful in Kennedy Class III partially edentulous situations where natural teeth remain both mesial and distal to the edentulous site, eliminating the possibility of lateral advancement of a full-thickness flap. In addition, this maneuver is useful in edentulous case types.

This surgical maneuver also involves contouring of the buccal flap tissues. Attached mucosa is taken from the top of the ridge and moved in a buccal direction while maintaining approximately 3 mm of attached lingual or palatal tissues. Subsequently, a fine scalpel is

Surgical maneuvers: Resective contouring

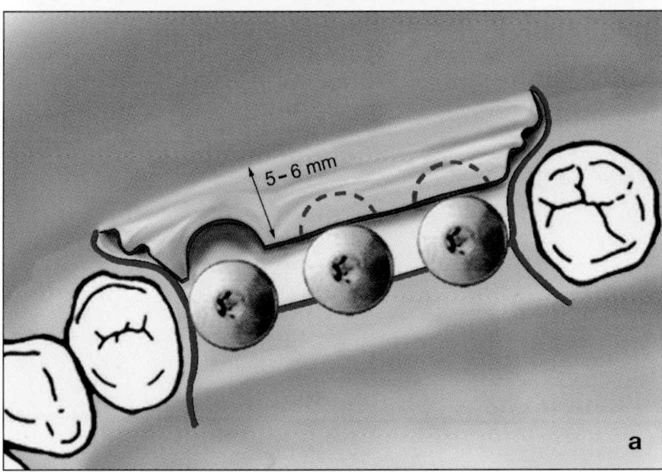

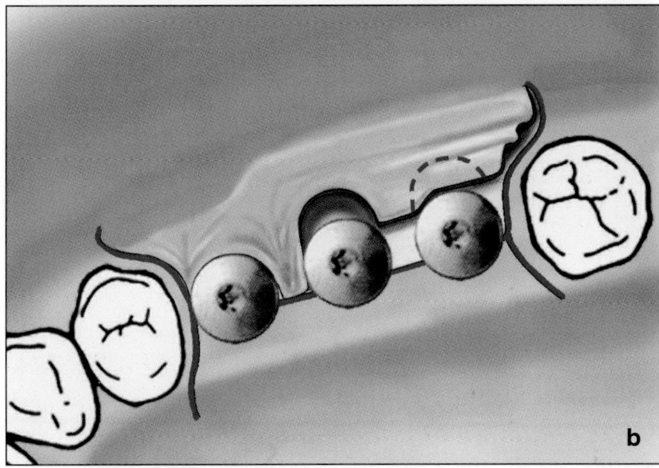

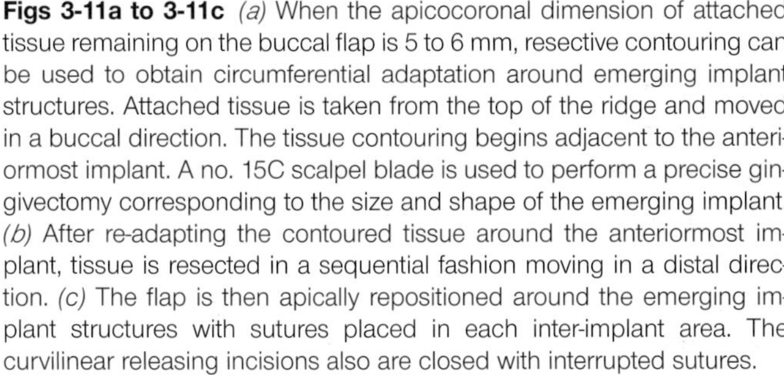

Figs 3-11a to 3-11c *(a)* When the apicocoronal dimension of attached tissue remaining on the buccal flap is 5 to 6 mm, resective contouring can be used to obtain circumferential adaptation around emerging implant structures. Attached tissue is taken from the top of the ridge and moved in a buccal direction. The tissue contouring begins adjacent to the anteriormost implant. A no. 15C scalpel blade is used to perform a precise gingivectomy corresponding to the size and shape of the emerging implant. *(b)* After re-adapting the contoured tissue around the anteriormost implant, tissue is resected in a sequential fashion moving in a distal direction. *(c)* The flap is then apically repositioned around the emerging implant structures with sutures placed in each inter-implant area. The curvilinear releasing incisions also are closed with interrupted sutures.

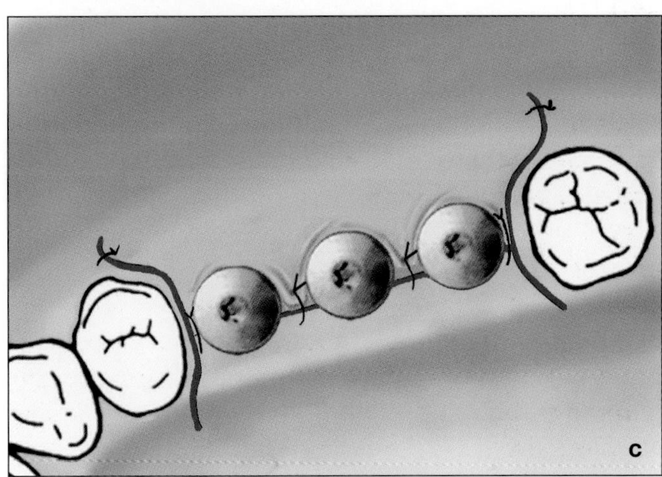

used to sharply dissect the tissues to create pedicles in the buccal flap, which are passively rotated to fill the inter-implant spaces (Figs 3-12a and 3-12b). In the author's experience, passive adaptation of the pedicles in the inter-implant space may require reverse cutback incisions made away from the base of the pedicle. The tissues are sutured, avoiding tension within the pedicles, usually using a figure-eight horizontal mattress suture (Fig 3-12c). Alternatively, a simple interrupted suture passed through the buccal flap in a fashion that passively advances the pedicle into the inter-implant space is effective in many situations. Care must be taken to avoid placement of the suture through the pedicle, as this would reduce circulation to the pedicle. This papilla regeneration maneuver facilitates circumferential adaptation around emerging implant structures with less tissue resection than is required in the resective contouring maneuver because the resulting soft tissue pedicle is used to obtain soft tissue coverage and primary closure in the inter-implant areas. This technique can be successfully applied to regenerate interdental papillae only if the underlying osseous scaffold and anatomic restorative contours support the soft tissue pedicles in the inter-implant area during their maturation. A variation of this technique that uses pedicles created in the palatal flap, which can also be rotated to fill the inter-implant spaces, is especially useful in maxillary situations where thick palatal tissues exist.

Lateral flap advancement

When the width of the gingival tissues remaining on the buccal flap is 3 to 4 mm, the author recommends the use of the lateral flap advancement maneuver to facilitate primary closure and circumferential adaptation of attached tissues around the emerging implant structures (Fig 3-13a). This maneuver is especially suited for completely edentulous or posterior partially edentulous implant case types where an adequate band of attached tissue exists adjacent to the implant site. The surgeon simply repositions the attached tissues available from adjacent areas in order to obtain primary closure with attached tissues around the emerging implant structures.

This maneuver requires that the flap be designed to extend beyond the area of implant placement to include the attached tissues present in adjacent edentu-

Surgical maneuvers: Papilla regeneration

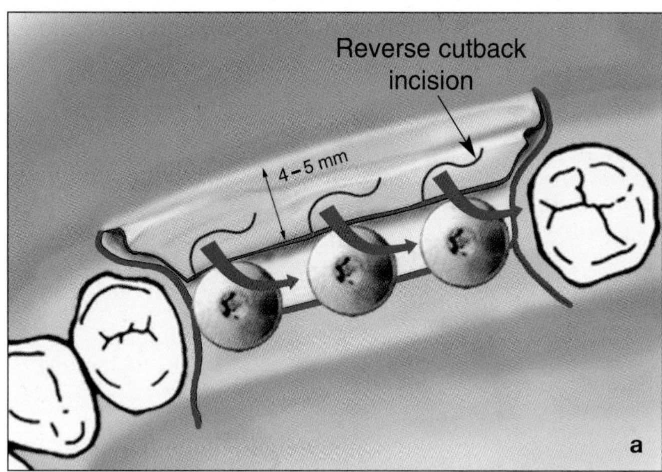

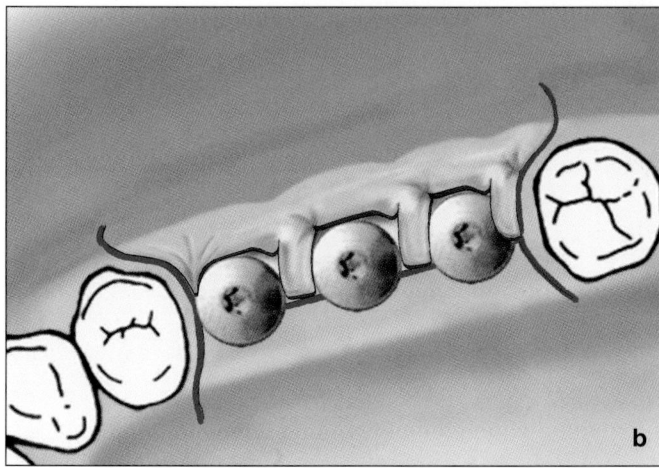

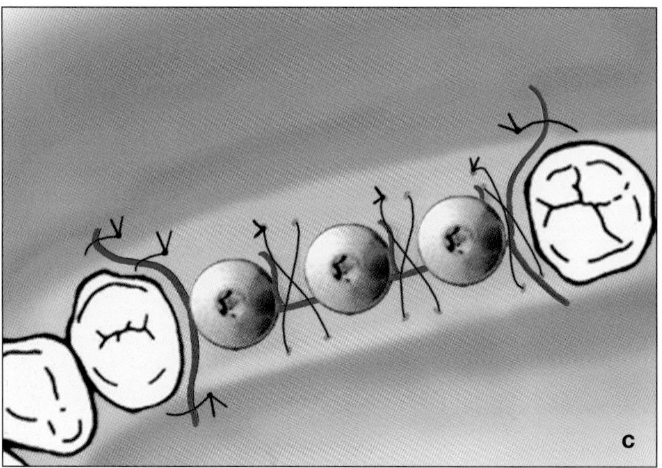

Figs 3-12a to 3-12c *(a)* When the apicocoronal dimension of attached tissue remaining on the buccal flap is 4 to 5 mm, the papilla regeneration technique can be used to obtain circumferential closure of attached tissue around the permucosal implant elements. Attached tissue is taken from the top of the ridge and moved in a buccal direction. Pedicles are created in the margin of the buccal flap adjacent to the emerging implants. The thickness of the pedicles corresponds to the size of the inter-implant space. *(b)* The pedicles are rotated into the inter-implant spaces. Extension of the incision away from the flap margin in the form of a "reverse cutback" facilitates passive positioning and advancement of the pedicles to the interdental spaces. *(c)* The flap is re-adapted and secured to obtain circumferential adaptation around emerging implant structures. Figure-eight or interrupted sutures are placed so as to avoid creating tension in the pedicles, which could embarrass their circulation.

lous areas. Subsequent to abutment connection or nonsubmerged implant placement, the closure usually begins around the mesialmost implant at the site and proceeds in a distal direction (Fig 3-13b). As the closure progresses, the flap will advance in a mesial direction to obtain primary closure around the implants while creating a denuded area that will heal by secondary intention at the distal extent of the dissection (Fig 3-13c). Alternatively, if warranted by the clinical situation, the closure may begin around the distalmost implant and advance in a distal direction, leaving a denuded area at the anterior releasing incision. The important concept is to reposition the attached tissues from adjacent areas to allow primary closure and circumferential adaptation around the permucosal implant structures. When adjacent areas are edentulous, the author recommends that full-thickness flap elevation be performed in these areas. This surgical maneuver is useful in both edentulous situations and Kennedy Class I and Class II partially edentulous situations. In addition, in certain Kennedy Class III situations, where an abundant volume of attached keratinized tissue is available around the adjacent dentition, the flap design can be modified to include partial-thickness dissection in these areas. This will facilitate primary closure and circumferential adaptation of attached keratinized tissue around the emerging implant structures with minimal risk of recession on the adjacent dentition.

Soft tissue augmentation

When the apicocoronal dimension of attached tissue remaining on the buccal flap is less than 3 mm, the surgeon should consider buccal soft tissue augmentation. Other factors to consider in the decision to proceed with soft tissue augmentation include tissue thickness, tissue quality, the presence of soft tissue inflammation or pathology, and the type of implant restoration planned.

In preparation for simultaneous soft tissue grafting, the horizontal incision is made at the mucogingival junction. The existing attached tissue is then preserved and, if needed, reflected and re-adapted to the lingual or palatal aspect of the emerging implant components. Alternatively, the surgeon can use the various surgical maneuvers described above to obtain primary closure and re-evaluate the need for soft tissue grafting based on the health and volume of peri-implant attached tissues obtained after initial healing.

Surgical maneuvers: Lateral flap advancement

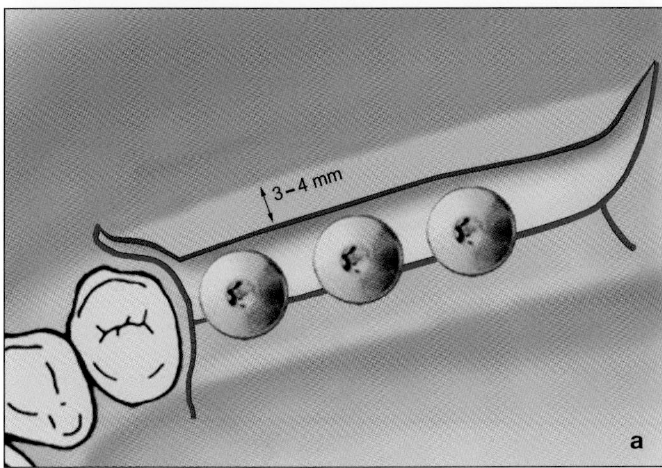

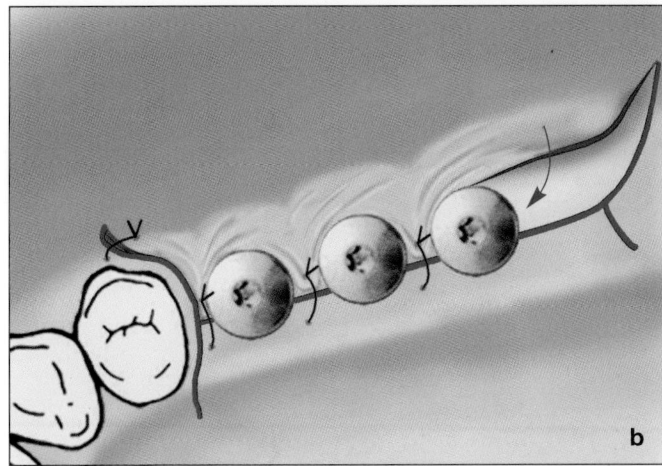

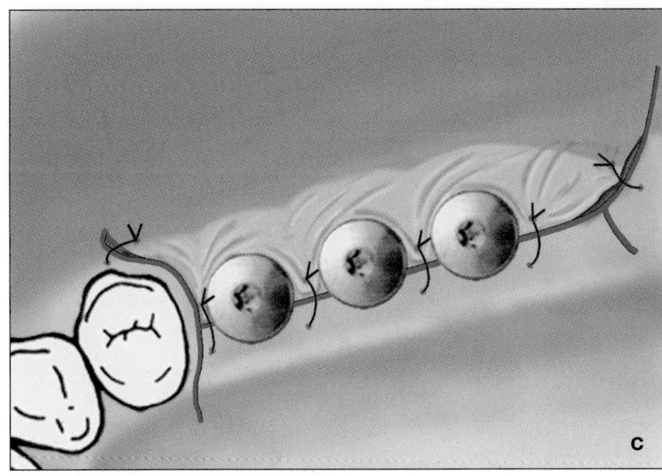

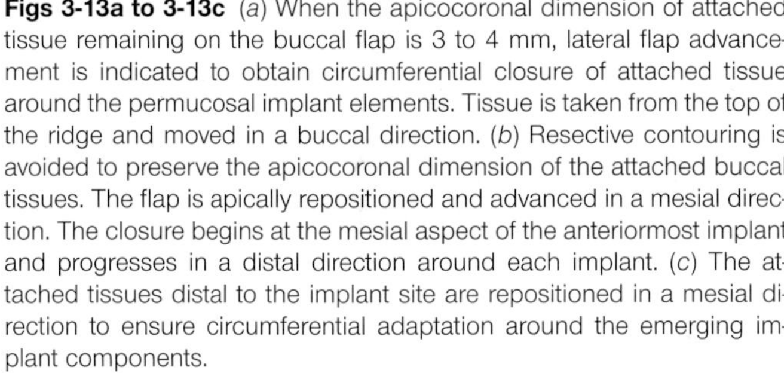

Figs 3-13a to 3-13c (*a*) When the apicocoronal dimension of attached tissue remaining on the buccal flap is 3 to 4 mm, lateral flap advancement is indicated to obtain circumferential closure of attached tissue around the permucosal implant elements. Tissue is taken from the top of the ridge and moved in a buccal direction. (*b*) Resective contouring is avoided to preserve the apicocoronal dimension of the attached buccal tissues. The flap is apically repositioned and advanced in a mesial direction. The closure begins at the mesial aspect of the anteriormost implant and progresses in a distal direction around each implant. (*c*) The attached tissues distal to the implant site are repositioned in a mesial direction to ensure circumferential adaptation around the emerging implant components.

Flap Design and Management Considerations for Mandibular Implant Surgery

When working in the mandible, the buccal access flap should be designed and the existing soft tissues manipulated in order to maintain approximately a 3-mm apicocoronal dimension of attached tissue lingual to the planned implant emergence. Failure to do so often results in a compromised lingual soft tissue environment, which is extremely difficult to correct once it has occurred. The surgeon varies the location and bevel of the pericrestal incision in each individual case to achieve this. The flap outline is completed with curvilinear-beveled releasing incisions that join the mesial and distal extent of the pericrestal incision. These releasing incisions are initiated in the mucosal tissues beyond the mucogingival junction and extended through the attached tissues that envelop the alveolar ridge crest to join the mesial and distal extent of the pericrestal incision. For submerged implant placement, the buccal flap is elevated and retracted to provide access for implant placement. Elevation of the lingual tissues is minimized or, in certain cases, avoided altogether. Subsequently, the flap is re-adapted and anchored to the attached lingual tissues. For abutment connection and nonsubmerged implant placement, the buccal access flap is elevated and retracted. Subsequently, the tissues are apically repositioned and carefully re-adapted around the permucosal implant structures. Frequently, lingual releasing incisions are also necessary to improve the adaptation of the lingual tissues around the emerging implant structures. When working posterior to the first molar area, lingual releasing incisions should be abbreviated to avoid damage to the lingual nerve.

Edentulous mandible

A simple variation of the buccal flap is used for implant surgery performed in the edentulous mandible. This approach is practical and effective for both standard and atrophic situations. With minor modifications, the flap becomes suitable for placement of both submerged and nonsubmerged implants as well as for abutment connection procedures.

Flap design and management for the edentulous mandible

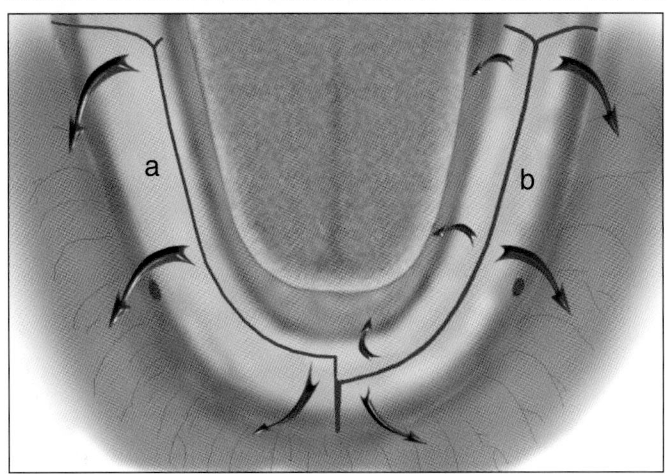

Fig 3-14a Flap design for implant placement in the edentulous mandible. *(a)* Line representing the flap outline used for submerged implant placement. This design minimizes the need for reflection of lingual tissues. *(b)* Line representing the flap outline for abutment connection and nonsubmerged implant placement. This design ensures the maintenance of approximately 3-mm apicocoronal dimension of attached tissues lingual to the implant emergence site.

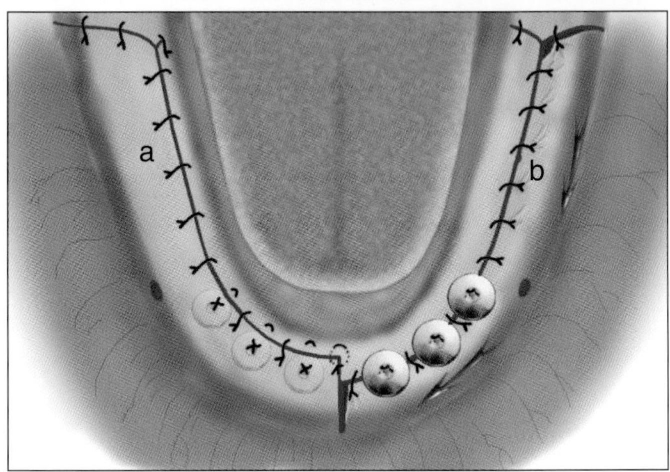

Fig 3-14b Flap management for implant placement in the edentulous mandible. *(a)* After submerged implant placement, closure begins by anchoring the buccal flaps to the attached midline lingual tissues with a three-point horizontal mattress suture. Horizontal mattress sutures are then alternated with interrupted sutures to obtain aligned wound margins and tension-free closure over the implants. The topography of the alveolar ridge and muccobuccal fold are preserved, thus simplifying the use of a provisional restoration. *(b)* After abutment connection or nonsubmerged implant placement, the buccal flap is apically repositioned and the appropriate surgical maneuvers are used to obtain circumferential closure around the emerging implants.

The flap outline includes a pericrestal incision that extends well beyond the area planned for implant placement or exposure. Posterior releasing incisions and a midline vertical incision complete the flap outline (Figs 3-14 and 3-15a). This flap design provides excellent access for surgical instrumentation and facilitates the use of surgical guides. Posterior extension of the pericrestal incision facilitates initial reflection of the buccal flap as the periosteum is quickly and easily elevated in the area of the posterior releasing incisions. Extending the dissection beyond the area of implantation also provides access for local bone harvest and lateral soft tissue advancement when needed for primary closure around emerging implant structures through the lateral flap advancement maneuver.

The subperiosteal dissection begins in the area of the posterior releasing incisions and moves in a mesial direction toward the area of the mental foramen. The dissection then is resumed at the midline vertical releasing incision, and the tissues are elevated distally toward the mental foramen. The Buser periosteal elevator facilitates elevation of the adherent fibrous tissue that is often encountered in underlying bony alveolar ridge defects resulting from previous tooth extractions. The Adson tissue forceps are used to carefully hold the flap as it is gently elevated to expose the mental nerve, which is then protected as the flap is gently reflected in an apical direction.

Reflection of the lingual tissues is minimized to preserve the circulation derived from the lingual periosteum and to provide an anchor for the buccal tissues during wound closure. Adherence to this surgical technique improves the stability of the wound complex and decreases the incidence of postoperative wound dehiscence (Figs 3-15b to 3-15f).

When submerged implant placement is planned, a lingual-crestal incision is performed through the attached tissue on the top of the ridge (Figs 3-14 and 3-16a). The scalpel blade is held in a vertical orientation to create a slight lingual bevel on the flap margin. The lingual-crestal incision minimizes the need for lingual reflection during osteotomy preparation.

After implant placement, wound closure begins with a three-point horizontal mattress suture placed through the anterior corners of each flap and the attached lingual tissues (see Fig 3-14b). This single suture properly aligns and reapproximates the buccal flaps. Horizontal mattress or simple interrupted sutures are then used to quickly obtain closure over the implants. Mattress sutures are less vulnerable to disruption by a provisional prosthesis worn in the immediate postoperative period. The author recommends

Flap design and management for nonsubmerged implants in the edentulous mandible

Fig 3-15a A pericrestal incision is beveled to the buccal and extended well beyond the area planned for implant placement.

Fig 3-15b Four nonsubmerged implants have been placed. Note that approximately 3 mm of attached lingual tissues were minimally reflected and will act as an anchor for the buccal flaps during wound closure.

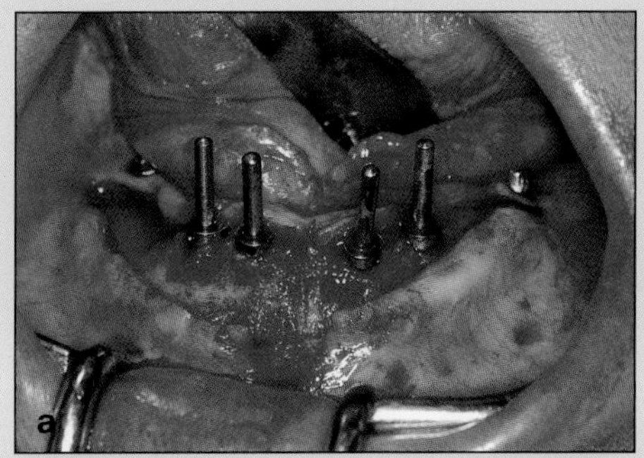

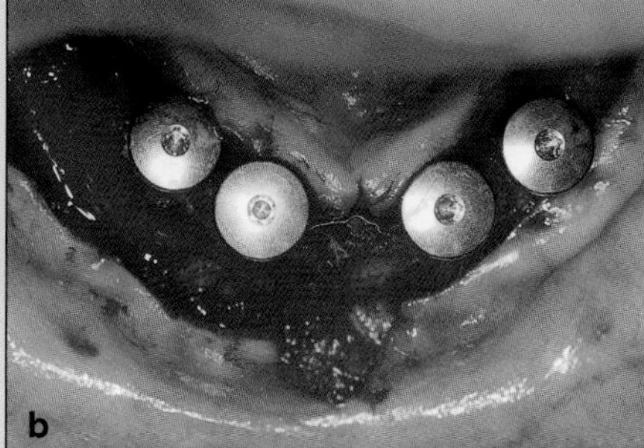

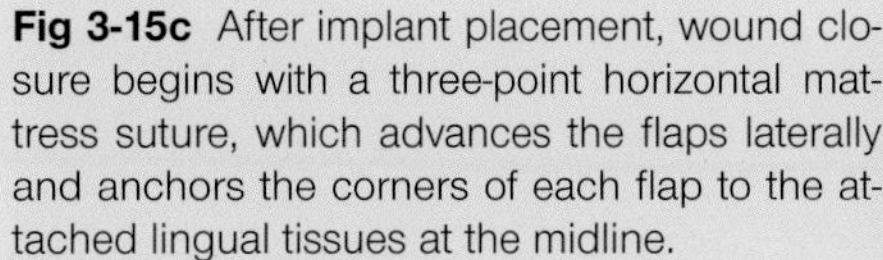

Fig 3-15c After implant placement, wound closure begins with a three-point horizontal mattress suture, which advances the flaps laterally and anchors the corners of each flap to the attached lingual tissues at the midline.

Fig 3-15d After lateral advancement of buccal flaps, interrupted sutures are used to ensure primary soft tissue closure and circumferential adaptation of attached tissues around the permucosal portion of the nonsubmerged implants.

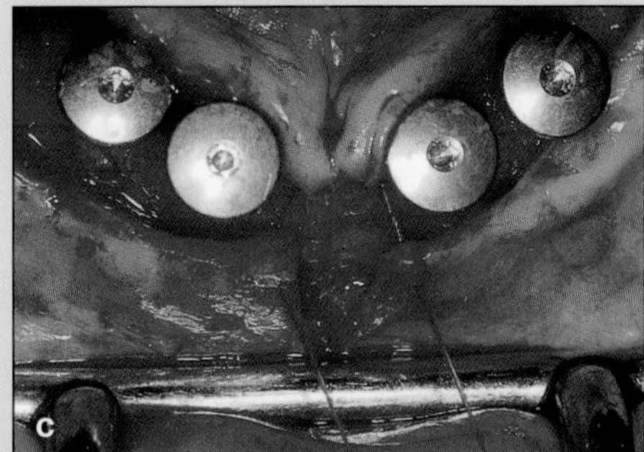

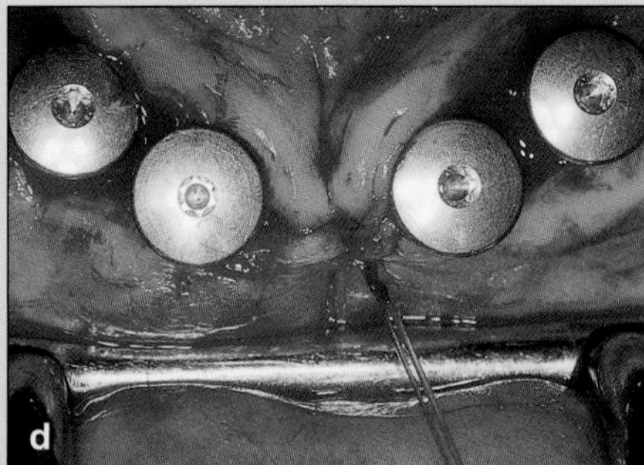

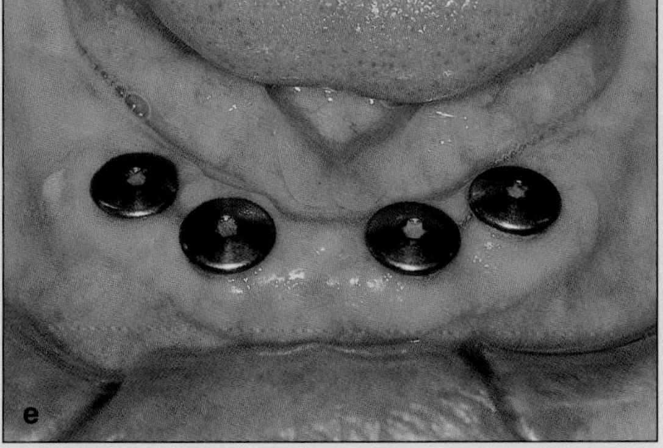

Fig 3-15e Use of the recommended flap design and lateral flap advancement maneuver resulted in circumferential adaptation of attached tissue surrounding each implant and an adequate band of attached tissue on the lingual and facial aspects of the implants.

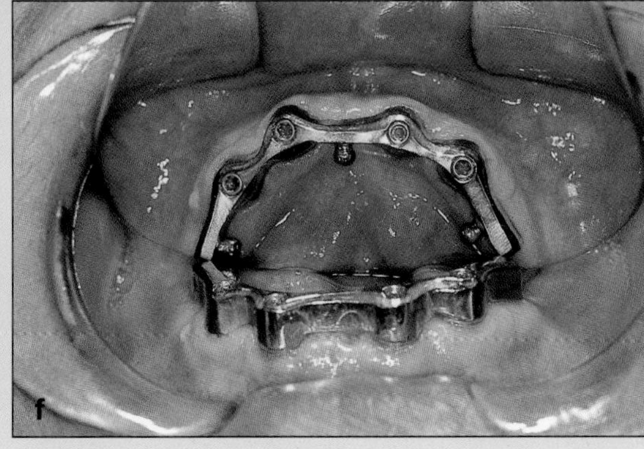

Fig 3-15f Two-year postoperative view showing no evidence of recession. Oral hygiene has been facilitated by the maintenance of an adequate band of attached soft tissues around the emerging implants. (Prosthetics and final restoration by Dr Larry Lesperance, Miami, FL.)

Flap design and management for abutment connection to submerged implants in the edentulous mandible

Fig 3-16a The pericrestal incision is extended beyond the area where the implants were placed.

Fig 3-16b Lateral flap advancement maneuver is used during wound closure to ensure circumferential adaptation of attached tissues around the emerging implant abutments.

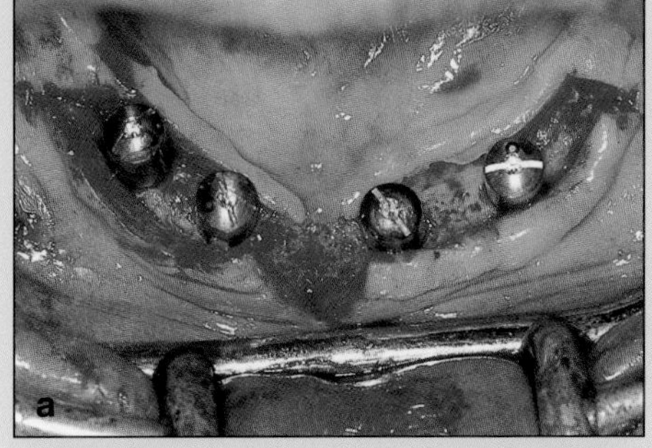

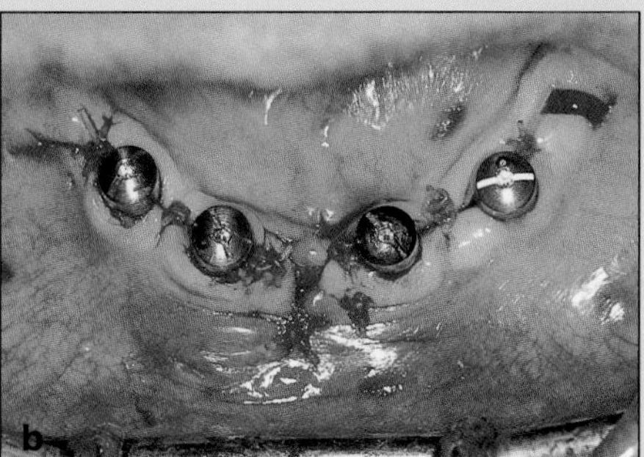

Fig 3-16c Facial view of implant bar 4 years after delivery of final restoration. Health and stability of soft tissue environment are evident.

Fig 3-16d Four-year postoperative view. A minimum of 3 mm of attached tissue was maintained on the lingual aspect of the emerging implants. (Prosthetics and final restoration by Dr Jose Gurevich, Miami, FL.)

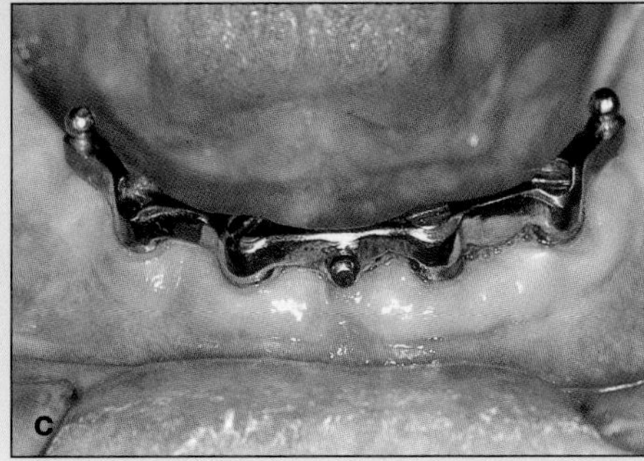

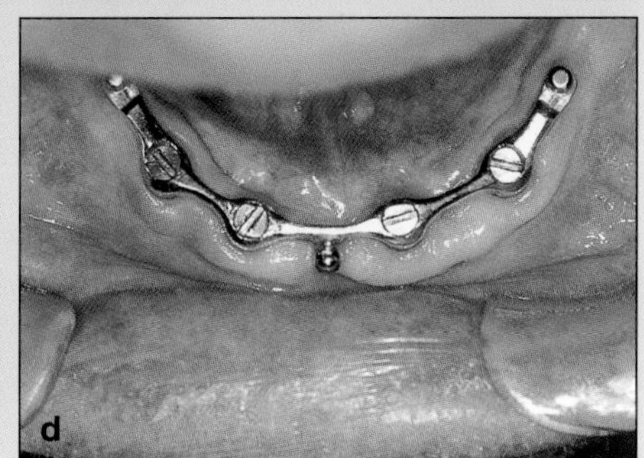

Flap design and management for the partially edentulous mandible

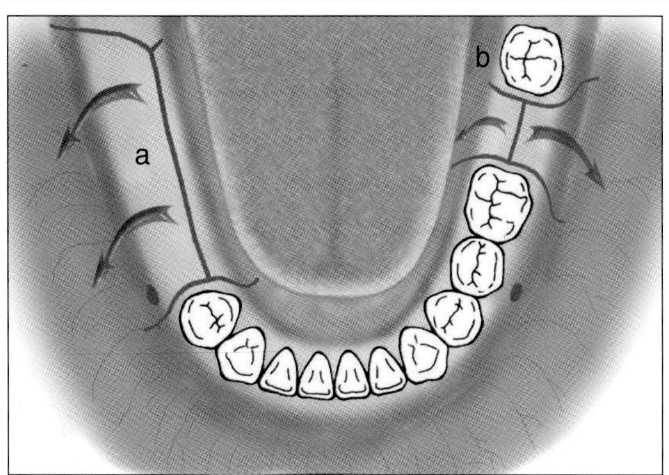

Fig 3-17a Flap design for implant placement in the partially edentulous mandible. *(a)* Line representing flap outline for submerged implant placement in a Kennedy Class I situation. The flap is extended beyond the site planned for implant placement. A lingual-crestal incision with a lingual bevel is used. The vertical releasing incisions are curvilinear and beveled toward the center of the flap. The papillary and col tissues are not included in the flap. *(b)* Line representing flap outline for nonsubmerged implant placement in a Kennedy Class III situation. The full-thickness flap cannot be extended beyond the site planned for implant placement. The location of the crestal incision ensures maintenance of approximately 3-mm apicocoronal dimension of lingual attached tissue. The papillary and col tissues are not included in the flap. The releasing incisions are curvilinear and beveled toward the center of the flap. Note that lingual releasing incisions are abbreviated posteriorly.

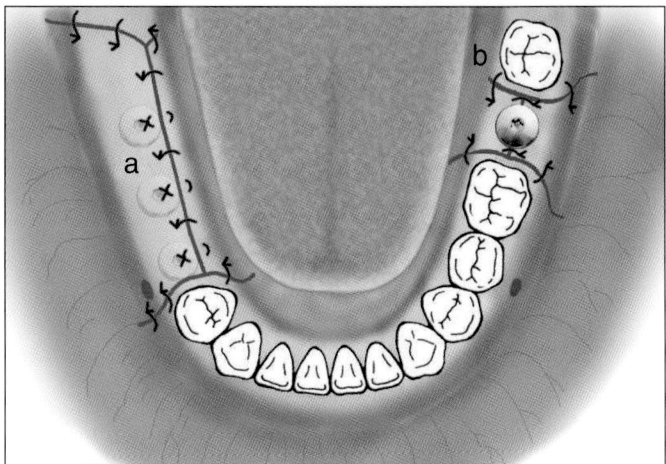

Fig 3-17b Flap management for implant placement in the partially edentulous mandible. *(a)* Flap management for submerged implant placement in a Kennedy Class I situation. The flap is re-adapted and secured to the attached lingual tissues over the submerged implants. Horizontal mattress sutures are alternated with interrupted sutures to ensure a tension-free closure. *(b)* Flap management for abutment connection and nonsubmerged implant placement in a Kennedy Class III situation. The buccal flap is apically repositioned and prepared with either resective contouring or the papilla regeneration technique to obtain circumferential closure around the emerging implant. Apical repositioning of the lingual tissues is sometimes necessary.

alternating simple interrupted and mattress sutures to obtain wound closure in the area where the implants have been placed. After tension-free closure has been obtained over the submerged implants, the wound closure is completed in a similar fashion at the distal extent of the dissection.

When preparing for abutment connection to a submerged implant or when placing a nonsubmerged implant, the pericrestal incision is usually located closer to the crest of the alveolar ridge. This will ensure maintenance of approximately a 3-mm apicocoronal dimension of attached tissue for re-adaptation to the lingual aspect of the emerging permucosal implant structures (see Fig 3-14b). The scalpel blade is oriented to create a slight buccal bevel so as to maximize the amount of attached tissue transferred with the buccal flap and minimize the lingual reflection needed for osteotomy preparation or abutment connection. Subsequently, the buccal and lingual flaps are both apically repositioned and manipulated as previously described in order to obtain circumferential adaptation around the permucosal implant structures (Figs 3-16b to 3-16d).

In summary, use of a flap design that maintains approximately a 3-mm apicocoronal dimension of lingual attached tissue and circumferential adaptation of attached tissues around emerging implant structures are key elements for successful management of edentulous mandibular implant case types.

Partially edentulous mandible

In partially edentulous mandibular situations, the location and bevel of the pericrestal incisions are adjusted as needed for submerged or nonsubmerged implant placement or for abutment connection (Fig 3-17a). Whenever possible, the flap is extended beyond the area planned for implant placement in either a mesial or a distal direction. The releasing incisions should always be of a curvilinear design and beveled toward the center of the flap. Care must be taken to avoid elevating the interdental papilla or col tissue adjacent to the natural teeth, since doing so not only compromises the vascular supply to the site but also creates an undesirable portal of entry for bacteria that will remain until the periodontal soft tissues reestablish a functional attachment to the tooth. This is an extremely important consideration when guided bone regeneration procedures are performed in conjunction with implant placement. Additionally, the flaps should be designed to minimize lingual tissue reflection and to maintain approximately a 3-mm apicocoronal dimension of attached lingual tissue for readaptation to the lingual aspect of the emerging implant structures (Fig 3-17b). The buccal flap is then managed with the surgical maneuvers as previously described for submerged and nonsubmerged implant surgery (Figs 3-18 to 3-21).

Flap design and management for abutment connection in the posterior partially edentulous mandible

Fig 3-18a Location of crestal incision ensured maintenance of approximately a 3-mm apicocoronal dimension of attached lingual tissues. The papillary and col tissues were not included in the flap. Lateral flap advancement facilitated circumferential adaptation of attached tissues around emerging implants.

Fig 3-18b Healthy peri-implant soft tissue environment 2 months after implant exposure. Flap design created a prosthetic-friendly environment and natural soft tissue architecture.

Fig 3-18c Stable soft tissues with natural restorative emergence 5 years after final restoration.

Fig 3-18d Maintaining approximately a 3-mm apicocoronal dimension of lingual attached tissues facilitated a healthy soft tissue environment and oral hygiene maintenance. The lingual tissues are healthy and recession has not occurred. (Restoration by Dr Fred Hart, Miami, FL.)

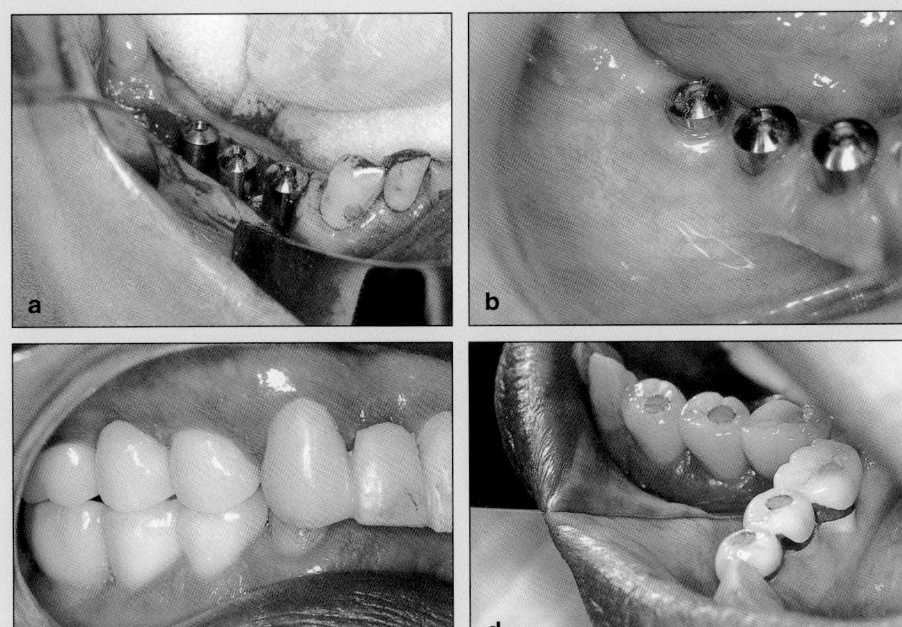

Flap design and management for placement of a nonsubmerged single-molar implant

Fig 3-19a Crestal incision ensured approximately a 3-mm apicocoronal dimension of lingual attached tissue. The papillary and col tissues were not included in the flap. Curvilinear releasing incisions were beveled toward the center of the flap. Resective contouring on the buccal and lingual flaps facilitated passive flap coaptation and circumferential adaptation around emerging implant collar *(arrow)*.

Figs 3-19b and 3-19c Soft tissue health and stability 3 months postoperatively. Single-stage surgery has allowed sufficient time for soft tissue integration.

Fig 3-19d Use of curvilinear-beveled releasing incisions and meticulous closure resulted in maintenance of positive gingival architecture and inconspicuous incision lines. Flap design and management have created a self-cleansing environment. Collection of food debris around implant restoration does not occur. (Restoration by Dr Alicia Abella-Torrente, Coral Gables, FL.)

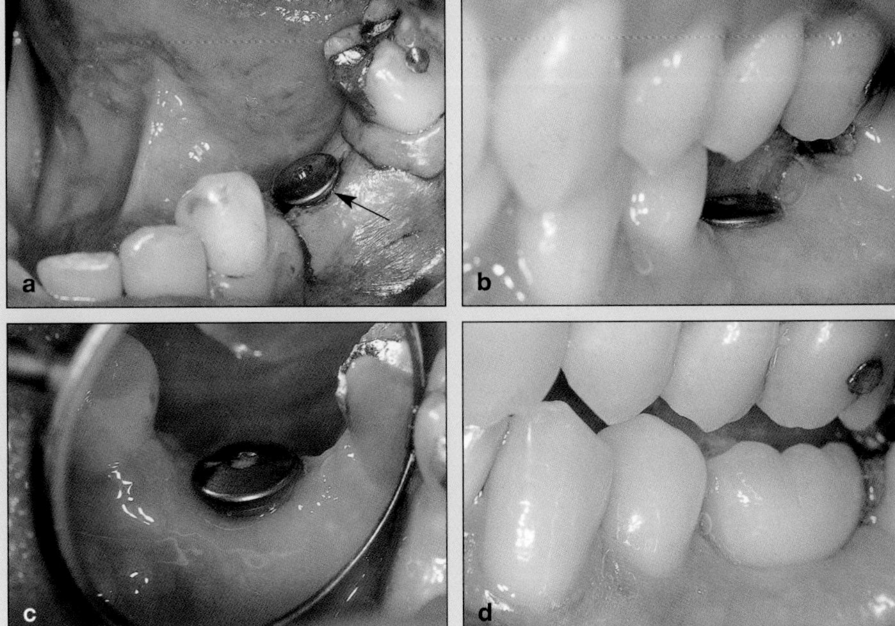

Flap design and management for ridge augmentation in Kennedy Class III posterior partially edentulous mandible

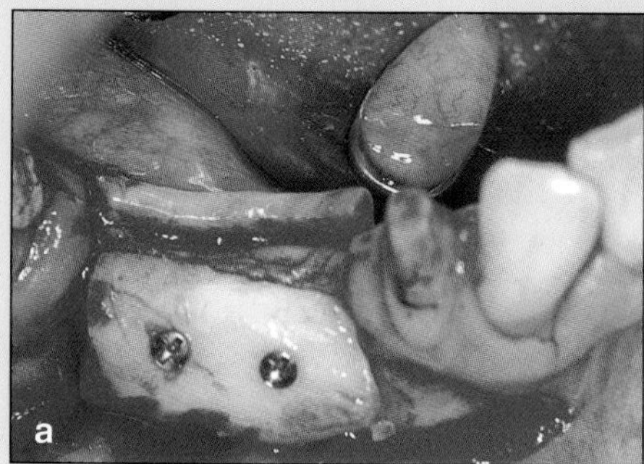

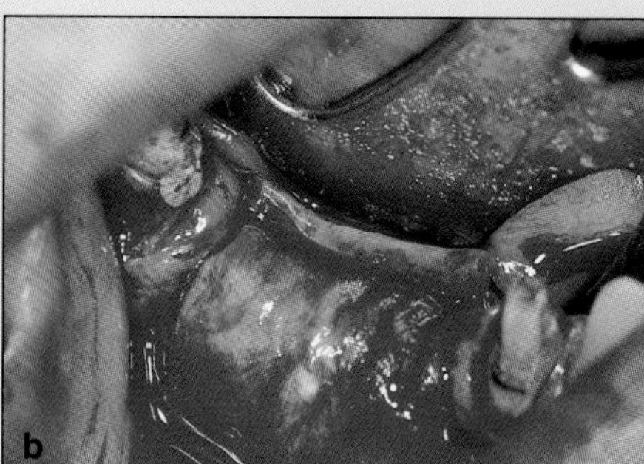

Fig 3-20a Lingual-crestal incision and exaggerated curvilinear-beveled releasing incisions outline flap. Minimal lingual reflection has been performed. After hard tissue recipient-site preparation, corticocancellous block graft secured in place with two rigid fixation screws (Osteomed, Addison, TX).

Fig 3-20b After compacting particulate bone around the periphery of the block graft, a resorbable collagen membrane (Bio-Gide; Osteohealth, Shirley, NY) is gently tucked under the edge of the lingual flap and adapted over the graft. When the buccal flap is properly developed with exaggerated curvilinear-beveled incisions, fixation of the membrane is not necessary since it will not be displaced upon flap coaptation.

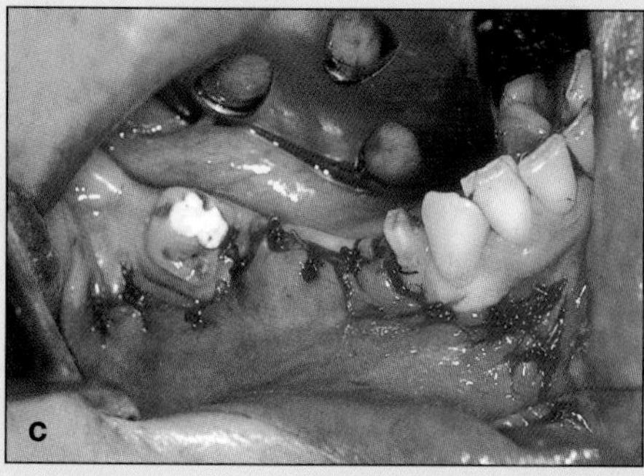

Fig 3-20c Tension-free closure obtained with 4-0 chromic gut suture. Note that the flap was extended well beyond the graft site.

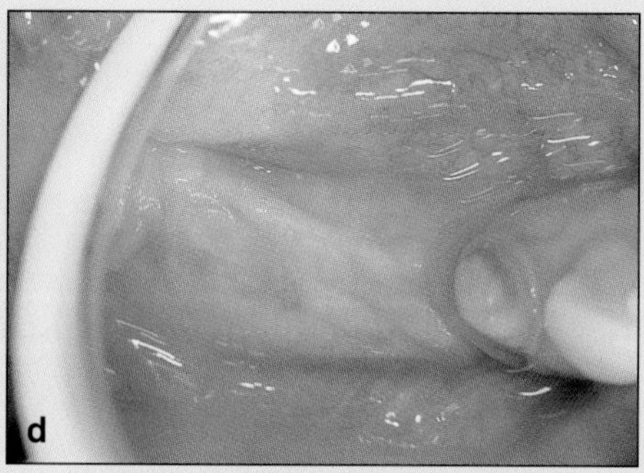

Fig 3-20d Excellent soft tissue healing 6 weeks after graft procedure.

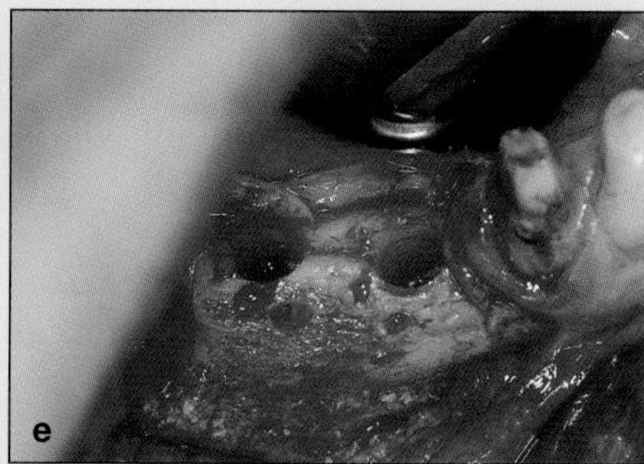

Fig 3-20e After 4 months, site is re-entered for implant placement. Proper soft tissue management at the time of grafting resulted in excellent volume yield from hard tissue site development, enabling preparation of the osteotomy for placement of wide-body molar implants.

Flap design and management for ridge augmentation in Kennedy Class I posterior partially edentulous mandible

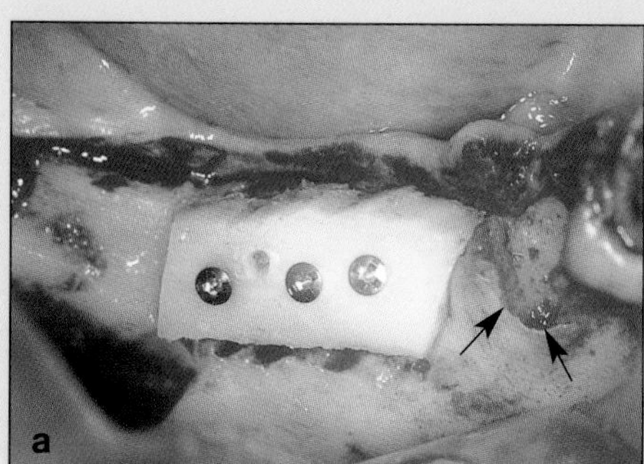

Fig 3-21a Flap outlined by lingual-crestal incision extended posteriorly beyond graft recipient site and curvilinear-beveled releasing incisions, which are initiated in the mucosal tissues and converge to meet the crestal incision. The second premolar was removed after the flap was elevated. Note buccal defect after extraction *(arrows)*. Corticocancellous block graft has been secured to prepared recipient site.

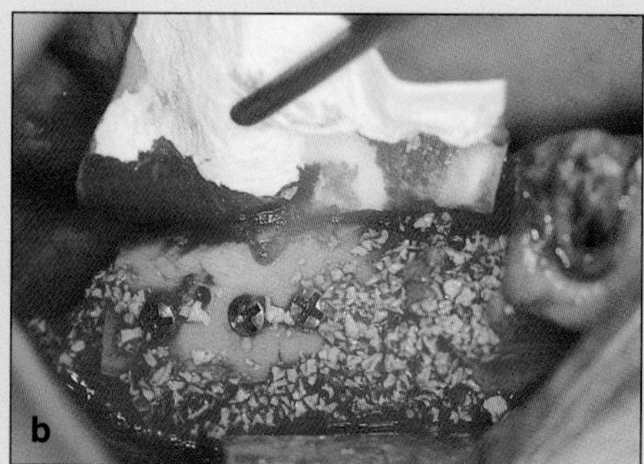

Fig 3-21b Particulate graft consisting of 50% autogenous cancellous and marrow bone and 50% Bio-Oss (Osteohealth) has been compacted around the periphery of the block graft. A resorbable Bio-Gide membrane has been tucked under the edge of the lingual flap prior to its adaptation over the graft site.

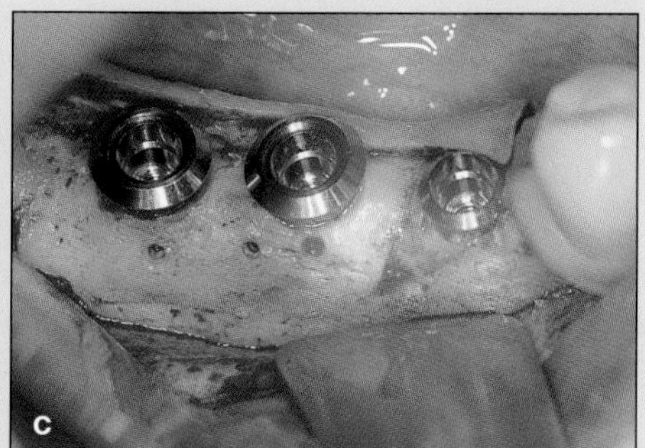

Fig 3-21c Four months after grafting, use of a curvilinear-beveled flap design effectively increased elasticity of the flap, thereby preserving circulation to flap margins after closure over the large-volume bone graft. Proper soft tissue management contributed to excellent bone regeneration from block and particulate bone grafts in molar areas as well as regeneration of the buccal wall defect at the premolar site.

Flap Design and Management Considerations for Maxillary Implant Surgery

The surgeon should be mindful of certain flap management considerations that are particular to working in the maxilla. These considerations include the occasional need for preoperative tissue conditioning to improve palatal soft tissue tone and the need for intraoperative reduction of palatal soft tissue thickness in certain situations.

Whenever possible, preoperative tissue conditioning should be performed to resolve any existing inflammation of the palatal tissues. Poor tissue tone is often encountered in patients with severe maxillary resorption secondary to an ill-fitting prosthesis or in patients who seldom remove an existing removable prosthesis. When mobile palatal tissues persist and demonstrate poor tissue tone despite efforts at preoperative tissue conditioning, a CO_2 laser can be used to excise and resurface the tissues to improve the situation prior to commencing implant therapy.

Intraoperative thinning of the palatal tissues is indicated when excessive palatal soft tissue thickness exists or when tissue tone is less than ideal. This is accomplished by means of sharp dissection with a scalpel to excise subepithelial fatty or glandular tissues in the area of concern. Subsequent scarring at the site improves the palatal tissue tone, while the reduction of tissue thickness avoids discrepancies in the height between the buccal and palatal soft tissue surrounding the permucosal implant structures. Failure to do so results in soft tissue irregularities in the inter-implant areas and excessive palatal tissue height, both of which promote the collection of food debris and hinder routine oral hygiene needed in these areas. When vertical releasing incisions are necessary in the palatal mucosa to allow access for reduction of tissue thickness, they should be abbreviated to avoid damage to neurovascular structures and to minimize postoperative tissue sloughing. In certain cases it is also necessary to excise connective tissue in the area.

When the palatal tissues are healthy, soft tissue flaps are designed and the existing soft tissues manipulated in such a manner as to obtain firm palatal soft tissues of appropriate thickness adjacent to the implant emergence site. Failure to do so results in a compromised palatal soft tissue environment, which is difficult to correct. The location and bevel of the crestal incision must be varied and the palatal tissue thickness reduced when necessary. The buccal flap outline is completed with curvilinear-beveled vertical releasing incisions, which are initiated in the mucosal tissues beyond the mucogingival junction and extended through the attached tissues to join the mesial and distal extent of the pericrestal incision.

For submerged implant placement, the flap is elevated and retracted during implant placement. Care is taken to minimize reflection of the palatal tissues. Wound closure is facilitated because the palatal tissues serve to anchor the buccal flap, thus improving the stability of the postoperative wound complex. Subsequent use of a removable provisional restoration is also facilitated because the palatal and vestibular anatomy have not been altered.

For abutment connection and nonsubmerged implant placement, the buccal flap is elevated just beyond the mucogingival junction to facilitate subsequent apical or lateral repositioning and adaptation of tissues around the emerging implant structures. Because the dissection is extended beyond the mucogingival junction, the surgeon should anticipate a small amount of recession and should therefore manage the flap with this in mind.

Edentulous maxilla

A simple variation of the buccal flap also is used for implant surgery in the edentulous maxilla. The author uses a flap that is specifically designed to avoid reflection of the soft tissues in the maxillary midline. Instead, buccal flaps are outlined and elevated bilaterally (Fig 3-22a). This approach preserves premaxillary anatomy and facilitates flap elevation, retraction, and subsequent wound closure. In addition, postoperative patient comfort is greatly improved and the use of an interim removable provisional restoration is facilitated because the topography of the alveolar ridge and mucobuccal fold is maintained.

The flaps are outlined as follows. A pericrestal incision is initiated in the tuberosity area and extended to the anterior maxillary area. The area planned for implant placement determines the mesial extent of the pericrestal incision. Releasing incisions are initiated in the mucosal tissues and join the mesial and distal extent of the pericrestal incision to complete the flap outline. These curvilinear releasing incisions are beveled toward the center of the flap. Flap elevation is initiated at the distal releasing incision as the periosteum is quickly and easily elevated in this area. The dissection is carried mesial to the premolar region. Flap reflection resumes at the mesial releasing incision and is carried distally to expose the underlying alveolar ridge anatomy. Because one often encounters adherent fibrous tissue in under-

Flap design and management for the edentulous maxilla

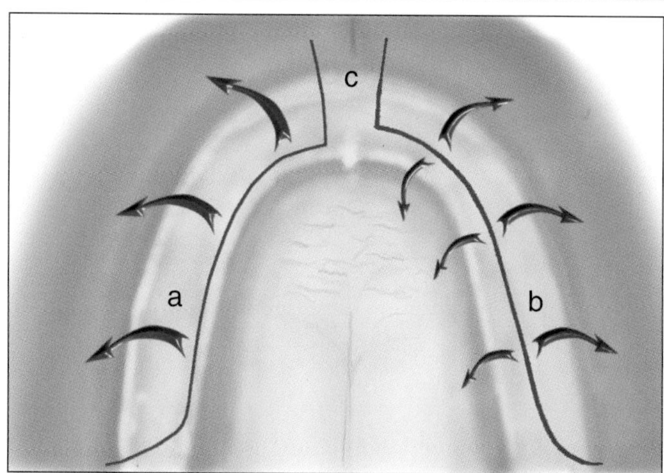

Fig 3-22a Flap design for implant placement in the edentulous maxilla. *(a)* Line representing flap design for submerged implant placement. A palatal-crestal incision with a palatal bevel is used to allow visualization of the alveolar crest with minimal elevation of the palatal flap. *(b)* Line representing flap design for abutment connection and nonsubmerged implant placement. The incision is placed so as to ensure adequate width of good-quality palatal tissues (free of rugae). *(c)* The tissues in the maxillary midline are not included in the flap. This improves patient comfort and facilitates the use of a provisional restoration postoperatively.

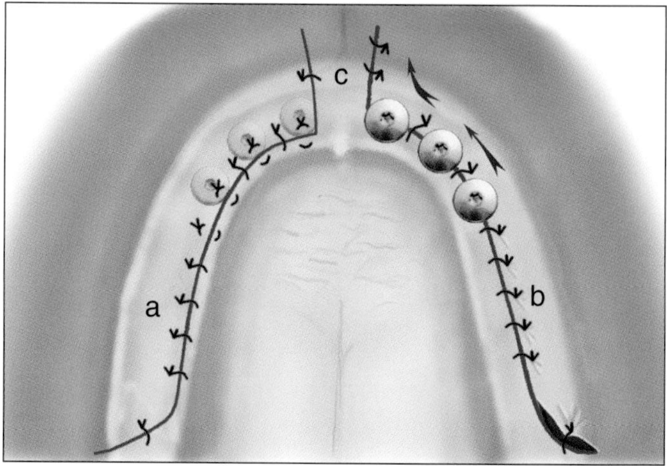

Fig 3-22b Flap management for implant placement in the edentulous maxilla. *(a)* Flap management for submerged implant placement. *(b)* Flap management for abutment connection and nonsubmerged implant placement. *(c)* When submerged implants are placed, the buccal flap is anchored to the unreflected tissues at the midline. Closure is then rapidly obtained by alternating mattress and simple interrupted sutures over the implant cover screw. For abutment connection or nonsubmerged implant placement, the buccal flap is apically repositioned and anchored to the unreflected maxillary tissues at the midline, and indicated surgical maneuvers are used to obtain circumferential adaptation of attached tissues around the emerging implant structures.

lying bony defects resulting from previous tooth extractions, sharp dissection with a Buser periosteal elevator or a no. 15C scalpel may be needed to initiate flap reflection in this area. Using the Adson tissue forceps to carefully hold the flap, gently elevate it so that the anatomy of the alveolar ridge and buccal aspect of the maxilla are clearly visible. The flap reflection is then carried apically.

When submerged implant placement is planned, a palatal-crestal incision with a palatal bevel is used (see Figs 3-5 and 3-22a). The beveled palatal-crestal incision exposes the entire alveolar ridge and minimizes the palatal reflection needed for osteotomy preparation. After implant placement, wound closure begins by re-adapting and anchoring the buccal flap to the attached palatal and premaxillary tissues. Horizontal mattress and simple interrupted sutures are then used to obtain tension-free closure over the implant site(s). Wound closure is quickly completed distally (Fig 3-22b).

When preparing to uncover a submerged implant for abutment connection or when nonsubmerged implant placement is planned, the pericrestal incision is usually located closer to the midcrest and beveled to the buccal. In these instances, care must be taken to maintain smooth palatal tissues for re-adaptation to the palatal aspect of the permucosal implant structures. The buccal bevel maximizes the amount of attached tissue that remains on the buccal flap. A small amount of palatal reflection may be necessary for osteotomy preparation or abutment connection, or to provide access for thinning of the palatal flap prior to its re-adaptation to emerging implant structures. Subsequently, the buccal flap is apically repositioned and managed with the surgical maneuvers previously described to obtain circumferential adaptation around the permucosal implant structures. Anchoring the flap to the attached premaxillary tissues facilitates lateral advancement, apical repositioning, and adequate immobilization of the buccal flap. The sutures are oriented to avoid coronal displacement of the buccal tissues over the implant components during healing and to aid in the maintenance of adequate vestibular depth after healing. Interrupted sutures are used for precise re-adaptation of the soft tissues around the implant components and to complete the wound closure (Figs 3-23 to 3-26).

A variation of this approach has proven useful in the management of atrophic maxillary cases where inadequate vestibular depth presents a significant soft tissue management problem for the surgeon and restorative dentist. At abutment connection or nonsubmerged implant placement, the flap design should allow for vestibular extension to accommodate the flange of the final prosthesis and to provide access for oral hygiene. In addition, the flap should be designed to prevent mobility of the tissues around the emerging implant structures during early wound healing. This will ensure the creation of a stable soft tissue environment during the period of soft tissue integration. To accomplish these goals, the author recommends a modification that employs the use of full- and partial-thickness flap dissec-

Flap design and management for nonsubmerged implant placement in the edentulous maxilla

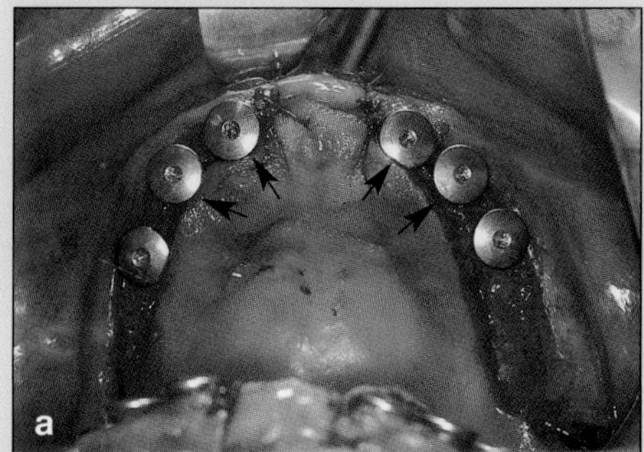

Fig 3-23a Palatal-crestal incision with buccal bevel was extended distally well beyond the area of implant placement. Curvilinear-beveled vertical releasing incisions complete the outline of the flap. After implant placement, a scalpel was used to perform submucosal excision, thereby reducing excessive palatal tissue thickness in the anterior palatal areas *(arrows)*.

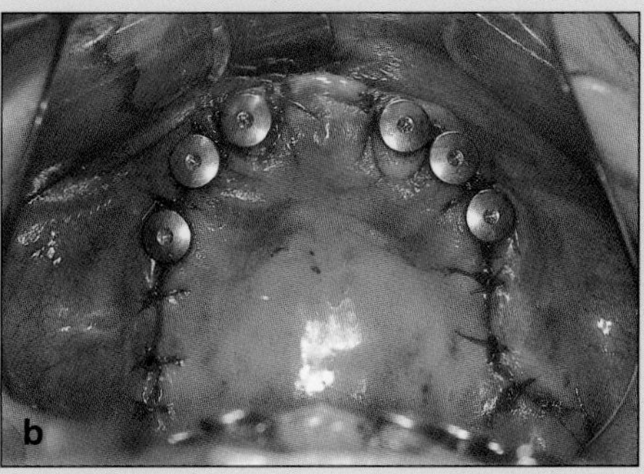

Fig 3-23b A combination of lateral flap advancement and resective contouring was used to accomplish circumferential closure around emerging transmucosal implant collars.

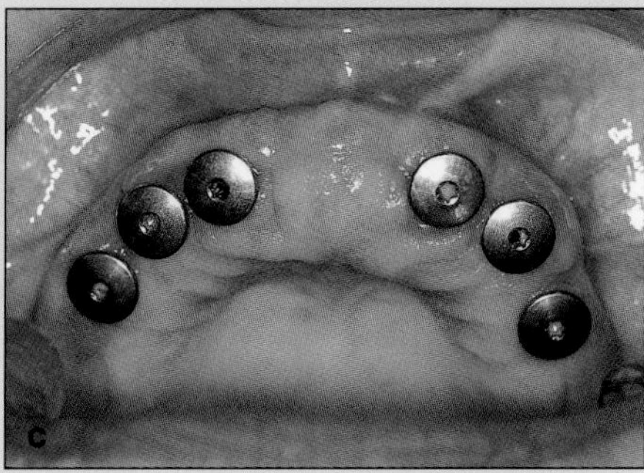

Fig 3-23c Six weeks after surgery, initial maturation of peri-implant soft tissues has occurred. Flap management has resulted in a soft tissue topography that will simplify subsequent restorative procedures and oral hygiene maintenance.

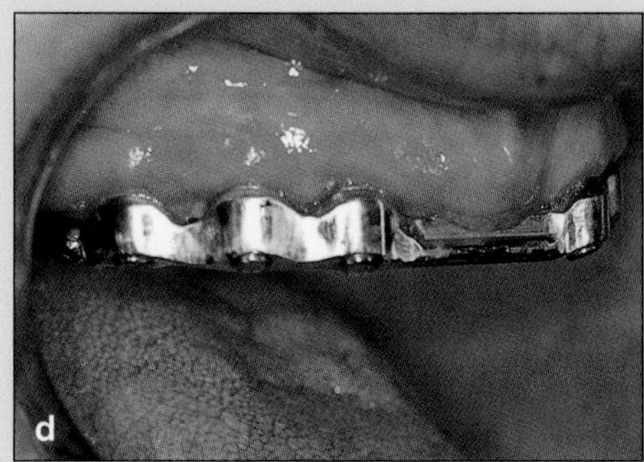

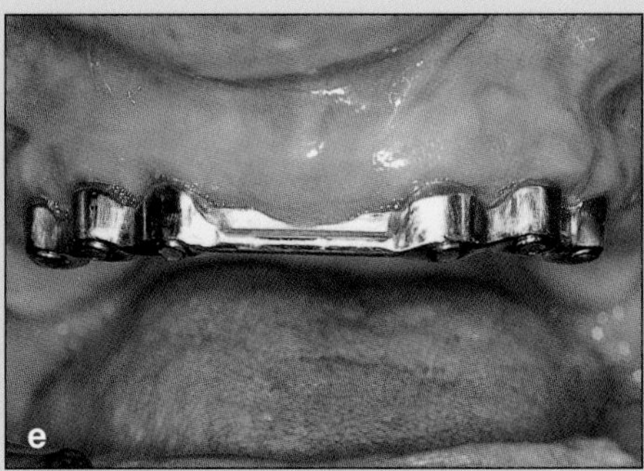

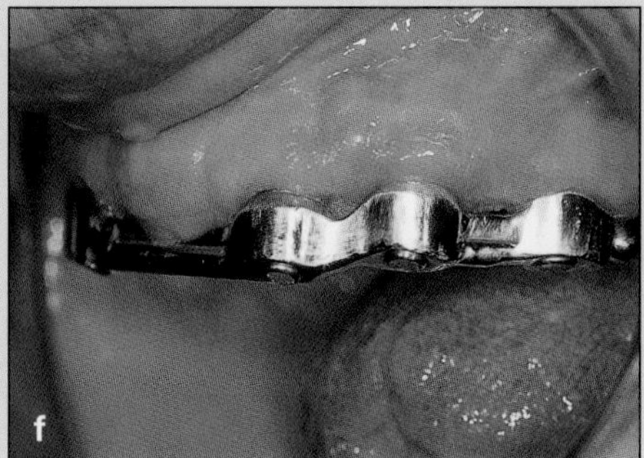

Figs 3-23d to 3-23f One year after delivery of final restoration, excellent peri-implant soft tissue health is evident. The apical repositioning of the buccal flaps and the reduction of palatal soft tissue thickness has created a healthy and stable peri-implant soft tissue environment. (Prosthetics and final restoration by Dr Cecil Abraham, Miami, FL.)

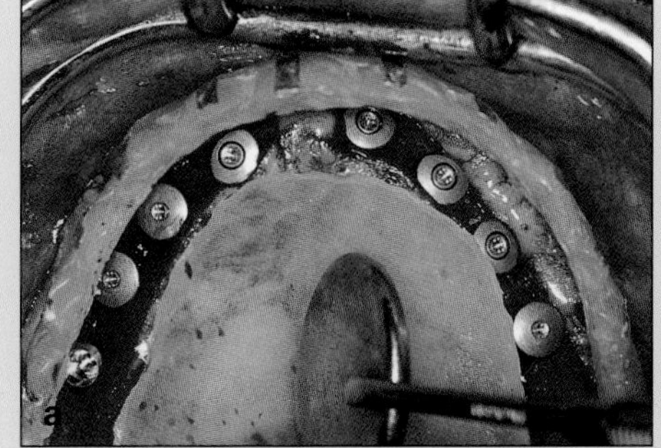

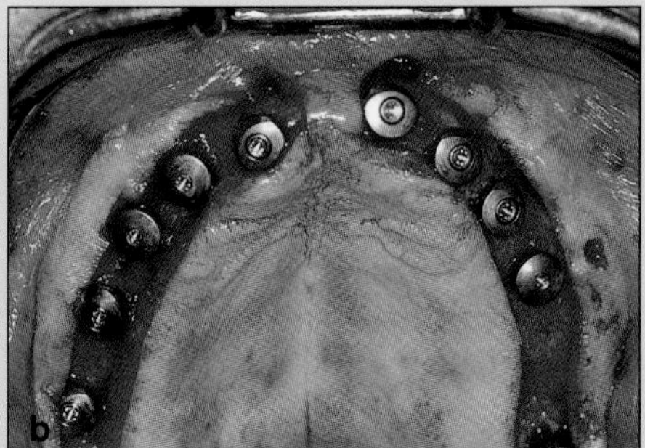

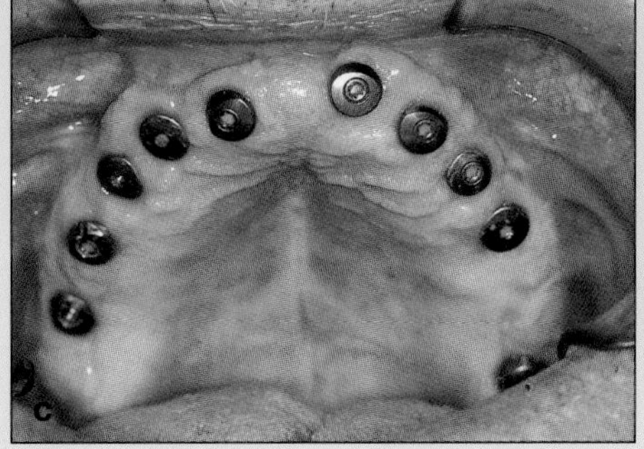

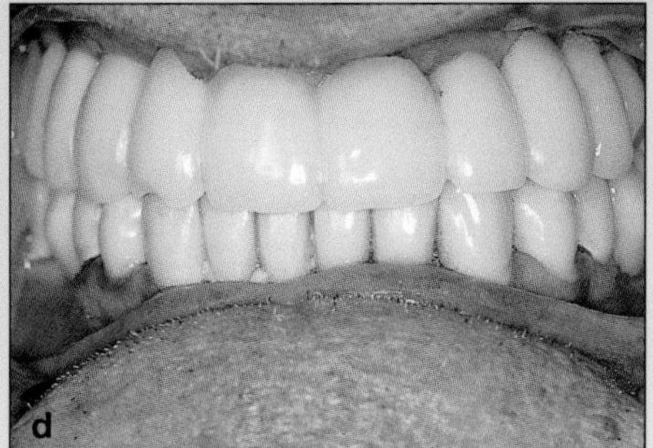

Fig 3-24a Flap design does not interfere with the use of a surgical placement guide.

Fig 3-24b Flap for nonsubmerged implant placement outlined by palatal-crestal incision with a buccal bevel to maximize width of attached tissue on the buccal flap. Curvilinear releasing incisions are located so as to allow access to all planned implants. Ten ITI implants (Straumann USA, Waltham, MA) have been placed in preparation for a fixed restoration.

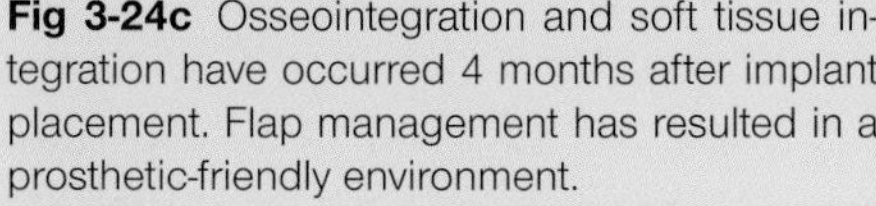

Fig 3-24c Osseointegration and soft tissue integration have occurred 4 months after implant placement. Flap management has resulted in a prosthetic-friendly environment.

Fig 3-24d Delivery of final restoration has been facilitated by the circumferential adaptation of attached tissues around emerging implants. Nonsubmerged technique avoided disruption of protective soft tissue seal during prosthetic procedures. One year following delivery of the restoration, stable soft tissues and excellent esthetics are evident. (Restoration by Dr John P. Cartledge, Hallandale, FL.)

Flap design and management for submerged implant placement in the edentulous maxilla

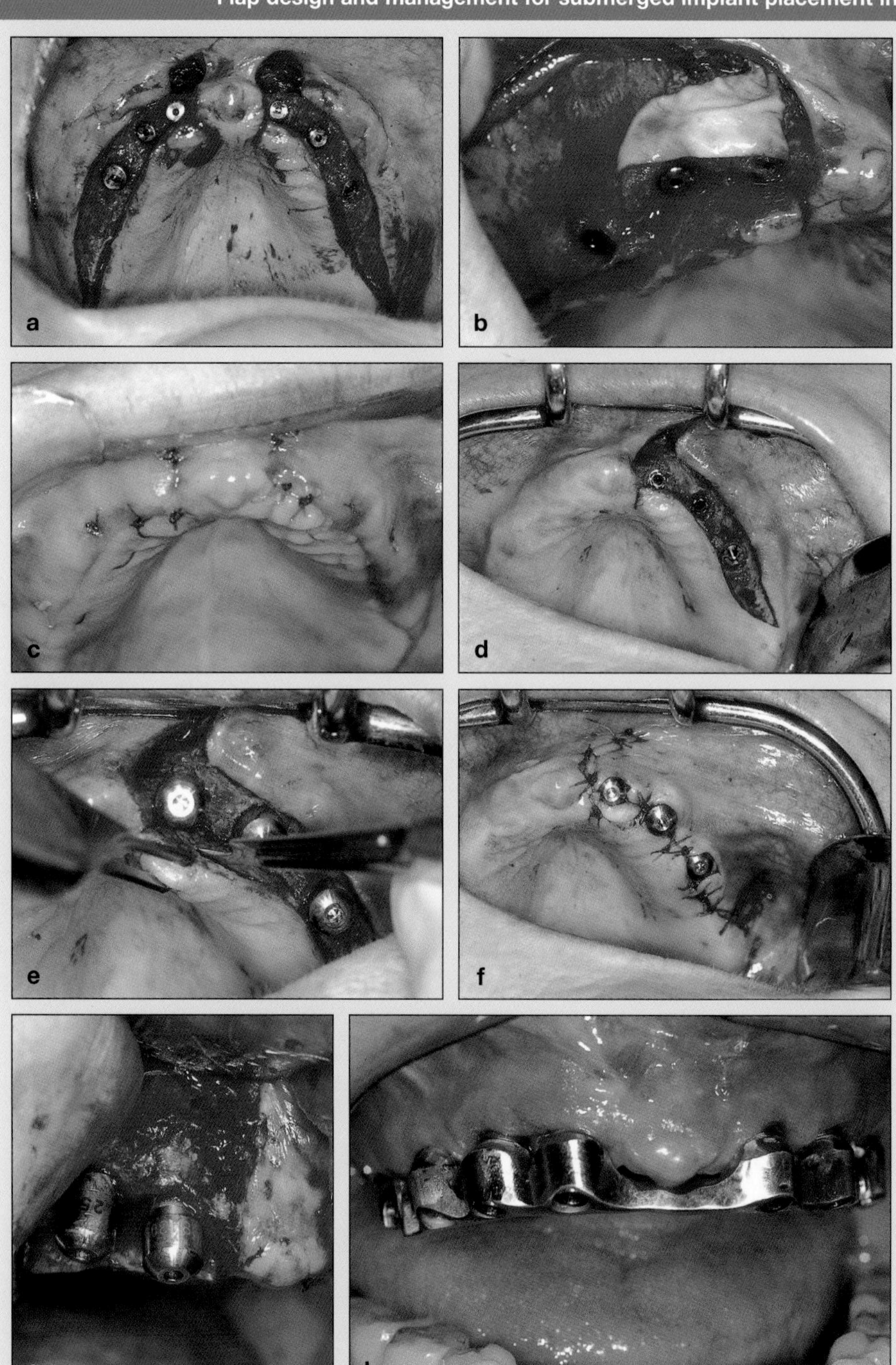

Fig 3-25a Palatal-crestal incision with palatal bevel and curvilinear-beveled vertical releasing incisions outline the flap. Six submerged Spline implants (Centerpulse Dental, Carlsbad, CA) have been placed.

Fig 3-25b Small-volume buccal dehiscence defect is treated with guided bone regeneration procedure using a mixture of autogenous bone harvested from local areas, Bio-Oss, and a Bio-Gide membrane.

Fig 3-25c Interrupted sutures secure buccal flaps to anterior maxillary tissues. Horizontal mattress sutures reapproximate the buccal and palatal tissues at the crest. The palatal bevel extends the wound margin by creating a split-thickness–full-thickness buccal flap that slides under the beveled palatal tissues during closure, thereby improving stability of the wound complex.

Fig 3-25d Implant exposure and abutment connection performed 4 months after initial surgery. Palatal-crestal incision with buccal bevel maximized the amount of attached tissue on the buccal flap.

Fig 3-25e A scalpel is used to reduce excess palatal soft tissue thickness.

Fig 3-25f Lateral flap advancement is used to obtain circumferential adaptation of attached tissues around emerging implant abutments. Apical repositioning of the flap was facilitated by securing it to unreflected tissues at the midline.

Fig 3-25g Successful bone regeneration on the buccal aspect of the anterior implant during abutment connection to implants on the right side of the maxilla. Soft tissue management mirrored that performed around the implants in the left maxilla.

Fig 3-25h Nine months after restoration delivery, excellent peri-implant health is evident. Apical repositioning of buccal flaps and reduction of palatal soft tissue thickness facilitates the excellent level of hygiene demonstrated by this patient. (Prosthetics and final restoration by Dr Larry Grillo, Aventura, FL.)

tion. The flap is outlined as previously described: full-thickness subperiosteal dissection is performed from the alveolar crest apically to the level of the mucogingival junction. Partial-thickness supraperiosteal dissection is then initiated with a scalpel and carried further apically to expose the lateral face of the maxilla. Care must be taken to avoid damage to the infraorbital nerve. After abutment connection or nonsubmerged implant placement, horizontal mattress sutures are used to lift and secure the flap apically to the periosteum of the extended recipient bed. The sutures pass through the mucosal tissues at the mucogingival junction, engaging the periosteum further apically, and then back through the flap at the mucogingival junction. Usually two or three sutures are passed in this fashion and clamped with a hemostat before tying. As the individual sutures are tied, the flap is lifted apically in a fashion analogous to the raising of a curtain in a theater. In effect, the surgeon performs a submucosal vestibuloplasty from an open flap approach. Subsequently, the coronal portion of the flap is secured around the emerging implant structures as previously described. This approach minimizes soft tissue complications by re-establishing vestibular depth, which allows adequate room for oral hygiene and accommodates an appropriate prosthesis flange that prevents chronic collection of food debris under the prosthesis while providing lip support for excellent esthetics (Fig 3-27).

Flap design and management to preserve soft tissue esthetics in the edentulous maxilla

Fig 3-26a Preoperative panoramic radiograph demonstrating advanced periodontal disease of maxillary dentition. Treatment plan included removal of remaining maxillary dentition and alveolar ridge preservation with the Bio-Col technique in preparation for delayed implant placement.

Fig 3-26b Successful ridge preservation is evident 6 months after tooth removal. Remaining maxillary ridge height and width have been preserved.

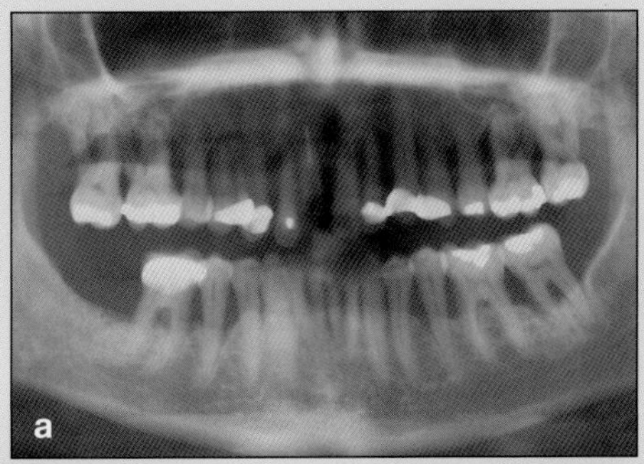

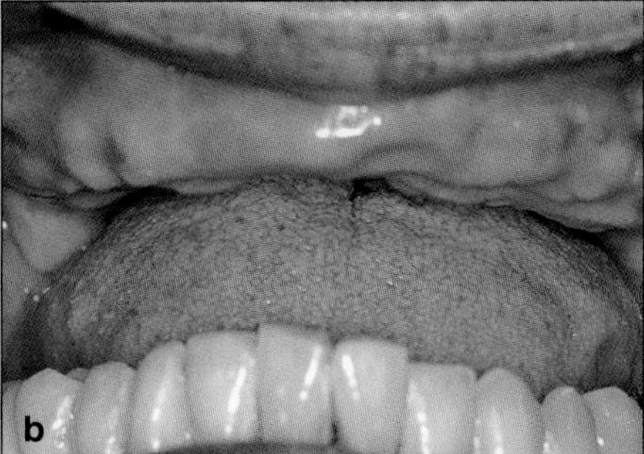

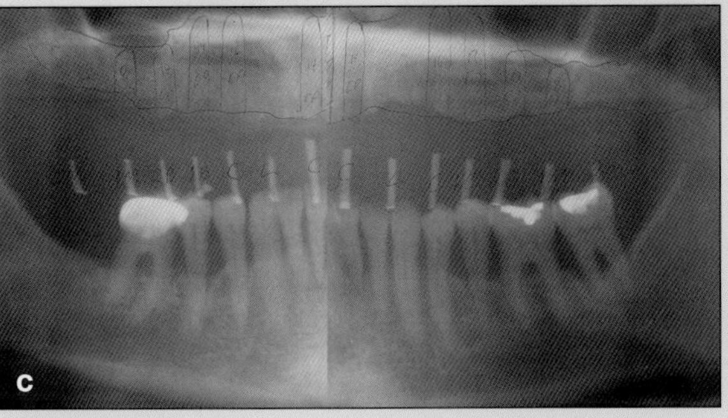

Fig 3-26c Panoramic radiograph prior to implant placement. Adequate bone volume is available to proceed with implant placement. Further bone grafting will not be necessary despite pre-existing severe periodontal bone loss with uncorrectable angular defects.

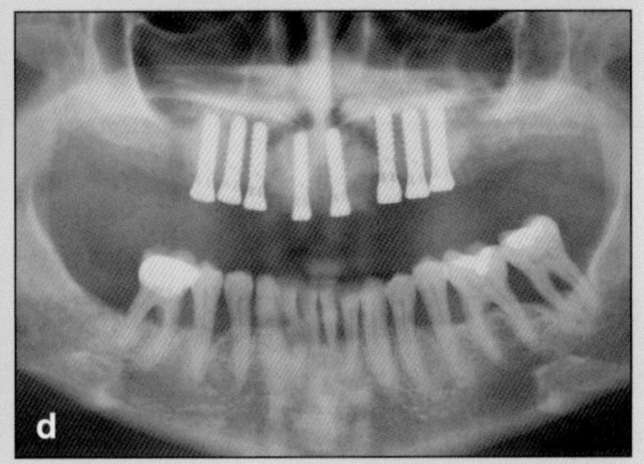

Fig 3-26d Eight nonsubmerged implants have been placed in preparation for fixed restoration.

Fig 3-26e Four months after placement of eight nonsubmerged ITI implants, flap management as previously described has resulted in a stable peri-implant soft tissue environment.

Fig 3-26f Use of one-piece nonsubmerged implants has allowed sufficient time for soft tissue integration. Subsequent restorative procedures will not disrupt junctional epithelium or connective tissue adaptation because they are limited to the superficial aspect of the peri-implant sulcus.

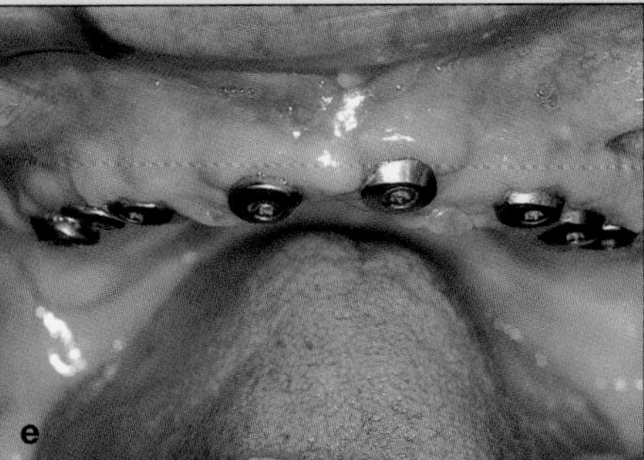

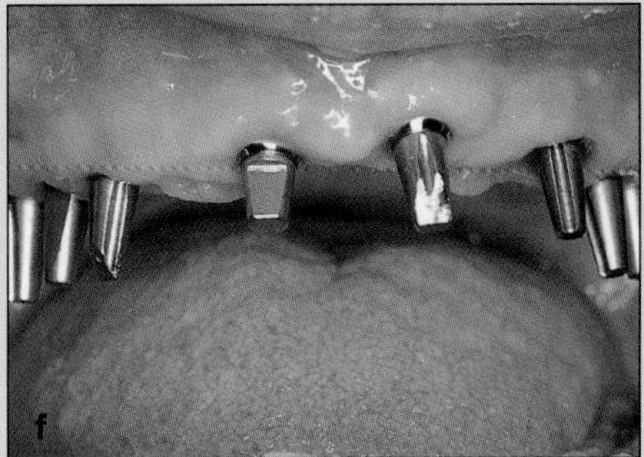

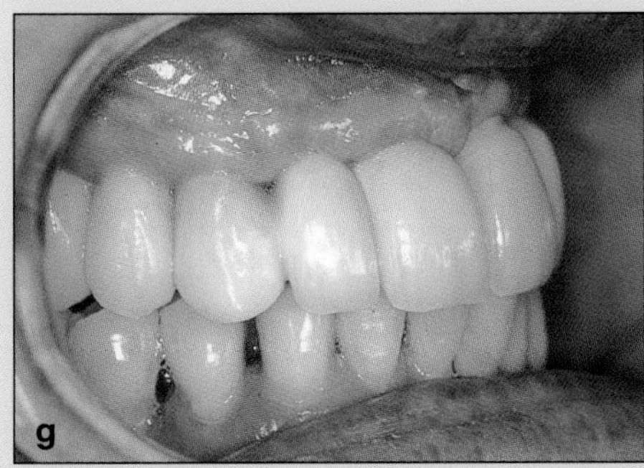

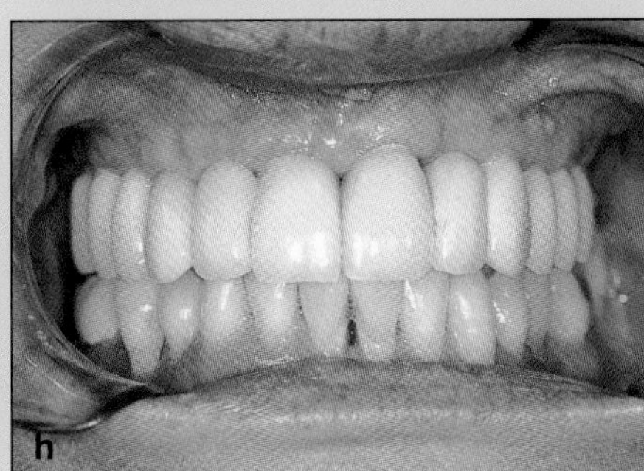

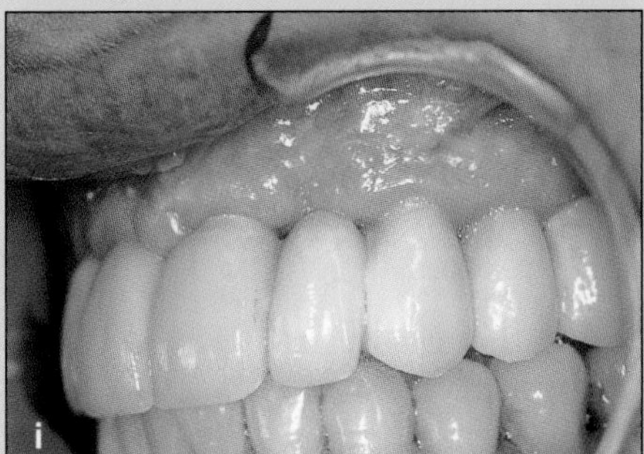

Figs 3-26g to 3-26i Soft tissue health is excellent 1 year following final restoration. A combination of alveolar ridge preservation following tooth removal, proper soft tissue management during implant placement, and use of one-piece nonsubmerged implants has resulted in functional and esthetic rehabilitation of the maxillary dentition in spite of pre-existing severe periodontal disease.

Fig 3-26j Harmonious tooth proportions have been restored. (Restoration by Dr Larry Stein, Miami, FL.)

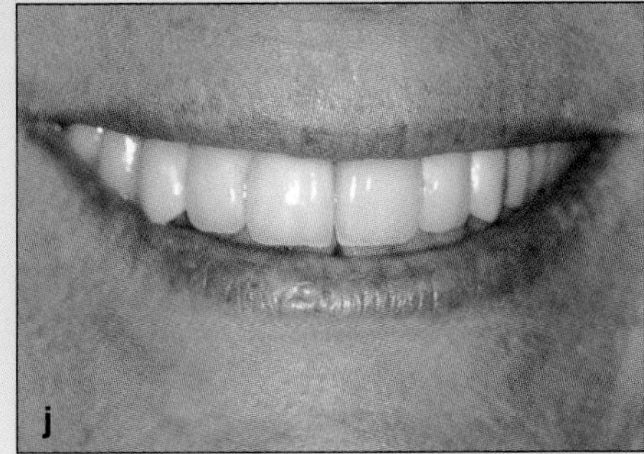

Flap design and management for hard tissue site development and subsequent placement of nonsubmerged implants in the edentulous maxilla

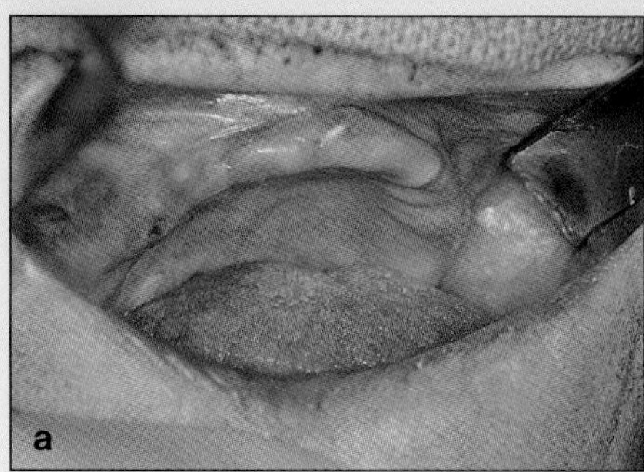

Fig 3-27a Preoperative view of atrophic maxilla. Resorption has reached the nasal floor in the maxillary anterior area. Sinus lift bone grafting and onlay bone grafting will be performed in preparation for implant placement for support of a fixed-removable restoration.

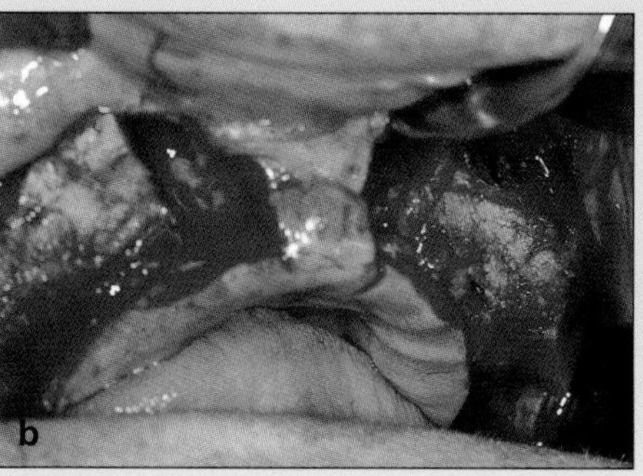

Fig 3-27b Flap design is identical to that used for submerged implant placement in the edentulous maxilla. Palatal-crestal incision is extended beyond the area planned for bone grafting. A palatal bevel ensures extension and overlapping of crestal wound margins upon closure. Curvilinear-beveled incisions with tension-releasing cutback incisions enable passive flap coaptation and tension-free closure over large-volume iliac bone grafts while minimizing periosteal releasing incisions that can jeopardize circulation to flap margins.

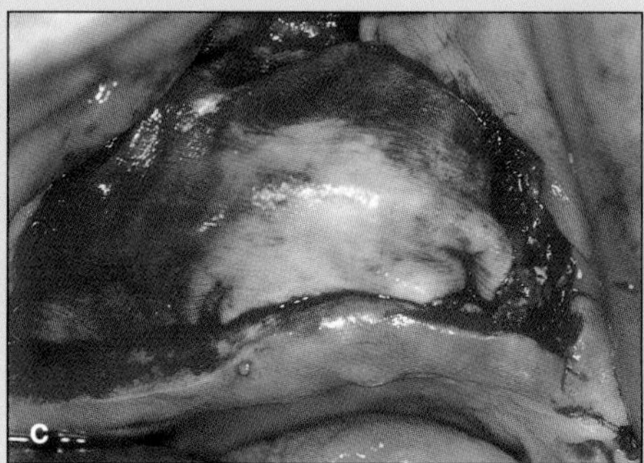

Fig 3-27c Particulate bone graft consisting of equal mixtures of autogenous marrow and Bio-Oss have been condensed around block grafts, and a large Bio-Gide resorbable membrane has been adapted over the graft. When the flap has been properly developed, securing the membrane is unnecessary as reapproximation of the flap will not displace the membrane.

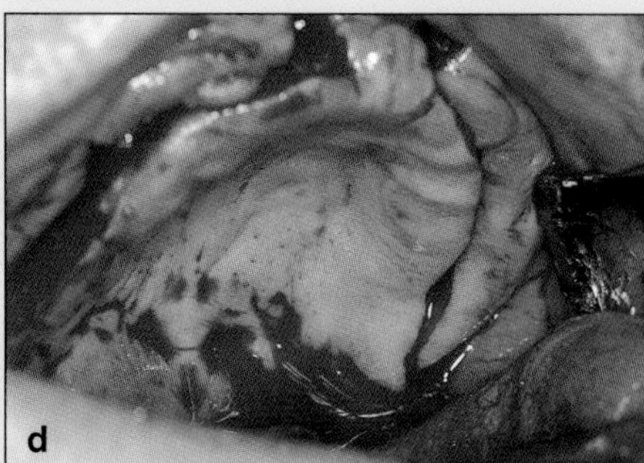

Fig 3-27d Flap design accommodates large-volume iliac bone graft augmentation. Passive coaptation over the bone grafts is evident.

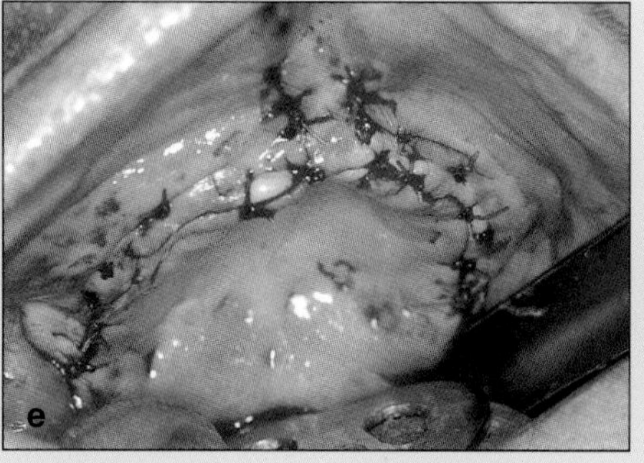

Fig 3-27e Primary closure begins with placement of sutures, which anchor and secure the buccal flap to the unreflected soft tissues at the midline. Crestal incisions are closed with a combination of interrupted and horizontal mattress sutures.

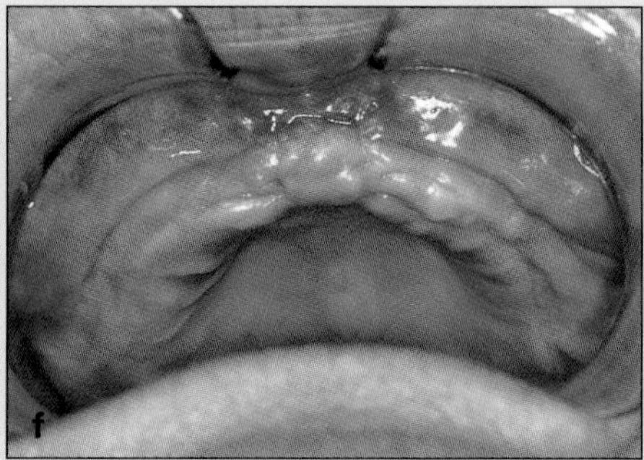

Fig 3-27f Two-week postoperative view demonstrates healthy soft tissue cover. Incision lines are sealed and significant ridge augmentation is evident.

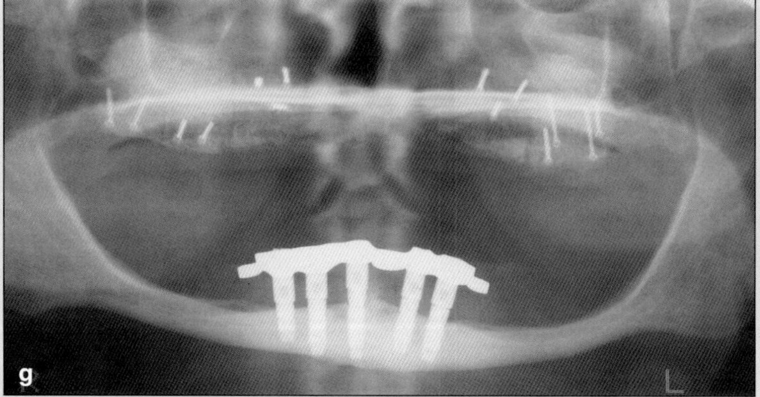

Fig 3-27g Four-month radiograph demonstrates consolidation of sinus lift bone grafts as well as integration of block bone grafts.

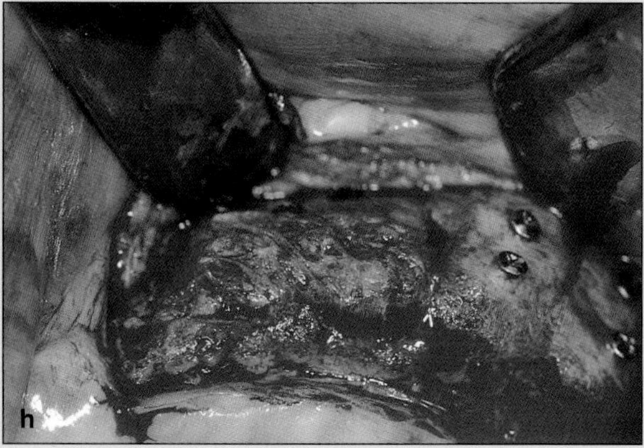

Fig 3-27h Site is entered for implant placement 4 months after bone graft procedure. Flap design differs only in the use of a buccal bevel on the crestal incision in preparation for nonsubmerged implant placement. Excellent volume yield and maturation of block and particulate bone grafts are evident.

Fig 3-27i Flap design accommodates the use of an implant-placement guide. The buccal flange of the guide has been reduced to improve visibility for the surgeon.

Fig 3-27j Four nonsubmerged one-piece implants with specially designed beveled Esthetic-Plus healing abutments (Straumann USA) are used bilaterally. The bevels are oriented toward the buccal to allow coronal advancement of the flap over the bevel, thereby preserving the width of attached tissue on the buccal flap and facilitating primary closure and circumferential adaptation of attached tissues around emerging implant structures. In this case a combination of lateral flap advancement and papilla regeneration maneuvers was used.

Fig 3-27k The buccal flap is first advanced laterally and secured to the unreflected tissues at the midline.

Fig 3-27l A no. 15C scalpel is used to create pedicles of attached tissue adjacent to each implant. Reverse cutback incisions *(arrows)* are made at the base of the pedicles to ensure passive rotation into inter-implant areas.

Fig 3-27m Interrupted sutures are passed through the buccal attached tissues apical and distal to the pedicle before passing through the palatal tissues. As the suture is loosely secured with a surgeon's knot, the flap advances laterally and the papillary pedicle passively occupies the inter-implant space. The suture should not be placed through the pedicle since this would compromise circulation.

Fig 3-27n Use of recommended flap design and lateral flap advancement and papilla regeneration maneuvers facilitated circumferential adaptation of attached tissue around emerging nonsubmerged implant collars and Esthetic-Plus healing abutments.

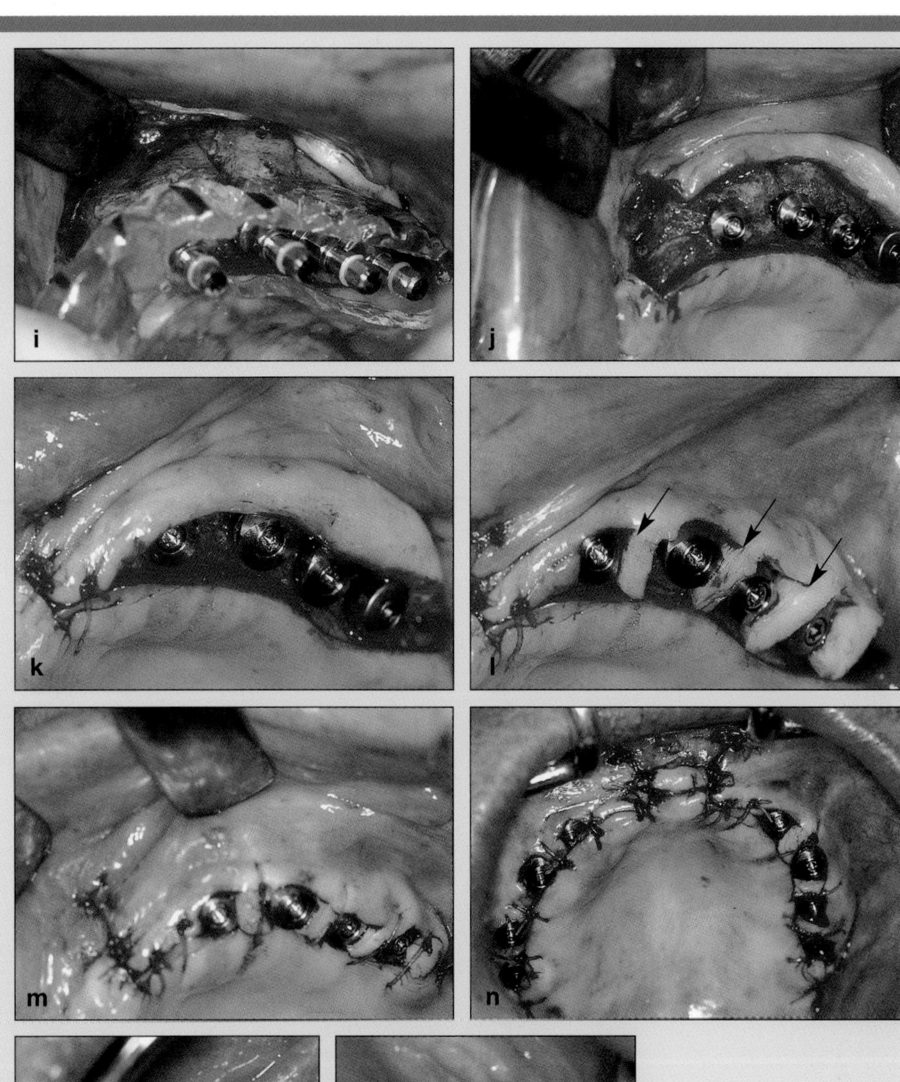

Figs 3-27o and 3-27p Clinical view 4 months after implant placement. Healing abutments have been removed in preparation for abutment connection. A "prosthetic-friendly" environment has been created. Peri-implant soft tissues are firm and free of inflammation. A connective tissue seal has formed around the transmucosal collar of the one-piece nonsubmerged implants. Restorative procedures will be limited to the superficial sulcular area, theoretically avoiding violation of biologic width.

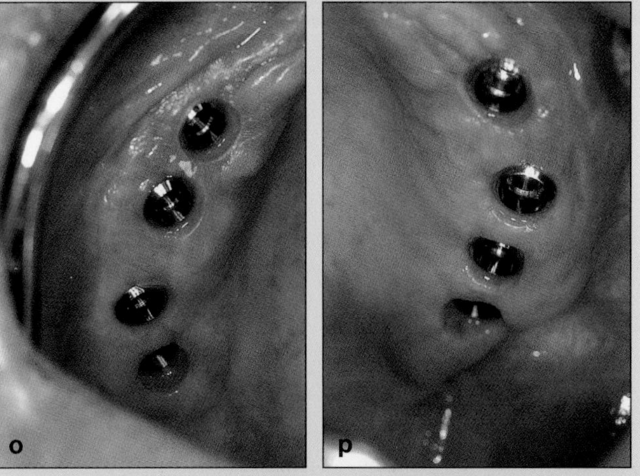

Fig 3-27q Panoramic radiograph 1 year after delivery of final restoration. A split-bar design provided support for a fixed-removable restoration. Avoiding grafting procedures in the premaxillary area enhanced patient comfort, facilitated the interim restoration, and provided maximum flexibility for functional restoration without esthetic or phonetic compromise. Crestal bone levels around implants are stable. (Prosthetics by Dr Gregory Tarantola, Miami, FL.)

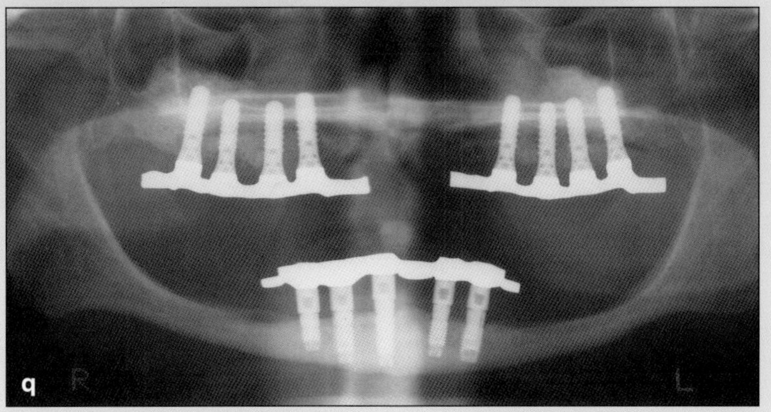

Flap design and management for the partially edentulous mandible

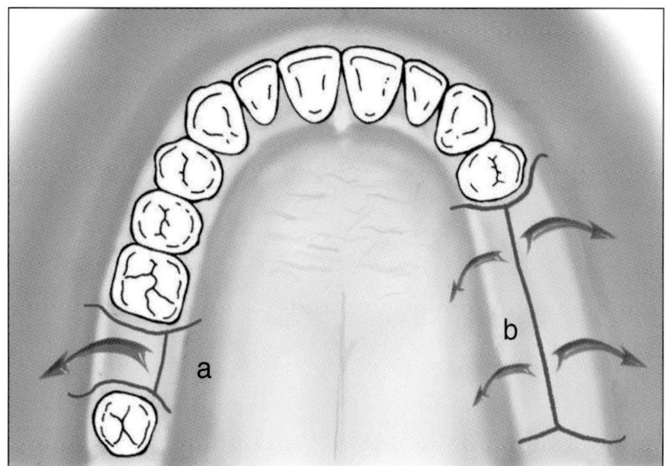

Fig 3-28a Flap design for the partially edentulous maxilla. *(a)* Line representing the flap design for submerged implant placement in a Kennedy Class III situation. *(b)* Line representing the flap design for abutment connection and nonsubmerged implant placement in a Kennedy Class I situation.

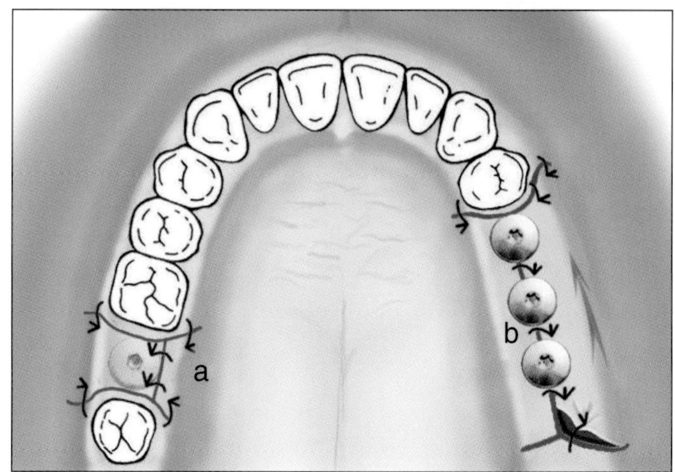

Fig 3-28b Flap management for the partially edentulous maxilla. *(a)* Flap management for submerged implant placement in a Kennedy Class III situation. *(b)* Flap management for abutment connection and nonsubmerged implant placement in a Kennedy Class I situation.

Flap design and management for submerged implant placement and abutment connection in the partially edentulous maxilla

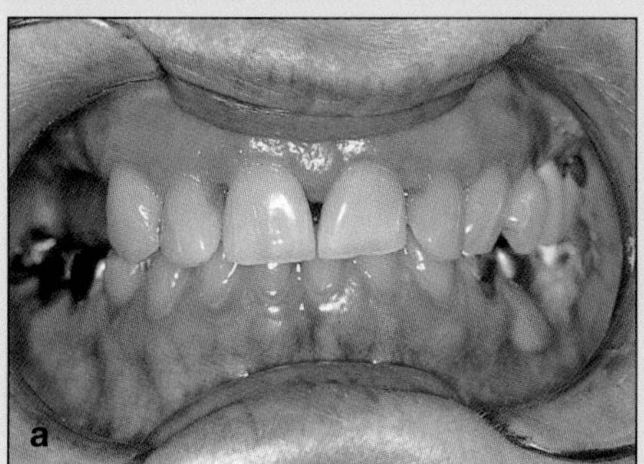

Fig 3-29a Preoperative frontal view. The treatment plan is to restore the maxillary right posterior quadrant with three submerged implants. Note the soft tissue deficiency in the edentulous area.

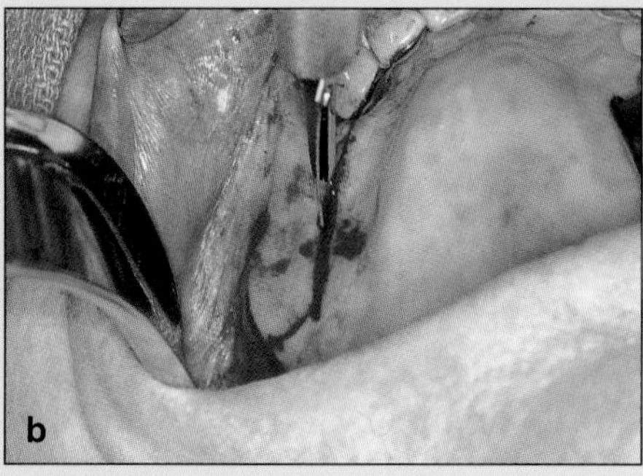

Fig 3-29b The flap outline included curvilinear-beveled releasing incisions and a palatal-crestal incision with a palatal bevel to ensure overlapping of palatal and buccal wound margins upon wound closure over the submerged implants.

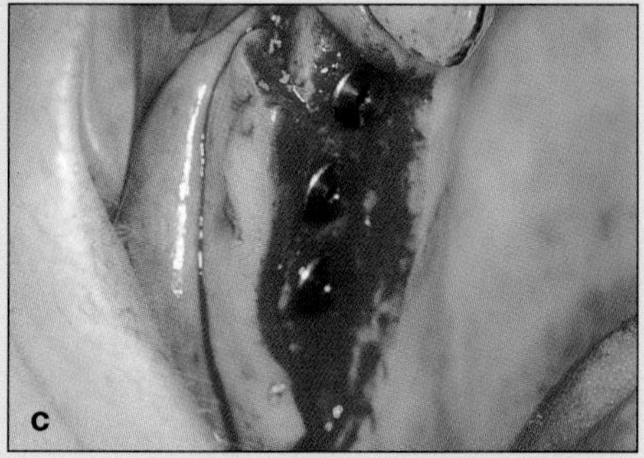

Fig 3-29c Cover screws have been placed. Note the palatal bevel, creating a split-thickness–full-thickness buccal flap margin that will be tucked under the palatal flap upon closure.

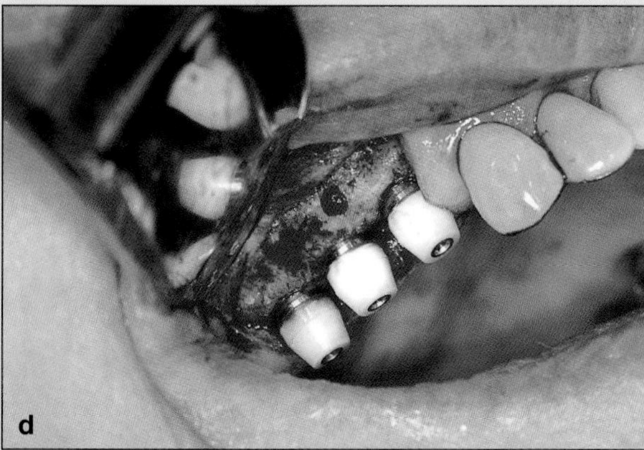

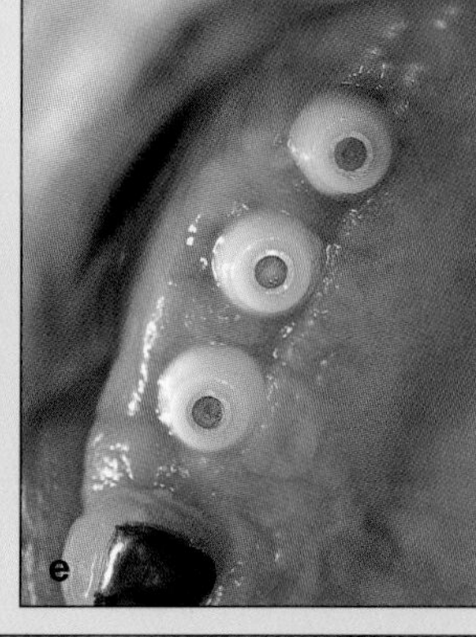

Fig 3-29d Flap design for abutment connection is similar except that the pericrestal incision incorporates a buccal bevel. Permanent abutments with protective caps have been installed.

Fig 3-29e Papilla regeneration maneuver was used along with lateral flap advancement to obtain primary closure and circumferential adaptation around emerging implant abutments. Two-week postoperative view demonstrates healing by primary intention and survival of inter-implant pedicle.

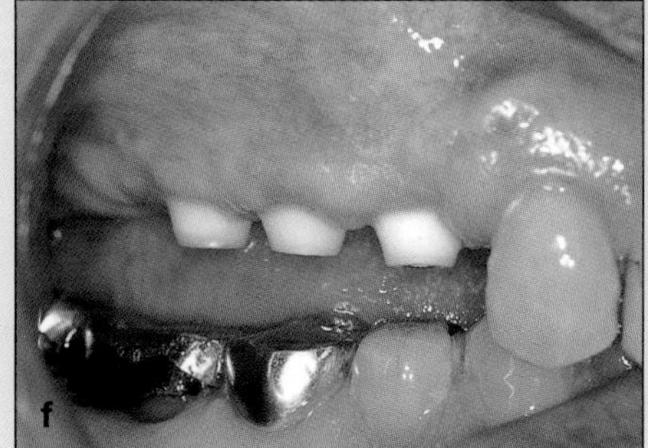

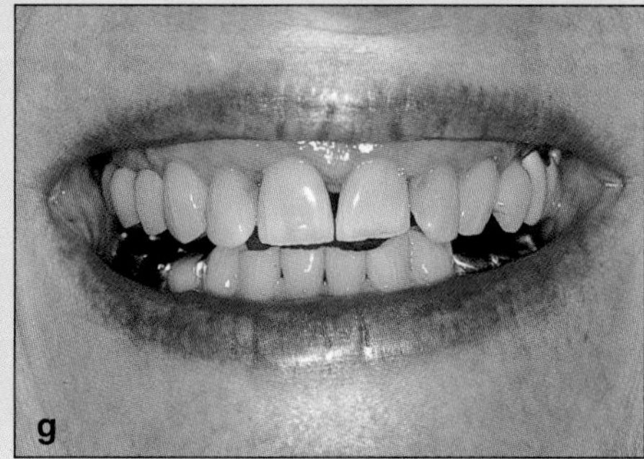

Fig 3-29f Scalloped gingival architecture evident 8 weeks after abutment correction.

Fig 3-29g Five years after final restoration, soft tissues are healthy and stable. Esthetic improvement is evident when compared to the natural dentition on the contralateral side. (Restoration by Dr Doug Deam, Coral Gables, FL.)

Flap design and management for simultaneous nonsubmerged implant placement and sinus lift bone graft in the partially edentulous posterior maxilla

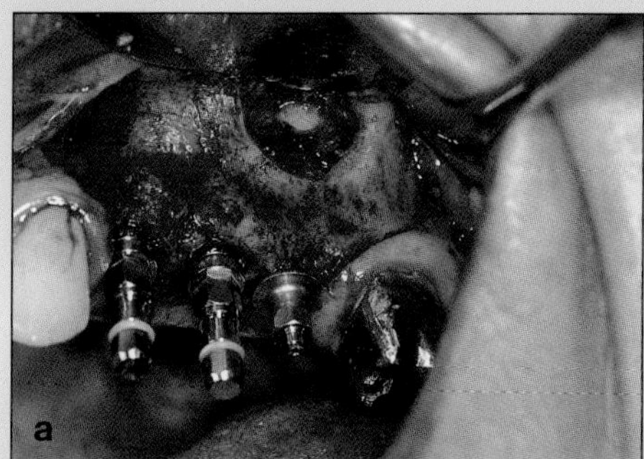

Fig 3-30a Exaggerated curvilinear-beveled flap design with pericrestal incision beveled to the buccal. Three one-piece nonsubmerged implants have been placed following a sinus lift procedure.

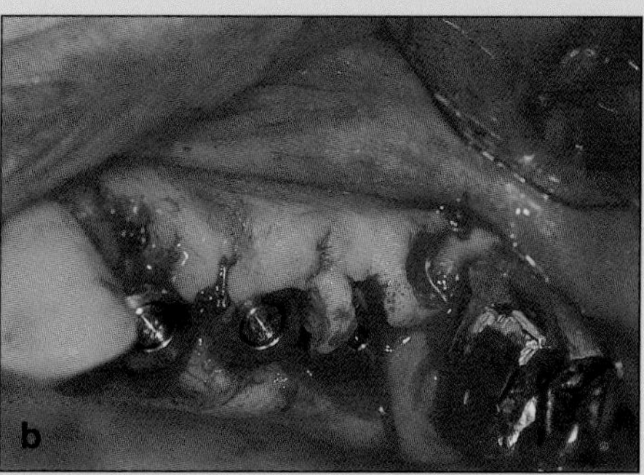

Fig 3-30b Papilla regeneration maneuver performed to establish primary closure and circumferential adaptation around emerging implants. Closure begins on the mesial, and pedicles are created to rotate into distal inter-implant spaces. Reduction of the distalmost papilla is often needed to obtain passive positioning of the flap in this area.

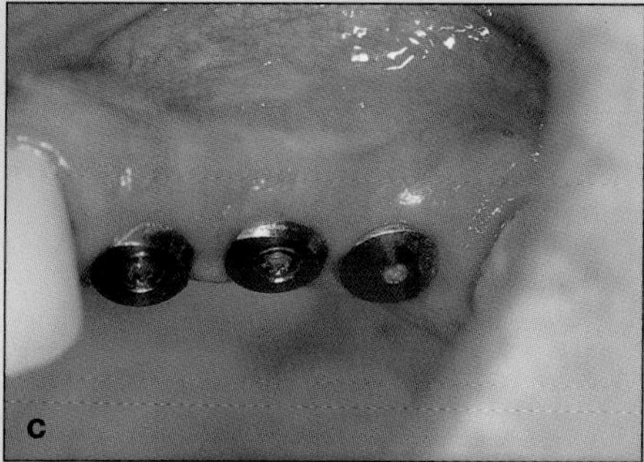

Fig 3-30c Use of the papilla regeneration maneuver provided the epithelial and connective tissue elements for a stable peri-implant soft tissue environment during the integration period. Combined with support from healing abutments, soft tissue management resulted in natural soft tissue architecture at the site.

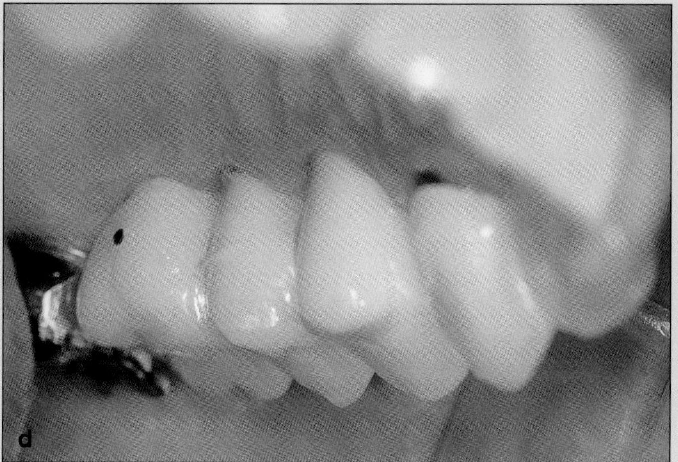

Fig 3-30d Palatal view of final restoration 1 year after delivery.

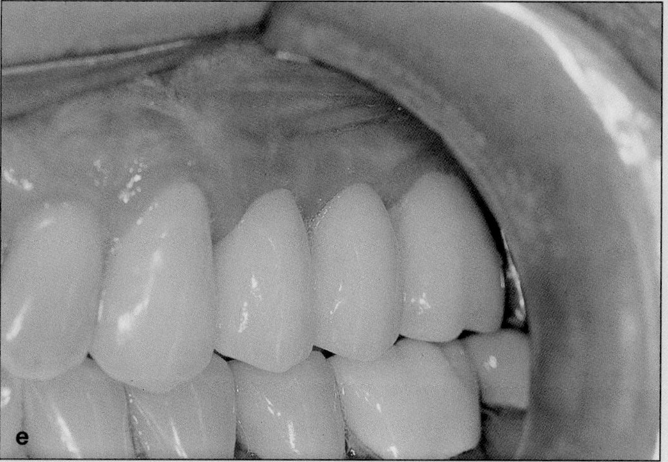

Fig 3-30e Buccal view of final restoration 1 year after delivery. Use of papilla regeneration maneuver allowed harmonious restorations with natural emergence. Oral hygiene is facilitated by circumferential adaptation of attached tissues around the implant restoration. (Restoration by Dr Larry Stein, Miami, FL.)

Partially edentulous maxilla

The location and bevel of the pericrestal incisions are adjusted as needed for submerged or nonsubmerged implant placement or for abutment connection in partially edentulous situations (Fig 3-28). Whenever possible, the flap is extended beyond the area planned for implant placement (Fig 3-29). The vertical releasing incisions should always be curvilinear and beveled toward the center of the flap. Initiating the releasing incisions further apically and laterally away from the implant site facilitates tension-free closure when buccal hard or soft tissue augmentation is needed. If used, palatal releasing incisions should be abbreviated to avoid damage to adjacent neurovascular structures. Care must be taken to avoid elevating the col tissue adjacent to the natural teeth, since doing so not only compromises the vascular supply to the site but also creates an unwanted portal of entry for bacteria until the periodontal soft tissues are able to re-establish a functional attachment to the tooth. As previously discussed, this is an important consideration when guided bone-regeneration procedures are performed prior to or in conjunction with implant placement. After elevation, the buccal flap is managed with one or more of the maneuvers previously described for abutment connection to a submerged implant or for nonsubmerged implant placement (Fig 3-30; see also Figs 3-11 to 3-13).

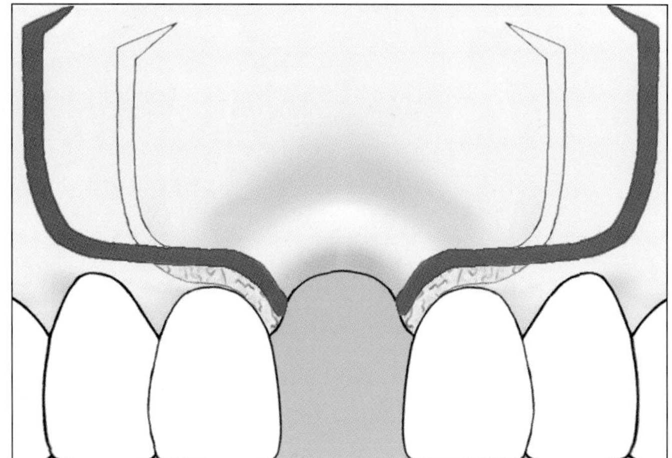

Fig 3-31 When an exaggerated curvilinear flap design is used for site-development procedures, the vertical leg of the incision is placed in an interdental area further away from the site, thereby incorporating even more elastic mucosal tissue. The exaggerated flap design dramatically increases the width of the base of the flap. This allows the surgeon greater extension of the tension-releasing cutback incisions for accommodation of large-volume hard and soft tissue grafts without embarrassing circulation to the flap margin. In such situations, de-epithelialization of the adjacent papillary areas is necessary not only to provide a connective tissue base for flap coaptation but to avoid incision line complications resulting from entrapment of epithelium.

Flap Design and Management Considerations for Esthetic Implant Therapy

Although the principles and flap designs for management of peri-implant soft tissues in edentulous and partially edentulous case types have already been described in detail, a discussion of flap modifications and techniques that enable the surgeon to manage the soft tissues in an inconspicuous fashion is pertinent. In areas of esthetic concern, the author uses three distinct approaches for inconspicuous management of the soft tissues: an exaggerated curvilinear beveled flap, a U-shaped peninsula flap, and a tissue punch. Each of these approaches has particular indications and is suitable for management of soft tissues around submerged and nonsubmerged implants placed in esthetic areas.

Exaggerated curvilinear flap

The buccal flap approach, as previously described, is indicated when exposure of the facial aspect of the alveolar ridge is necessary for visualization of the buccal anatomy or when hard or soft tissue augmentation is indicated as part of site development. When buccal exposure is necessary in esthetic areas, the author uses a flap design outlined by incisions that follow an exaggerated curvilinear path. The incisions are carefully beveled and directed through or parallel to existing anatomic landmarks such as the mucogingival junction and interdental grooves in order to provide esthetic camouflaging (Fig 3-31). Moving the incisions further away from the implant site immediately makes them less conspicuous. In addition, the flap base becomes wider and the overall elasticity of the flap is improved secondary to the incorporation of additional elastic mucosal tissues in the flap base. Tension-releasing cutback incisions can then be used without compromising the width ratio of the flap base to its margin. Although these cutback incisions are full thickness, pass through periosteum, and are directed into the base of the flap, circulation is preserved because the periosteum is not incised across the entire base of the flap, as is commonly necessary with previously described techniques to achieve tension-free closure. In addition, tension-absorbing mattress sutures, which stretch the mucosal tissues at the base of the flap and often compromise circulation by exceeding the elastic limit of the flap, are not necessary with this approach, as the cutback incisions are made at the point of greatest flap tension at the apical extent of the curvilinear releasing incision.

In the author's experience, using the exaggerated curvilinear flap with tension-releasing cutback incisions as a standard procedure ensures passive flap coaptation and improved esthetics even when multiple procedures are necessary for reconstruction of large-volume hard and soft tissue defects at esthetic implant sites.

Once outlined, full-thickness dissection is performed when hard tissue augmentation is planned prior to implant placement or when small-volume osseous defects will be reconstructed in conjunction with implant placement (Fig 3-32). A split-thickness supraperiosteal dissection is performed when soft tissue augmentation is planned. This allows immobilization of a soft tissue graft to a periosteal recipient bed. Prior to flap closure, the attached tissue on the facial aspect of the alveolar ridge and the adjacent papilla are de-epithelialized. This provides a greatly extended wound margin to accommodate overlapping of the flap as it is coronally advanced over the hard or soft tissue graft. This greatly enhances early wound stability and final soft tissue esthetics.

In summary, the use of an exaggerated curvilinear flap design in esthetic implant therapy minimizes flap retraction and wound dehiscence and maximizes vol-

Use of exaggerated curvilinear-beveled flap for hard tissue esthetic implant site development

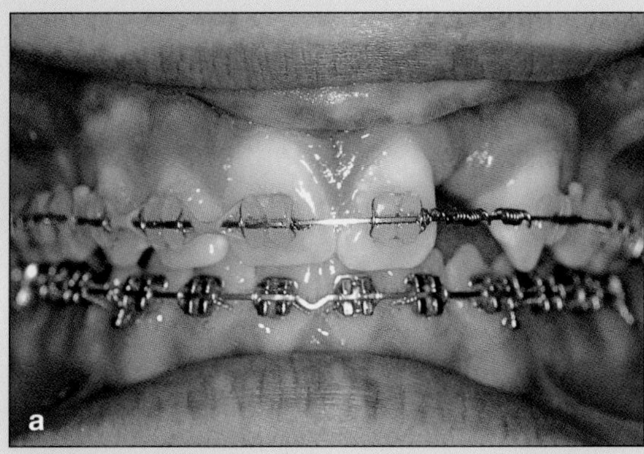
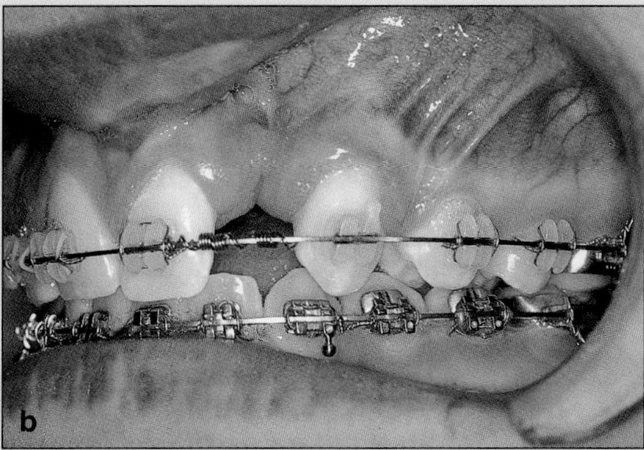

Figs 3-32a and 3-32b Preoperative views of maxillary left lateral incisor with alveolar cleft. A large-volume hard tissue defect is present at this site. Soft tissue scarring resulted from a previous attempt at bone grafting. Preoperative orthodontics was used to diverge roots in order to facilitate rigid fixation of a block bone graft.

Fig 3-32c Exaggerated curvilinear-beveled flap was used to gain access for bone grafting. Note that the cleft defect extends through the palatal bone. Flap design incorporates elastic mucosal tissues beyond the graft site and tension-releasing cutback incisions to allow passive accommodation of a large-volume hard tissue graft.

Fig 3-32d Corticocancellous bone graft has been harvested from the mandibular symphysis.

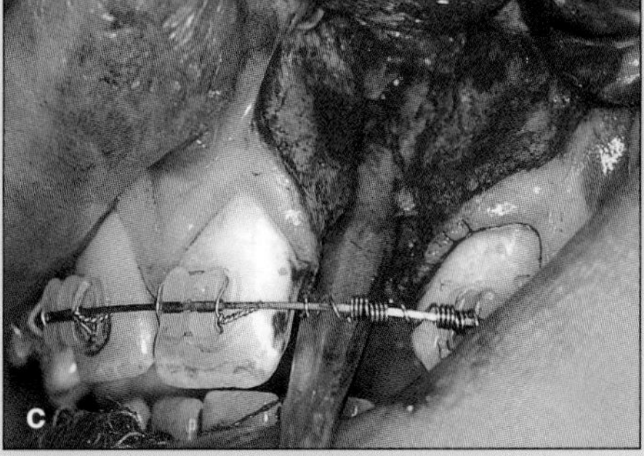
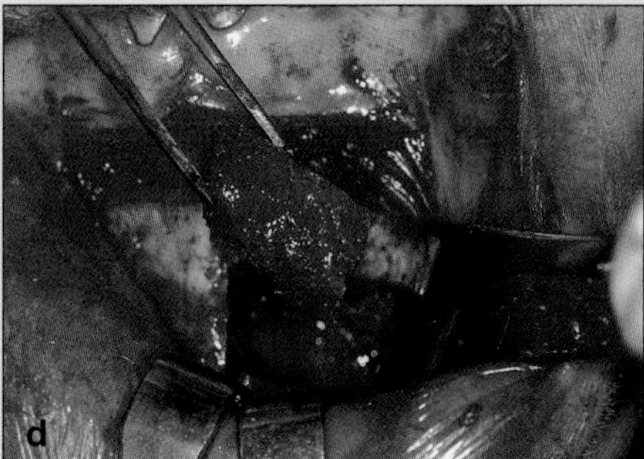

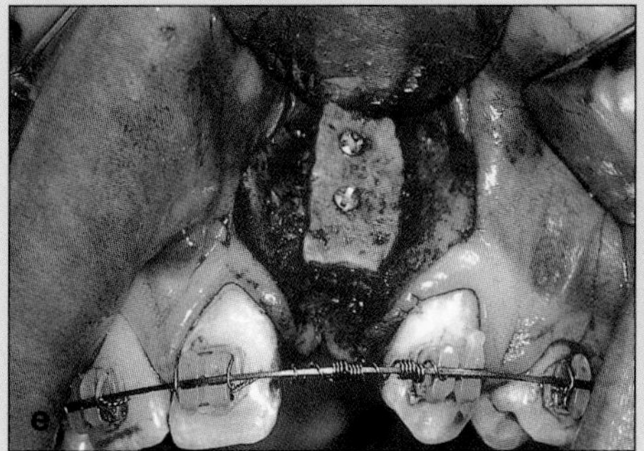
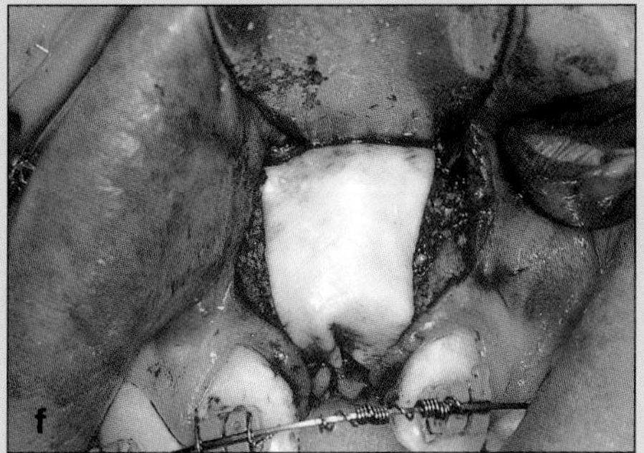
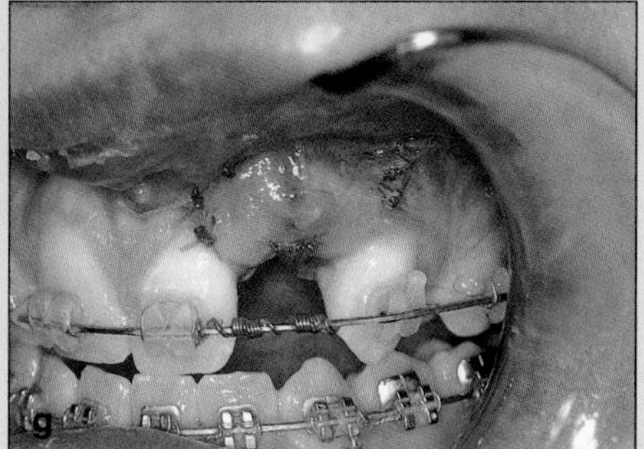

Fig 3-32e Recipient site was prepared to ensure a precise fit of graft prior to placement of rigid fixation screw (Osteomed, Addison, TX). The screws were angulated so as to engage palatal bone.

Fig 3-32f After the particulate graft is condensed around the periphery of the block graft, a Bio-Gide resorbable collagen membrane is adapted over the graft.

Fig 3-32g Exaggerated curvilinear-beveled flap design with apical cutback incisions allowed passive coronal advancement of the flap over the bone graft. Elastic limit of flap was not exceeded and circulation to flap margin was preserved. Adjacent papillary areas were de-epithelialized prior to closure with 4-0 chromic gut sutures.

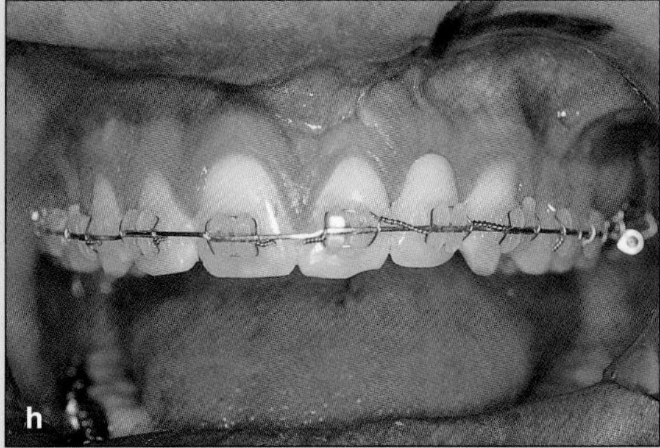
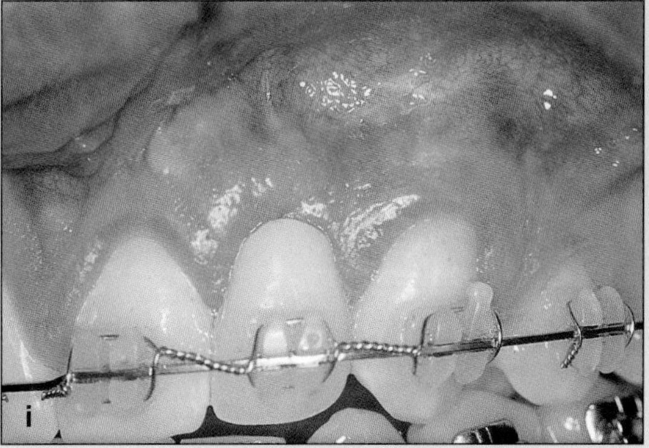

Figs 3-32h and 3-32i Excellent volume yield from bone graft is evident 6 months after procedure. Although soft tissue volume and esthetics have been preserved through the use of an exaggerated curvilinear-beveled flap design, soft tissue augmentation is indicated to offset the predictable loss of soft tissue volume that will occur following implant placement and subsequent restorative procedures. (Orthodontics by Dr Idalia Lastra, Coral Gables, FL.)

Use of U-shaped peninsula flap in esthetic implant therapy

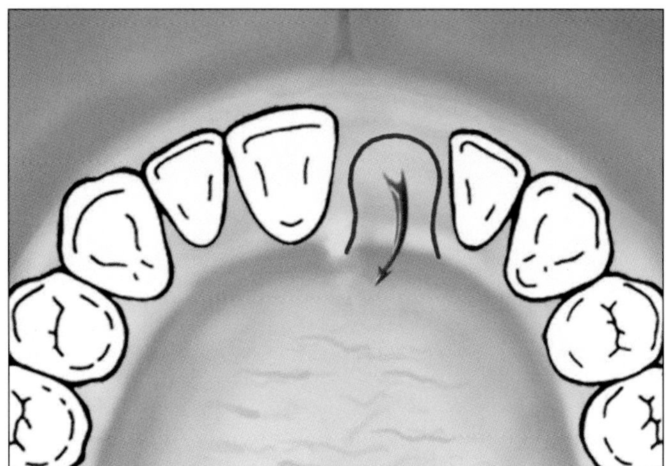

Fig 3-33a Peninsula flap design for esthetic implant therapy. This flap design allows visualization of the palatal, lingual, and buccal bone crests without the need for buccal flap elevation and is useful for submerged, nonsubmerged, and semisubmerged approaches.

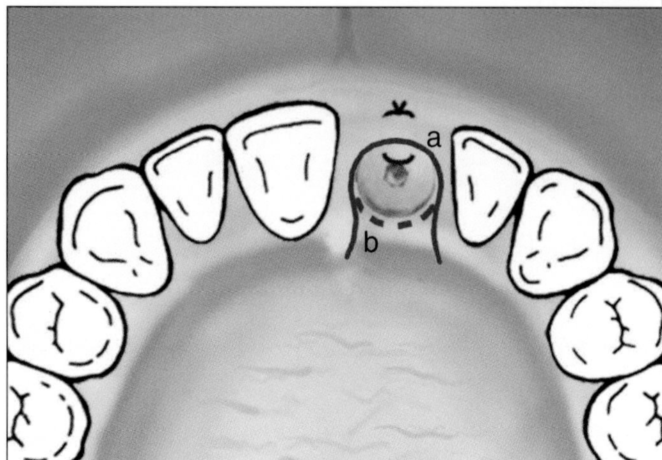

Fig 3-33b Peninsula flap management for esthetic implant therapy. *(a)* Line representing flap reapproximation after submerged implant placement. *(b)* Dotted line indicating location of incision for resective contouring of the soft tissue peninsula following nonsubmerged implant placement to allow the soft tissues to adapt to the palatal aspect of the emerging implant.

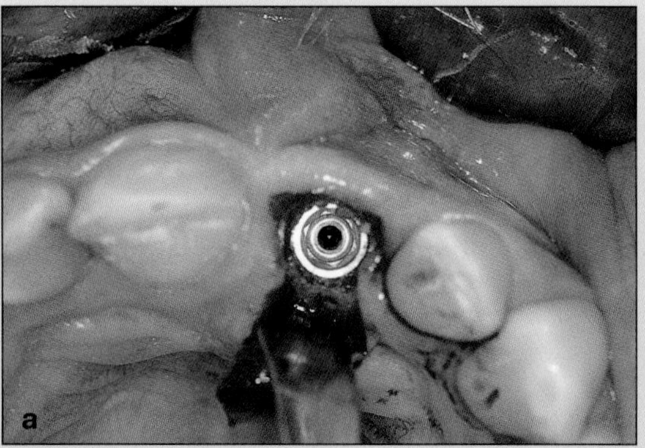

Fig 3-34a Palatal peninsula flap used for implant placement allowed direct visualization of palatal and buccal crests, thereby facilitating implant placement without the need for a buccal flap.

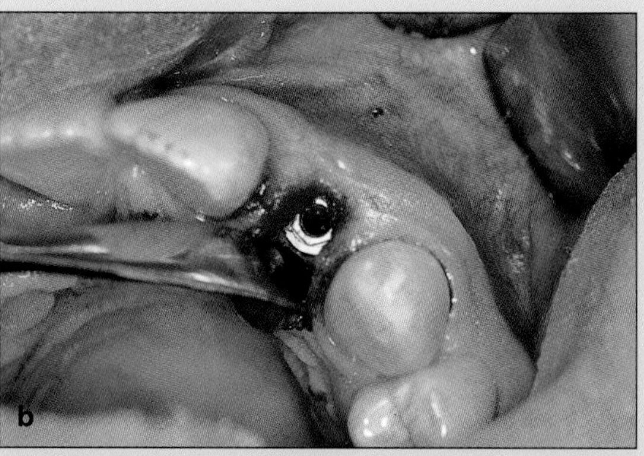

Fig 3-34b A palatal peninsula flap was used to expose this submerged implant for abutment connection. Note that slight tissue excess is intentionally left on the buccal aspect of the implant to ensure an esthetic emergence.

ume yields obtained from site-development procedures by preserving flap circulation in a fashion superior to previously described approaches, resulting in inconspicuous reconstructions of esthetic implant sites. An additional benefit to the surgeon is decreased procedure time, since the soft tissues are managed in a predictable and inconspicuous fashion.

U-shaped peninsula flap

The author uses a palatal- or lingual-based peninsula flap for access to an esthetic implant site when visualization of the buccal aspect of the alveolar ridge is unnecessary (Fig 3-33a). This is the case when hard or soft tissue augmentation is not necessary or desired or when site development has been previously accomplished (Figs 3-34 and 3-35). Incisions through the buccal tissues are avoided to minimize scarring and to prevent soft tissue recession at the site. This conservative flap design preserves circulation and soft tissue volume at the implant site by avoiding reflection of both the col tissue and the buccal mucoperiosteal tissues. This not only preserves the circulation derived from the longitudinal vessels of the periodontal ligaments of adjacent teeth and the interseptal vessels arising from the alveolar bone but also preserves the perforators that emanate from the buccal supraperiosteal vessels. Additionally, the anastomosis between the alveolar perforators and the other periodontal vasculature is maintained. These potential anastomotic channels become an important consideration when the clinician desires to maintain or reconstruct interdental papillae in esthetic situations. This approach also exposes the palatal or lingual aspect of the alveolar ridge crest, which is advantageous during osteotomy preparation, implant placement, and abutment connection because the surgeon can visualize the crestal bone preparation, depth of implant placement, and implant-abutment interface.

The peninsula flap follows a U-shaped path over the area where the implant restoration will eventually emerge. The incision is made with a no. 15C scalpel

Use of peninsula flap for submerged implant placement and subsequent abutment connection in an esthetic area

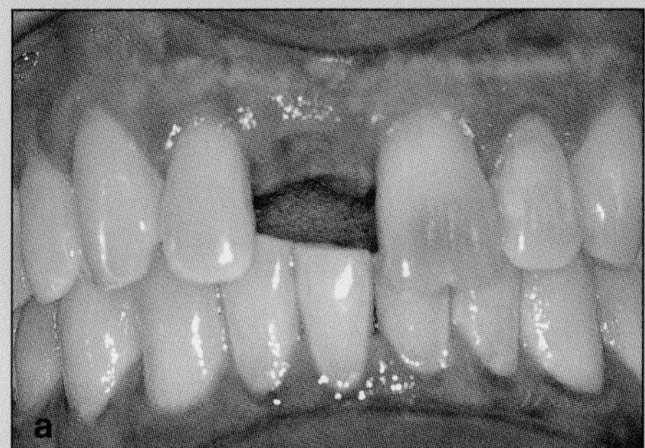

Fig 3-35a Besides a missing right central incisor, the patient has a thin, scalloped periodontium but declines recommended esthetic soft tissue graft procedure.

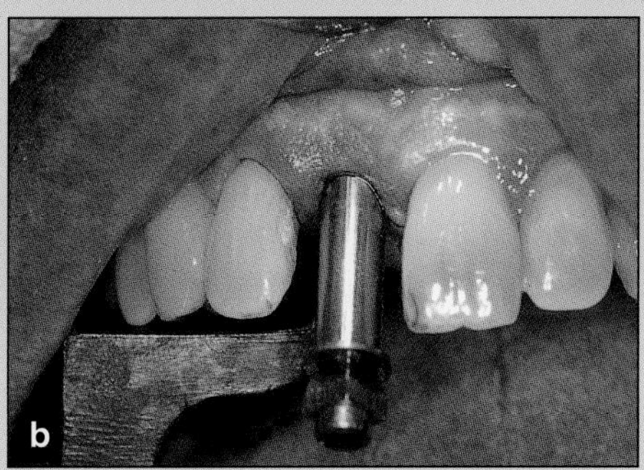

Fig 3-35b Submerged implant placed via conservative U-shaped peninsula flap to avoid further loss of soft tissue height and volume. Note that adjacent papillae are not included in the flap.

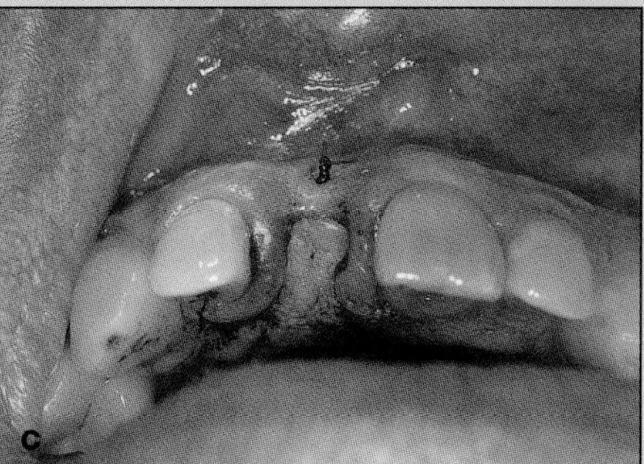

Fig 3-35c Cover screw placed and closure obtained with a single horizontal mattress suture.

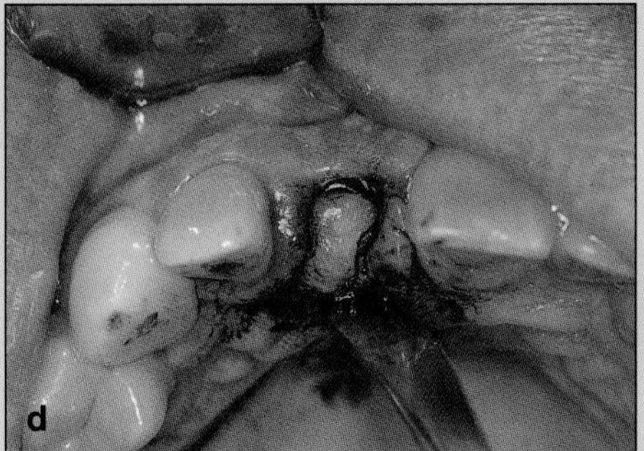

Fig 3-35d Implant exposure performed 6 months later, again using peninsula flap.

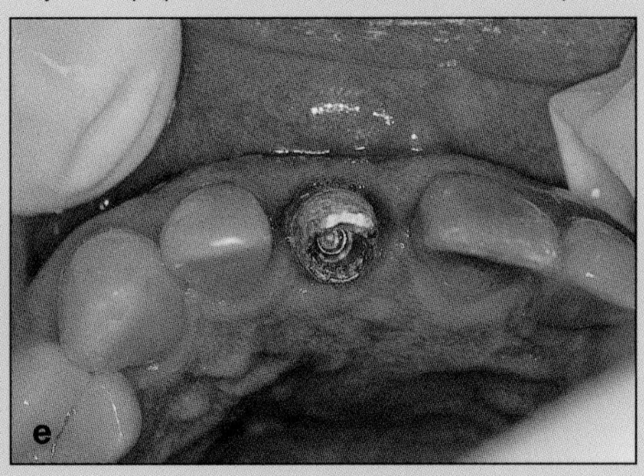

Fig 3-35e Occlusal view of abutment 3 months after it was placed via peninsula flap. Use of a surgical index at the time of implant placement allowed the delivery of a custom permanent abutment and provisional restoration at the time of implant exposure.

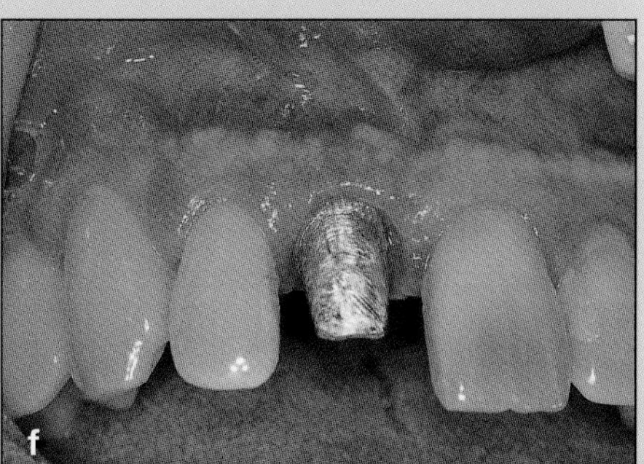

Fig 3-35f Frontal view 3 months after abutment connection. Use of U-shaped peninsula flap preserved existing soft tissue volume and architecture. Note that adjacent papillae are intact.

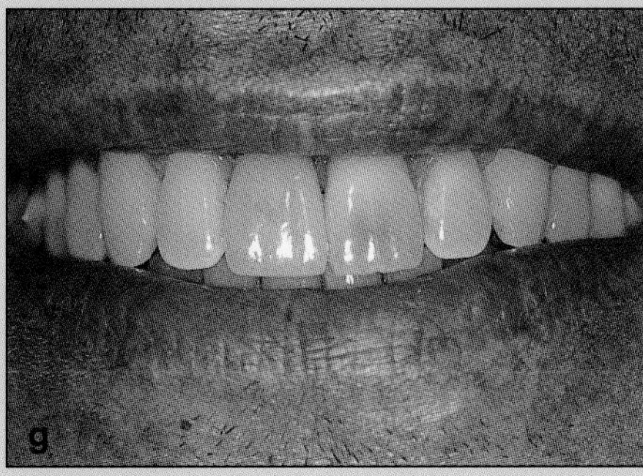

Fig 3-35g Final restoration has a natural appearance 2 years after delivery. Papillary volume has been preserved. (Restoration by Dr Faustino Garcia, Coral Gables, FL.)

blade in a round handle. The incision follows a path just palatal or lingual to the ideal buccal emergence of the implant restoration. The scalpel blade is oriented to create a bevel toward the center of the flap. When a submerged implant is placed, the flap is re-adapted over the cover screw and secured with a single horizontal mattress suture (Fig 3-33b). When nonsubmerged or semisubmerged implant placement is performed, the soft tissue peninsula is excised with a no. 15C scalpel blade, and the remaining soft tissues are readapted to the palatal aspect of the implant (see Fig 3-33b).

Tissue punch

The use of a tissue punch in esthetic implant therapy is primarily indicated for exposure of a submerged implant when the volume and architecture of the peri-implant soft tissues are ideal in the area critical for prosthetic emergence. In areas of esthetic concern, the punch is oriented with a palatal or lingual inclination as it is used to expose the implant (Fig 3-36). This technique preserves excess soft tissue volume on the facial aspect of the provisional healing abutment or provisional restoration, counteracting any tissue recession that might occur as a result of procedures required for fabrication and delivery of the final prosthesis. If necessary, this excess tissue can be carefully removed from the cervical area of the implant restoration to create harmony with the adjacent natural dentition prior to final restoration. The tissue punch is available in a variety of diameters to accommodate different implant sizes.

Use of tissue punch for implant exposure

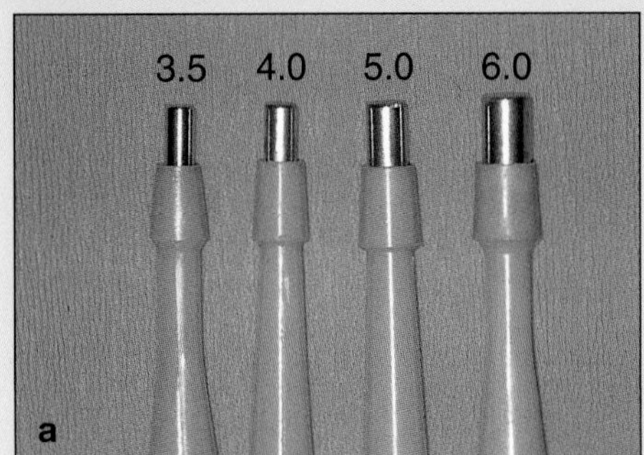

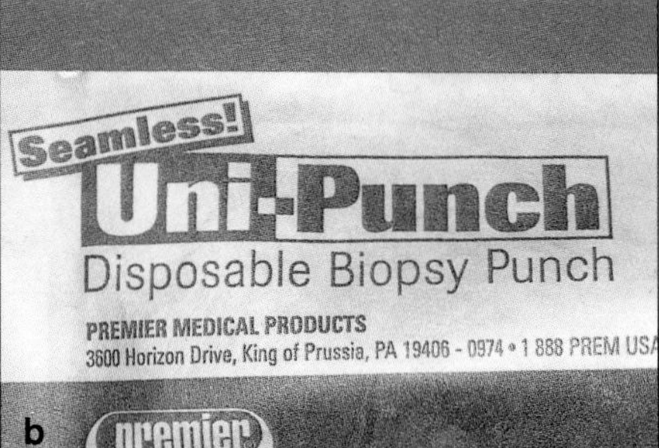

Figs 3-36a and 3-36b Disposable tissue punches are available in a variety of diameters (Uni-Punch, Premier Medical, King of Prussia, PA).

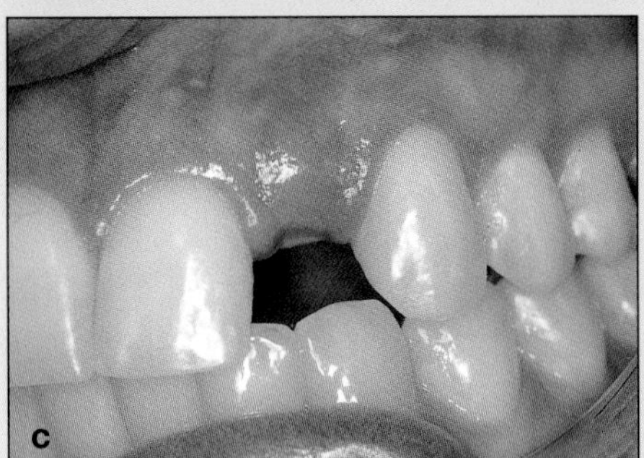

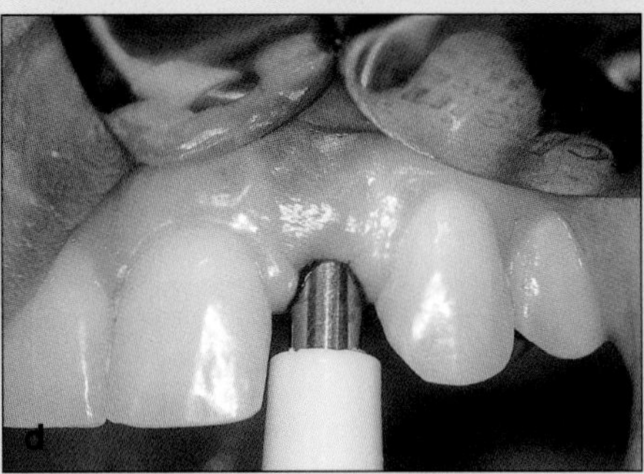

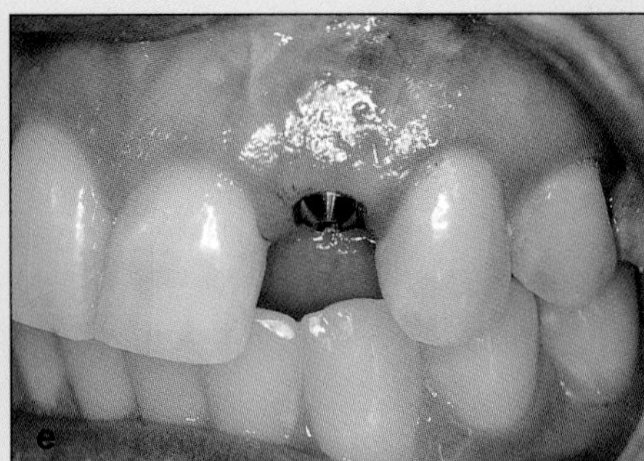

Fig 3-36c Subepithelial connective tissue graft performed simultaneously with submerged implant placement in the left lateral maxillary incisor area. The tissue punch approach was selected to preserve the soft tissue volume during abutment connection.

Fig 3-36d A 3.5-mm punch is oriented palatally during exposure to maximize the tissue remaining in the area, which is critical for prosthetic emergence.

Fig 3-36e Six weeks after placement of temporary healing abutment, soft tissue volume and architecture are intact.

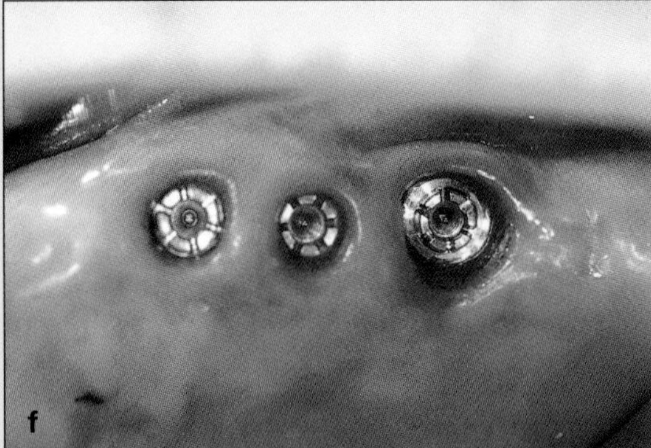

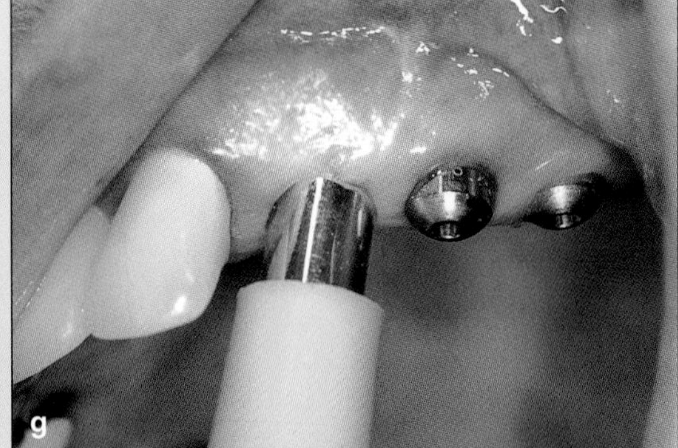

Fig 3-36f Occlusal view of maxillary implant site. The left canine was removed and an immediate submerged implant (Spline) was placed with the Bio-Col technique. The "flapless" approach for placement preserved soft tissue volume at the canine site. Soft tissue regeneration at the site was ideal. Three additional Spline implants were also used in a nonsubmerged approach to replace the premolars and first molar. Healing abutments have been removed, revealing stable peri-implant soft tissues after 4 months of healing.

Fig 3-36g A 5.0-mm-diameter tissue punch is used to expose the implant.

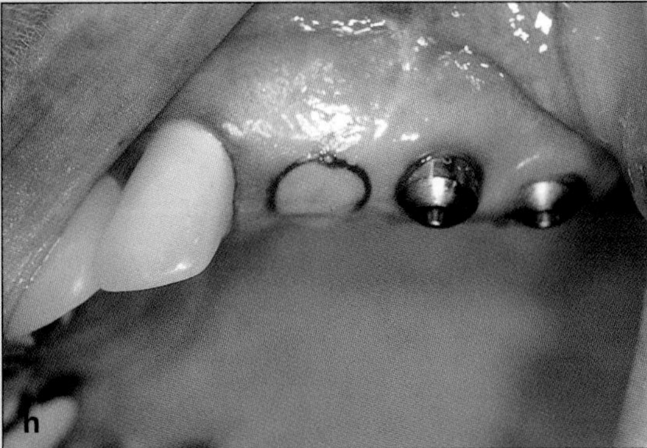

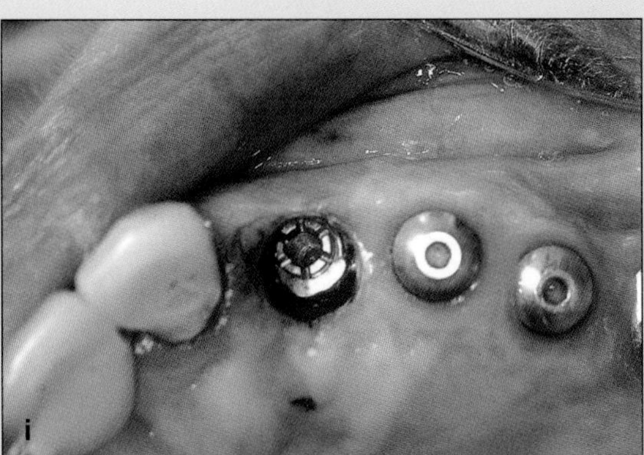

Fig 3-36h The involved tissue is carefully elevated with a small periosteal elevator or extracted with a mini rangeur.

Fig 3-36i Occlusal view with cover screw removed. Note that palatal orientation of tissue punch maximizes the attached tissue remaining in the area critical for prosthetic emergence. This will avoid unexpected compromise due to soft tissue recession occurring after placement of abutment or final restoration.

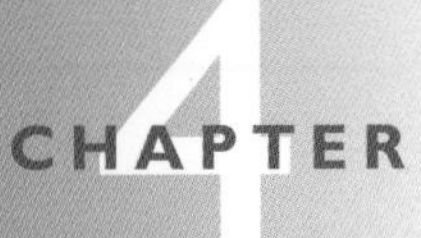

CHAPTER 4 The Bio-Col Technique

The Bio-Col alveolar ridge preservation technique takes advantage of the synergistic effect of combining surgical and prosthetic site-preservation protocols. The surgical protocol ensures the preservation of both hard and soft tissues at the time of tooth removal, and it diminishes or eliminates the bone resorption that normally follows. The prosthetic protocol uses interim provisional restorations to support the soft tissues surrounding the extraction site, thereby preventing their collapse during maturation. The result is the preservation at the extraction site of the natural hard and soft tissue anatomy, which, when lost, is extremely difficult to re-create.

This chapter presents the rationale, biologic basis, clinical goals, indications, and long-term results of the Bio-Col alveolar ridge preservation technique for patients undergoing tooth removal in conjunction with implant therapy. The technique and its applications in implant therapy are presented in a detailed, step-by-step fashion.

The Importance of Site Preservation

After removing a tooth, the dental implant team faces the formidable challenge of creating a prosthetic restoration that is in harmony with the surrounding natural dentition. To consistently meet this challenge, the implant team and the patient must appreciate the importance of site preservation. In its simplest terms, site preservation involves the use of surgical and prosthetic techniques to preserve both the volume and architecture of the hard and soft tissues at an implant site. While the term *site preservation* is most often associated with techniques designed to preserve alveolar ridge anatomy following tooth removal, the author believes that site preservation also plays an important role in all of the surgical and restorative phases involved in implant therapy. For example, the flap designs and surgical approaches described in chapter 3, which preserve circulation to the soft tissues at an implant site and thereby minimize their shrinkage, can be considered to be surgical site-preservation techniques. Similarly, prosthetic techniques that provide anatomic support to the soft tissues, thereby preventing their collapse throughout the various phases of implant therapy, are considered to be prosthetic site-preservation techniques.

In the author's experience, careful attention to site preservation at the time of tooth removal often reduces or eliminates the need for subsequent site-development procedures (ie, hard and soft tissue grafting) in preparation for an implant restoration. Furthermore, and possibly of greater significance, failure to use site-preservation techniques at the time of tooth removal, even when additional grafting procedures will be unavoidable (eg, in the case of an unfavorable socket wall defect), increases the complexity of subsequent reconstructive efforts because of collapse of the soft tissues into the osseous defect. Subsequent contraction of the reconstructed soft tissue envelope and loss of elasticity of the soft tissue cover often necessitates additional soft tissue grafting procedures to provide adequate soft tissue coverage for the hard tissue reconstruction that will be required to re-create natural alveolar ridge anatomy at the site. Finally, the use of site-preservation techniques is especially important for patients with thin, scalloped periodontal biotype because of their predisposition for soft tissue shrinkage and concurrent alveolar bone resorption, which can jeopardize the long-term esthetic and functional success initially realized with an implant restoration.

Alveolar ridge collapse after tooth removal

Although the healing that follows the removal of a tooth is usually uneventful, only partial bone fill of the alveolar socket generally occurs.[1,2] Concurrent with bone growth into the socket, there is also well-documented, predictable resorption of the alveolar ridge in the buccal-lingual and apicocoronal dimensions.[1,3,4] This resorption results in a narrower and shorter ridge. Studies have shown that 3 to 4 mm of both buccal-lingual and apicocoronal ridge resorption occurs within 6 months of extraction of anterior teeth.[1,3,4] This amount of ridge resorption leads to an esthetic compromise in implant therapy because of osseous contours that cannot properly support the overlying soft tissues or inadequate bone volume for ideal implant placement. In addition, implant restoration may be conspicuous at these deficient sites despite the use of various hard and soft tissue reconstructive techniques.

The eventual shrinkage of the alveolar ridge after tooth removal seems to be related not only to the trauma of tooth removal but also to the environment within which the natural healing process takes place within the tooth socket. Early clot contraction and accumulation of oral debris in the socket may limit the potential of the alveolus to fully exhibit its regenerative potential.[2] Epithelium proliferates over newly regenerated connective tissue at a level apical to oral debris collecting within the socket. As a consequence, the natural process of healing in the oral environment results in bone fill of the socket that falls short of the original alveolar crest height. Subsequently, loss of ridge height and width occur secondary to the remodeling process.

Preliminary studies by Lekovic et al[1,4] demonstrated that the use of barrier membranes over extraction sockets significantly decreases the loss of alveolar bone height and width and simultaneously increases the level of bone fill in the socket. In addition, when dental implants are placed into fresh extraction sockets and the sites are isolated according to the principles of guided bone regeneration, the crestal levels of bone regeneration have been shown to improve significantly but are dependent on the maintenance of soft tissue coverage over the membrane.[5,6]

In clinical practice, however, use of a barrier membrane to enhance healing of an extraction site requires the advancement of a large full-thickness flap. While this facilitates tension-free closure and minimizes complications associated with membrane exposure, it permanently disfigures the soft tissue architecture at the site, limiting its use in esthetic areas. Flap elevation also compromises the vascular supply to the area, contributing to soft tissue recession and possibly limiting future regenerative potential. These considerations are critical in planning tooth removal and implant replacement in an area of esthetic concern.

Clinical goals and biologic considerations for ridge preservation

The primary clinical goal of any alveolar ridge preservation technique should be to preserve both the hard and soft tissue volume and architecture, especially the interdental papillae, in order to optimize function and esthetics. It is essential to maintain a stable osteoconductive environment or scaffold within the entire area of the socket or in the void existing between the socket walls and the immediately placed implant, as well as to isolate this scaffold from the deleterious effect of oral debris during healing. Another important biologic consideration is to maximize the supply of osteoprogenitor cells and their ability to invade the area occupied by the osteoconductive scaffold. In implant therapy, this scaffold should be slowly resorbed and replaced by vital mineralized bone to contribute to osseointegration and thus provide support for the implant restoration. Whenever esthetics is important, the advancement of large mucoperiosteal flaps should be avoided to preserve the periodontal circulation and the natural soft tissue anatomy at the site. The key elements in obtaining an optimal esthetic rehabilitation with implant therapy are the avoidance of postextraction bone resorption and the preservation of the natural soft tissue volume and architecture at the site. This enables the restorative dentist to create an inconspicuous restoration free of prosthetic compensation.

Rationale for the Bio-Col technique

The rationale for the Bio-Col technique's surgical site-preservation protocol was based on the author's understanding that postextraction bone resorption could be reduced or eliminated by *(1)* minimizing trauma to surrounding tissues during tooth removal, *(2)* preparing and grafting a bleeding socket with an ideal osteoconductive material (Bio-Oss; Osteohealth, Shirley, NY) that is slowly resorbed and replaced by vital bone, and *(3)* using a technique to isolate the surgical site that avoids the esthetic disfigurement commonly associated with advancement and closure of a large mucoperiosteal flap over a membrane, but yields results similar to those obtained with traditional membrane-assisted guided bone regeneration procedures. Knowing that the use of absorbable collagen material (CollaPlug; Centerpulse Dental, Carlsbad, CA) would act as a matrix for connective tissue growth, the author theorized that when this material was condensed within the soft tissue confines of the bleeding socket and sealed with impervious tissue cement (Isodent; Ellman International, Hewlett, NY), the grafted site would be isolated from the deleterious effects of the oral environment. This combination offered the potential for guided bone regeneration while avoiding the limitations associated with the use of a nonresorbable membrane and primary flap closure. The conceptualization of this approach and the combined surgical-prosthetic protocol that followed represented a significant departure from the then-accepted protocols recommended for obtaining guided bone regeneration at extraction sites in conjunction with immediate or delayed implant placement.

Similarly, the rationale for the Bio-Col's prosthetic site-preservation protocol was based on the author's understanding that supracrestal gingival tissue morphology is totally dependent upon support from the emerging dentition, and that the soft tissue collapse that occurs following tooth removal could be eliminated by immediately supporting these tissues with anatomically correct provisional restorations that replicate the natural tooth contours.

Finally, the rationale for combining the surgical and prosthetic site-preservation protocols was based on the author's understanding of the potential synergistic effects that result when surgical and prosthetic management are closely linked and coordinated. Specifically, the provisional restoration must be delivered immediately after completion of the grafting and isolation of the socket to protect the site from mechanical trauma during initial healing. This would ensure the maintenance and undisturbed healing of the osseous graft (Bio-Oss + blood clot *or* Bio-Oss + autogenous bone + blood clot) within the socket. Ideally, the provisional restoration would be designed with an ovate pontic that replicates the cervical anatomy of the extracted tooth. The pontic would extend approximately 3 mm into the soft tissue socket to provide both support for the surrounding soft tissues and protection for the underlying grafted socket. A provisional prosthesis that was designed and properly adjusted to avoid the transmission of micromotion to the site, which would otherwise interfere with the integration of the graft complex, would promote maximum bone regeneration. Rapid epithelialization over newly formed connective tissue within the superficial aspect of the socket would be enhanced because the site was immediately protected from the deleterious effects of the oral environment, and soft tissue regeneration would be limited to more superficial levels than commonly seen at untreated sites, where connective tissue is known to occupy the coronal third of the socket.

Whereas scientific evidence supported the selection of materials for use in the Bio-Col technique, the conceptualization and theoretical premise—that the combined surgical and prosthetic protocols would create an ideal environment for bone regeneration and soft tissue healing at extraction sites, thereby facilitating immediate or delayed implant rehabilitation—would have to be proven with long-term follow-up in clinical practice. Furthermore, the author understood that host response and anatomic limitations such as residual socket defects would be the critical factors in determining the outcome of the procedure on a case-by-case basis, providing that the procedure was performed consistently in all cases. This understanding allowed the author to use this technique in good faith in clinical practice. Improved clinical results were immediately observed, and subsequent long-term follow-up better defined the potential benefits for patients in implant therapy.

Biologic basis for the Bio-Col technique

The biologic basis for the selection of Bio-Oss as an ideal osteoconductive scaffold for grafting the extraction sockets is well supported in the literature. In a study by Klinge et al,[7] Bio-Oss provided an excellent scaffold for new bone growth when placed in experimental defects in rabbit bone. In a study using Bio-Oss as a grafting material in simultaneous sinus elevation–implant placement procedures in beagle dogs, Wetzel et al[8] found abundant new lamellar bone formation and bone apposition to the implant surfaces. Human histologic evidence in sinus augmentation procedures also supports the biologic basis for the use of Bio-Oss as an ideal osteoconductive matrix.[9,10] Valentini and Abensur[9] performed a study using a composite graft of Bio-Oss and demineralized freeze-dried bone in 20 patients requiring sinus lift procedures and found abundant amounts of bone formation integrated with the grafted Bio-Oss particles. The authors concluded that Bio-Oss showed excellent osteoconductive properties. Another sinus elevation–implant study found that the force required to pull out implants placed in sinuses grafted with Bio-Oss was at least equal to the force required to pull out implants placed into sinuses grafted with autogenous bone.[11]

Furthermore, in an animal study conducted by Berglundh and Lindhe,[12] Bio-Oss was shown to be an effective osteoconductive material that gradually undergoes replacement with normal bone through a slow resorption process. Specifically, these investigators demonstrated that Bio-Oss integrated with newly formed bone when grafted into extraction sites where defects were experimentally created. They also demonstrated that implants placed 3 months later at these grafted sites osseointegrated to the same degree as implants placed at control sites. Of special significance was the finding that the graft particles were consistently separated from the implant surface by vital mineralized bone and were gradually resorbed and replaced with bone. The significance of this study is that its findings validate the use of Bio-Oss for grafting extraction sites to preserve or augment the alveolar ridge in preparation for delayed implant placement. The study also supports the use of this material to fill the voids between an implant placed immediately after tooth removal and the residual socket walls.

Finally, Boyne[13] demonstrated that Bio-Oss is an ideal osteoconductive graft material because it is highly porous; it undergoes early revascularization, thereby inviting the ingress of neoangiogenic tissue and prodromal osteoblasts; and it is slowly resorbed, thus participating in phase-two bone graft healing, formation of the outer cortex of the defect, and enhancement of the thickness of the trabecular pattern of the new cancellous bone within the defect. Furthermore, Boyne reported the remarkable observation that guided bone regeneration could be obtained without the use of a membrane system, which he discovered when he grafted alveolar ridge defects with a mixture of autogenous particulate marrow and cancellous bone with Bio-Oss. He emphasized that nonporous osteoconductive materials do not yield this inclusive barrier effect when mixed with autogenous particulate bone since they do not biodegrade physiologically under the influence of osteoclast resorption and are not subsequently replaced by osteoblastic activity.

It is important for the implant surgeon to recognize that bone regeneration within an extraction socket depends more on the genetic makeup and general health of a patient and the regenerative potential of a particular site than on the "magical" properties of a bone graft material. Although positive outcomes of the Bio-Col technique depend on the surgeon's care in following the details and individual steps presented in this chapter, the host and individual site factors will always be the primary determinants of the degree of osteoconduction and vital bone regeneration at a particular site. The one exception appears to be the lack of graft integration observed at sites where micromotion is transmitted by an unstable provisional restoration. During initial healing, micromotion diminishes the volume yields of any graft system in the same way it interferes with osseointegration of a dental implant; that is, it results in connective tissue encapsulation rather than bone-to-implant contact. Similarly, even when Bio-Oss is grafted in a biologically ideal extraction site and host, exposing the site to micromotion interferes with revascularization, osteoconduction, and ultimately, bone regeneration.

For the purposes of predicting the outcome of the Bio-Col technique at a particular extraction site, it is helpful for the surgeon to classify the site as either a healthy site with good regenerative potential or as a compromised site with poor regenerative potential. A healthy site is one that is free of hard or soft tissue pathology and that demonstrates abundant bleeding within the socket following tooth removal. A compromised site is one where the regenerative potential is diminished secondary to decreased circulation to the area as a result of a history of trauma such as subluxation, intrusion, or avulsion with reimplantation of the tooth; infections; endodontic procedures; or multiple surgical procedures. In most instances, little bleeding is noted following tooth removal (see Site-Preservation Algorithm in the Appendix).

Bio-Col Technique for Delayed Implant Placement

There are numerous clinical situations in which delayed implant placement is indicated following tooth removal. In these situations, the goal of the Bio-Col site-preservation technique is to minimize loss of alveolar ridge contours secondary to osseous remodeling, increase bone regeneration within the extraction socket, and prevent soft tissue collapse associated with tooth removal.

In general, delayed implant placement is indicated when primary implant stability is not feasible; when an acute infection is accompanied by edema, cellulitis, or abscess of the periodontal tissues; when a socket wall defect threatens predictable osseointegration; and when a patient is contemplating but not committed to proceeding with an implant replacement. Additional criteria for delaying implant placement in esthetic areas include dehiscence defects, fenestration defects that jeopardize the integrity of the buccal ridge crest by their size or location, and tooth mobility or chronic irritation secondary to a violation of biologic width or recurrent decay under an existing restoration that is accompanied by edema of the marginal soft tissues. The implant surgeon should recognize that considerable esthetic risk is associated with immediate implant replacement under these conditions, each of which can compromise the esthetic outcome secondary to soft tissue recession and early or late osseous remodeling.

In these instances, re-evaluation of the site approximately 3 months after performing the Bio-Col technique allows the surgeon an opportunity to inspect the alveolar ridge contours at the site, to classify any residual esthetic ridge defect that may have developed, and to select and sequence any site-development procedures needed to ensure an inconspicuous restoration. This also gives the patient an opportunity to visualize the deficient ridge contours at the site, which often reinforces their understanding and acceptance of necessary site-development procedures.

When the Bio-Col technique is performed in preparation for delayed implant placement at a site with an intact socket, the author routinely proceeds with implant placement 2 to 3 months following tooth removal. Additional healing time is allowed for sites deemed to be compromised based on the history or on clinical observation at the time of tooth removal. In addition, sites with very large sockets (ie, molar sites) also require additional healing time prior to implant placement.

When the Bio-Col technique is performed in preparation for delayed implant placement at a site where there is an osseous defect, the implant surgeon should recognize that in addition to all of the considerations previously mentioned, the predictability and outcome of the procedure is largely determined by the morphology of the defect.

The author distinguishes osseous defects at extraction sites as either favorable or unfavorable based on their morphology. Favorable defect morphology exists when the width of a socket wall defect at an extraction site is less than one third the mesiodistal distance between the adjacent teeth (Fig 4-1a). The remaining interdental bone volume at these sites generally has sufficient cellularity and vascularity (ie, regenerative potential) to provide for repair across the gap when treated with a modified Bio-Col technique, as described later in this chapter. Unfavorable defect morphology exists when the width of the socket wall defect is greater than one third the mesiodistal distance between adjacent teeth (Fig 4-1b). The diminished volume of interdental bone generally does not have the regenerative potential to provide for complete osseous repair across the gap, even when osteoconductive graft material and barrier membranes are used, as described later in this chapter.

Favorable defects at esthetic sites are managed with a modified Bio-Col technique followed by a 4- to 6-

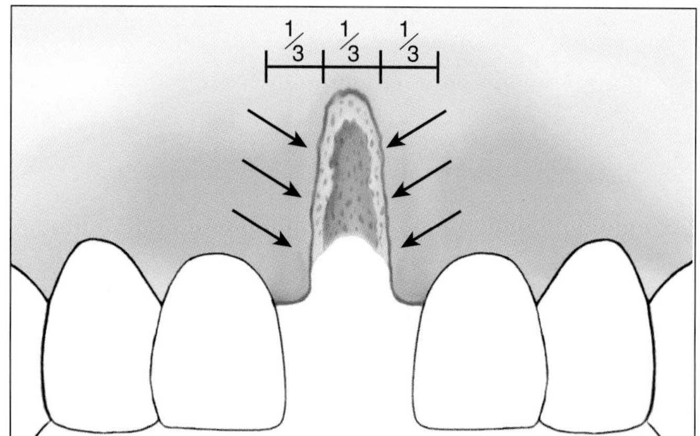

Fig 4-1a Favorable defect morphology. When the width of a socket wall defect is less than one third the mesiodistal dimension between the adjacent teeth, the remaining interdental bone volume generally has the potential to provide for osseous repair across the gap when the Bio-Col technique is performed, provided the site is not compromised by a history of trauma, infection, previous surgery, or multiple endodontic procedures.

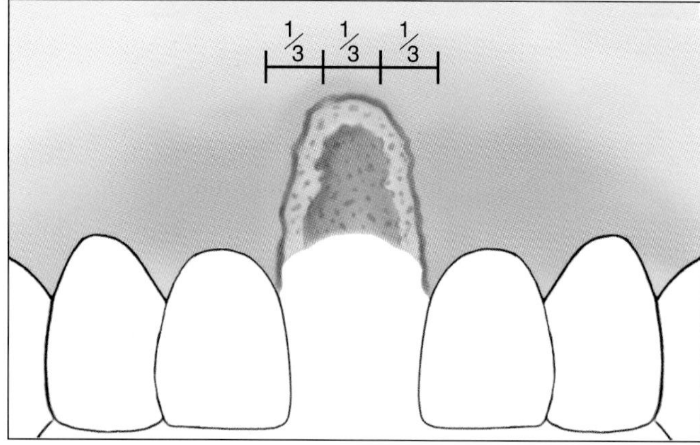

Fig 4-1b Unfavorable defect morphology. When the width of a socket wall defect exceeds one third the mesiodistal dimension between the adjacent teeth, staged reconstruction with autogenous block and particulate bone grafts, as well as necessary soft tissue grafting, will yield the most predictable esthetic results. Despite the use of the Bio-Col technique, the resultant diminished interdental bone volume will not predictably provide for osseous repair across the gap.

month healing period prior to implant placement. The site is then re-evaluated in order to verify maintenance of ideal ridge contour before proceeding with implant placement. At the same time, the patient is informed that additional bone grafting may be necessary should it be discovered upon re-entry to the site that incomplete repair of the osseous defect will not allow ideal implant placement. The author uses a conservative peninsula flap approach and observes the integrity of the repaired socket wall defect during implant osteotomy preparation. If the repair maintains its integrity, the implant is placed in an ideal position. Should there be any doubt as to the integrity of the repair, a curvilinear flap is used to obtain buccal access to the site for further hard tissue site development, and in most instances implant placement is delayed. If the surgeon determines that ideal ridge contours have not been maintained following the initial site-preservation procedure, further site-development procedures are planned as indicated.

In contrast, favorable defects at nonesthetic sites are often successfully managed in conjunction with immediate implant placement. A full-thickness mucoperiosteal flap is elevated, the peri-implant defect is grafted with Bio-Oss or a mixture of autogenous particulate bone and Bio-Oss, and a resorbable collagen membrane is adapted over the grafted defect. The flap is then advanced to obtain closure over a submerged implant or to obtain circumferential soft tissue adaptation around the transmucosal portion of a nonsubmerged implant.

For unfavorable defects at esthetic sites, the Bio-Col technique is used to maintain space and prevent soft tissue collapse and scarring at the site, thus facilitating subsequent site-development procedures performed prior to implant placement. Staged hard and soft tissue site development with autogenous block bone grafts and a series of soft tissue augmentation and refinement procedures, or simultaneous hard and soft tissue site development are required in order to prepare these sites for esthetic implant restoration. The author usually allows a 3-month healing period for sufficient maturation of the soft tissues at these sites before proceeding with the indicated site-development procedures, as described in chapters 6 and 7.

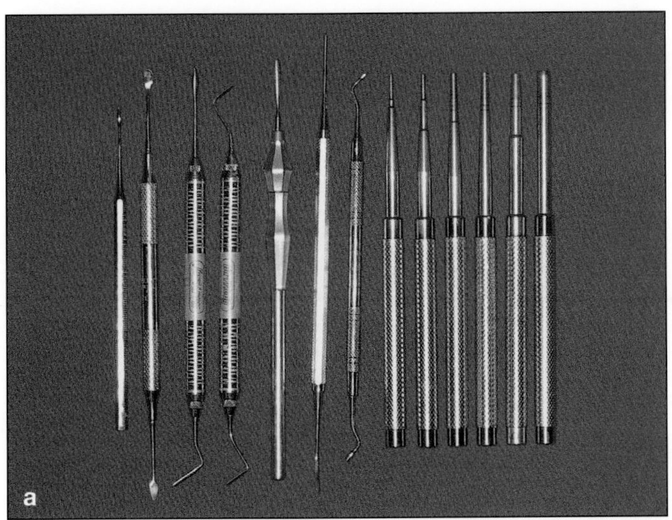

Fig 4-2a Surgical instrumentation. A sharpened dissector or Buser periosteal elevator and an assortment of periotomes are used to carefully sever the periodontal attachments to the tooth. A Lucas surgical curette is used to thoroughly debride the socket to initiate bleeding. A Freer elevator is used to deliver the Bio-Oss graft to the site, and an amalgam plugger or tapered osteotomes are used to condense the graft within the socket.

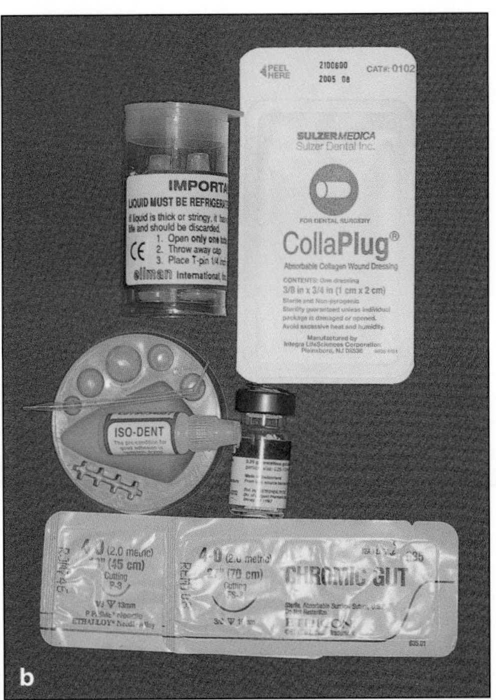

Fig 4-2b Materials used in the Bio-Col technique. On average, 0.25 g of Bio-Oss particulate cancellous bone graft material is used to graft a single extraction site. CollaPlug absorbable collagen dressing and Isodent tissue cement are used to isolate the grafted site from the oral cavity. To prevent coronal displacement of the CollaPlug dressing, 4-0 chromic gut suture is used on a P3 or FS2 needle.

In contrast, unfavorable defects at nonesthetic sites that are limited to the buccal socket wall are usually managed via a traditional guided bone regeneration procedure in preparation for delayed implant placement. After elevation of a full-thickness mucoperiosteal flap outlined with curvilinear-beveled releasing incisions, the site is grafted either with Bio-Oss alone or mixed with autogenous particulate bone and then isolated with a resorbable barrier membrane. The flap is then advanced, and tension-free closure is obtained. In these instances, re-entry to the site 4 to 6 months later usually allows placement of the implant without further need for hard tissue site development, although large-volume defects involving adjacent interdental bone will require autogenous block bone grafts in order to allow acceptable implant positioning.

Surgical protocol for intact sockets

In addition to the standard instrumentation required for the surgical removal of a tooth, the following instruments and materials should be included in the surgical setup: a sharpened dissector or Buser periosteal elevator, an assortment of periotomes, a Lucas surgical curette, a Freer elevator, an amalgam plugger or tapered osteotomes, Bio-Oss cancellous grafting material in a particle size of 0.25 to 1 mm, CollaPlug absorbable collagen wound dressing, and Isodent tissue cement (Fig 4-2).

When delayed implant placement is indicated at a site with an intact socket, the vascular supply to the hard and soft tissues at the extraction site is preserved by avoiding flap elevation during tooth removal. The soft tissue architecture is preserved by eliminating flap closure after socket grafting. A minimally traumatic technique is essential to preserve the surrounding periodontal soft tissues during tooth removal. A sharpened dissector or a Buser periosteal elevator is used to carefully incise the gingival attachments from the tooth to be extracted. The periodontal ligament attachment is then severed circumferentially using periotomes, which are carefully advanced toward the apex of the tooth within the periodontal ligament space. Care is taken to avoid splintering the thin buccal or lingual alveolar bone. When necessary, the tooth is care-

Bio-Col technique for delayed implant placement in the intact socket

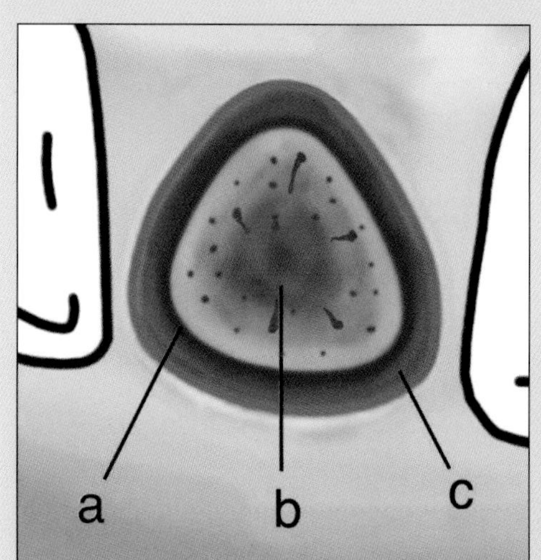

Fig 4-3a Bleeding extraction socket with intact bony walls. Tooth has been removed with minimal trauma, avoiding the need for flap elevation. This is achieved by carefully incising the dentogingival attachments with a periotome and, if necessary, removing the tooth in sections. Immediate implant placement is indicated when the selected implant will achieve primary stability and obliterate most of the socket. *(a)* Crestal bone level; *(b)* bleeding from perforations made in the socket walls; *(c)* unsupported soft tissues surrounding the extraction site.

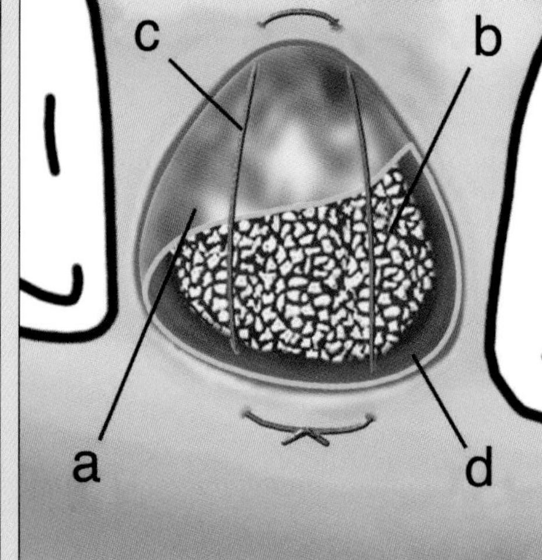

Fig 4-3b Bleeding socket with intact bony walls grafted to the level of the alveolar crest with Bio-Oss natural bone mineral. CollaPlug absorbable collagen dressing *(a)* is condensed over the grafted bone mineral *(b)*, and a horizontal mattress suture *(c)* is loosely secured to prevent its coronal displacement. A thin coat of Isodent tissue adhesive is applied to the surface of the collagen dressing within the confines of the soft tissue socket to seal the site from the oral cavity. *(d)* Soft tissues surrounding the extraction site.

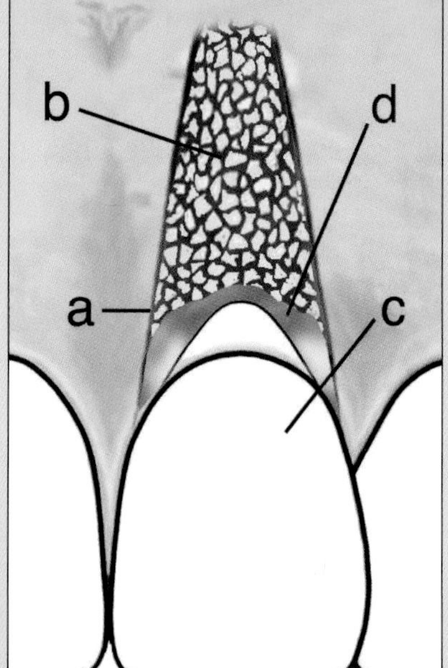

Fig 4-3c Bleeding socket with intact bony walls *(a)* grafted up to the level of the alveolar crest with Bio-Oss natural bone mineral *(b)*. A removable or fixed provisional restoration *(c)* is placed with an ovate pontic extending 3 to 4 mm subgingivally, compressing the CollaPlug *(d)* and supporting the surrounding soft tissues.

fully sectioned with high-speed rotary instrumentation, and the resultant tooth fragments are carefully removed while maintaining the integrity of the socket walls. A Lucas surgical curette is used to perform a thorough curettage of the socket so as to remove any granulation tissue, thus stimulating bleeding. The site is inspected for the presence of socket wall defects and for evidence of spontaneous bleeding. When spontaneous bleeding is not observed, the socket walls are perforated with a small carbide bur. This provides bleeding into the socket and enhances the ability of osteoprogenitor cells to invade the scaffold created by a mixture of the blood clot and the Bio-Oss material. A bleeding socket is essential for subsequent integration of the graft at the site (Figs 4-3a and 4-3d).

Next, the graft material is moistened slightly with sterile saline or blood from the extraction site and delivered in small quantities into the socket. A Freer elevator is used to transfer the graft to the bleeding socket. In a healthy site where abundant bleeding is present, the instrument is placed over the graft while the surgical assistant suctions the excess blood from the site. This prevents the graft material from being displaced by the flow of blood. Within seconds, the hydrophilic porous bone mineral readily absorbs the blood, stabilizing the graft within the socket. The graft material should be thoroughly condensed until the bony socket is completely filled. The author routinely uses tapered osteotomes or amalgam pluggers for this purpose. Condensing the particulate graft

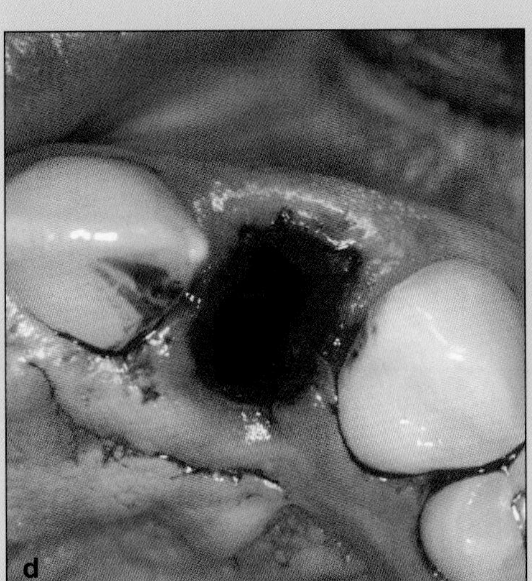

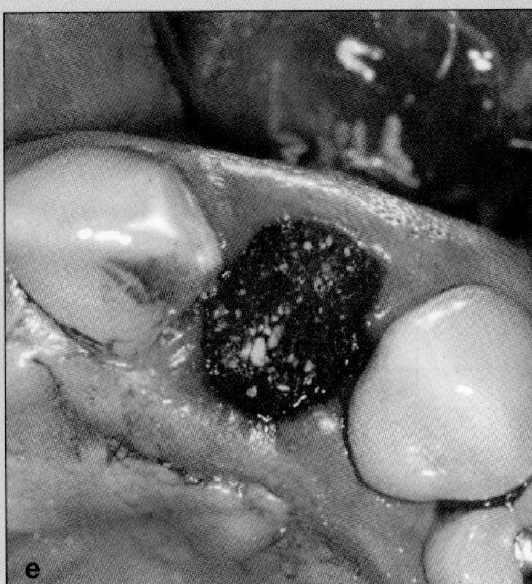

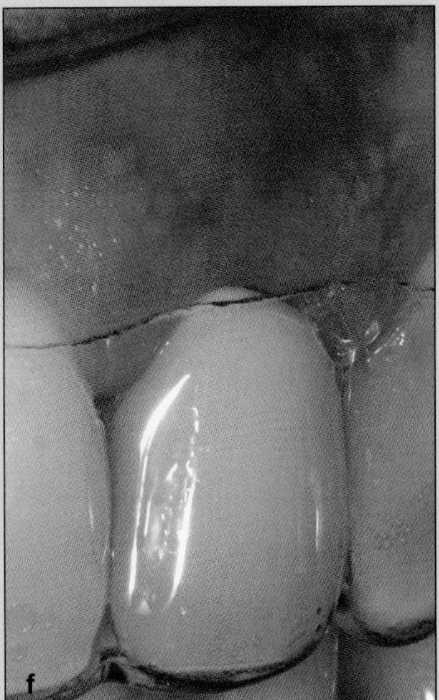

Figs 4-3d to 4-3f These clinical photos correspond to the illustrations shown in Figs 4-3a to 4-3c. Note that in this case an Essex provisional restoration that housed an ovate pontic was used for the initial healing period.

eliminates dead space, thereby favoring guided bone regeneration within the socket. It also avoids possible settling of the graft, which could jeopardize the ultimate height of the bone fill. Ideally, the surgeon should observe bleeding through the condensed Bio-Oss graft. The graft should be so thoroughly condensed that suctioning over the graft will remove only loose Bio-Oss particles displaced within the superficial soft tissue confines of the socket.

If necessary, a 30-gauge needle is then used to stimulate additional bleeding from the surrounding soft tissues. CollaPlug material is densely packed over the Bio-Oss graft until the level of the free marginal gingiva is reached (Figs 4-3b and 4-3e). The collagen dressing should be dry when taken to the site and should become saturated with blood as it is condensed over the graft. Again, bleeding is essential to ensure incorporation of the collagen dressing, which acts as a matrix for soft tissue healing at the site. In most instances the CollaPlug is cut in half and can be used at two sites.

At esthetic sites, a horizontal mattress suture (4-0 or 5-0 chromic gut on a P3 needle) is then loosely secured over the CollaPlug to prevent coronal displacement of the material without disfiguring the soft tissue architecture (see Fig 4-3b). At nonesthetic sites, a figure-eight suture can be used to better secure the CollaPlug within the socket; 4-0 chromic gut suture on an FS2 needle is used for this purpose. To seal the CollaPlug and complete the isolation of the site, a small amount of Isodent tissue adhesive is applied with a sterile pipette to coat the superficial aspect of the collagen material. When used in this manner, the collagen material becomes relatively impervious to oral liquids, and the surgical site becomes physically isolated from the oral environment. When bleeding continues through the CollaPlug, blotting with a dry gauze sponge will facilitate accurate application of the tissue cement. The application of the tissue cement should be limited to the collagen material within the perimeter of the surrounding soft tissues; excess tissue cement should not run over the adjacent soft tissues and thus hamper seating of the ovate pontic provisional restoration (Figs 4-3c and 4-3f). After a healing period of 2 to 3 months, these sites are reentered for implant placement, using the standard approaches described in chapter 3 (Figs 4-4 and 4-5).

Bio-Col technique for delayed implant replacement of ankylosed resorbing maxillary central incisors

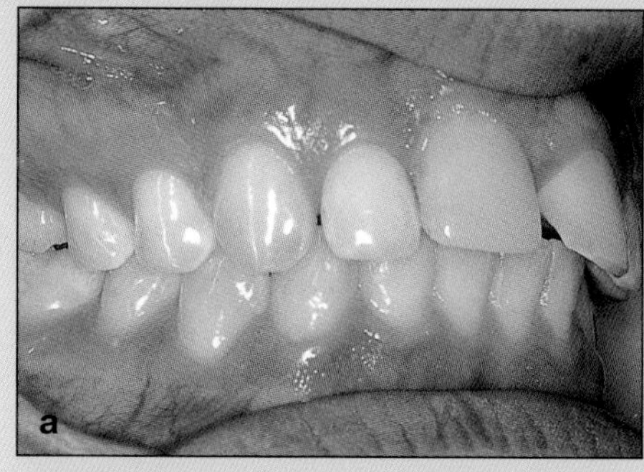
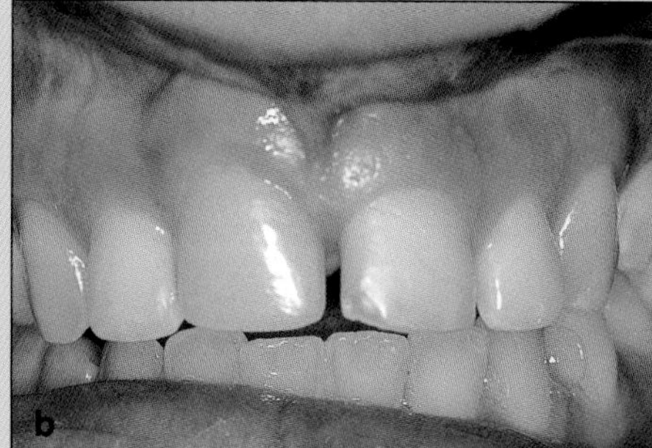

Figs 4-4a and 4-4b Unesthetic ankylosed maxillary incisors. Both central incisors are malposed secondary to trauma. Previous attempts at orthodontic correction were unsuccessful. Immediate implant placement was not indicated due to the large irregular socket that would result after removal of the right central incisor, which was traumatically intruded, and the risk for buccal wall defects upon tooth removal.

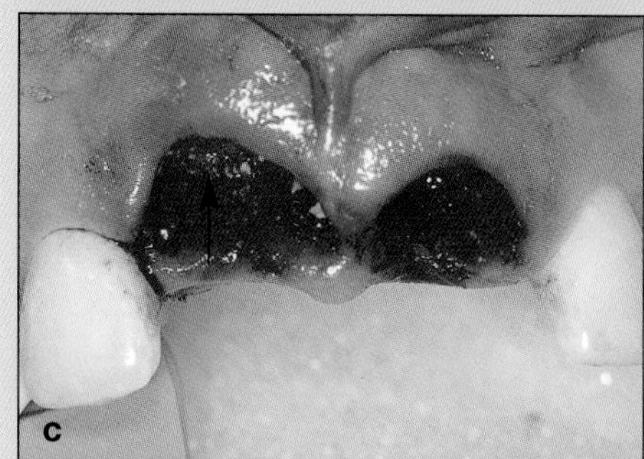
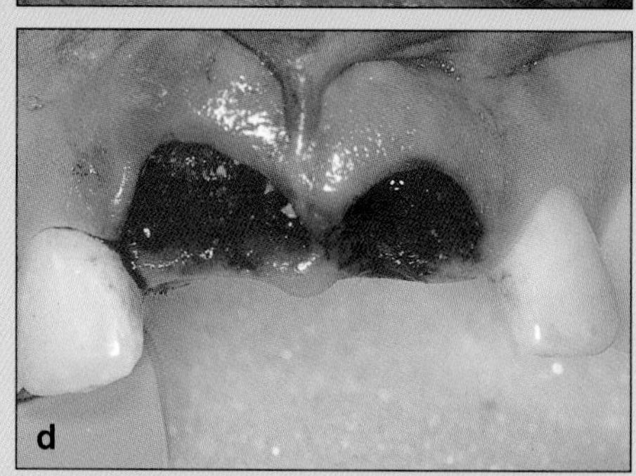

Fig 4-4c Both incisors were carefully removed via a minimally traumatic technique to preserve soft tissue architecture. Note that the palatal bone level of the right socket *(arrow)* is much more apical than that of the left socket.

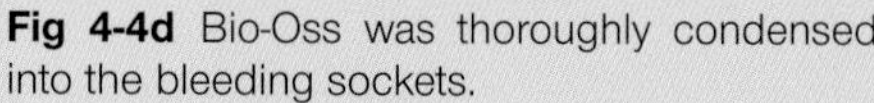

Fig 4-4d Bio-Oss was thoroughly condensed into the bleeding sockets.

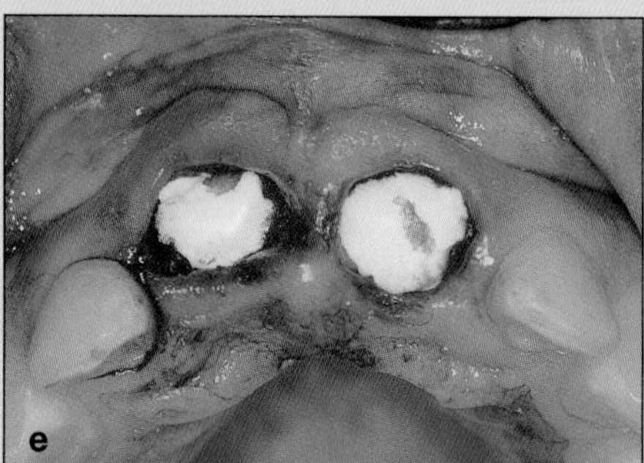
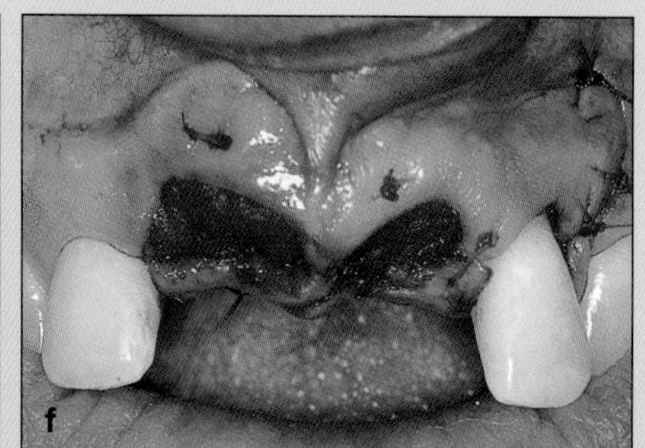

Fig 4-4e CollaPlug absorbable collagen dressing was delivered into the soft tissue socket. The dry material absorbs the blood at the site as it is gently condensed over the Bio-Oss graft.

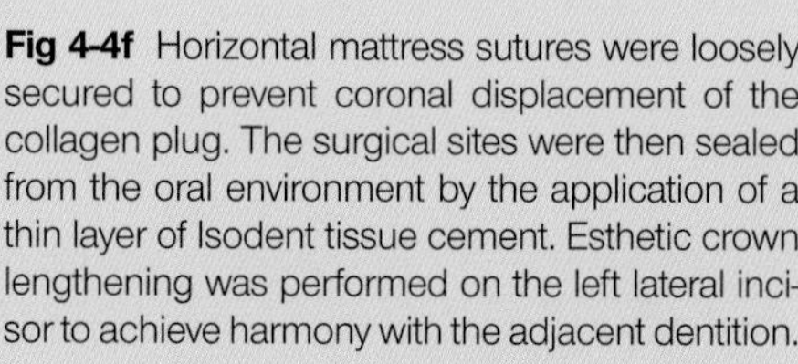

Fig 4-4f Horizontal mattress sutures were loosely secured to prevent coronal displacement of the collagen plug. The surgical sites were then sealed from the oral environment by the application of a thin layer of Isodent tissue cement. Esthetic crown lengthening was performed on the left lateral incisor to achieve harmony with the adjacent dentition.

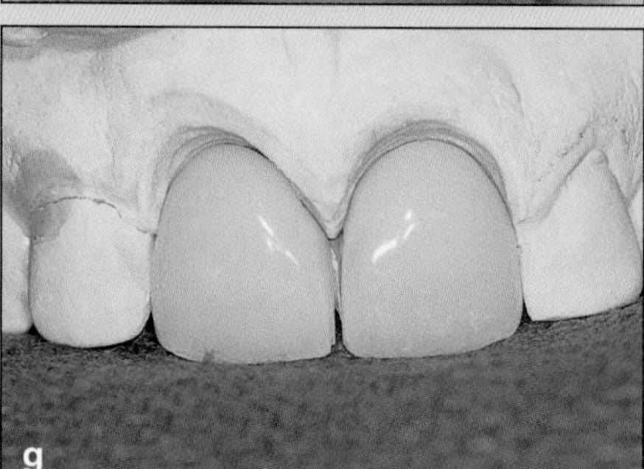
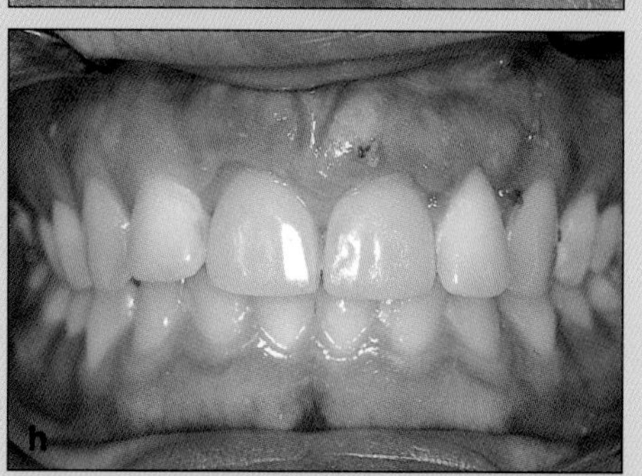

Fig 4-4g Ovate pontic removable provisional restoration was fabricated with symmetrical central incisor pontics. These pontics were not designed to follow the pre-existing, unesthetic soft tissue contours. Instead, the pontics were idealized in terms of their dimensions and contours.

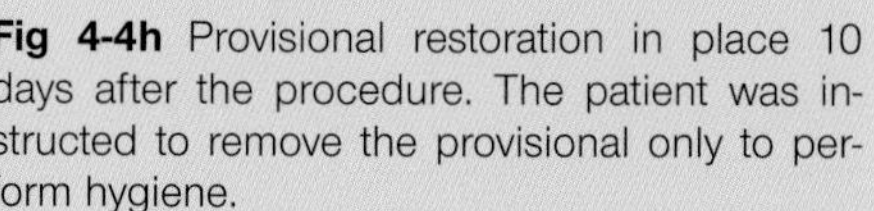

Fig 4-4h Provisional restoration in place 10 days after the procedure. The patient was instructed to remove the provisional only to perform hygiene.

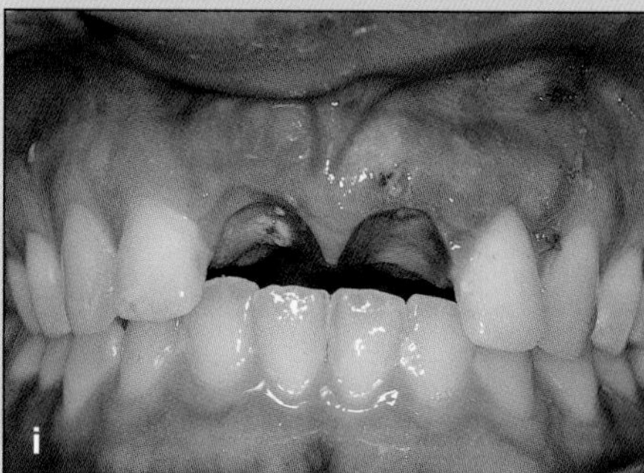
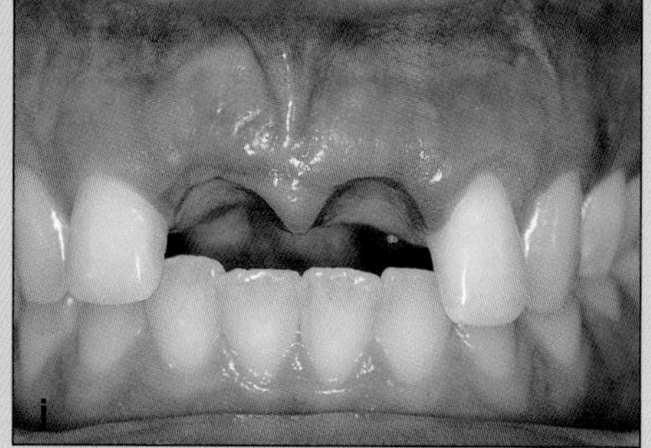

Fig 4-4i Surgical sites 10 days after the procedure. Note the rapid epithelialization of the sockets over the CollaPlug material and the preservation of soft tissue architecture and papillary morphology at the site.

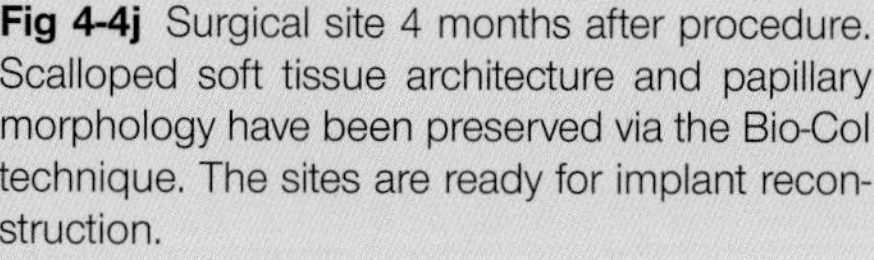

Fig 4-4j Surgical site 4 months after procedure. Scalloped soft tissue architecture and papillary morphology have been preserved via the Bio-Col technique. The sites are ready for implant reconstruction.

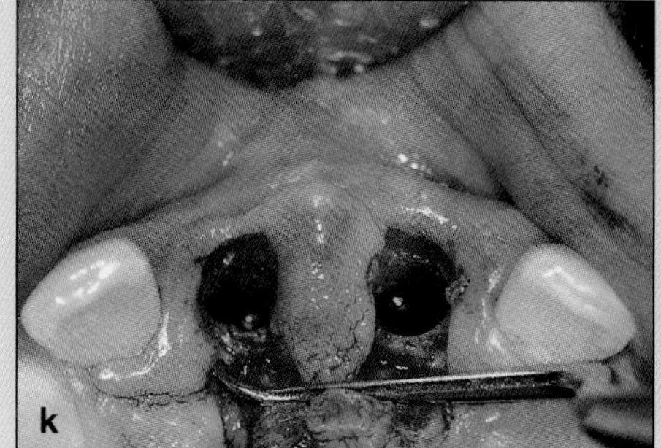
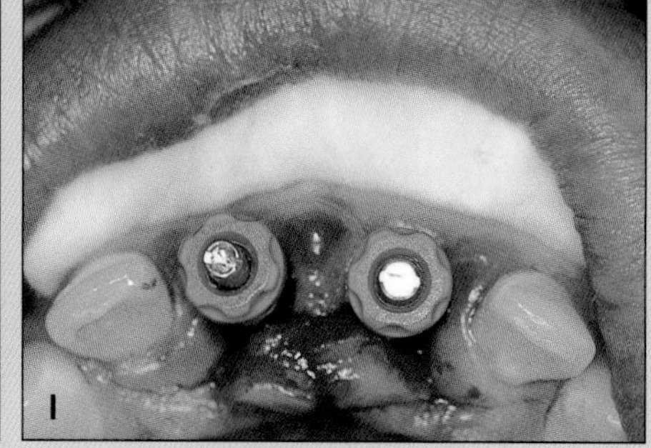

Fig 4-4k Palatal peninsula flaps, which allow for visualization of the crestal portion of the osteotomy preparation, were used to gain access for implant placement. Note that the preparation does not extend to the original socket walls; instead, the implants will be placed into preparations lined by partially integrated graft consisting of Bio-Oss and vital bone.

Fig 4-4l After placement of tapered root-analog implants (Frialit-2; Dentsply, York, PA), surgical indexing was performed and peninsula flaps reapproximated.

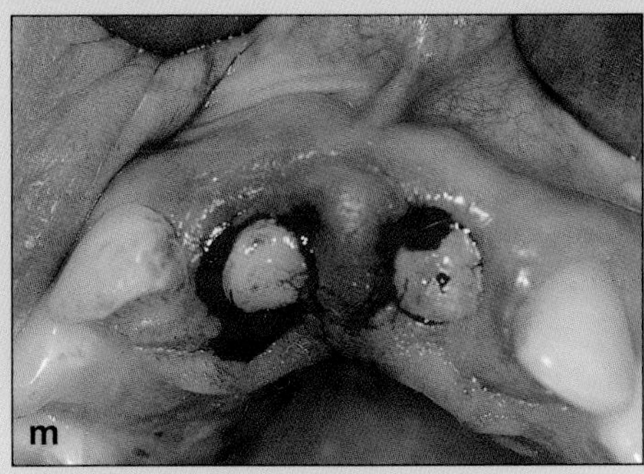

Fig 4-4m After a 4-month osseointegration period, implants were exposed by means of a disposable tissue punch.

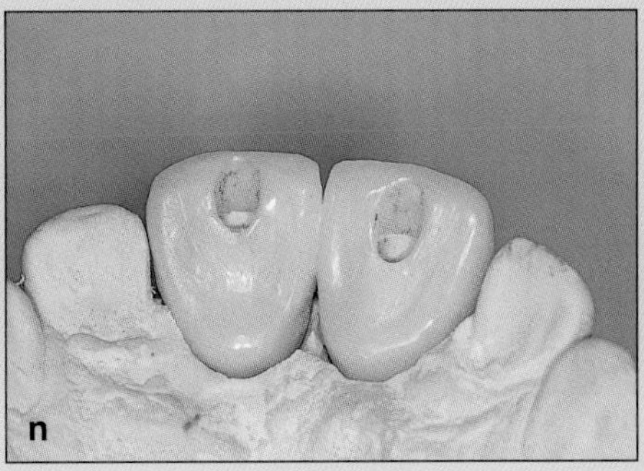

Fig 4-4n Provisional restoration fabricated on an altered cast fabricated from the surgical index.

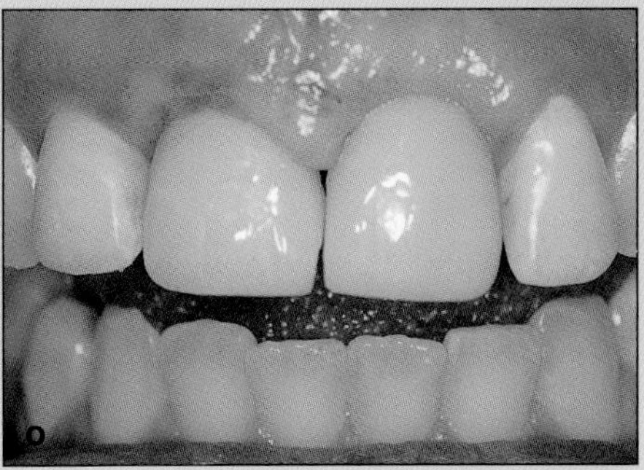

Fig 4-4o Screw-retained provisional restoration was delivered through conservative access provided by the tissue punch.

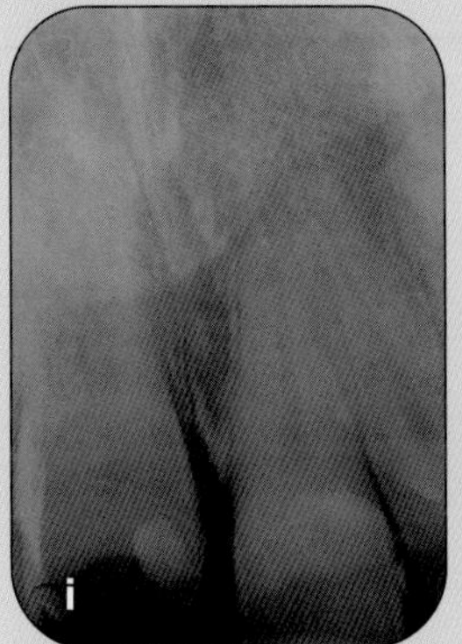

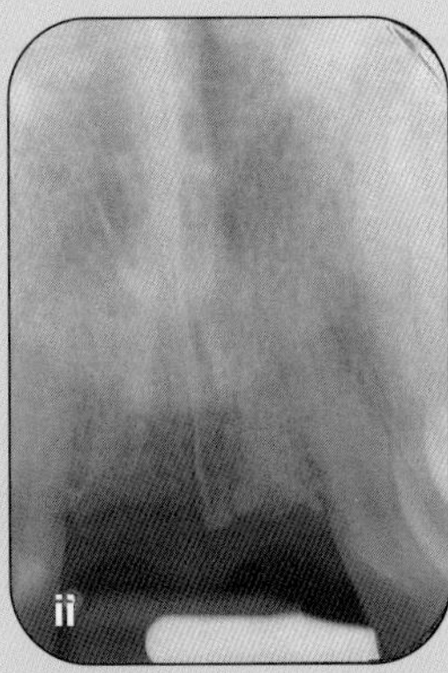

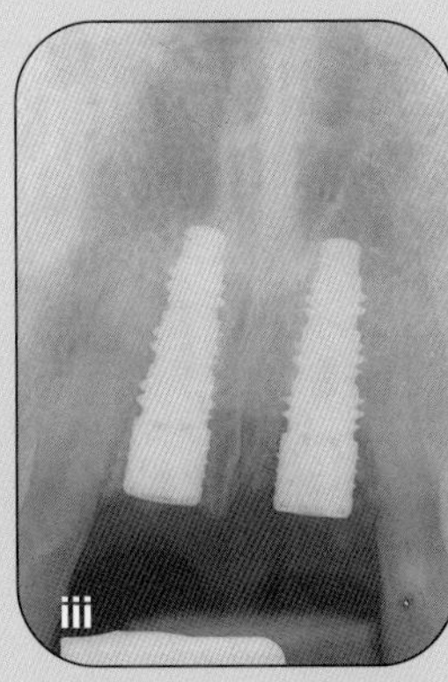

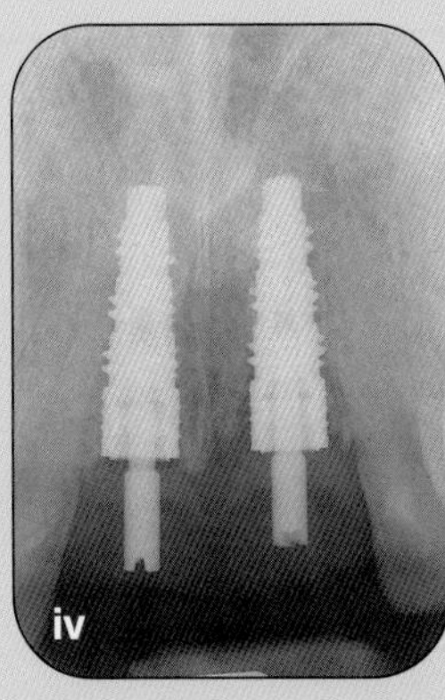

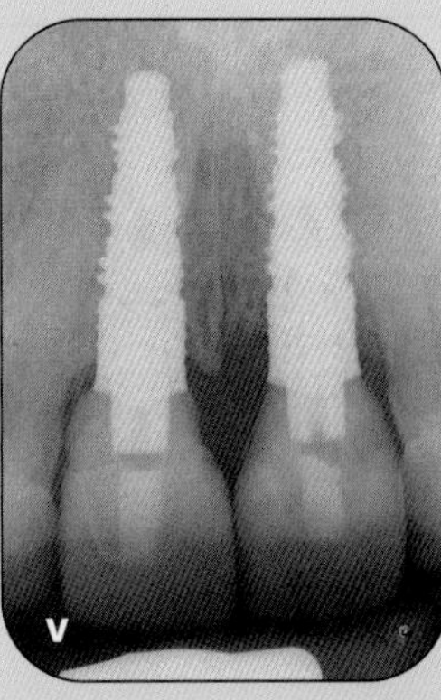

Fig 4-4p Series of radiographs demonstrating pretreatment condition *(i)*, postextraction condition *(ii)*, implant placement *(iii)*, delivery of provisional restoration *(iv)*, and final restoration *(v)*. Note the progression from initial integration of the graft at the site followed by the gradually increased difficulty of discerning the graft at its apical extent and the continued incorporation of the graft coronally.

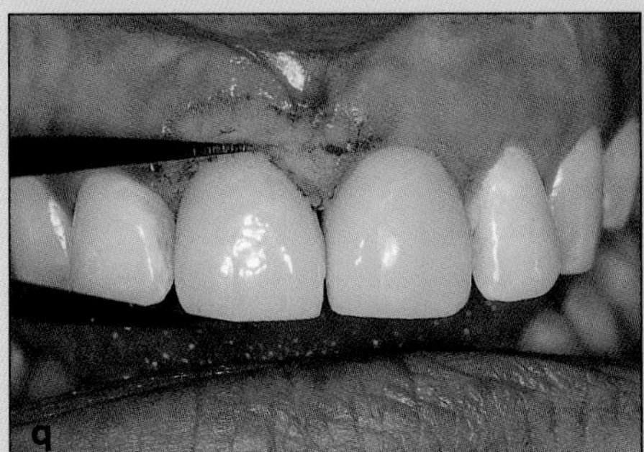

Fig 4-4q A CO_2 laser was used to perform esthetic soft tissue recontouring and resurfacing. Castroviello caliper is used to verify the symmetrical height of the central incisors.

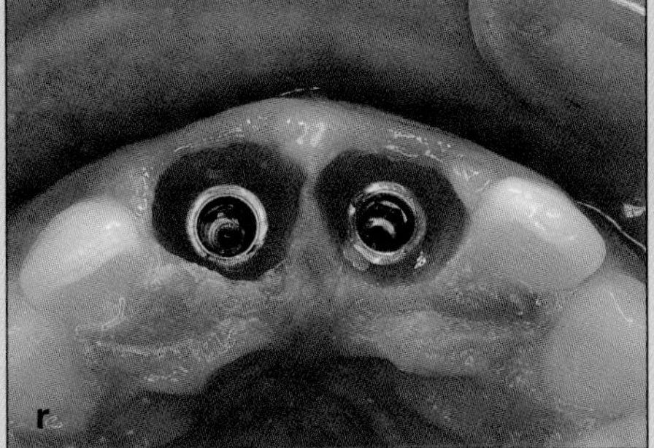

Fig 4-4r Two months after implant exposure, the provisionals were removed, revealing preservation of the soft tissue volume and architecture surrounding the implant sites. A "prosthetic-friendly" environment now awaits final impressions.

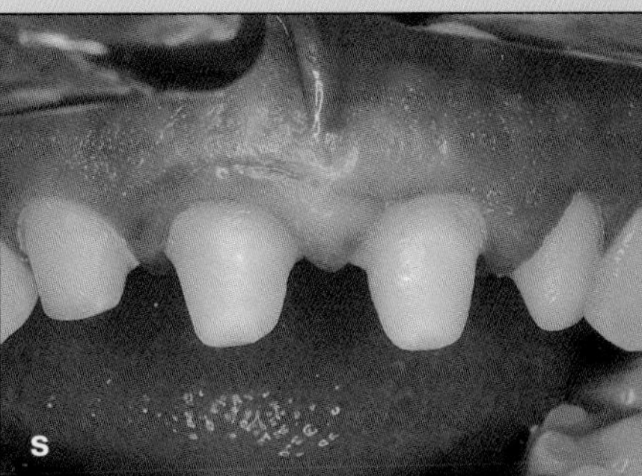

Fig 4-4s Seating of anatomically shaped ceramic abutments.

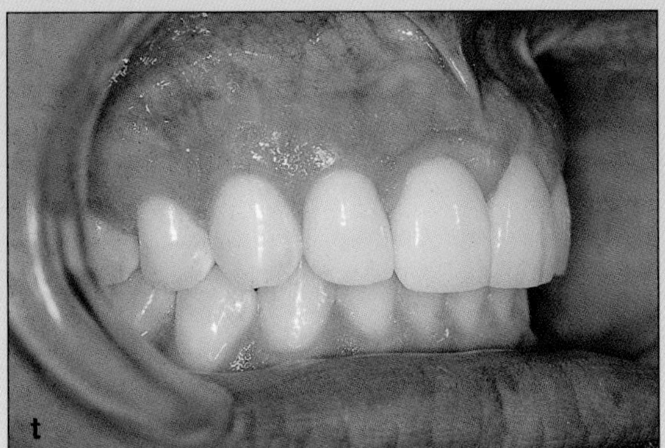

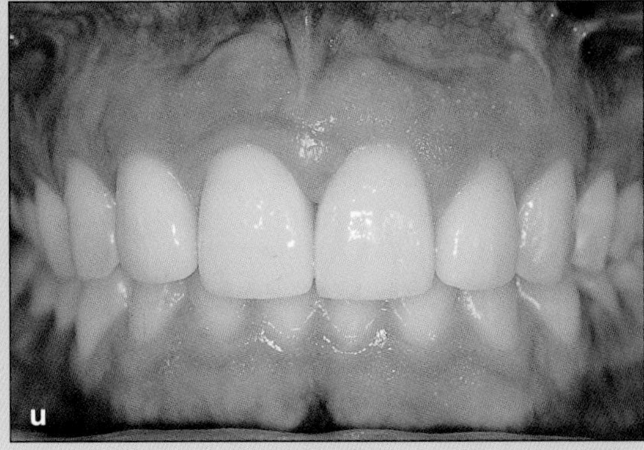

Figs 4-4t and 4-4u Final restorations are natural in appearance and demonstrate enhanced esthetics compared to the pretreatment condition. Hard and soft tissue preservation afforded by the Bio-Col technique ensured natural restorative emergence without prosthetic compensations. (Restoration by Dr Jorge Blanco, Miami, FL.)

Bio-Col technique in preparation for delayed implant replacement of fractured maxillary central incisors

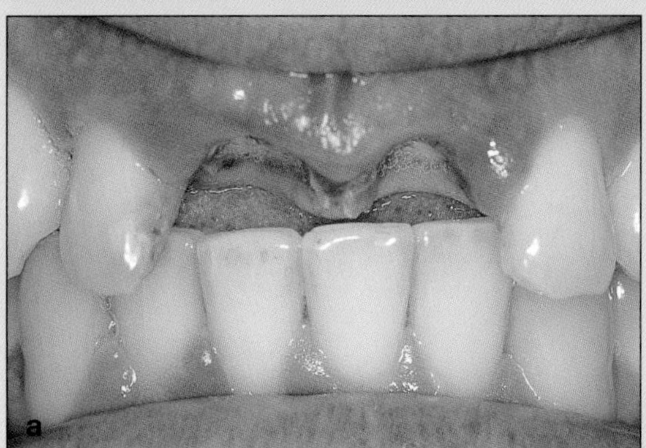

Fig 4-5a Preoperative view of trauma-induced fracture of maxillary central incisors, which necessitated their removal. Delayed implant placement was indicated due to periapical pathology as well as a possible defect of the buccal socket walls secondary to trauma.

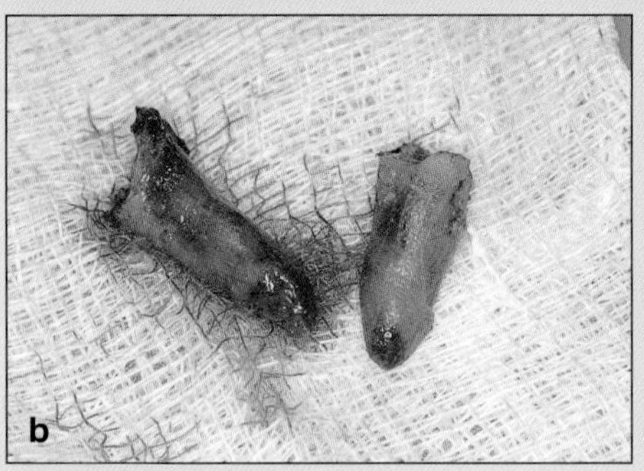

Fig 4-5b The residual roots were carefully removed. Oral-facial sectioning was required to maintain the integrity of the socket.

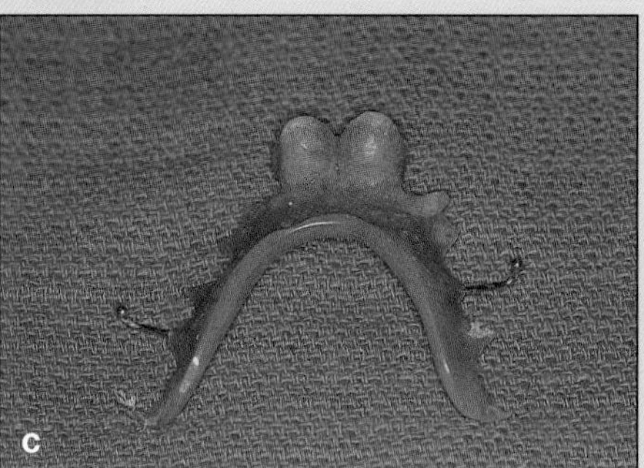

Fig 4-5c A removable partial denture with ovate pontics was prepared for immediate delivery. Clasp retainers prevent deleterious apicocoronal movement of the provisional restoration.

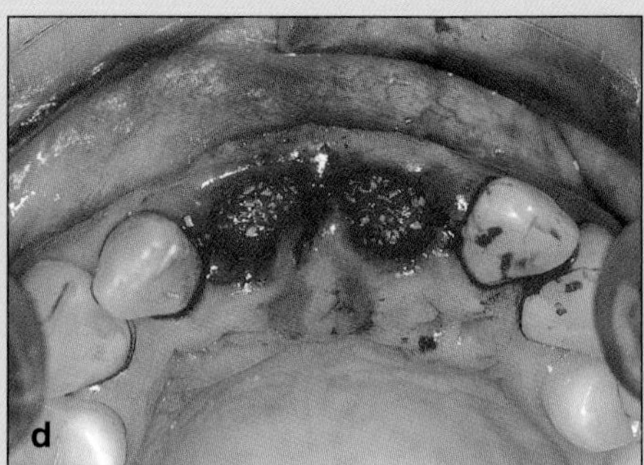

Fig 4-5d Extraction sockets grafted with Bio-Oss deproteinized bovine bone mineral. Thorough curettage and perforation of the socket walls was necessary to stimulate bleeding.

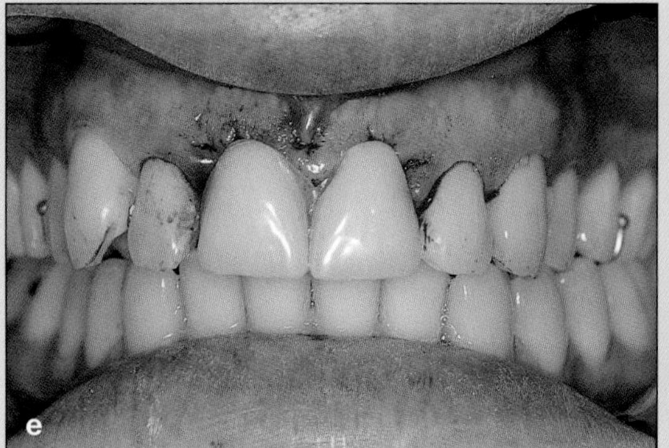

Fig 4-5e After the sockets were sealed with absorbable collagen dressing and tissue cement, the ovate pontics were adjusted to extend approximately 3 to 4 mm subgingivally. The patient was instructed to remove the provisional restoration only to perform oral hygiene for the first 2 weeks following tooth removal and for only brief daily periods thereafter.

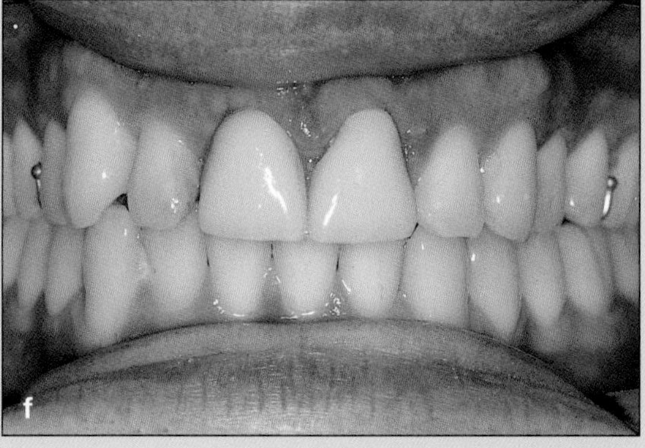

Fig 4-5f One-week postoperative appearance of surgical site. Note the soft tissue support provided by the ovate pontics.

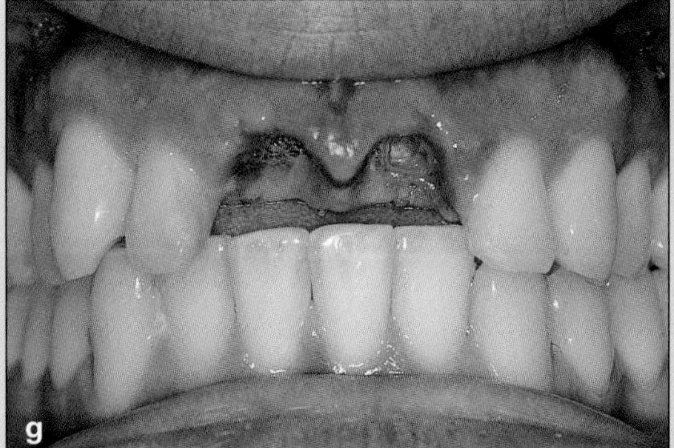

Fig 4-5g One-week postoperative appearance of surgical site. Note the maintenance of natural soft tissue architecture and the rapid re-epithelialization of the socket, which occurred further coronally than is typically observed.

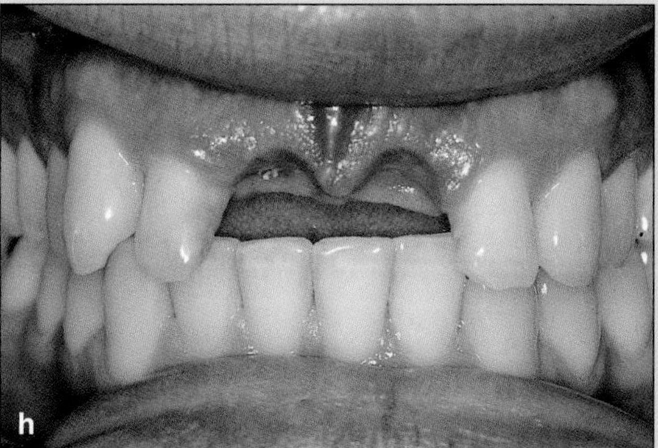

Fig 4-5h Appearance of site 3 months after tooth removal, showing no evidence of ridge collapse and an intact scalloped gingival anatomy.

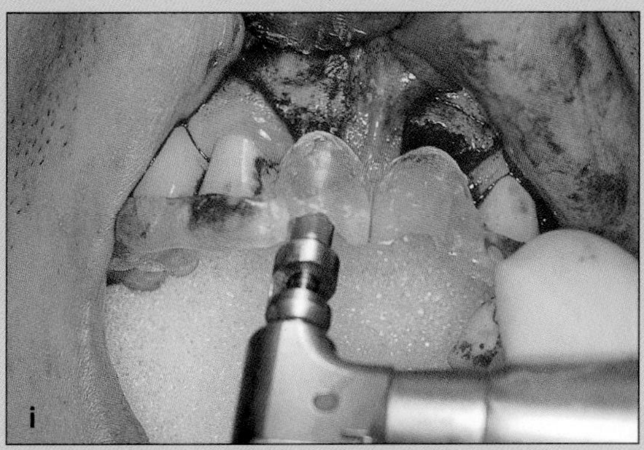

Fig 4-5i Implant placement as dictated by the surgical guide resulted in apical fenestration during osteotomy preparation for the right central incisor.

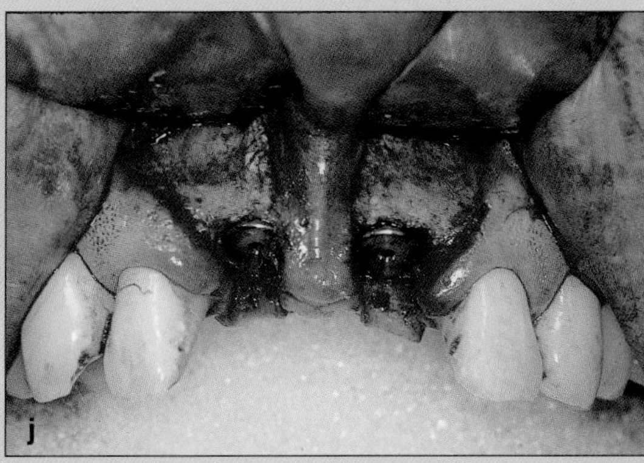

Fig 4-5j Submerged implants. The fenestration defect will be treated with a bone graft and guided bone regeneration procedure. Despite the use of the Bio-Col technique, unfavorable ridge morphology necessitated the use of buccal flaps for a correction of the resultant osseous defects. This may result in an esthetic defect secondary to the soft tissue shrinkage.

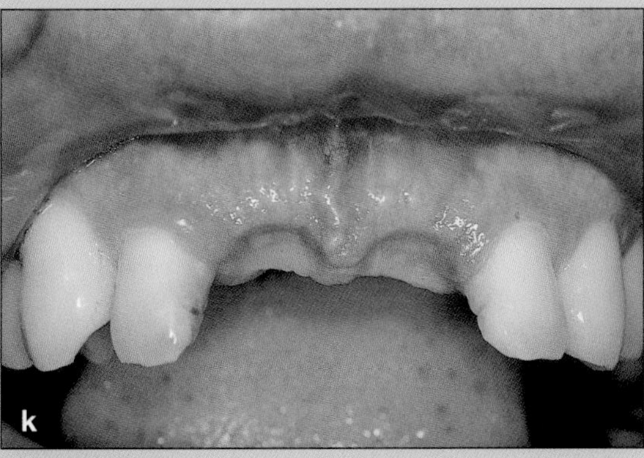

Fig 4-5k Four-month postoperative view. Despite some translucency of the thin buccal soft tissues, natural alveolar ridge anatomy and the central incisor interdental papilla are intact in the area critical for prosthetic emergence.

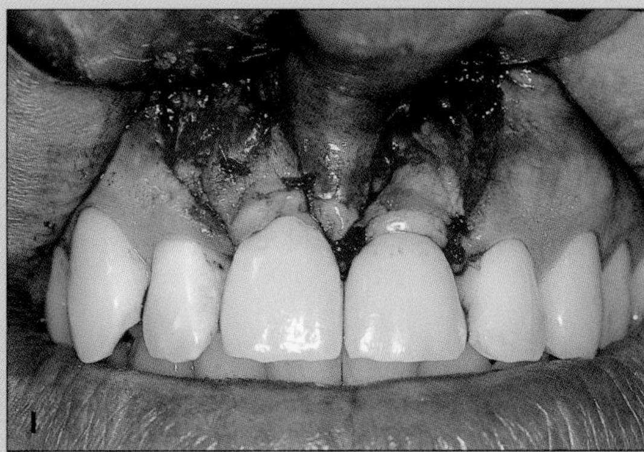

Fig 4-5l Subepithelial connective tissue grafts, performed in conjunction with delivery of custom abutments and provisional implant restorations to eliminate metal showthrough.

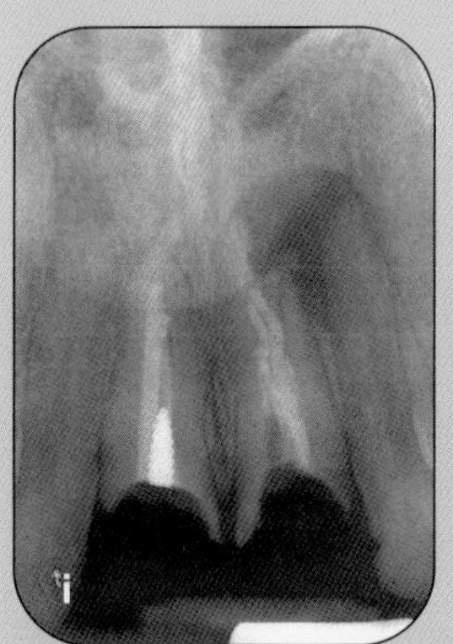

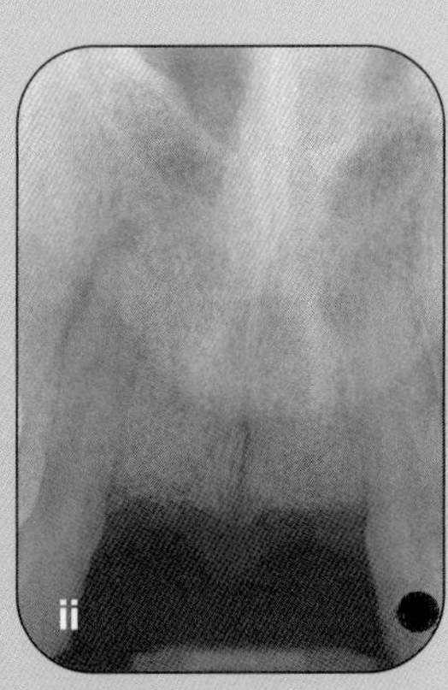

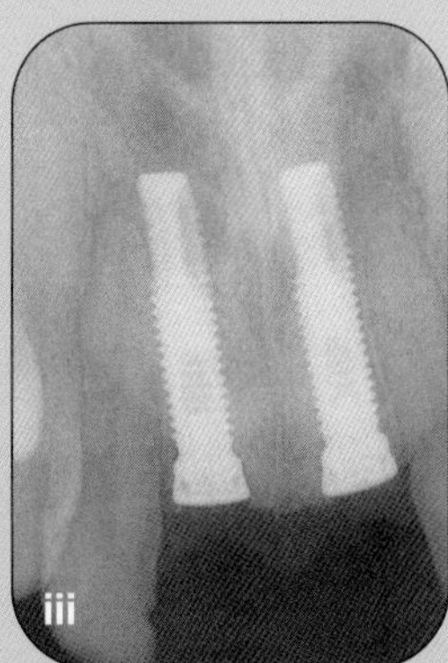

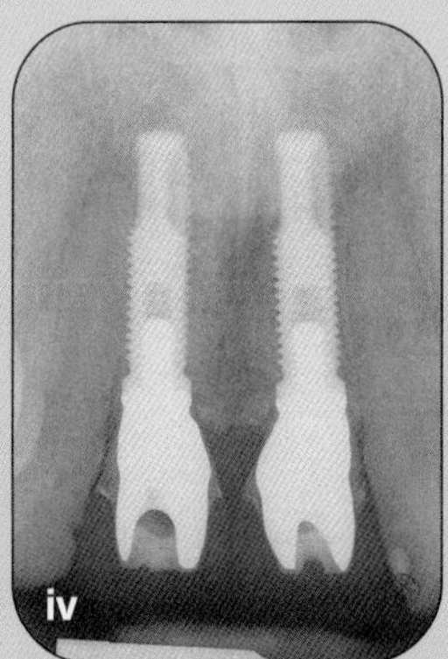

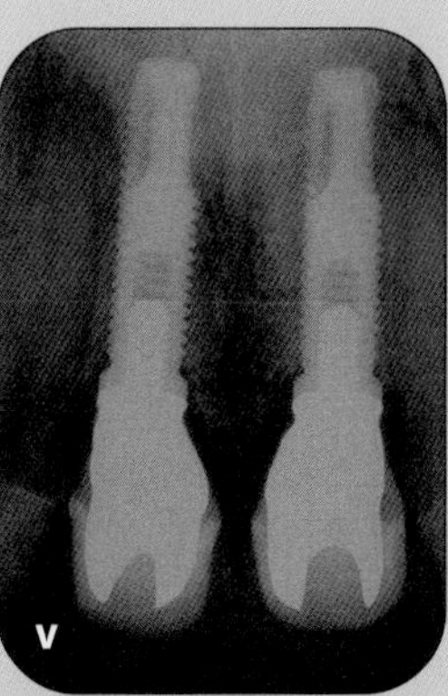

Fig 4-5m Series of radiographs demonstrating pretreatment condition *(i)*, postextraction condition *(ii)*, implant placement *(iii)*, delivery of provisional restoration *(iv)*, and final restoration *(v)*. Note the progression from initial integration of the graft at the site followed by the gradually increased difficulty of discerning the graft at its apical extent and the continued incorporation of the graft coronally.

Fig 4-5n Appearance of final restoration 1 year after delivery. Note the maintenance of the natural alveolar ridge contours and the presence of the interdental papilla between the central incisor implants. Preservation of the alveolar ridge anatomy following tooth removal enabled the creation of inconspicuous implant restorations with minimal adjunctive procedures. (Restoration by Dr Jorge Blanco, Miami, FL.)

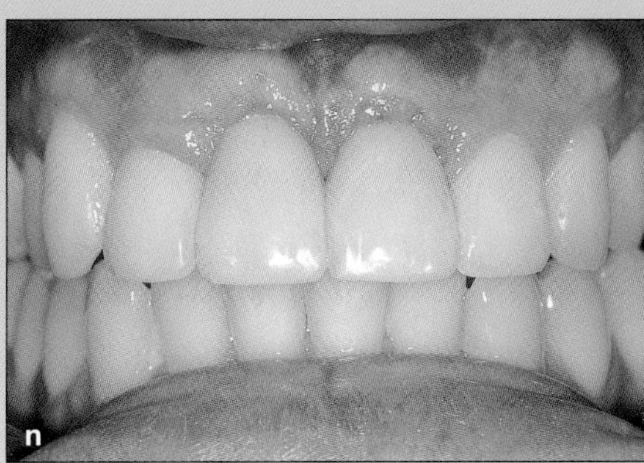

Surgical protocol for defect sockets

Inspection and probing of the socket after tooth removal will delineate the size and location of any existing bony defects. The socket is then thoroughly debrided while maintaining the integrity of the soft tissues overlying the bony defect (Fig 4-6a). Osseous defects most commonly occur in the buccal socket walls. The bone in the areas surrounding the socket is perforated with a small carbide bur to create bleeding and to maximize the ability of osteoprogenitor cells to invade the grafted socket. This is often necessary in extraction sites where circulation is compromised secondary to previous trauma, endodontic therapy, or multiple surgical procedures. Growth factors derived from autologous platelet-rich plasma (PRP) have been used by the author as an additional strategy to enhance osseous regeneration within defect sockets treated with the Bio-Col technique, as described later in this chapter.

Next, the periosteum is gently elevated approximately 2 mm beyond the periphery of the bony defect using both a Buser periosteal elevator and a Lucas surgical curette (Fig 4-6b). This creates a subperiosteal pocket that is slightly larger than the defect. A resorbable membrane (Bio-Gide; Osteohealth) is then carefully sized and fitted into this subperiosteal pocket. The blunt end of a membrane-placement instrument is moistened in sterile saline and used to precisely position the membrane within the pocket (Fig 4-6c). The membrane should extend beyond the periphery of the osseous wall defect in all areas.

The graft material (Bio-Oss alone or Bio-Oss + autogenous marrow bone) is then condensed into the defect. The defect is slightly overfilled, resulting in buccal expansion of the overlying mucoperiosteal tissues and bulging of the membrane buccally. Digital pressure should be maintained over the labial soft tissues while the graft is condensed to avoid compromising the circulation to the mucoperiosteal tissues through overdistention. Any excess membrane protruding coronally from the socket can be adapted over the graft material in the socket. Slight expansion of the overlying soft tissues will be noted. CollaPlug absorbable collagen dressing is then placed over the graft or graft-membrane complex and sealed with Isodent tissue cement, as previously described for the intact socket (Fig 4-7).

Following 4 to 6 months of healing, a conservative flap approach is used for implant placement. Both surgeon and patient must be prepared for the possible need for additional bone grafting despite the presence of favorable defect morphology at the time of tooth removal. If the osseous regeneration is incomplete, the surgeon must decide whether to proceed with additional bone grafting, implant placement, or both. This decision is based not only on the ability to stabilize the implant in an ideal position but also on how well the graft has integrated at the recipient site. The graft may demonstrate a bone-like consistency that is maintained during osteotomy preparation (Fig 4-8). If it does, no additional bone grafting is needed, and the implant is placed in a standard fashion. When the repair of the defect is complete, additional bone grafting is avoided despite the pre-existence of a significant buccal wall defect grafted at the time of tooth extraction. This is often the case when the defect morphology is favorable, as described above, and the regenerative potential of the site is optimal (healthy bleeding site). In other instances, the grafted material will have areas that are not completely integrated at the site but remain intact during osteotomy preparation and implant placement. If portions of the graft are soft or gelatinous, additional bone grafting may be performed simultaneously with implant placement. A mixture of autogenous bone and Bio-Oss, along with a long-lasting resorbable membrane, are used to obtain predictable guided bone regeneration at the site, as previously described.

Finally, in instances where the graft has failed to integrate at the site, additional bone grafting prior to implant placement is unavoidable despite the presence of favorable defect morphology following tooth removal, as described above. This usually occurs at an extraction site with decreased regenerative potential secondary to previous trauma, infection, periodontal disease, surgery, or multiple endodontic procedures. In addition, a graft at any site may fail to integrate solely as a result of transmission of micromotion to the site from an unstable provisional restoration. In these situations, a staged approach to reconstruction of the area becomes necessary. These scenarios can be distinguished from those at sites where unfavorable defect morphology immediately commits the surgeon to performing additional site development prior to implant placement in order to avoid long-term functional and esthetic compromises.

Prosthetic protocol for delayed implant placement

Soft tissue architecture at the extraction site is preserved by immediately supporting the soft tissues surrounding the extraction socket with an interim provisional restoration that extends approximately 3 to 4 mm into the socket. The provisional restoration should have an ovate pontic design. Upon delivery, the provisional restoration slightly condenses the collagen dressing and helps protect the surgical site from subsequent

Bio-Col technique for delayed implant placement in the defect socket

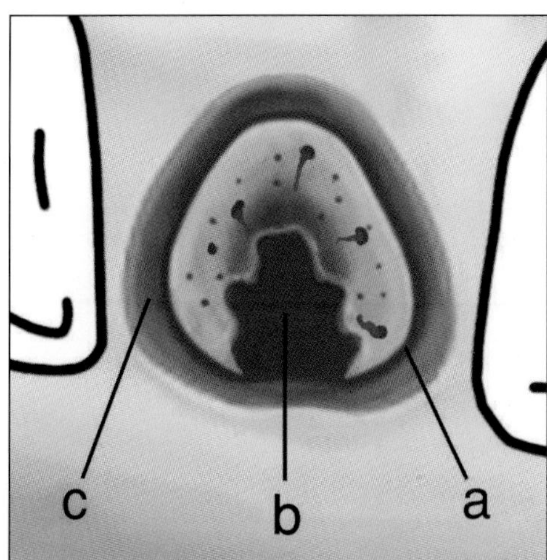

Fig 4-6a Following tooth removal, a buccal wall defect of favorable morphology is present. Thorough curettage of the socket is performed, and the socket walls are perforated, if necessary, to obtain bleeding. A subperiosteal pocket is created by carefully elevating the periosteum beyond the defect area. *(a)* Crestal bone level; *(b)* buccal wall defect of favorable morphology (ie, less than one third the mesiodistal dimension between the adjacent dentition); *(c)* soft tissues surrounding the extraction site.

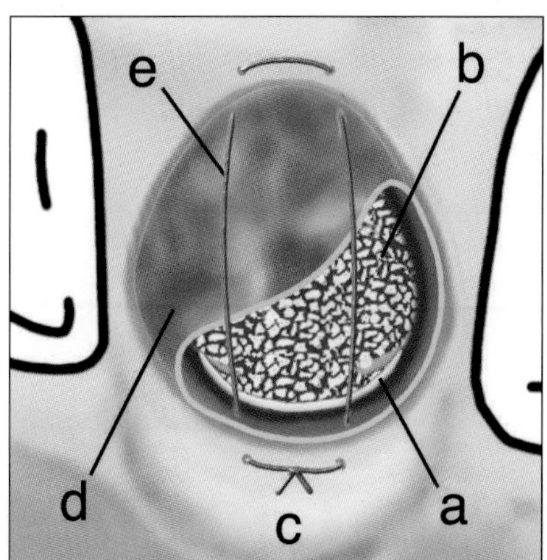

Fig 4-6b Prior to grafting the socket, a Bio-Gide resorbable collagen membrane *(a)* is placed in the prepared subperiosteal pocket. The membrane is sized to overlap the periphery of the bony socket wall defect. Bio-Oss bone mineral *(b)* is then grafted into the socket and defect area. The condensed graft material slightly expands the overlying soft tissues *(c)*. CollaPlug absorbable dressing *(d)* is placed over the graft and maintained with a horizontal mattress suture *(e)*. A thin coat of Isodent tissue cement is then applied to the surgical site to seal it from the oral cavity.

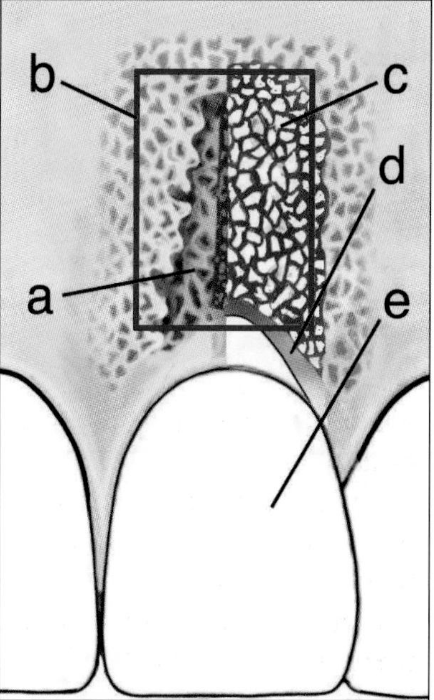

Fig 4-6c The Bio-Gide resorbable membrane has been accurately sized to overlap the periphery of the buccal wall defect by approximately 2 mm. *(a)* Buccal wall defect; *(b)* outline of appropriately sized Bio-Gide resorbable membrane placed in subperiosteal pocket; *(c)* condensed Bio-Oss graft with blood clot; *(d)* CollaPlug absorbable dressing; *(e)* ovate pontic provisional restoration extending 3 to 4 mm subgingivally, compressing the CollaPlug dressing and supporting the surrounding soft tissues.

mechanical trauma (see Figs 4-3c and 4-6c). A fixed or removable restoration can be used for this purpose. To ensure optimal soft tissue support, the restoration should be fabricated with contours identical to those of the extracted natural tooth. A removable provisional restoration must be designed to avoid apicocoronal movements over the site, which have been observed to cause the loss of a portion of the graft material, poor integration at the site, or chronic inflammation and disfigurement of the soft tissues. The addition of clasp retainers and occlusal rests, along with careful adjustments to traditional removable provisional restorations, eliminates these problems (see Figs 4-4 and 4-5). Nevertheless, the author favors the use of a fixed interim provisional restoration or tooth-borne removable prosthesis (see Figs 4-7 and 4-8). In certain cases, an Essex retainer with an ovate pontic may be used (see Fig 4-6c).

The crown of the extracted tooth can sometimes be modified into an ovate pontic, which is then bonded to the adjacent dentition or incorporated into an Essex retainer. The provisional restoration is periodically re-evaluated and adjusted to ensure optimal soft tissue support during healing. This results in an ideal prosthetic recipient site for esthetic emergence of the final restoration.

Bio-Col technique in preparation for delayed implant placement of maxillary central incisor with buccal wall defect

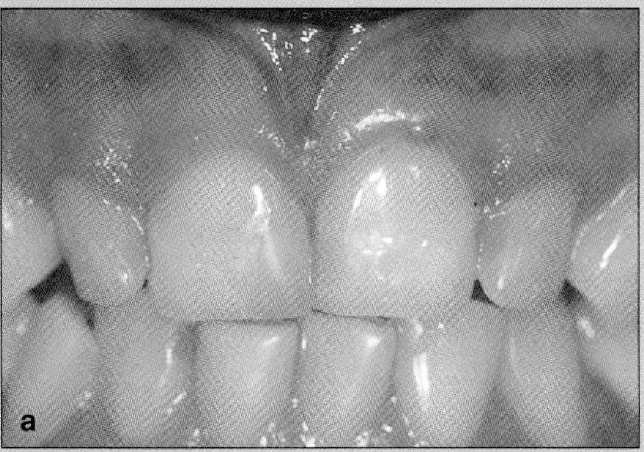

Fig 4-7a Preoperative view of ankylosed and resorbing maxillary left central incisor. No infection is present. Soft tissue pathology presents an esthetic risk for immediate implant placement.

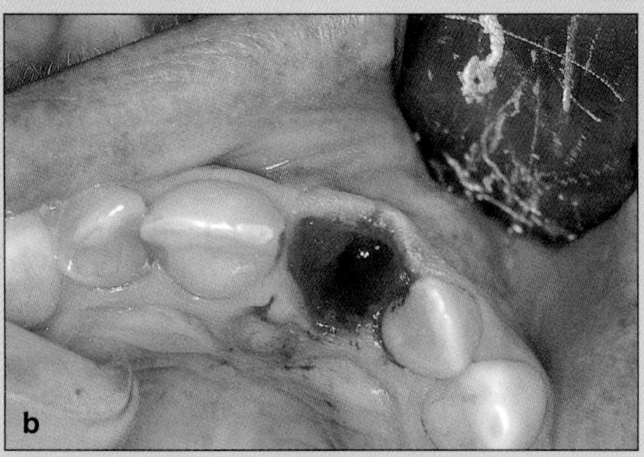

Fig 4-7b Despite the use of periotomes and careful sectioning of the tooth, a buccal wall defect resulted. The width of the defect is less than one third the mesiodistal dimension between the adjacent teeth, thus favoring possible regeneration.

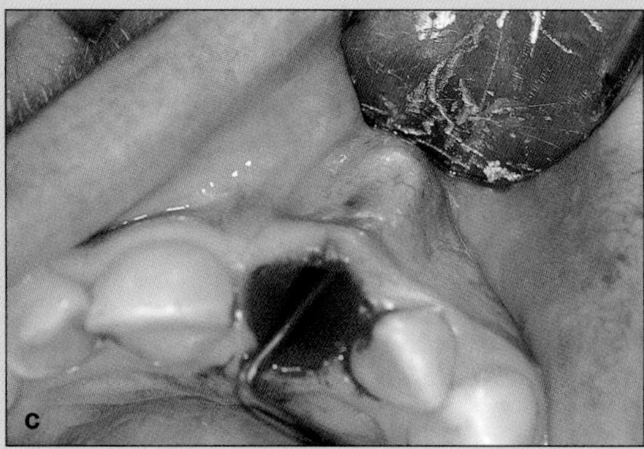

Fig 4-7c Use of a periodontal probe demonstrates that the height of the defect extends to the apex of the socket. Note the thickness of the adjacent osseous defect margin.

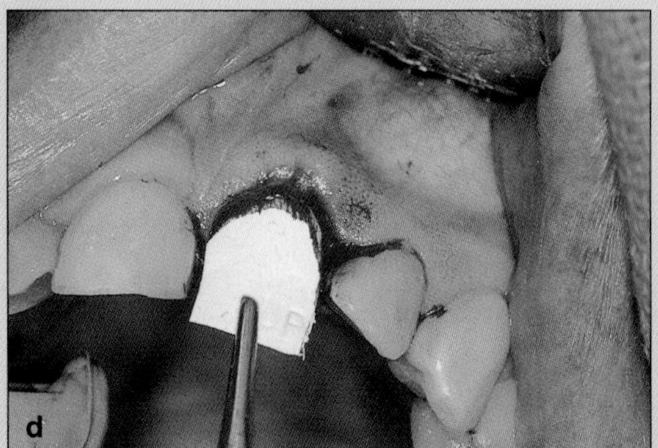

Fig 4-7d After thorough curettage and perforation of the socket walls to create bleeding, a pre-shaped Bio-Gide resorbable collagen membrane is stabilized in the subperiosteal pocket and extends around the periphery of the defect.

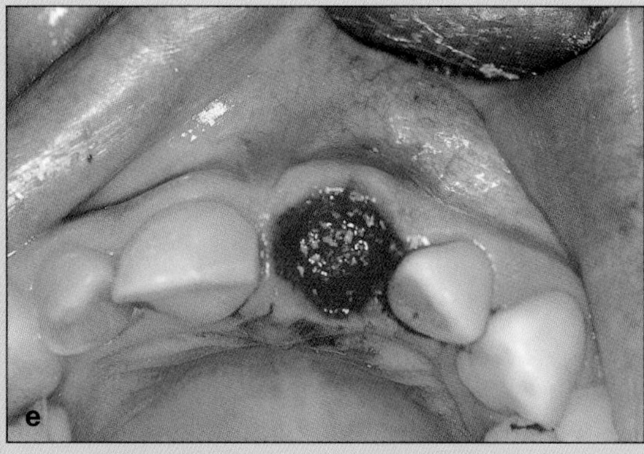

Fig 4-7e Bio-Oss has been condensed into the bleeding socket. Digital pressure over the buccal soft tissues prevents overdistention. The site was subsequently sealed with CollaPlug and Isodent tissue cement and provisionalized with a toothborne Essex retainer restoration.

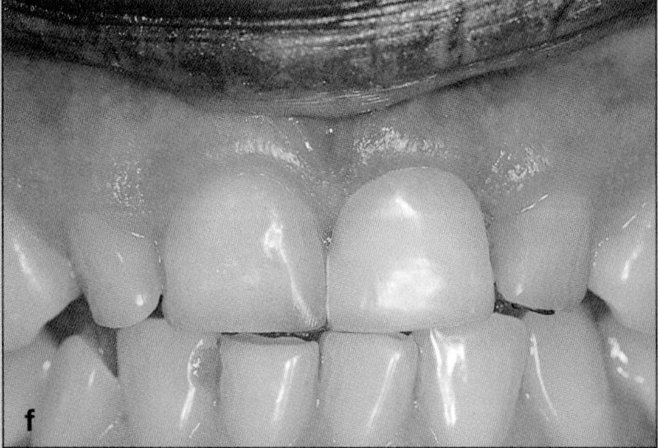

Fig 4-7f A provisional resin-bonded restoration was delivered after 10 days of healing to optimize tissue support and integration of the graft at the site.

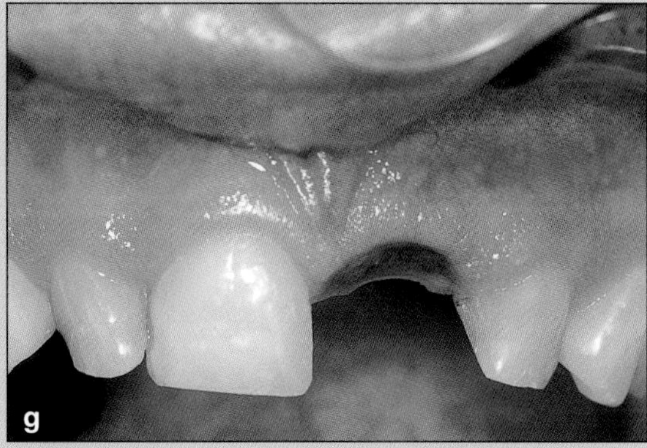

Fig 4-7g Clinical view 4 months after tooth removal demonstrates preservation of alveolar ridge contours at the site. Soft tissue health and appearance are ideal.

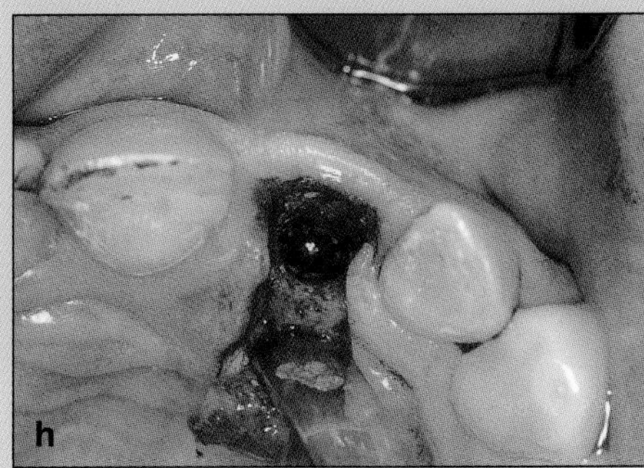

Fig 4-7h A palatal peninsula flap is used to access the site for osteotomy preparation. After preparation, the repaired buccal wall remains intact, and there is adequate bleeding for successful osseointegration in all areas of the socket. The preparation does not extend to the original socket walls.

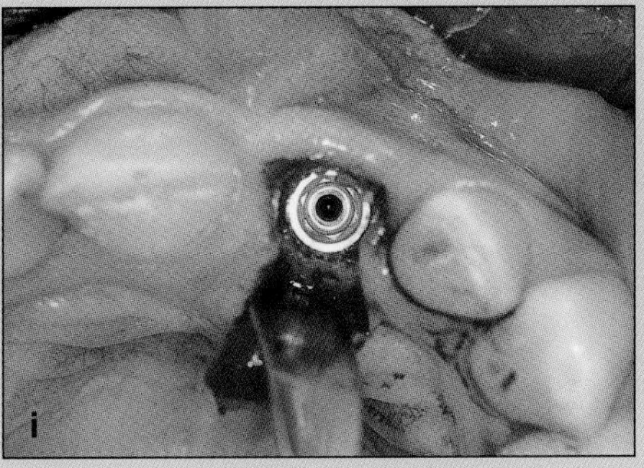

Fig 4-7i Placement of a tapered root-analog implant (Frialit-2). Although the Bio-Oss graft is only partially integrated at the site, the particles are reduced in size and have been partially replaced by viable bone.

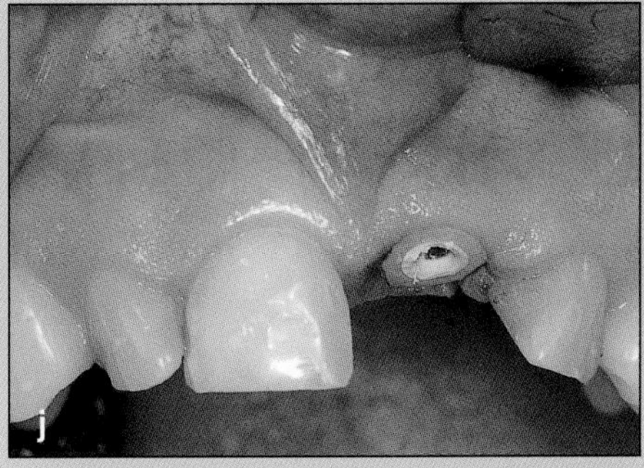

Fig 4-7j A customized tooth-form abutment is used for immediate support of the surrounding tissues with a one-stage approach.

Fig 4-7k Series of radiographs demonstrating pretreatment condition *(i)*, 1-week postoperative condition *(ii)*, 4-month postoperative condition *(iii)*, implant placement *(iv)*, final restoration *(v)*, and 1-year postfunction condition *(vi)*. Note the progression from initial integration of the graft at the site followed by the gradually increased difficulty of discerning the graft at its apical extent and the continued incorporation of the graft coronally.

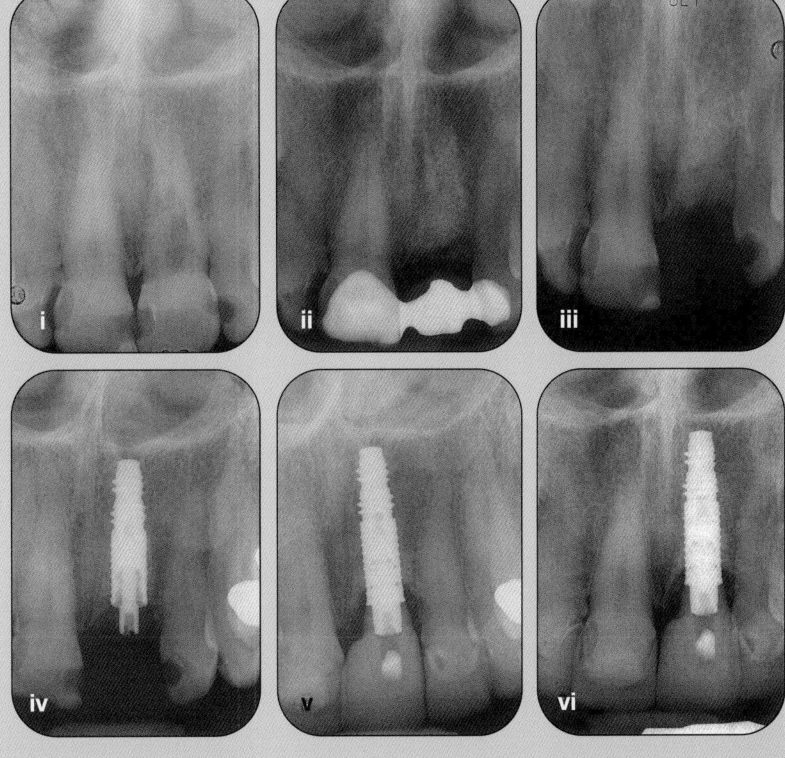

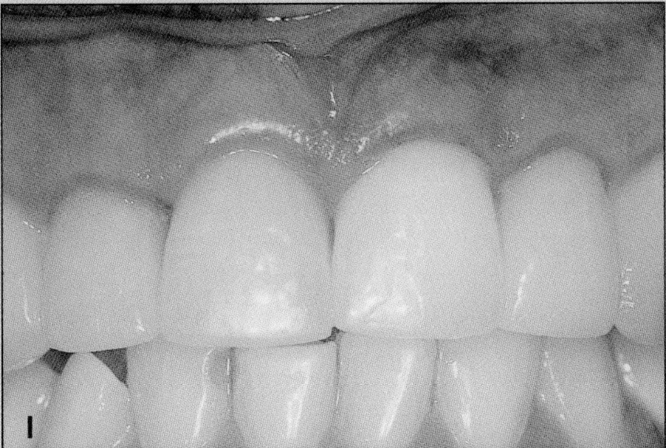

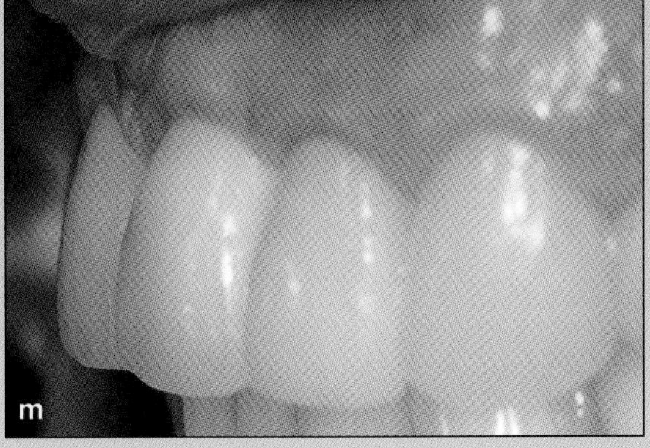

Figs 4-7l and 4-7m No evidence of resorption or collapse of the regenerated buccal plate defect is seen after 1 year of function. The restoration is natural in appearance and soft tissue esthetics are excellent. (Restoration by Dr Gordon Sokoloff, Coral Gables, FL.)

Bio-Col technique in preparation for delayed implant placement of maxillary central incisor with buccal wall defect

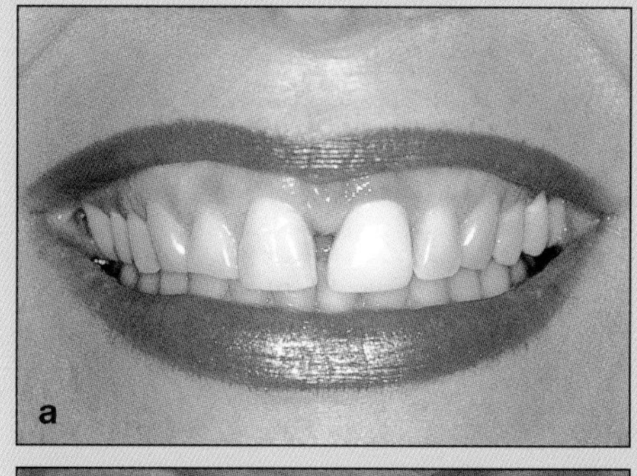

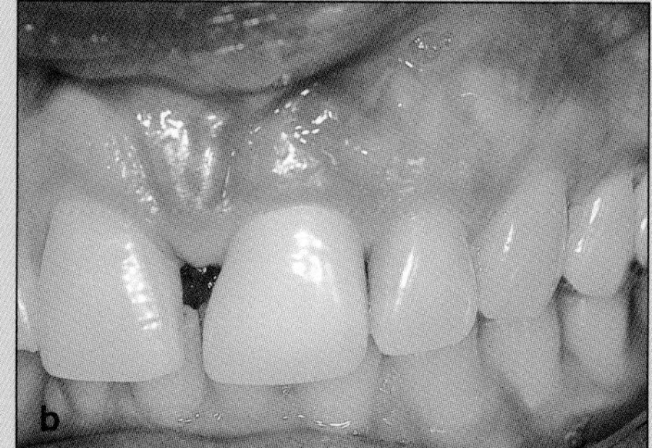

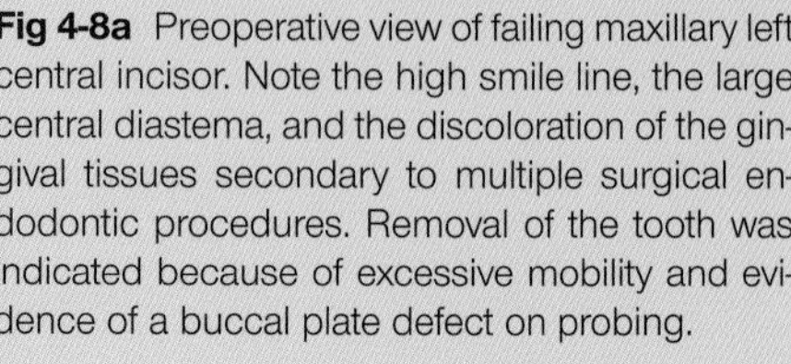

Fig 4-8a Preoperative view of failing maxillary left central incisor. Note the high smile line, the large central diastema, and the discoloration of the gingival tissues secondary to multiple surgical endodontic procedures. Removal of the tooth was indicated because of excessive mobility and evidence of a buccal plate defect on probing.

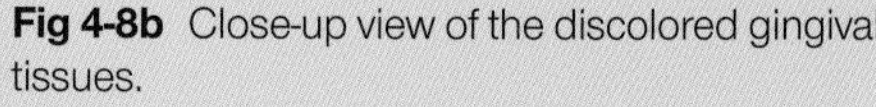

Fig 4-8b Close-up view of the discolored gingival tissues.

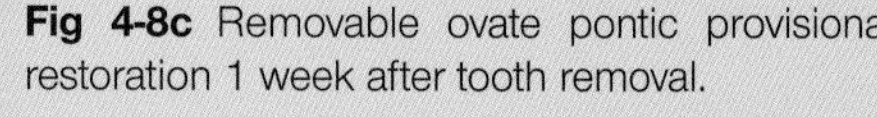

Fig 4-8c Removable ovate pontic provisional restoration 1 week after tooth removal.

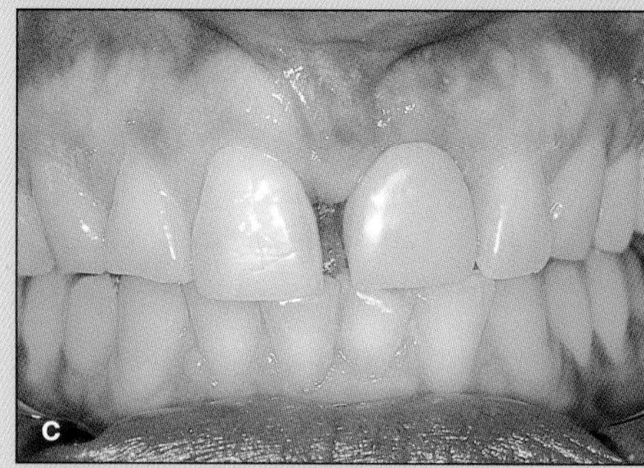

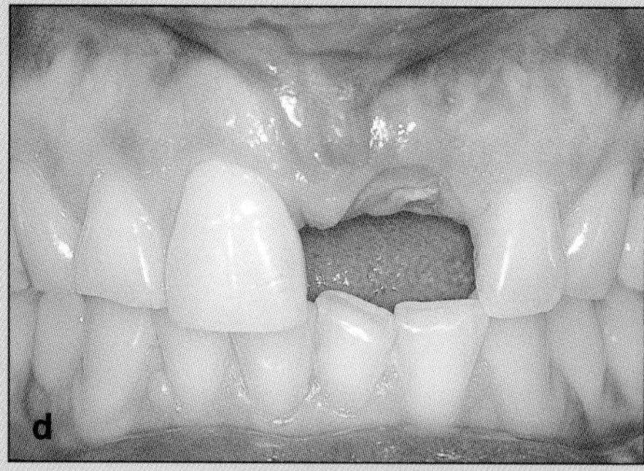

Fig 4-8d After tooth removal, a Bio-Gide membrane was stabilized in a subperiosteal pocket created around the periphery of the defect. The Bio-Col technique was then performed. Note the rapid re-epithelialization of the socket and the maintenance of the soft tissue architecture evident 1 week after tooth removal.

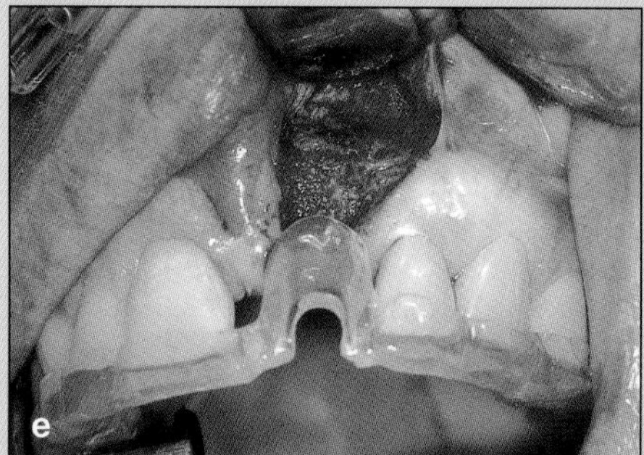

Fig 4-8e Four months after tooth removal, the site was re-entered and evaluated for an additional hard tissue grafting procedure, either in conjunction with or prior to implant placement. After elevation of a buccal flap, adequate integration of the graft at the site was noted, and the graft demonstrated a hard, bone-like consistency. The surgical guide also indicated adequate hard tissue volume for ideal fixture placement.

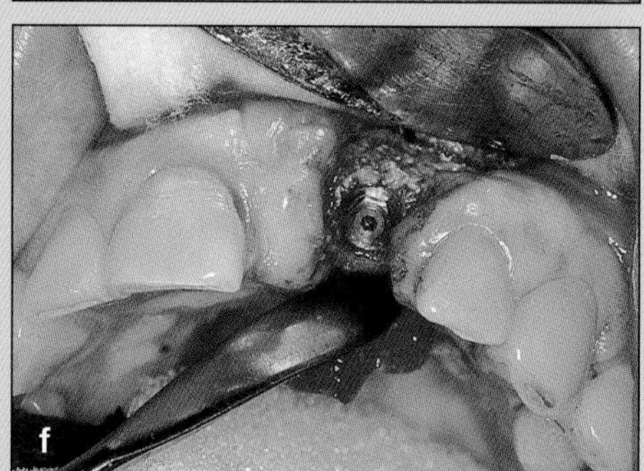

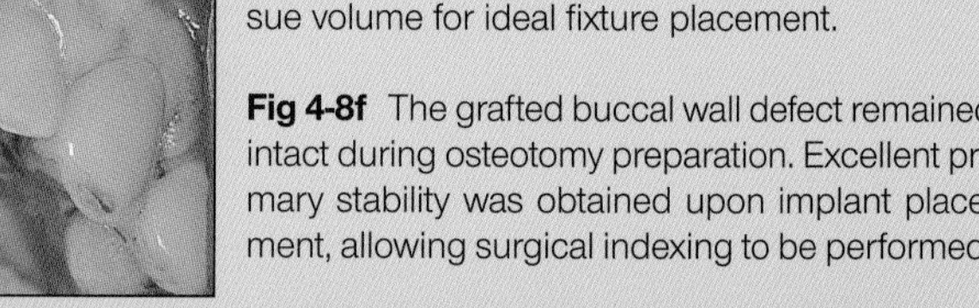

Fig 4-8f The grafted buccal wall defect remained intact during osteotomy preparation. Excellent primary stability was obtained upon implant placement, allowing surgical indexing to be performed.

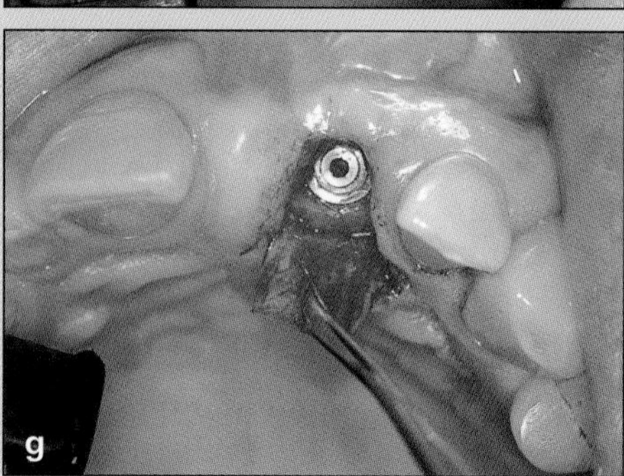

Fig 4-8g Implant exposure via a palatal peninsula approach. A custom abutment and provisional restoration were delivered to provide anatomically correct guided soft tissue healing.

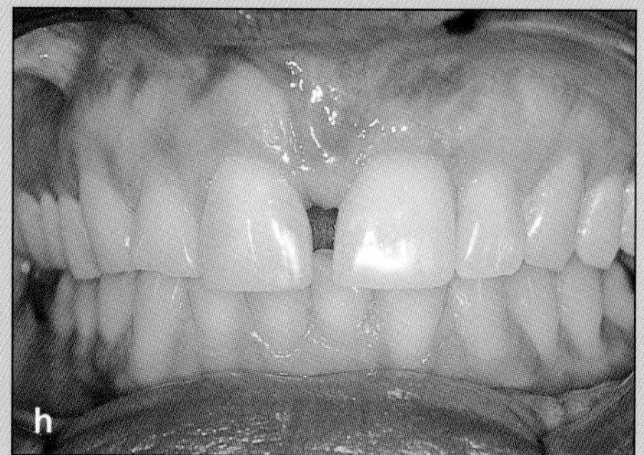

Fig 4-8h Provisional restoration in place 2 weeks after delivery. The restoration is inconspicuous, has harmonious proportions, and blends nicely with the adjacent dentition.

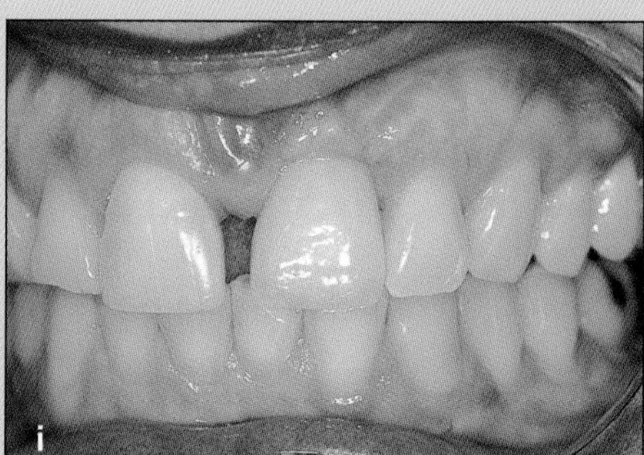

Fig 4-8i View 2 months after implant exposure. The provisional restoration has maintained the soft tissue architecture.

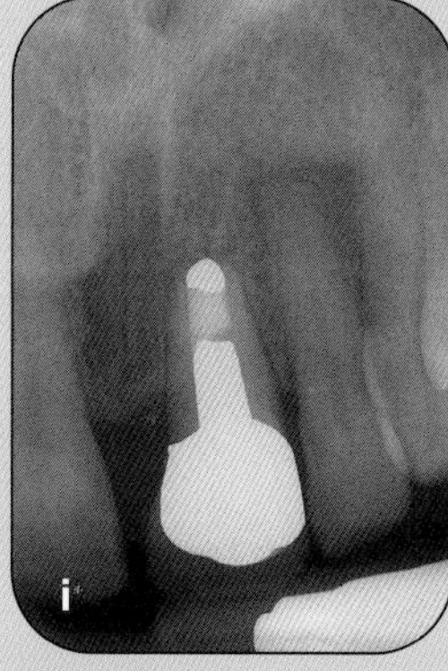

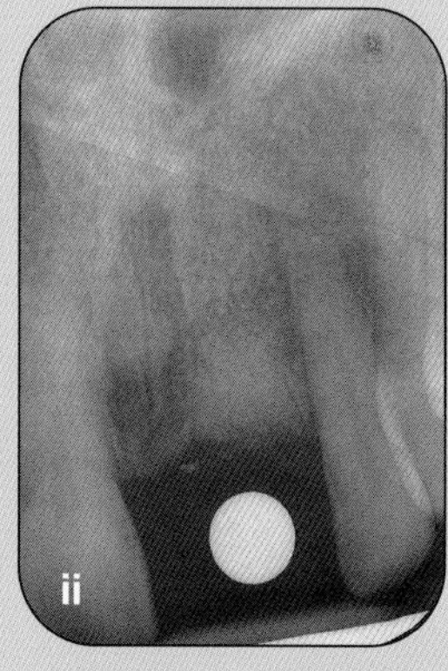

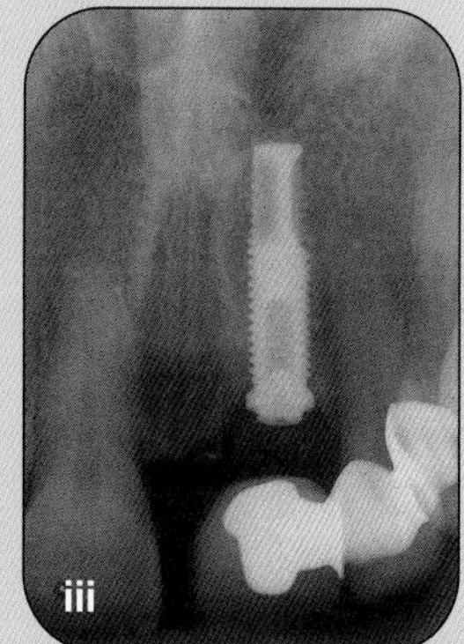

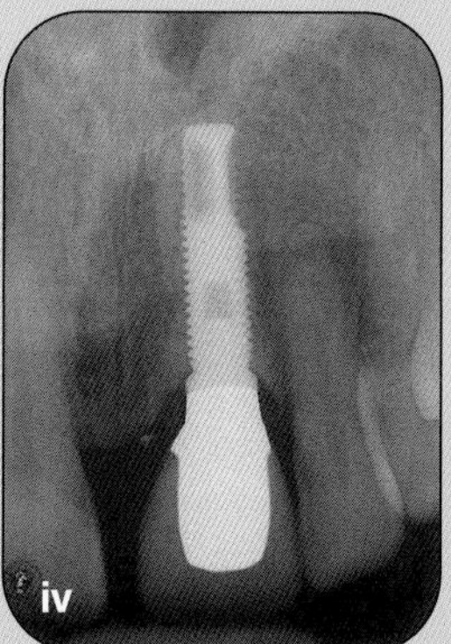

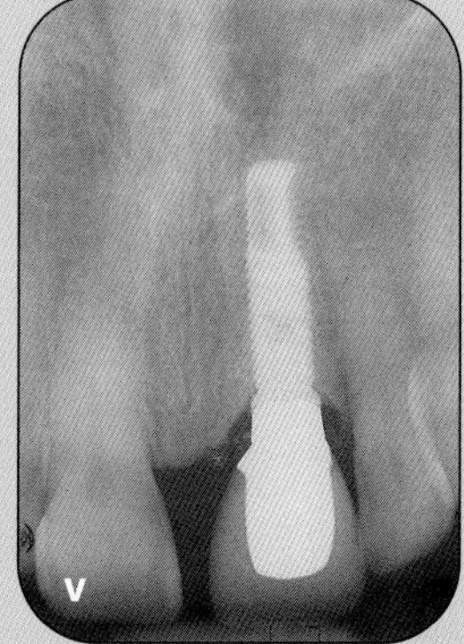

Fig 4-8j Series of radiographs demonstrating pretreatment condition *(i)*, 4-month postoperative condition *(ii)*, 4-month post–implant placement condition *(iii)*, 1-year postfunction condition *(iv)*, and 4-year postfunction condition *(v)*. Note the progression from initial integration of the graft at the site followed by the gradually increased difficulty of discerning the graft at its apical extent and the continued incorporation of the graft coronally.

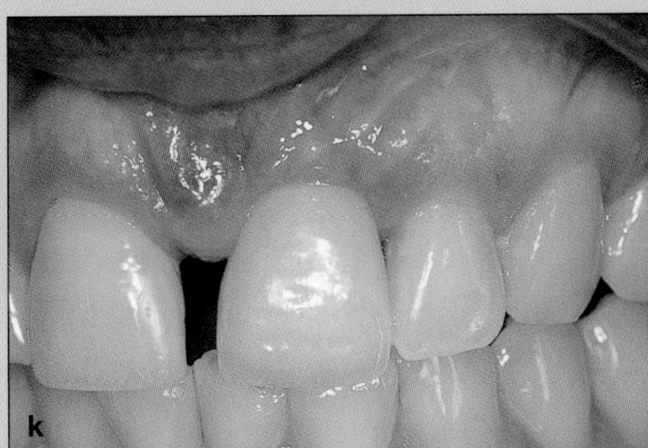

Fig 4-8k Final restoration demonstrates improved esthetics and soft tissue contours compared to the initial condition. The patient chose to preserve the central diastema and declined soft tissue augmentation to correct gingival discoloration.

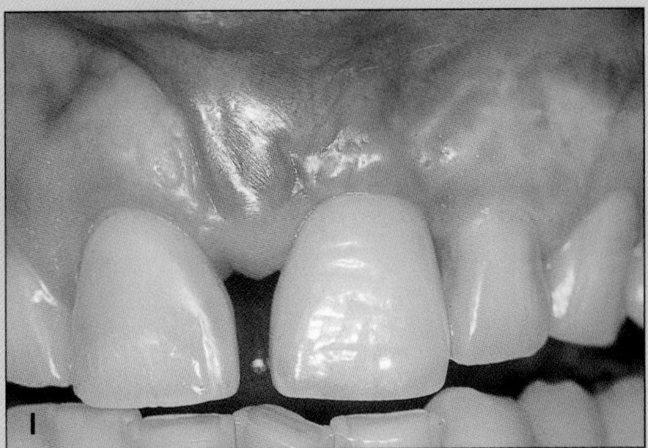

Fig 4-8l View of final restoration 4 years after delivery. Despite the presence of a significant buccal wall defect, use of the Bio-Col technique was successful in preserving alveolar ridge contours needed to maintain an esthetic restorative emergence. (Restoration by Dr Cecil Abraham, Miami, FL.)

Bio-Col Technique for Immediate Implant Placement

In esthetic areas, there are two conditions under which implants are placed immediately: when there are no bony defects in the socket walls and when primary stability of an ideally placed implant is possible. To obtain predictable esthetic results, the author delays implant placement in esthetic areas whenever an osseous defect threatens the buccal ridge crest or when tooth mobility or chronic irritation secondary to a violation of biologic width or recurrent decay under an existing restoration is accompanied by edema of the marginal soft tissues. Both of these situations present an esthetic risk, as detailed earlier.

In nonesthetic areas, defects involving the coronal socket walls can be predictably managed with guided bone regeneration procedures performed simultaneously with immediate implant placement, as long as the implant has been placed well within the alveolar housing. When an immediate implant is placed in these situations, flaps are elevated and advanced to obtain tension-free closure over the submerged implant and grafted defect. Similarly, when an immediate implant is placed in a nonsubmerged fashion at a site with a favorable osseous defect, flaps are elevated and advanced to obtain tension-free closure over the grafted defect and circumferential adaptation of the soft tissues around the transmucosal portion of the implant.

In esthetic areas, the surgeon should be aware that the implant should be placed so as to avoid loading of the buccal socket wall or excessive infringement of the adjacent interdental bone, either of which can result in unexpected late-appearing esthetic compromises. For this reason, the author routinely strives to obtain approximately a 1.0-mm void between the buccal socket wall and the immediately placed implant. This also facilitates the condensation of the Bio-Oss graft into the void. The graft material is used as a "bone-grouting" substance to fill these voids, providing an ideal osteoconductive environment to maximize future bone-to-implant contact as well as improved primary implant stability. Using a bone-grouting substance around press-fit orthopedic implants is a well-recognized means of improving primary stability. The author has exploited this finding in cases where implants were immediately placed into fresh extraction sites and immediately loaded with fixed prostheses. When the Bio-Col technique was used as described below with immediate placement of 10- and 12-mm standard-diameter implants, torque values measured at final sink depth routinely exceeded 35 Ncm in posterior maxillary and mandibular sites and commonly reached or exceeded 45 Ncm in anterior maxillary and mandibular sites. These torque values represent significant improvements over values previously measured in similar cases where 10- and 12-mm implants of the same type were immediately placed without Bio-Oss grafting.

Bio-Col technique for immediate implant placement

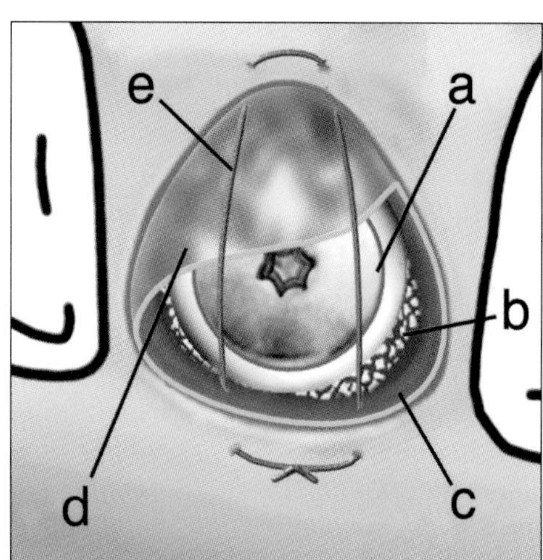

Fig 4-9a Semi-submerged implant placed immediately following tooth removal *(a)*. After the implant was placed to two thirds its final sink depth, Bio-Oss bone mineral *(b)* was condensed between the implant and bony socket walls. As it is fully seated, the anatomic cervical neck design effectively condenses the Bio-Oss in an apical and lateral direction. Additional grafting is seldom needed after the implant reaches final sink depth. The implant and Bio-Oss graft were covered with CollaPlug absorbable collagen dressing *(d)*, and the latter was maintained with a horizontal mattress suture *(e)*. Isodent tissue cement applied to the outer layer of the collagen dressing further secured and sealed the dressing.

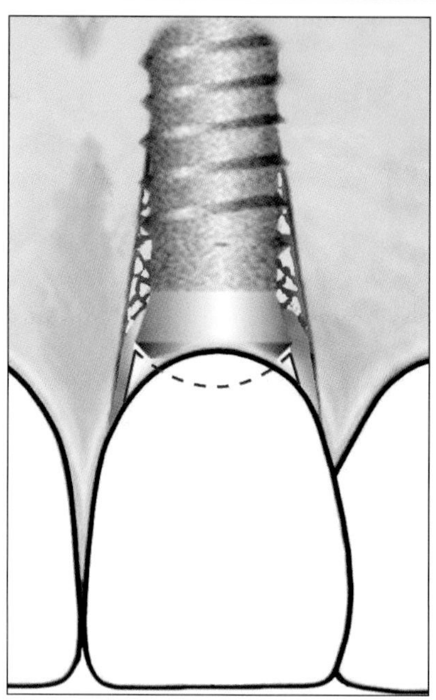

Fig 4-9b When a submerged implant is placed, the collagen dressing is condensed over the cover screw. When a semi-submerged implant is placed (shown here), the collagen dressing is carefully condensed between the permucosal portion of the implant and the surrounding soft tissues. Tissue cement is then applied with care so as not to contaminate the implant or abutment surfaces. The ovate provisional restoration is modified to avoid pressure over the implant while maintaining subgingival extension peripherally to support the surrounding soft tissues. The soft tissue support provided by the modified provisional restoration prevents soft tissue collapse and blunting of the interdental papillae.

Surgical protocol

The goal of the surgical protocol for immediate implant placement is to minimize trauma and maximize bone regeneration within the socket while preserving soft tissue architecture at the site. To preserve both the circulation and the soft tissue architecture at esthetic sites, flap elevation is avoided during tooth removal and implant placement.

Following minimally traumatic tooth removal, the osteotomy is carefully prepared according to a surgical guide. An osseous coagulum trap can be used to collect any autogenous bone available from the osteotomy preparation. The osseous coagulum is then mixed with the Bio-Oss graft material prior to delivery to the site. When used alone, Bio-Oss should be moistened slightly with sterile saline or blood from the socket to improve its handling characteristics. Once moistened, the Bio-Oss graft is easily carried to and condensed within the bleeding site (Fig 4-9).

Next, the selected implant is seated to approximately two thirds its final sink depth and the graft mixture is condensed into any voids that exist between the implant and the socket wall. Initial seating of the implant will avoid trapping graft material in the apical aspect of the osteotomy preparation, which otherwise could prevent complete seating of the implant when dense bone is encountered. Small amounts of the graft material are sequentially delivered and condensed using an amalgam plugger or small osteotome. The goal is to completely obliterate the void with thoroughly condensed graft material. While tedious and time-consuming, this procedure is essential in order to realize the full benefit of a guided bone regeneration effect and to enhance the primary stability of the immediately placed implant. As the implant is being fully seated, the graft is condensed between the implant and the socket walls.

Implant options include one-piece implants that incorporate an anatomically designed transmucosal collar and are designed to be placed in a nonsubmerged fashion and two-piece cylindrical threaded and tapered root-analog implants that are designed to be used in a submerged fashion.

When a one-piece nonsubmerged implant is used, the graft material is effectively condensed in an apical direction as the implant is fully seated, and additional grafting material is seldom needed. When either a two-piece large-diameter cylindrical implant or a root-analog implant is used, the implant usually closely approximates the mesial and distal socket walls in the cervical area and obliterates the socket apically. Grafting material is usually needed to fill voids that are present between the buccal, palatal, or lingual socket walls and the implant. When a standard-diameter two-piece cylindrical threaded implant is used, voids are often present around the circumference of the implant in the cervical area of the socket. Although the graft is condensed as the cylindrical threaded and root-analog implants are seated, some of the graft is usually displaced coronally. Subsequently, the cover screw is placed, and additional graft material should be carefully condensed around the periphery of the implant. The surgeon should avoid adding excess graft material coronal to the cover screw of a submerged implant or to the transmucosal surface of a one-piece nonsubmerged implant.

Next, if necessary, a 30-gauge needle is used to stimulate additional bleeding from the soft tissues. CollaPlug absorbable collagen dressing is densely packed over the Bio-Oss graft and submerged implant to the level of the free marginal gingiva. A horizontal mattress suture (4-0 or 5-0 chromic gut on a P3 needle) is then loosely secured over the socket to avoid coronal displacement of the collagen plug. If a one-piece nonsubmerged implant is used or if a two-piece implant is placed in a nonsubmerged fashion by immediately connecting an abutment, the collagen material is condensed over the Bio-Oss graft between the transmucosal portion of the implant and the surrounding soft tissues. The dry CollaPlug is cut into small pieces and delivered to the site, where it will become saturated with blood as it is condensed over the graft (see Fig 4-9b). A suture to resist coronal displacement of the collagen material is seldom necessary in these instances.

A small amount of Isodent tissue cement is then used to seal the surface of the exposed collagen material. When sealed in this manner, the collagen material becomes relatively impervious to liquids and thus completes the isolation of the surgical site. In nonsubmerged implant placement, care should be taken to prevent excess tissue cement from overflowing into the surrounding soft tissues, which will otherwise lead to dislodgment of the collagen dressing secondary to trauma within the oral cavity. The use of tissue cement may be unnecessary where a customized tooth-form healing abutment provides anatomically correct support for the surrounding soft tissues. In these instances, a small piece of absorbable collagen dressing is carefully introduced around the periphery of the custom tooth-form healing abutment, which is designed to completely obliterate the soft tissue socket (Figs 4-10 to 4-14).

Prosthetic protocol

The prosthetic protocol for immediate implant placement closely parallels the protocol previously described for delayed implant placement. In esthetic areas, the critical factor is to ensure that the provisional restoration or prosthetic element attached to the implant accurately replicates the contours of the extracted tooth. Excessive buccal contours often precipitate soft tissue recession, while under- or overcontoured interproximal zones can lead to blunting or elimination of adjacent interdental papillae. Soft tissue architecture at the site is preserved after completion of the surgical protocol by providing immediate support for the surrounding soft tissues using an interim provisional restoration, an anatomic healing abutment, or a custom tooth-form healing abutment.

When a nonsubmerged or semi-submerged approach is used, the interim provisional restoration is modified to ensure optimal soft tissue support while avoiding the possibility of premature implant loading (Fig 4-15; see also Fig 4-12). The ovate pontic is hollowed in the center to avoid contact with the transmucosal portion of the implant, but a thin shell is maintained peripherally to support the surrounding soft tissues and adjacent papillae. Either a fixed or a removable interim provisional can be used for this purpose, provided it is designed to avoid the transmission of micromotion to the site. Alternatively, a prefabricated anatomic healing abutment or custom tooth-form healing abutment that closely approximates the interproximal contours of the extracted tooth can be used to support the adjacent papillae, and the overlying provisional restoration can be designed as a facial veneer to support the buccal marginal gingival tissues. In esthetic areas, an Essex retainer provisional restoration can be used initially and then replaced after several weeks of healing with a resin-bonded provisional restoration. Alternatively, a custom tooth-form healing abutment can be shaped and polished chairside to closely replicate all of the cervical contours of the extracted tooth (see Figs 4-11 and 4-14). While effective, this process requires additional chair time in most instances.

Bio-Col technique for immediate replacement of resorbing right maxillary central incisor

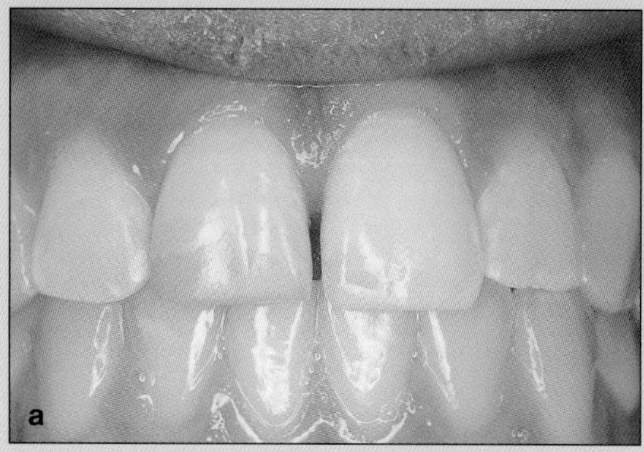

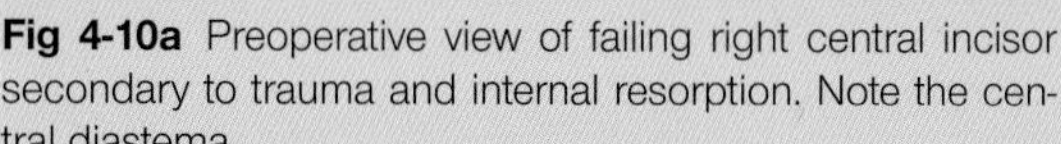

Fig 4-10a Preoperative view of failing right central incisor secondary to trauma and internal resorption. Note the central diastema.

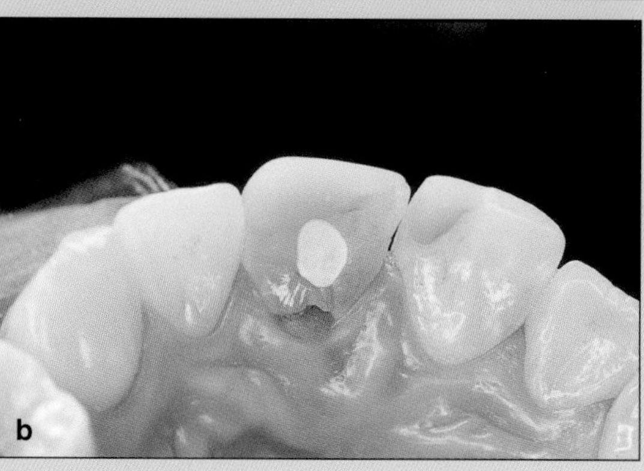

Fig 4-10b Palatal view demonstrating extensive internal resorption.

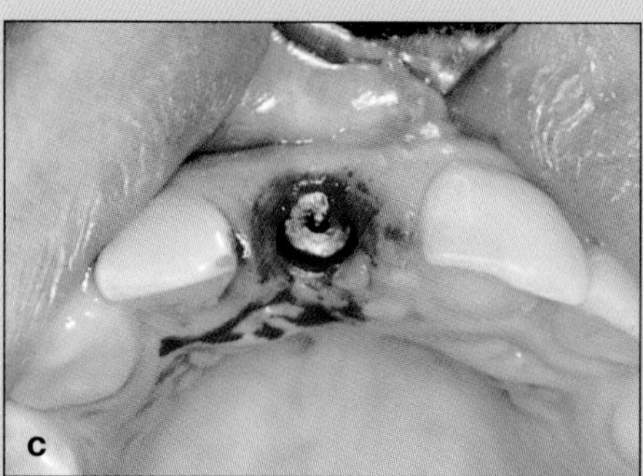

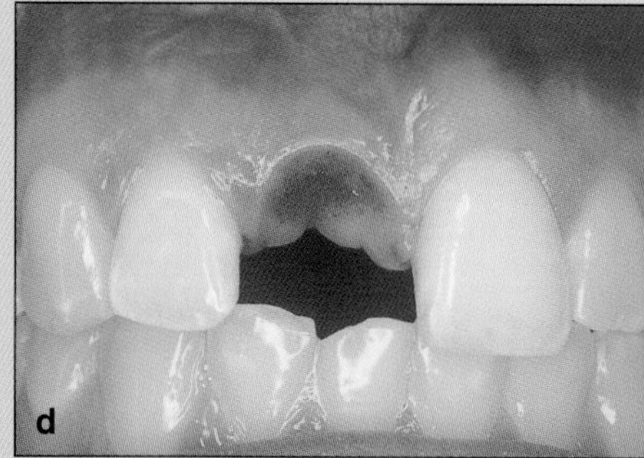

Fig 4-10c The tooth was removed in a minimally traumatic fashion, preserving surrounding hard and soft tissue anatomy. A cylindrical threaded implant was carefully placed to avoid contact with the fragile buccal plate. The circumferential void between the implant and the socket wall was grafted with Bio-Oss, and the socket was sealed with CollaPlug and Isodent tissue cement prior to delivery of a resin-bonded interim provisional restoration. The crown of the tooth was modified into an ovate pontic and bonded to the adjacent dentition.

Fig 4-10d The interim provisional was removed 6 months after tooth removal and immediate implant placement, revealing successful preservation of natural alveolar ridge anatomy at the site.

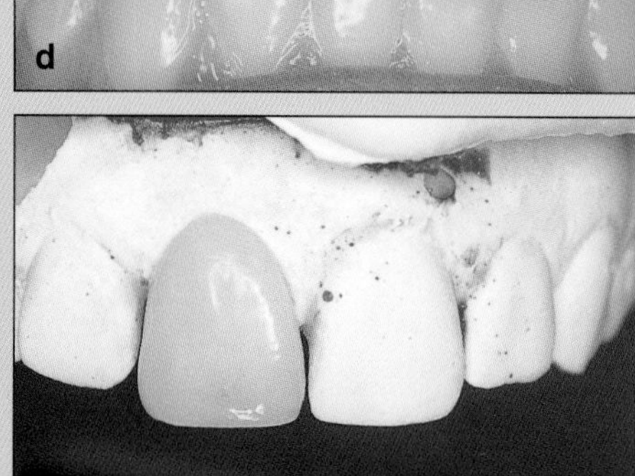

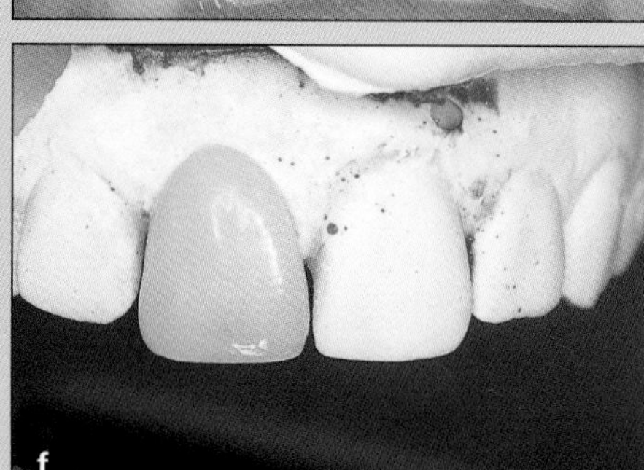

Fig 4-10e A tissue punch was used to expose the implant, and a prefabricated CeraOne (Nobel Biocare, Yorba Linda, CA) abutment was placed. The surrounding tissues have maintained the cross-sectional form of the extracted tooth.

Fig 4-10f A shell for fabricating a chairside provisional restoration via a direct technique was prepared in advance.

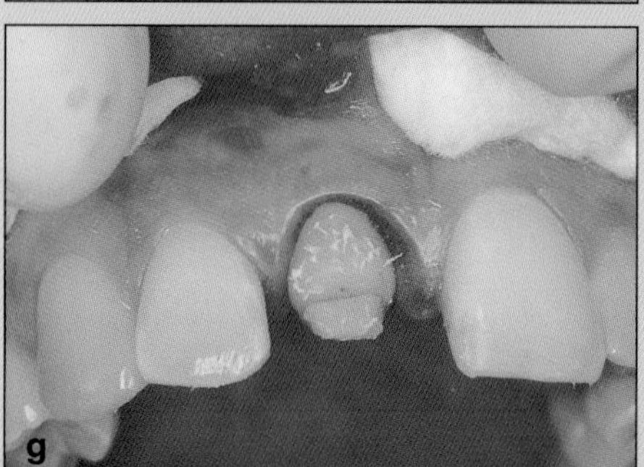

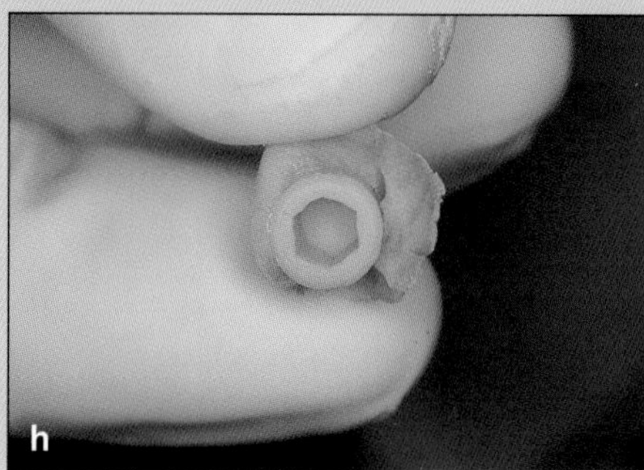

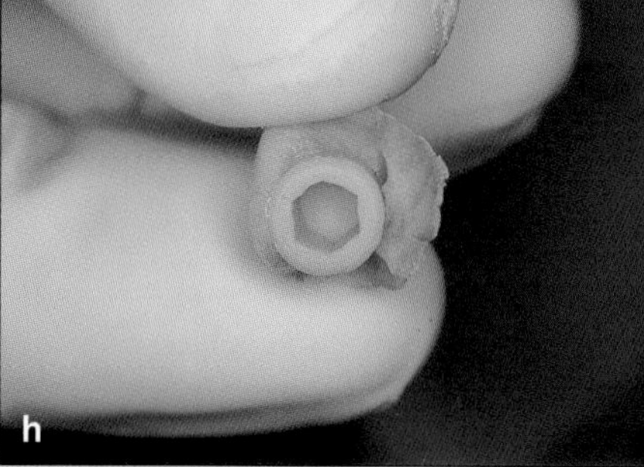

Fig 4-10g The abutment's protective cap was roughened with a bur to facilitate mechanical bonding of the acrylic resin.

Fig 4-10h The shell was filled with acrylic resin and seated over the roughened protective cap. After initial setting of the material, the crown shell–protective cap was removed for finishing and polishing.

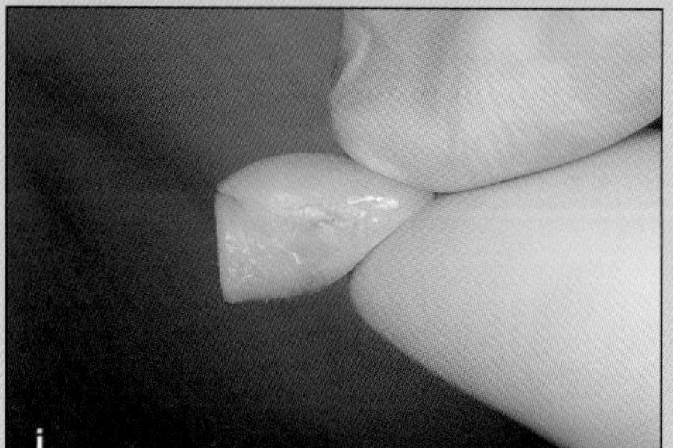

Fig 4-10i Finished and polished provisional crown. The contours mimic those of a natural tooth.

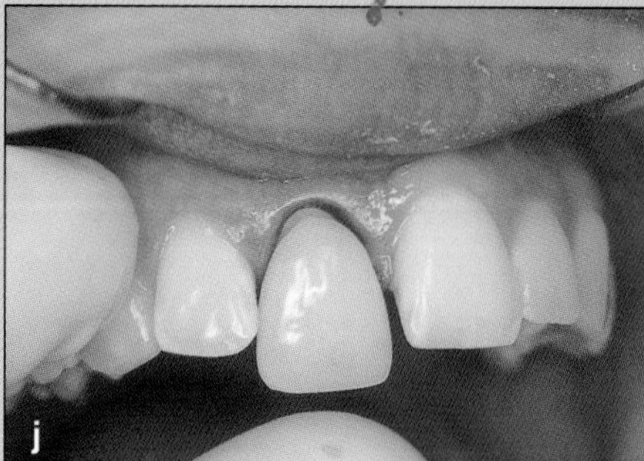

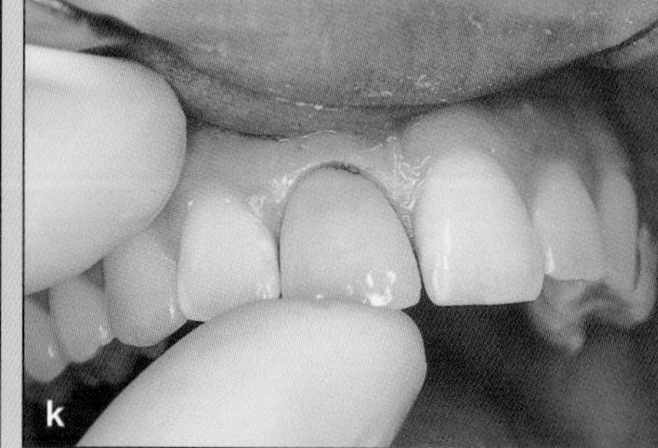

Figs 4-10j and 4-10k The provisional implant crown is delivered and stabilized in a press-fit fashion. No cement was necessary.

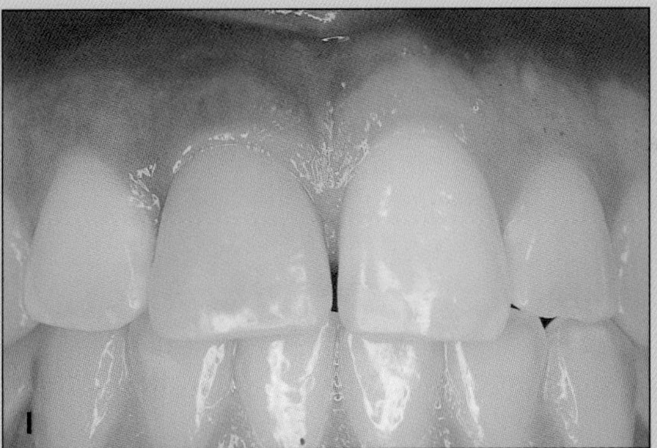

Fig 4-10l Provisional restoration 3 days after delivery, demonstrating a natural appearance. Alveolar ridge anatomy has been preserved following tooth removal and immediate implant replacement with the Bio-Col technique.

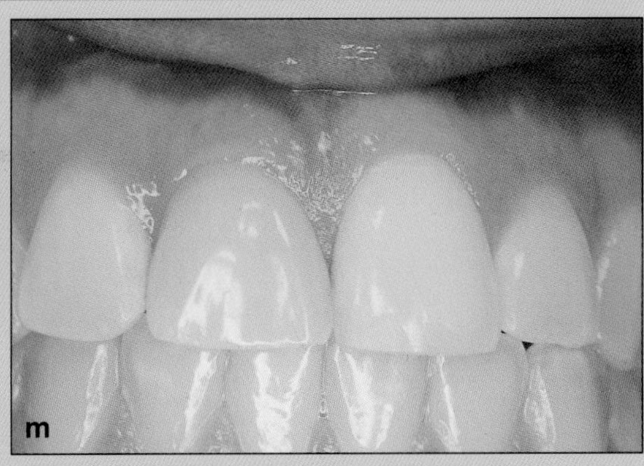

Fig 4-10m Final restoration 1 year after delivery. Soft tissue architecture is intact. The patient desired closure of the diastema but declined modification of the left central incisor. (Restoration by Dr Osvaldo Mayoral, Pinecrest, FL.)

Bio-Col technique for immediate replacement of resorbing left maxillary lateral incisor

Fig 4-11a Resorbing lateral incisor is carefully removed with a periotome.

Fig 4-11b Note the large area of external resorption.

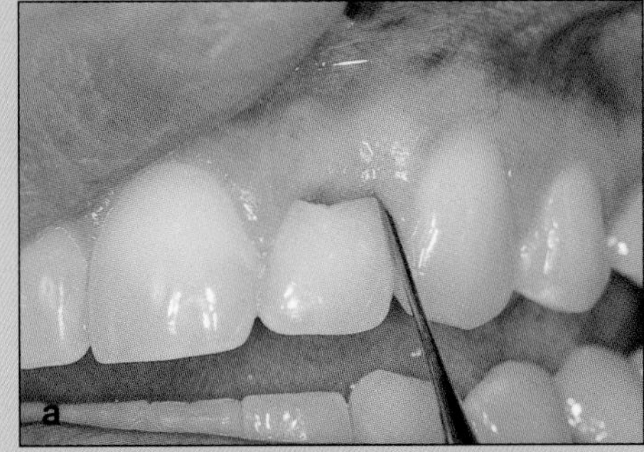

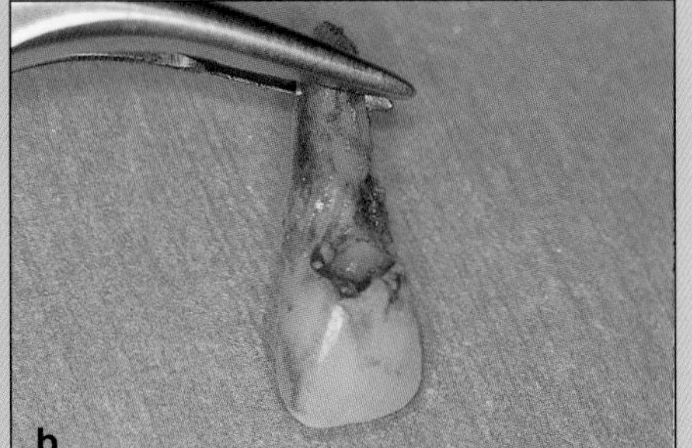

Fig 4-11c A tapered root-analog implant (Frialit) was placed to two thirds its final sink depth, and Bio-Oss was condensed into the socket around the implant. The implant was then seated to full sink depth. Note that a void was deliberately maintained between the implant body and the fragile buccal wall of the socket.

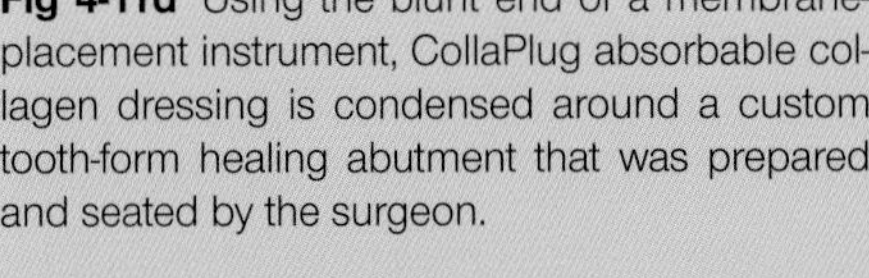

Fig 4-11d Using the blunt end of a membrane-placement instrument, CollaPlug absorbable collagen dressing is condensed around a custom tooth-form healing abutment that was prepared and seated by the surgeon.

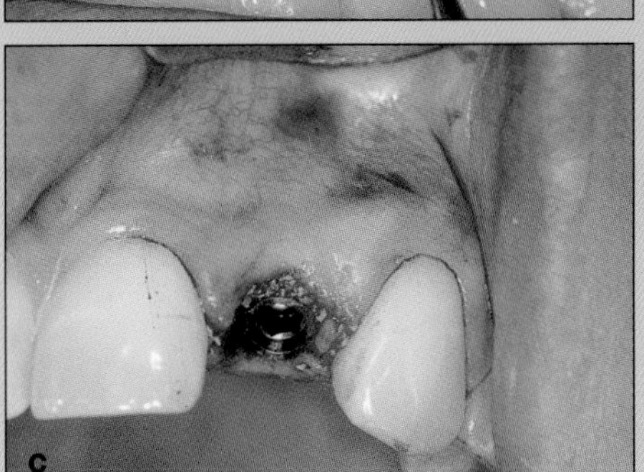

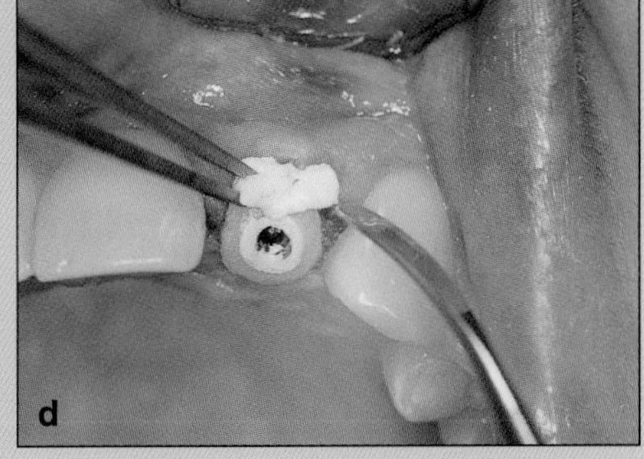

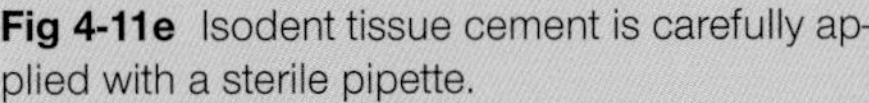

Fig 4-11e Isodent tissue cement is carefully applied with a sterile pipette.

Fig 4-11f The cross-sectional anatomy of the customized healing abutment replicates that of the natural tooth crown at the cervical level.

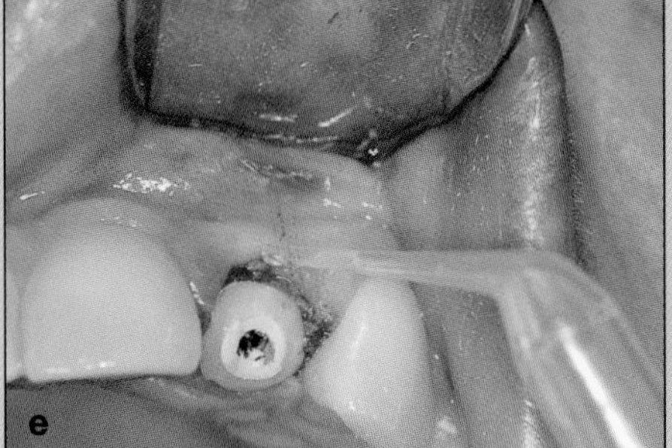

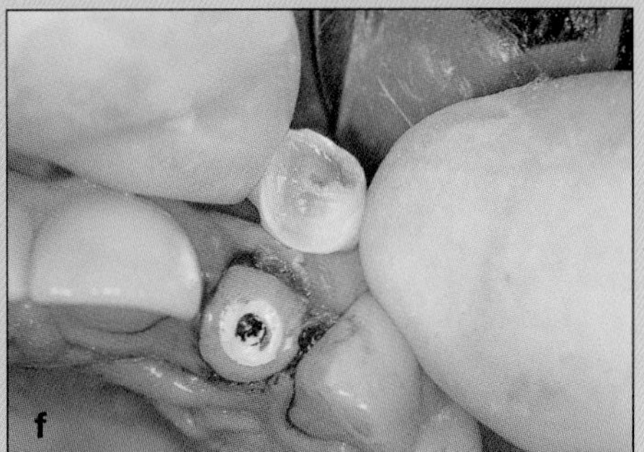

Fig 4-11g Successful preservation of highly scalloped gingival architecture is evident prior to restoration. Preservation of alveolar ridge anatomy at the site ensures a harmonious esthetic result.

Fig 4-11h Final restoration demonstrates excellent esthetics. The use of the Bio-Col technique has resulted in preservation of soft tissue architecture at the site; however, a risk remains of subsequent soft tissue recession in this patient with a thin, scalloped periodontium. (Restoration by Dr Faustino Garcia, Coral Gables, FL.)

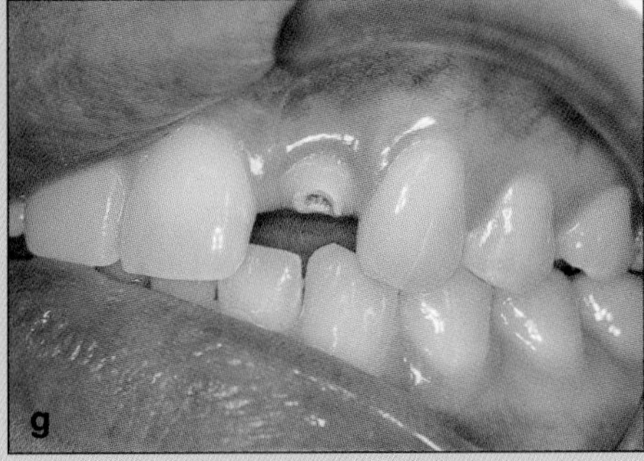

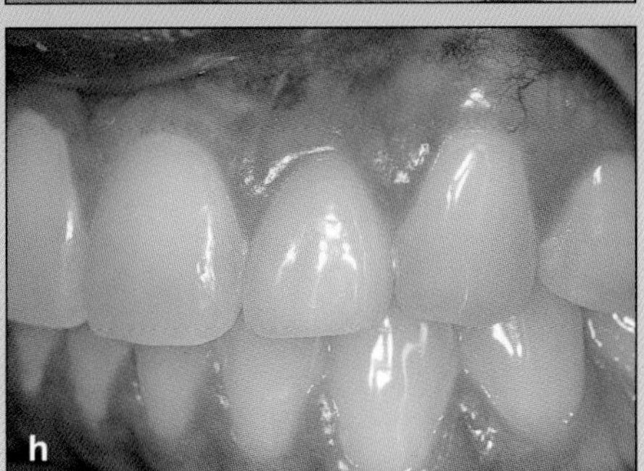

Bio-Col technique for immediate replacement of resorbing left maxillary central incisor

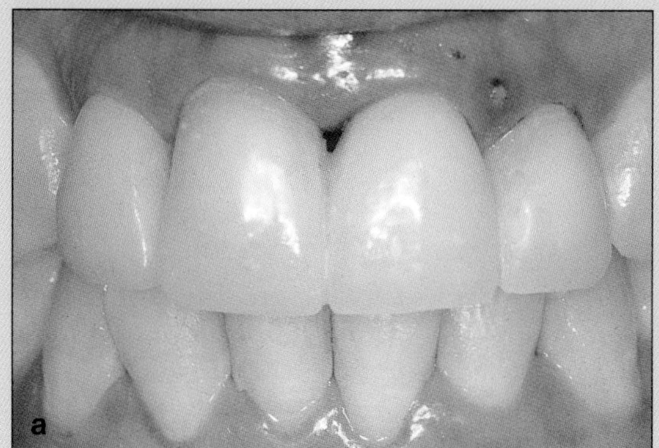

Fig 4-12a Preoperative view. The left central incisor has formed a fistula secondary to resorption. There is a fixed prosthesis extending from the right central incisor to the left lateral incisor. The failing tooth was reduced subgingivally, and a provisional restoration with an ovate left central incisor pontic was fabricated by the restorative dentist.

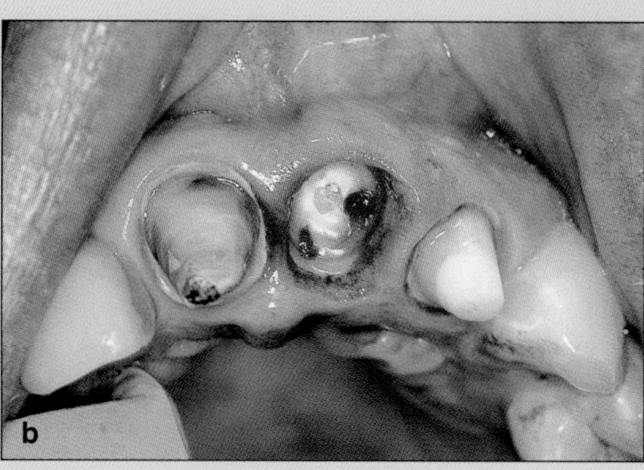

Fig 4-12b The provisional fixed partial denture has been removed, revealing that the area of resorption corresponds to the fistula. No infection is present.

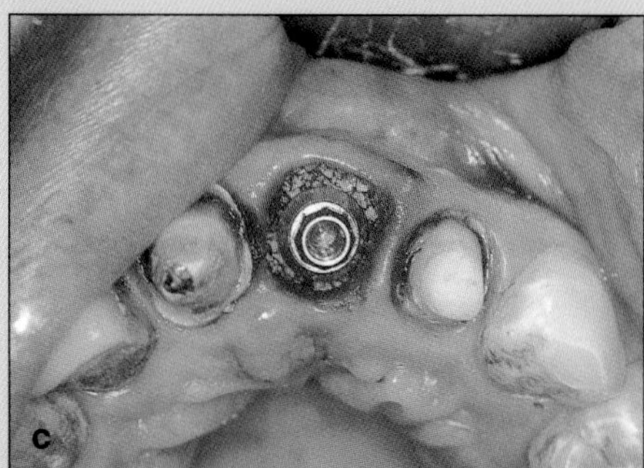

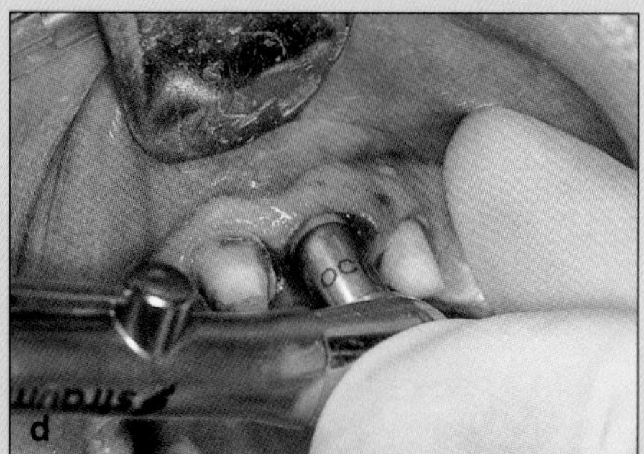

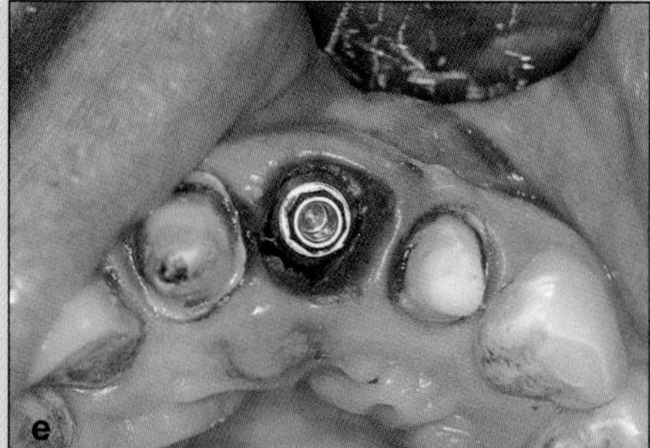

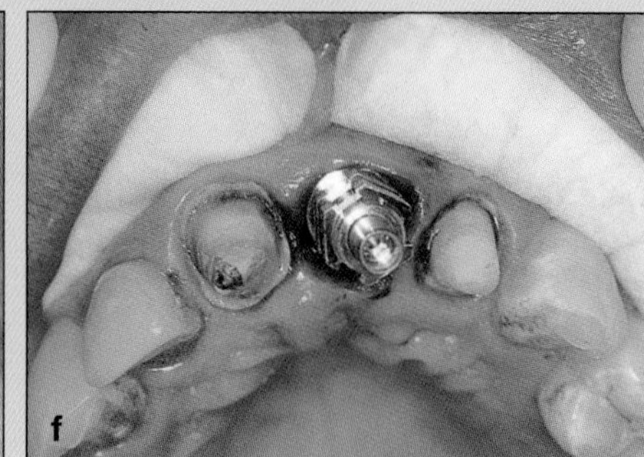

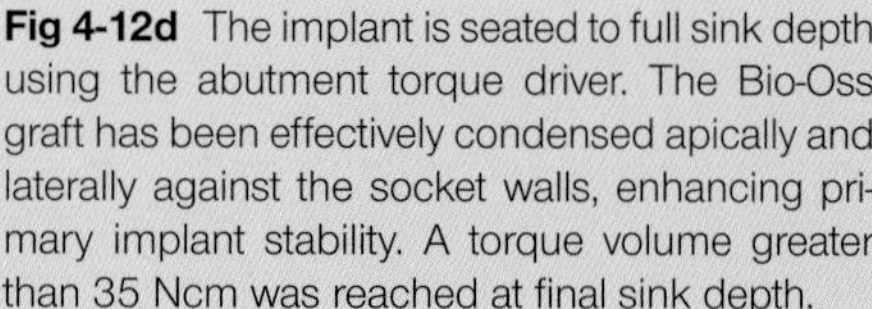

Fig 4-12c Following tooth removal with minimal trauma, a one-piece implant with an anatomic cervical area (Straumann USA, Waltham, MA) has been inserted to two thirds its final sink depth, and Bio-Oss has been grafted into the voids between the implant and the socket walls. A permanent Octa abutment (Straumann USA) has been delivered.

Fig 4-12d The implant is seated to full sink depth using the abutment torque driver. The Bio-Oss graft has been effectively condensed apically and laterally against the socket walls, enhancing primary implant stability. A torque volume greater than 35 Ncm was reached at final sink depth.

Fig 4-12e The implant has been conveniently seated so that the implant shoulder is located 2 mm below the buccal gingiva. Note that the graft material was not displaced coronally.

Fig 4-12f Surgical index coping in place. Excellent primary stability enabled the index to be performed without risk of implant movement. The position of the implant was registered relative to the adjacent dentition using Blue Velvet impression material (J. Morita, Irvine, CA). The laboratory technician uses the surgical index to fabricate a master cast for custom abutment fabrication.

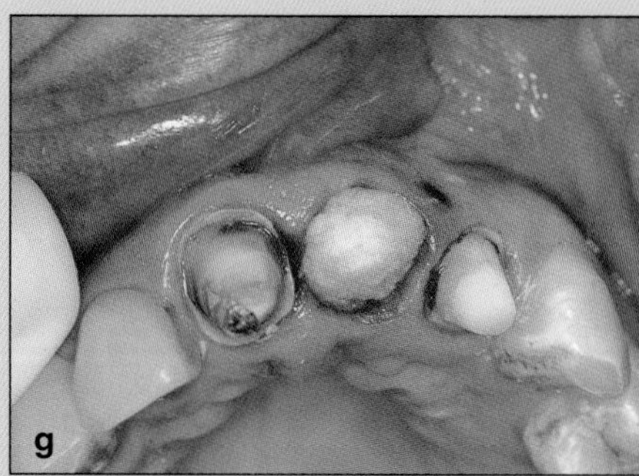

Fig 4-12g Implant and graft have been covered with condensed collating absorbable collagen dressing. The outer layer has been sealed with Isodent tissue cement.

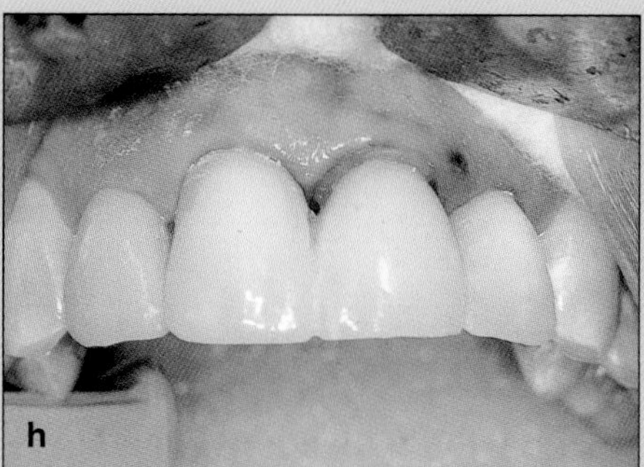

Fig 4-12h Provisional fixed partial denture modified to support the surrounding soft tissues while avoiding loading of the implant. Note the further compression of the absorbable collagen dressing against the surrounding soft tissues.

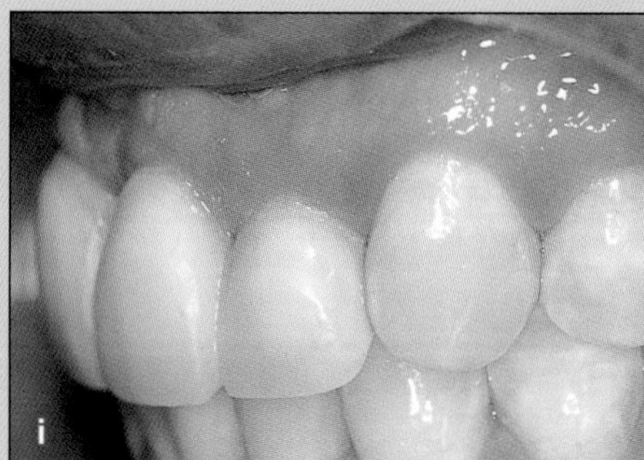

Fig 4-12i Six-week postoperative view. The modified ovate pontic provisional restoration has preserved the natural soft tissue anatomy at the site.

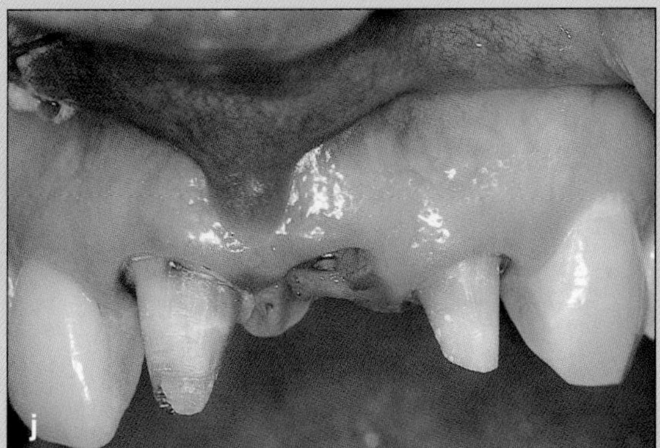

Fig 4-12j Eight-week postoperative view with fixed partial denture removed. Semi-submerged implant is visible. Soft tissue architecture has been preserved.

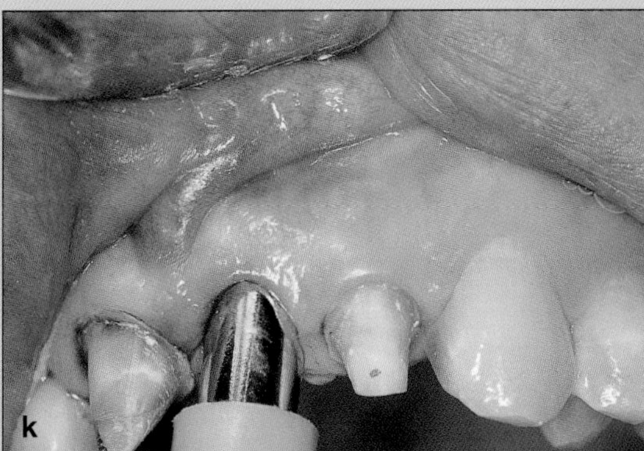

Fig 4-12k A tissue punch is used to remove the regenerated soft tissues covering the margins of the implant. Excess buccal tissues are intentionally maintained to offset any recession that may occur after delivery of the provisional restoration.

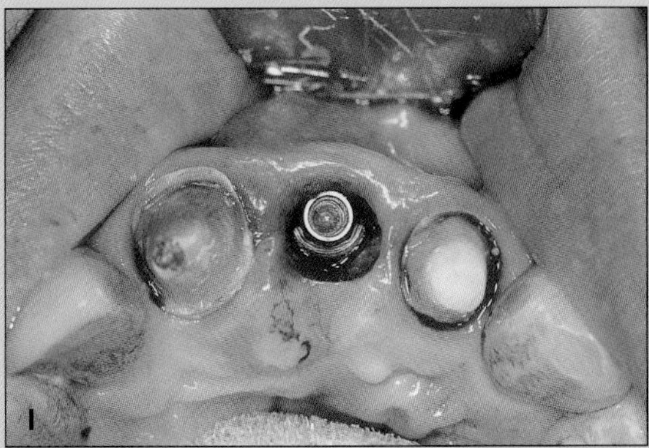

Fig 4-12l Occlusal view of integrated implant prior to delivery of the custom abutment. Note the excess buccal tissue.

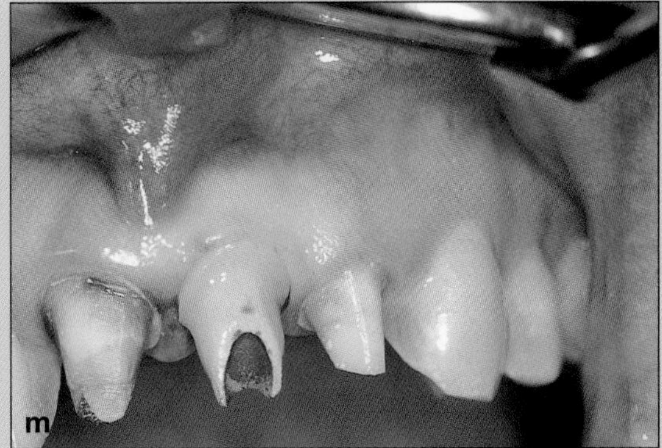

Fig 4-12m The custom abutment slightly blanches the gingival tissues upon delivery. Early employment of guided soft tissue healing will improve the soft tissue esthetic result.

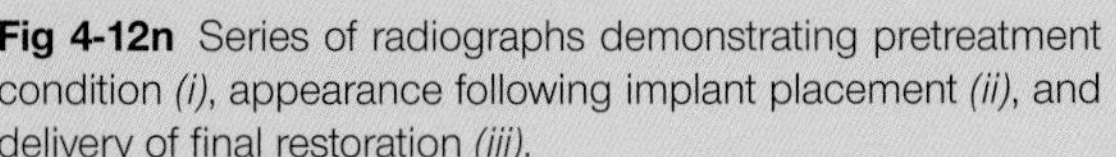

Fig 4-12n Series of radiographs demonstrating pretreatment condition *(i)*, appearance following implant placement *(ii)*, and delivery of final restoration *(iii)*.

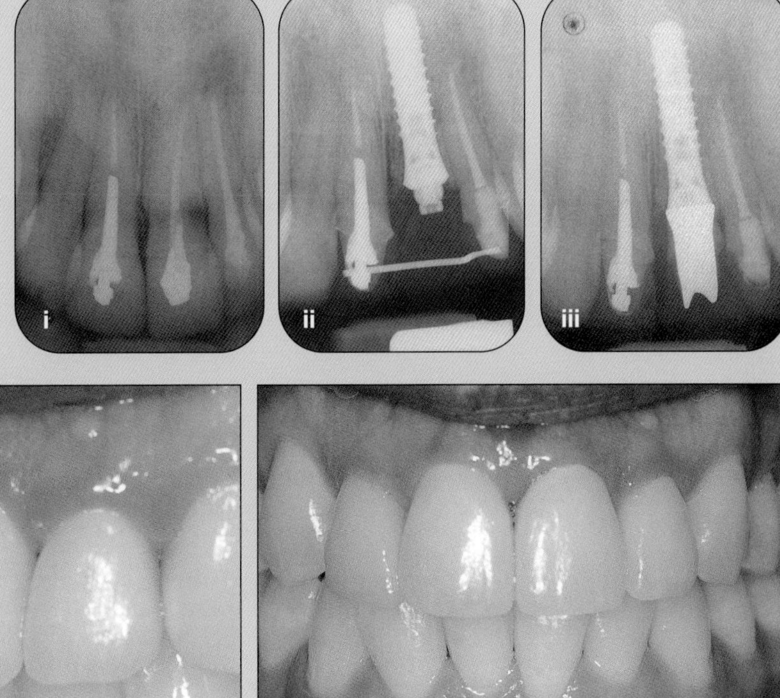

Figs 4-12o and 4-12p The final restoration emerges naturally from the preserved alveolar ridge tissues. The restoration is harmonious in form and indistinguishable from the adjacent dentition. Note the improved appearance of the soft tissues and interdental papilla when compared to the patient's preoperative condition. This result was achieved in a 10-week period without the need for additional site-development procedures. (Restoration by Dr Stephen J. Parr, Coconut Grove, FL.)

Bio-Col technique for immediate replacement of failing mandibular first molar

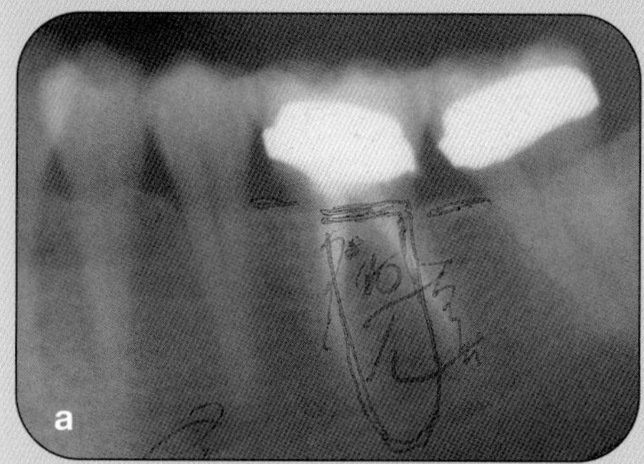

Fig 4-13a Preoperative radiograph of failing mandibular molar. Immediate replacement is planned based on assessment of adequate volume of interdental bone to provide for initial implant stability without risk of impinging on the inferior alveolar nerve.

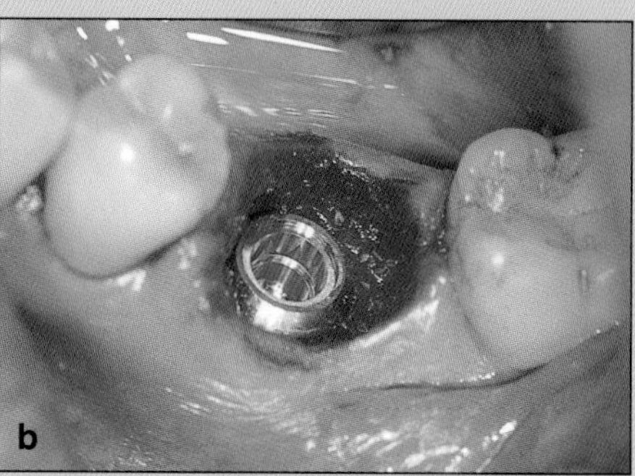

Fig 4-13b After carefully removing the molar, a one-piece, nonsubmerged, wide-neck implant (Straumann USA) was placed to full sink depth following grafting with Bio-Oss.

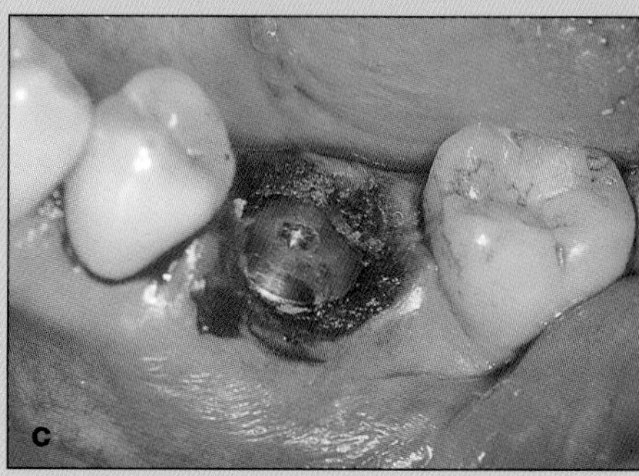

Fig 4-13c After placement of the closure screw, CollaPlug absorbable collagen dressing was condensed into the soft tissue confines of the socket and sealed with Isodent tissue cement.

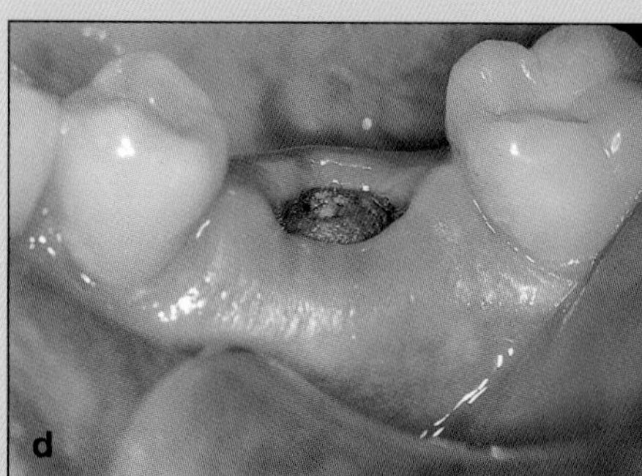

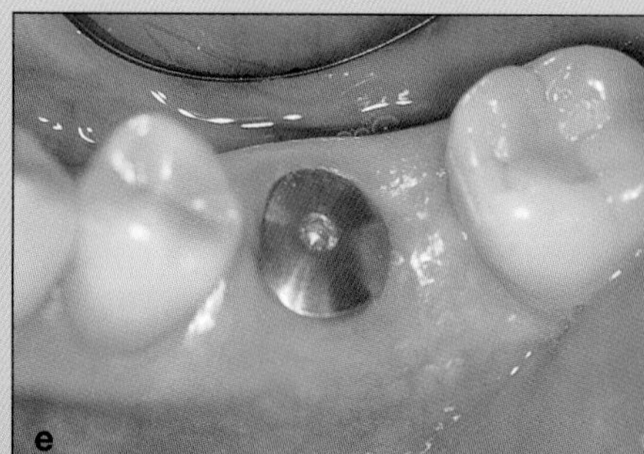

Fig 4-13d One-week postoperative view demonstrating rapid epithelialization of the socket.

Fig 4-13e Ten-week view of immediately placed molar implant demonstrating excellent soft tissue health and contours.

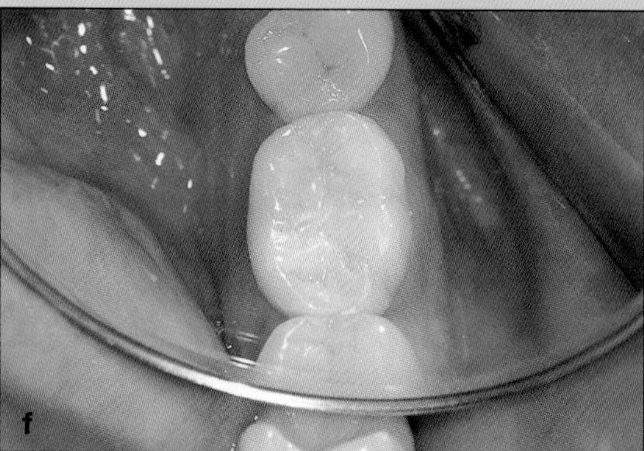

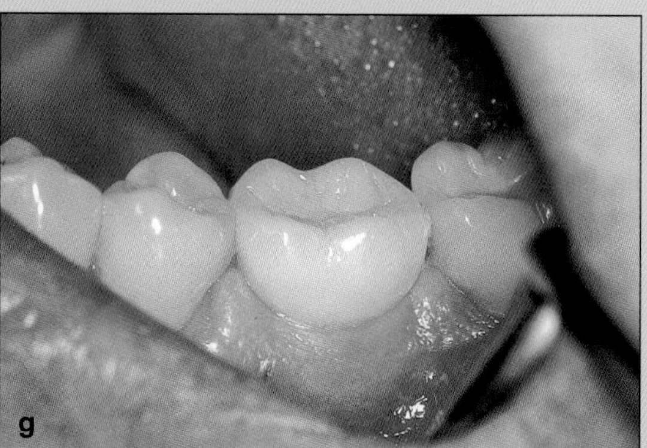

Figs 4-13f and 4-13g Final restoration with natural molar contours and full occlusal table. Preservation of soft tissue architecture prevents collection of food debris at the gingival embrasures. Use of a wide-neck implant allows for natural restorative emergence. (Restoration by Dr Roy Greenberg, Miami, FL.)

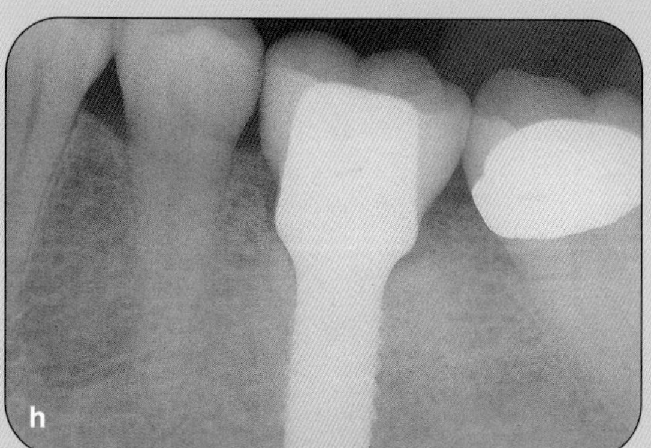

Fig 4-13h Postoperative radiograph demonstrates good bone apposition. Bio-Oss is barely discernible within the socket.

Bio-Col technique for immediate implant replacement of fractured maxillary canine

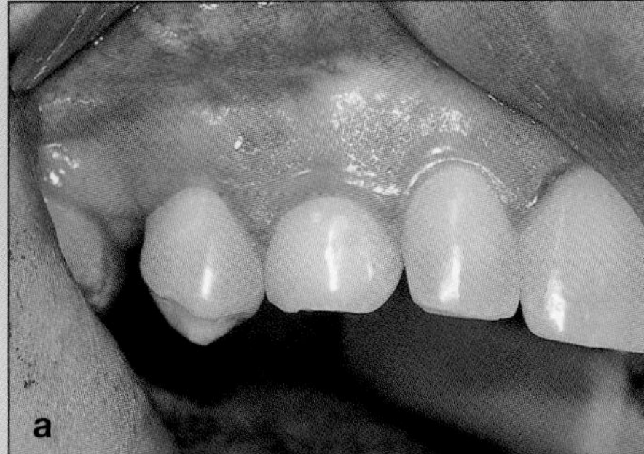

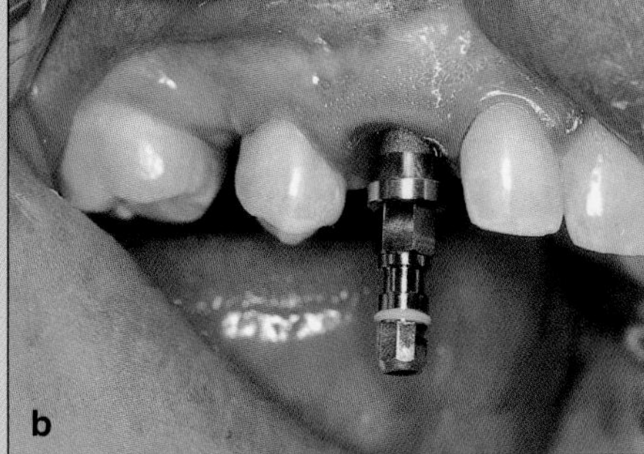

Fig 4-14a Preoperative view of fractured maxillary canine. Removal and immediate replacement with a one-piece nonsubmerged implant and customized tooth-form healing abutment are planned.

Fig 4-14b Tooth removal was accomplished with minimal trauma using periotomes, and a nonsubmerged implant (Straumann USA) has been placed at two thirds its final sink depth. Note the anatomic design of the cervical aspect of the implant body.

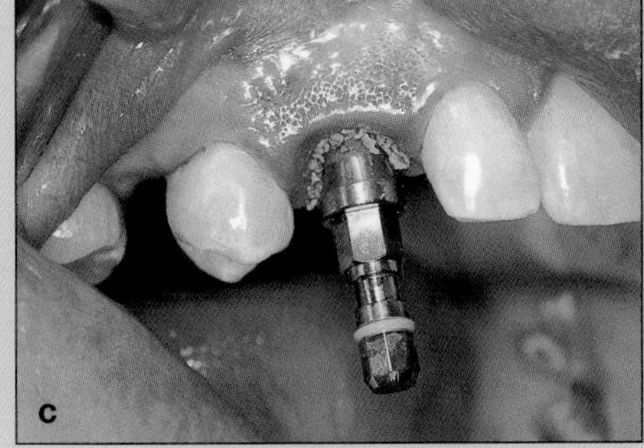

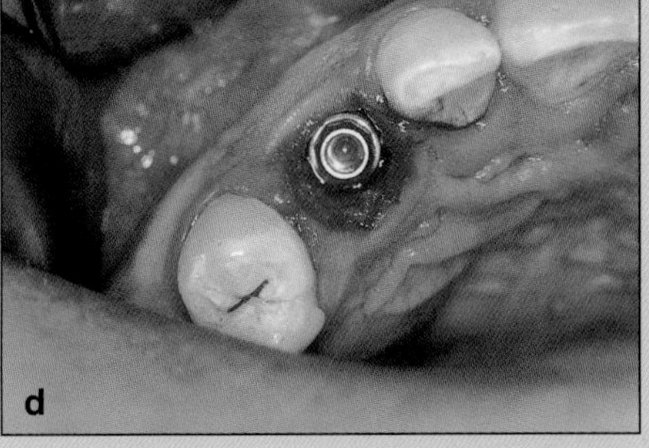

Fig 4-14c Bio-Oss deproteinized bone mineral has been condensed into the voids between the implant and the socket walls. As the implant is seated to its final depth, the graft is condensed apically and laterally, enhancing primary stability.

Fig 4-14d The fixture is at its final sink depth. Excellent primary stability was obtained, enabling the permanent abutment to be secured with 35-Ncm torque. CollaPlug was then condensed around the periphery of the transmucosal portion of the implant prior to the delivery of the customized healing abutment.

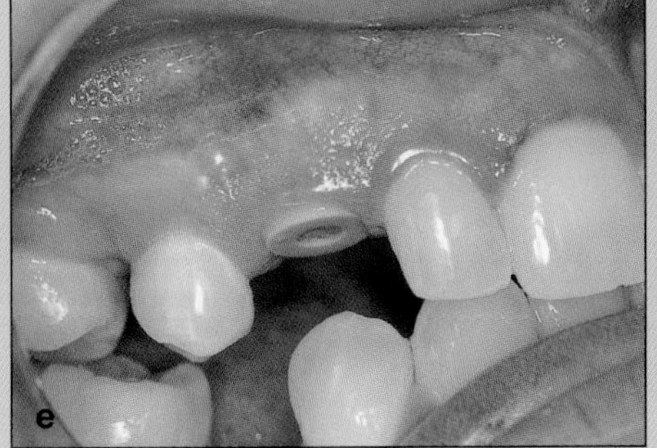

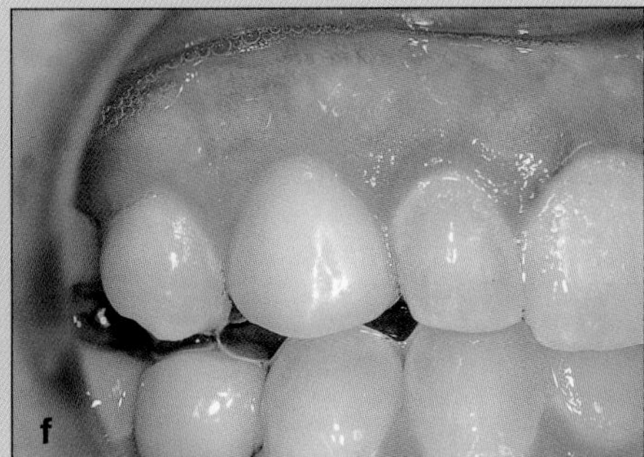

Fig 4-14e Four-week postoperative view. Customized healing abutment was modified chairside and delivered at the time of implant placement. The contours of the customized healing abutment replicate the cervical contours of the extracted tooth. The peri-implant soft tissues are free of inflammation and the natural soft tissue anatomy has been preserved.

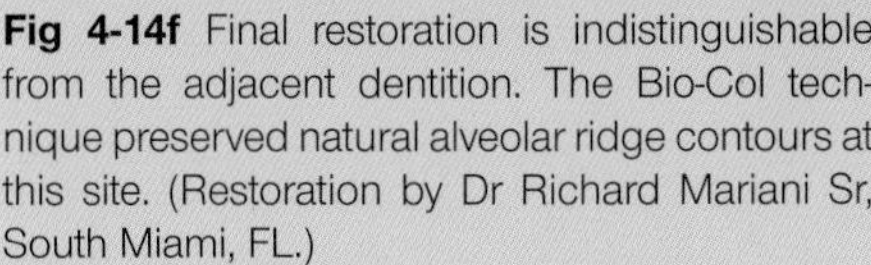

Fig 4-14f Final restoration is indistinguishable from the adjacent dentition. The Bio-Col technique preserved natural alveolar ridge contours at this site. (Restoration by Dr Richard Mariani Sr, South Miami, FL.)

In nonesthetic areas, a traditional cylindrical healing abutment with an enlarged diameter is used at the time of immediate implant placement to provide generous access for the restorative dentist (see Fig 4-14).

For a submerged implant approach, an interim provisional restoration is used initially, as previously described for a delayed implant approach. Following an appropriate osseointegration period, a conservative peninsula flap or tissue punch approach is used to expose the implant for abutment connection. Once again, the goal is to introduce anatomically correct prosthetic contours immediately upon transmucosal emergence of the implant in order to take advantage of the benefits provided by prosthetic guided soft tissue healing. When a surgical index is used to register implant position at the time of placement, the laboratory technician can provide either a custom implant provisional restoration or a custom tooth-form healing abutment. Alternatively, the surgeon can use an anatomic healing abutment or custom tooth-form healing abutment that is shaped and polished chairside, as described above, or a permanent abutment can be delivered and a provisional restoration fabricated chairside via a direct technique.

Bio-Col technique for multiple immediate implant replacements in a failing maxillary dentition

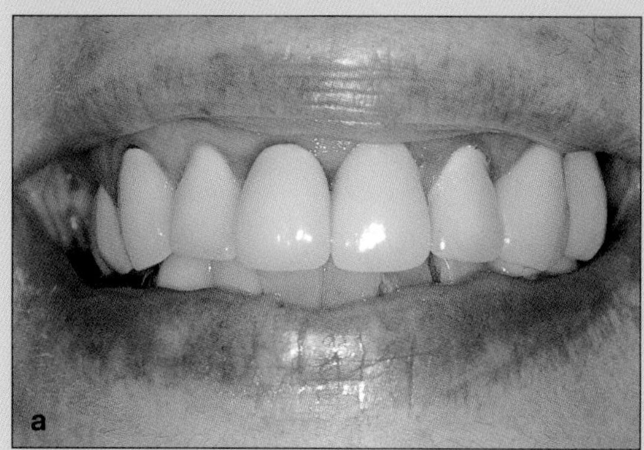

Fig 4-15a Preoperative view of failing maxillary fixed partial denture. Biologic width impingements are evident by marginal tissue discoloration.

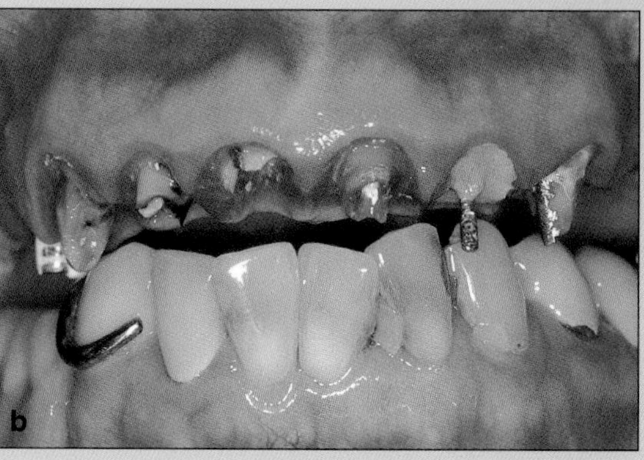

Fig 4-15b Frontal view of failing maxillary dentition demonstrates recurrent subgingival decay.

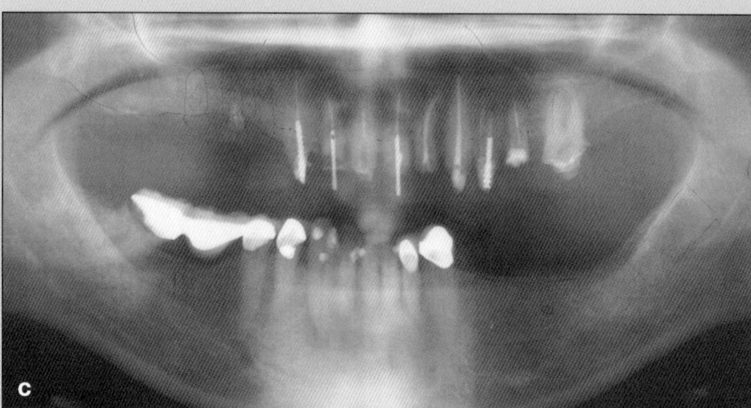

Fig 4-15c Preoperative radiograph demonstrates the compromised maxillary dentition and the amount of alveolar bone available for primary implant stabilization. Three strategic abutments will be retained to support an interim provisional fixed partial denture with ovate pontics at immediate replacement sites.

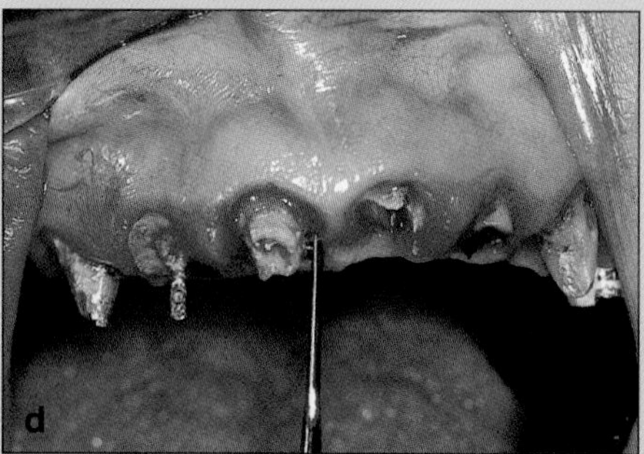

Fig 4-15d Periotomes were used during tooth removal to minimize trauma to surrounding hard and soft tissues.

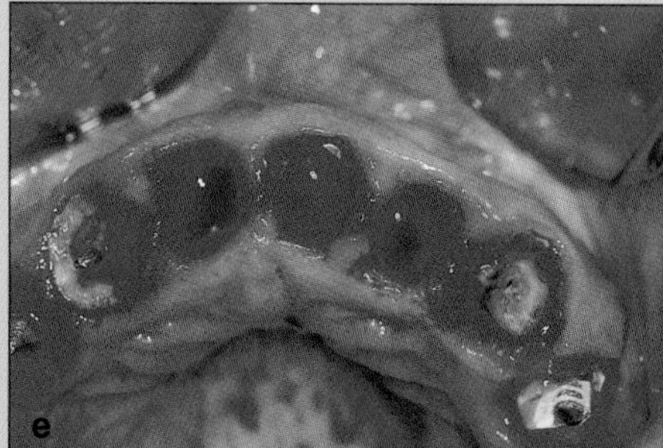

Fig 4-15e Bleeding is observed within the intact extraction sockets after osteotomy preparations were completed. Note that surrounding soft tissue anatomy has been preserved. This is an extremely important consideration in esthetic areas.

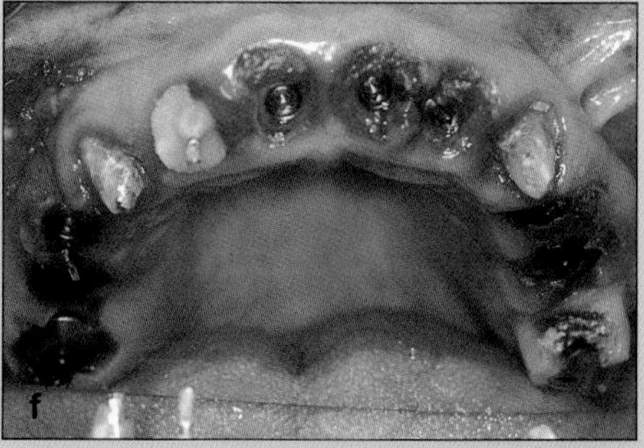

Fig 4-15f Nonsubmerged one-piece implants (Straumann USA) have been placed in conjunction with the Bio-Col technique. The implants were positioned to avoid engaging the fragile buccal plate to prevent subsequent resorption, which could jeopardize esthetics.

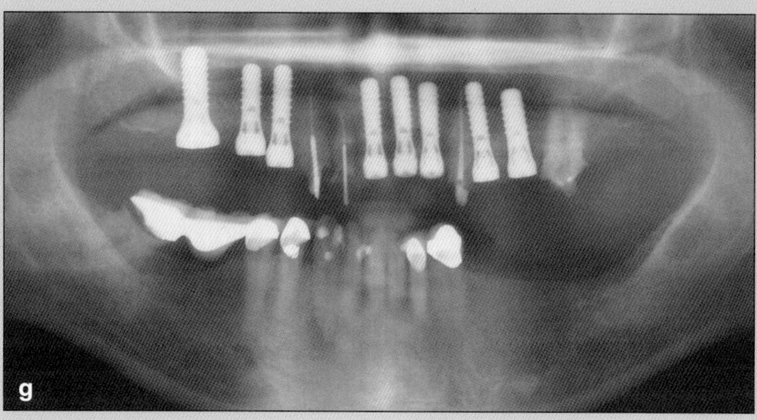

Fig 4-15g Postoperative panoramic radiographic view of immediate nonsubmerged implants.

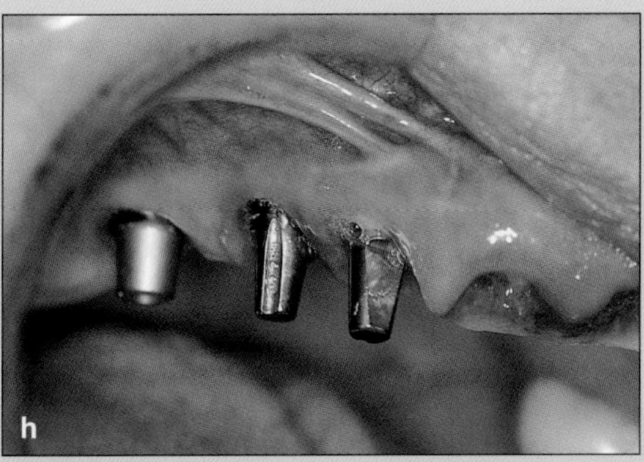

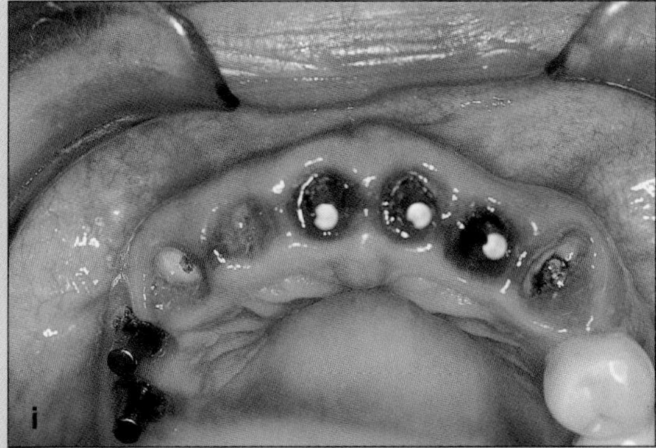

Figs 4-15h and 4-15i After 4 months, solid abutments were placed, and the provisional restoration was modified in preparation for removal of the remaining failing maxillary teeth.

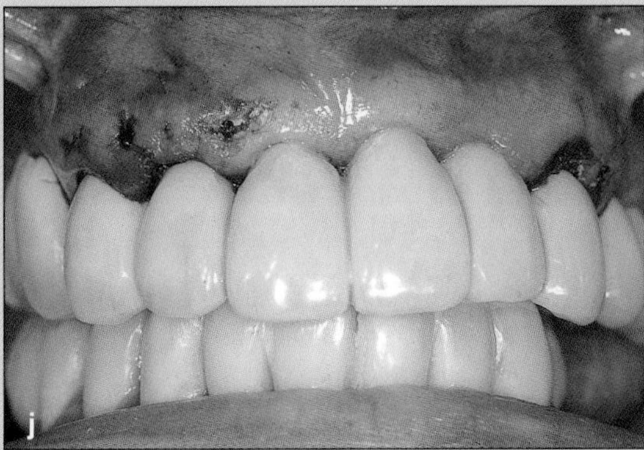

Fig 4-15j Provisional bridge adjusted and cemented over implant abutments following removal of the previously retained strategic abutments.

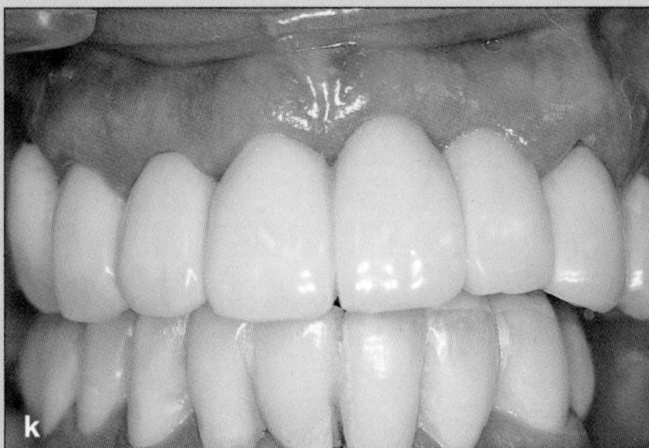

Fig 4-15k Several months later, surgical sites are healed and ready for the final restoration. The Bio-Col technique enabled an acceptable esthetic result to be obtained.

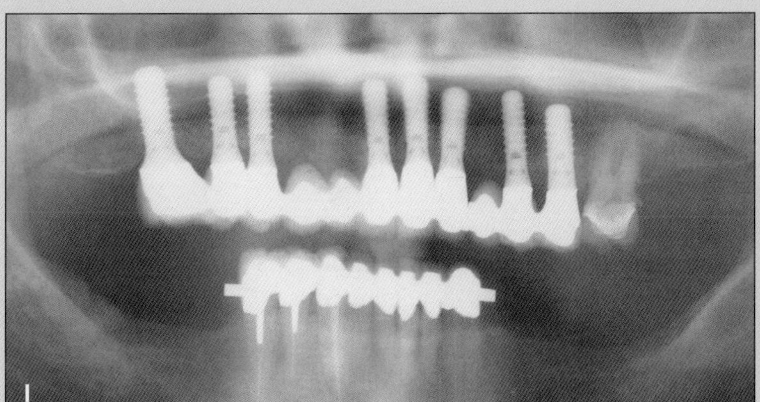

Fig 4-15l Panoramic radiograph of the final implant-supported restoration.

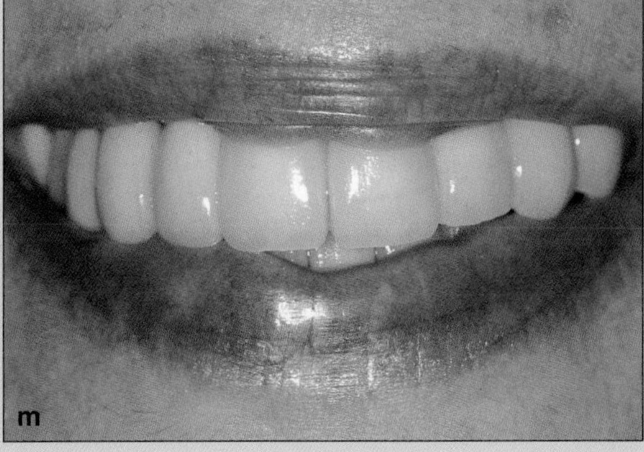

Fig 4-15m Final restoration several months later. Natural esthetics have been obtained. Total treatment time was reduced to 7 months, including time allotted for healing of pontic sites after removal of previously retained strategic abutments. (Restoration by Dr Juan Diego Cardenas, Coral Gables, FL.)

Long-Term Clinical Results Obtained with the Bio-Col Technique

The Bio-Col alveolar ridge preservation technique is a clinically proven approach that has been used by the author for more than a decade to enhance both functional and esthetic outcomes in implant therapy. Application of this technique greatly diminishes post-extraction bone resorption and consistently preserves hard and soft tissue ridge anatomy. Moreover, it often eliminates the need for additional site-development procedures commonly required in esthetic implant therapy, resulting in reduced treatment times and increased patient satisfaction. Finally, in cases where site-development procedures are unavoidable, this technique may be used to maintain the volume of the reconstructive soft tissue envelope, thus facilitating subsequent hard and soft tissue site-development procedures.

The Bio-Col technique has consistently enhanced esthetic and functional results in both delayed and immediate implant placements following tooth removal. In 423 extraction sites in 187 patients treated from March 1992 to January 2000, the technique was used to preserve alveolar ridge anatomy and to potentiate future sites when delayed implant placement was indicated. Retrospective analysis revealed a successful osseointegration rate of 95.8% with a follow-up period ranging from 12 to 93 months. Where osseous crestal defects of favorable morphology, as described above, were encountered at the time of tooth extraction in areas of high esthetic importance, additional bone-grafting procedures prior to implant placement were avoided in an initial series of 15 of 21 sites. This is an impressive statistic considering that, in extraction sites with defects in the coronal aspect of the buccal socket wall, obtaining harmonious implant esthetics usually requires a staged approach with bone grafting prior to implant placement.

The Bio-Col technique was also used in conjunction with immediate implant placement (as described above) in 512 extraction sites in 117 patients from July 1992 to January 2000. Retrospective analysis revealed successful osseointegration in 97.2% of the sites, with a follow-up time ranging from 12 to 85 months. Semiannual radiographic evaluations demonstrated stable crestal bone levels under function. In addition, it was noted that the graft material could no longer be discerned from the surrounding socket walls in the apicalmost portions of the socket between 6 and 12 months, on average, in the majority of cases. The graft also was no longer discernible in the coronal portions of the socket between 24 and 36 months after the procedure. Clinical examinations demonstrated healthy peri-implant soft tissues that appeared natural. Of special interest is the consistent preservation of the peri-implant papillary form, which is commonly lost and extremely difficult to regain following the use of conventional implant techniques.

Suggested Refinements

Use of a resorbable barrier membrane over the Bio-Oss graft

Epithelial or connective tissue downgrowth around an immediately placed implant, a concern expressed by implant surgeons in response to the author's initial presentation of clinical results of the Bio-Col technique, has not materialized. Histologic examination of tissue excised at the time of exposure of submerged implants placed immediately after tooth removal with the Bio-Col technique demonstrated an intact connective tissue base over the implant cover screws without evidence of epithelium in the deeper portions of punch biopsies taken over the cover screws. In addition, vital bone tissue was repeatedly observed over the cover screws upon re-entry for abutment connections when submerged implants were immediately placed with this technique. Biopsies of the bone tissue over the cover screws 6 months after implant placement found no connective tissue and revealed tissue primarily composed of Bio-Oss particles and vital bone (Fig 4-16). These findings are consistent with the results of animal studies discussed earlier in this chapter. Furthermore, stable osseous levels and uniform trabecular bone patterns were consistently noted on evaluation of follow-up radiographs of sites treated with the Bio-Col technique in conjunction with immediate implant replacement.

Although excellent long-term clinical results have been obtained with the Bio-Col technique as described in this chapter, there is a rationale for the incorporation of a resorbable collagen barrier membrane to cover the osseous graft within the socket. Initially, a barrier membrane was not included in the technique to avoid the well-documented complications reported to occur when primary soft tissue closure was not obtained over the nonresorbable membranes available at the time. The use of a nonresorbable barrier membrane was not considered compatible with the Bio-Col technique in esthetic areas because flap elevation and closure were intentionally avoided to preserve the vascular supply and soft tissue anatomy at the site. Instead, the author used condensed absorbable collagen dressing sealed with tissue cement to function as a barrier and isolate the healing socket from the oral environment. In conjunction with a provisional restoration, this collagen material also aided in the support of the surrounding soft tissues and thus prevented their collapse. The introduction of resorbable collagen barrier membranes has diminished the risk of complications from membrane exposure. Consequently, the use of the improved resorbable barrier membranes currently available may be appropriate in the Bio-Col technique.

A resorbable membrane, if used, should be interposed between the Bio-Oss graft and the absorbable collagen dressing and should extend at least 1 to 2 mm over the buccal and palatal socket borders. The clinician should avoid elevation of adjacent col or papillary tissue during membrane adaptation, as this would compromise the circulation to the site and could have a negative effect on the soft tissue contour and esthetics. Although the author's experience with this modification has not been unfavorable, it has not yielded any discernible clinical improvement over the original technique. Therefore, the author has not added the use of a resorbable collagen membrane to the surgical protocol for immediate or delayed implant placement. Histologic comparisons of extraction sockets grafted with and without the use of a resorbable membrane as well as of bone-to-implant contact obtained with and without the resorbable barrier membrane following immediate implant placement are needed to quantify any improvement and verify the biologic merit of the Bio-Col technique and its modifications.

An additional question to consider is whether Bio-Oss or a mixture of Bio-Oss and autogenous particulate bone marrow grafts condensed into a bleeding socket actually is able to provide guided bone regeneration in and of itself when protected from trauma within the oral cavity, as suggested by Boyne,[13] or whether the key to the reproducible success achieved by clinicians who routinely use the Bio-Col technique is the result of isolating the site with an absorbable collagen dressing that is sealed with tissue cement and then protected by a provisional restoration. The author believes that the different elements involved in this technique combine to deliver consistent results within the limitations imposed by the variations in host response to be expected from different individuals.

Although significant improvements were originally noted when a resorbable membrane was used in the treatment of defect sockets, no appreciable improvements have been observed as a result of including a resorbable membrane in the treatment of healthy intact sockets. On the other hand, early experience with a mixture of autogenous bone and Bio-Oss, with and without PRP as described below, has shown promise in the treatment of compromised sites.

Use of PRP

At compromised sites where previous trauma, infection, endodontic procedures, or surgical procedures may have decreased the regenerative potential, the author has used PRP to improve osteoconduction within the graft and to potentially realize the theoretical benefits that the growth factors contained in PRP may have on bone regeneration within the socket. The author has also taken advantage of this technology when the Bio-Col technique is used at compromised sites, at defect sites, and at sites where implants have previously failed to integrate (Fig 4-18). PRP has also been used as an aid to wound healing when the Bio-Col technique is performed in conjunction with immediate implant placement. In particular, when multiple immediate-placement sites are treated with the Bio-Col technique as part of a full-arch immediate-load technique (Figs 4-17 and 4-19), the use of PRP has become a routine part of the author's surgical protocol.

The rationale of including PRP as part of the surgical protocol includes the technical advantage of facilitating the delivery to and maintenance of the graft material at the sites. In addition, the wound-sealing effect helps maintain the position of the CollaPlug material and aids healing by improving early tensile strength when soft tissue flaps and guided bone regeneration procedures are involved.

At compromised and defect sites, the author has used PRP with Bio-Oss alone as well as with 1:1 mixtures of Bio-Oss and autogenous particulate bone marrow grafts. Theoretically, the growth factors (platelet-derived growth factor and transforming growth factor β) contained within the PRP have the ability to improve bone regeneration within the graft by enhancing the invasion of healing-capable cells into the grafted socket through chemotaxis and through the response of the viable bone graft cells included in the graft itself.

Most importantly, the use of PRP ensures the presence of a blood clot in the socket, thus facilitating osteoconduction within the graft. For delayed implant placement, the author recommends injecting the graft

Bio-Col technique for immediate replacement of fractured maxillary first premolar

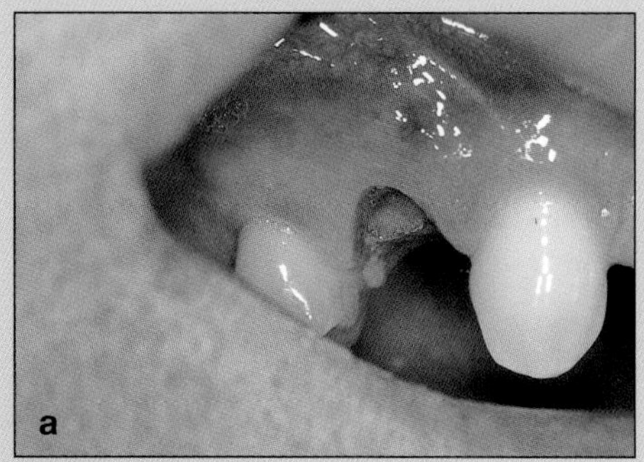

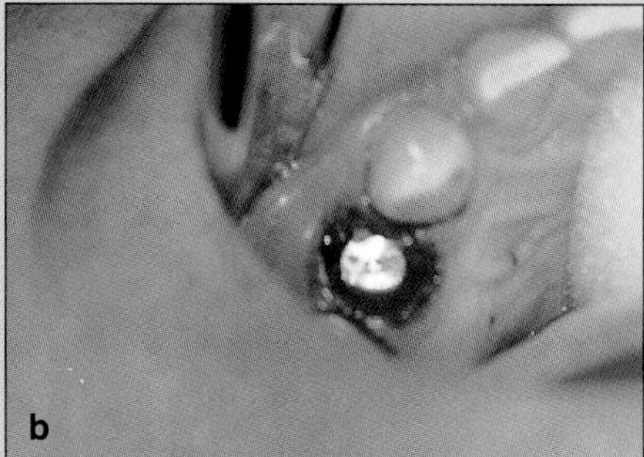

Fig 4-16a Preoperative view of fractured maxillary first premolar.

Fig 4-16b Cylindrical threaded implant has been placed. Note the circumferential void between the implant and the socket walls.

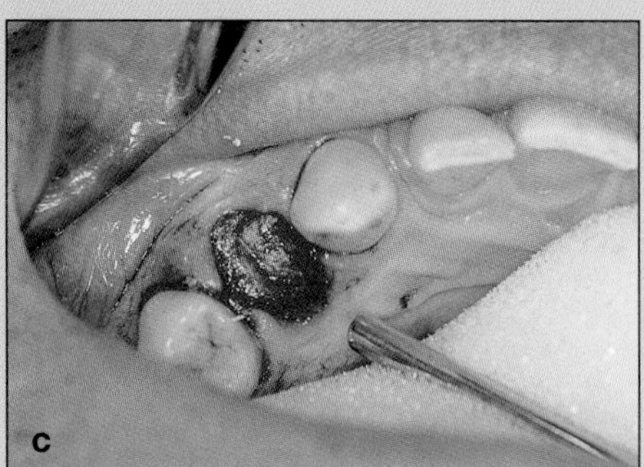

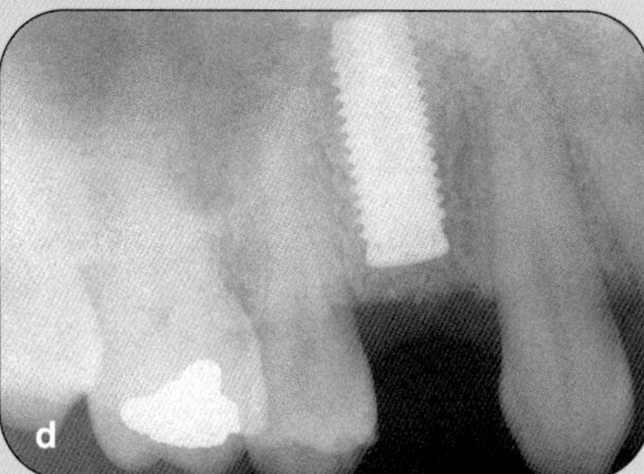

Fig 4-16c Bio-Oss has been grafted into the void surrounding the implant, and CollaPlug has been condensed over the graft and cover screw.

Fig 4-16d Six-month postoperative radiograph demonstrates osseous regeneration over the cover screw.

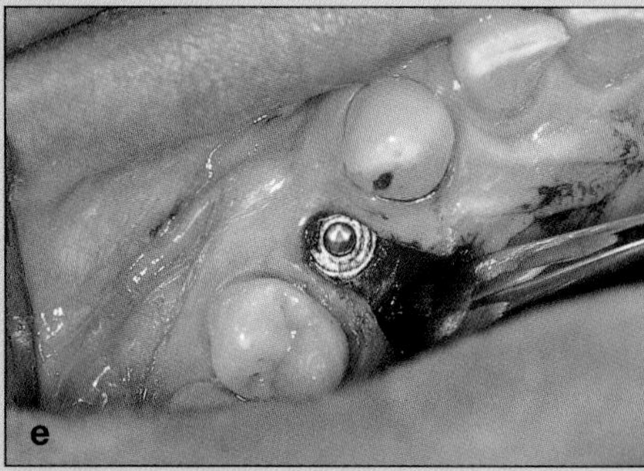

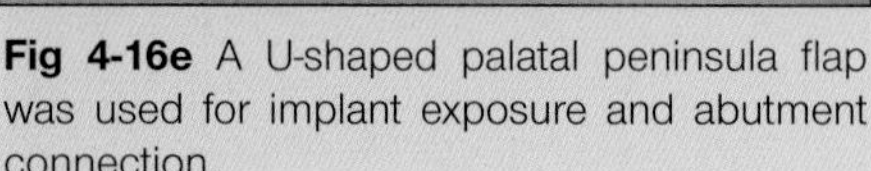

Fig 4-16e A U-shaped palatal peninsula flap was used for implant exposure and abutment connection.

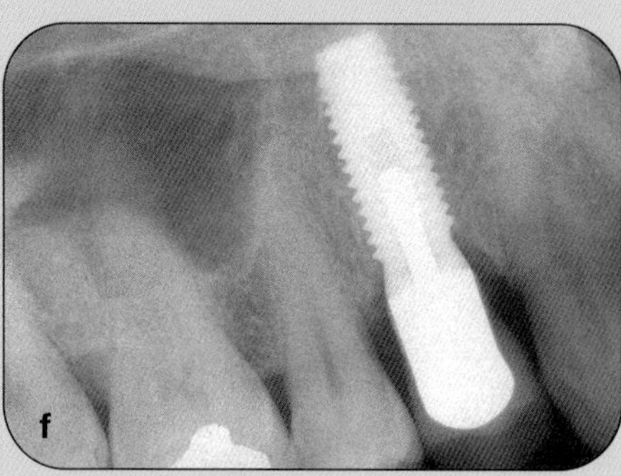

Fig 4-16f Post-restoration radiograph demonstrates stable osseous levels, positive osseous architecture, and further integration of the graft at the site.

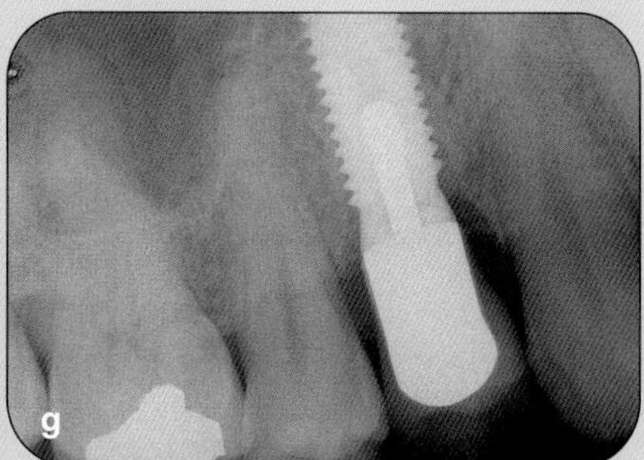

Fig 4-16g Radiographic view 31 months after delivery of the final restoration, demonstrating the long-term stability of the osseous levels under function and complete integration of the graft at the site. A uniform trabecular pattern surrounding the implant is evident.

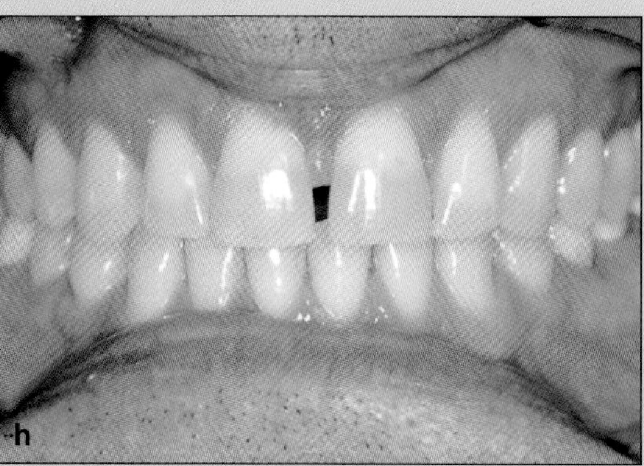

Fig 4-16h Follow-up view 31 months after delivery of the final restoration. Esthetics and soft tissue health have been maintained, and the restoration continues to be indistinguishable from the adjacent dentition. (Restoration by Dr Faustino Garcia, Coral Gables, FL.)

Modified Bio-Col technique for full-arch immediate-load mandibular restoration

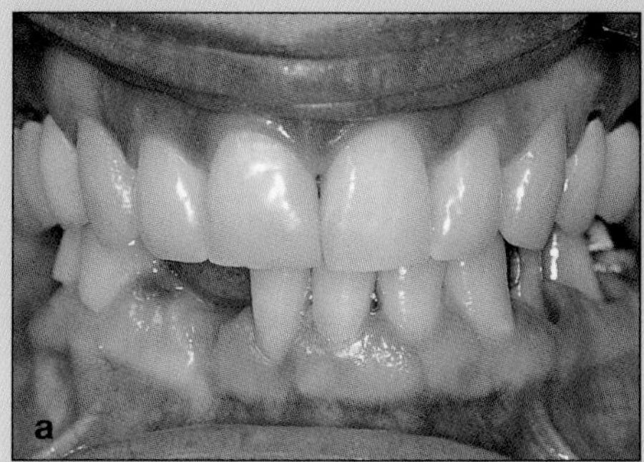

Fig 4-17a Full-mouth view demonstrates good alignment of mandibular and maxillary dentition and adequate interocclusal dimension for immediate delivery of an implant-supported provisional restoration.

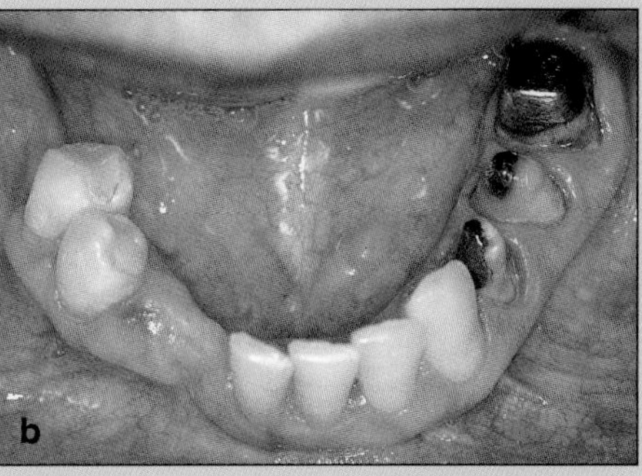

Fig 4-17b Preoperative view of failing mandibular dentition secondary to recurrent root caries. Note the undercuts on the buccal aspect of the alveolar ridge.

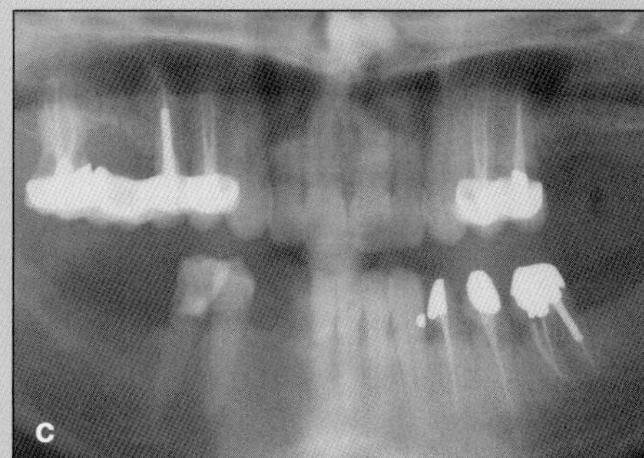

Fig 4-17c Preoperative radiograph demonstrating recurrent root caries of remaining mandibular dentition. Treatment plan included removal of remaining mandibular dentition and immediate implant replacements in conjunction with a modified Bio-Col technique.

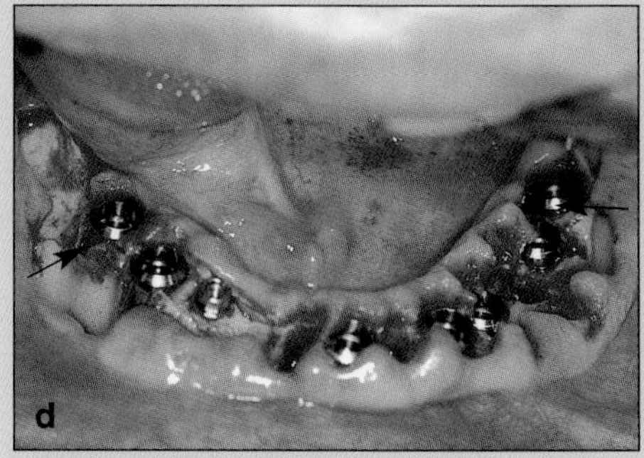

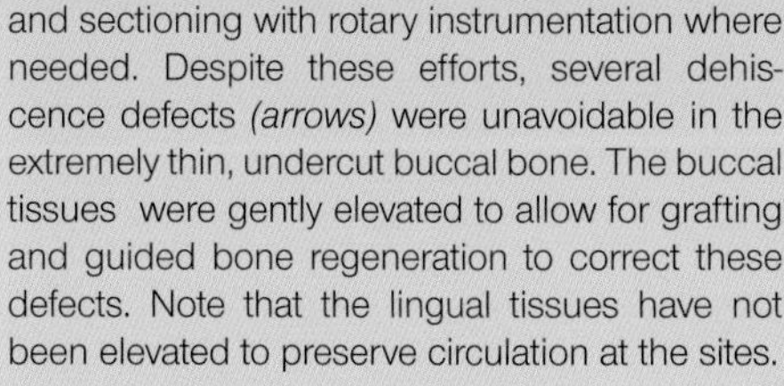

Fig 4-17d The remaining mandibular dentition has been carefully removed using periotomes and sectioning with rotary instrumentation where needed. Despite these efforts, several dehiscence defects *(arrows)* were unavoidable in the extremely thin, undercut buccal bone. The buccal tissues were gently elevated to allow for grafting and guided bone regeneration to correct these defects. Note that the lingual tissues have not been elevated to preserve circulation at the sites.

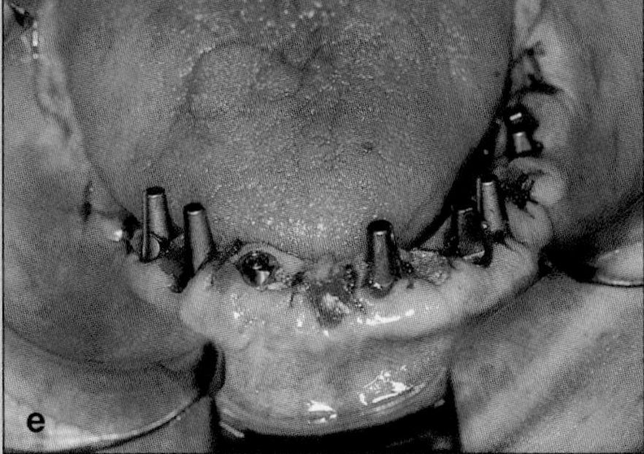

Fig 4-17e The voids between the immediately placed implants (Straumann USA) and the intact socket walls were grafted and isolated in the standard fashion. Dehiscence defects were grafted with a mixture of autogenous bone, Bio-Oss, and PRP. A Bio-Gide membrane was adapted over the grafted areas prior to tension-free soft tissue closure.

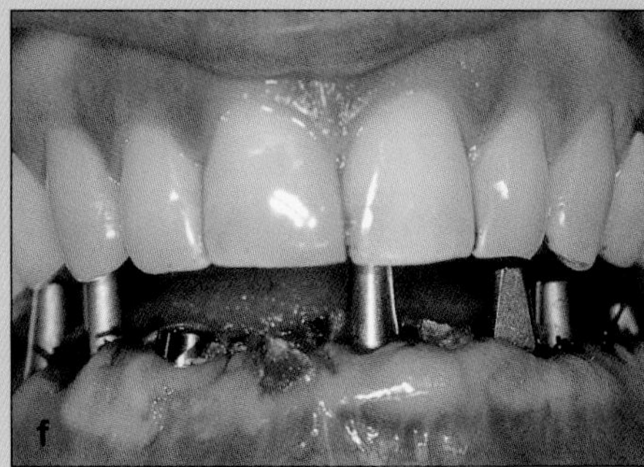

Fig 4-17f Solid abutments were placed on seven of the eight implants. Note excellent alignment of abutments with opposing dentition.

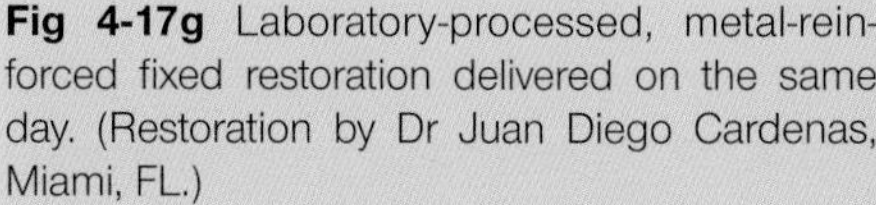

Fig 4-17g Laboratory-processed, metal-reinforced fixed restoration delivered on the same day. (Restoration by Dr Juan Diego Cardenas, Miami, FL.)

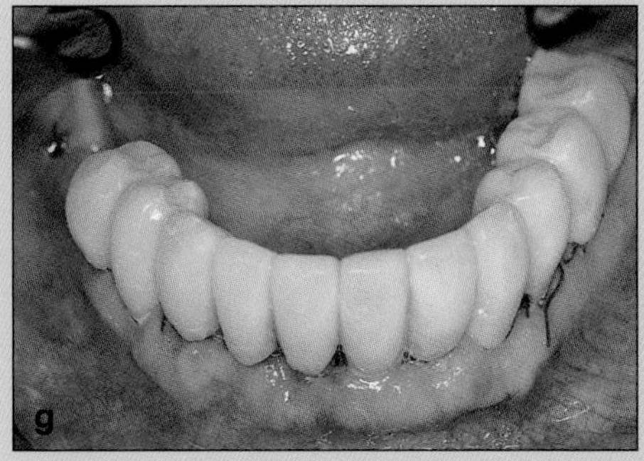

Fig 4-17h Three months after extraction and immediate implant placement, the provisional fixed partial denture was removed, and all implants were integrated. Note health and stability of peri-implant tissues.

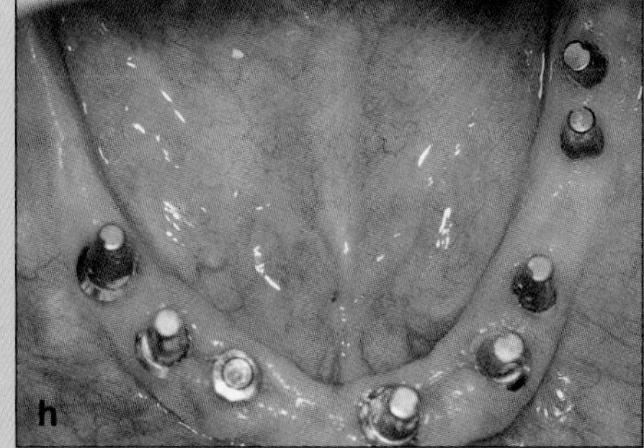

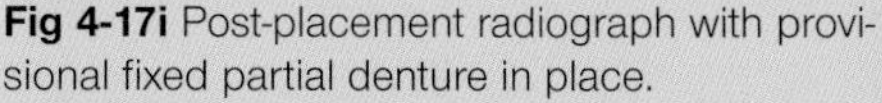

Fig 4-17i Post-placement radiograph with provisional fixed partial denture in place.

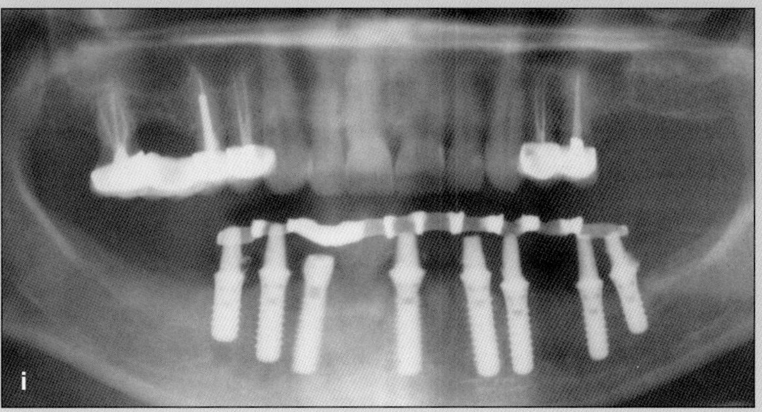

Bio-Col technique with PRP to prepare a compromised site for delayed implant placement following two previous failures

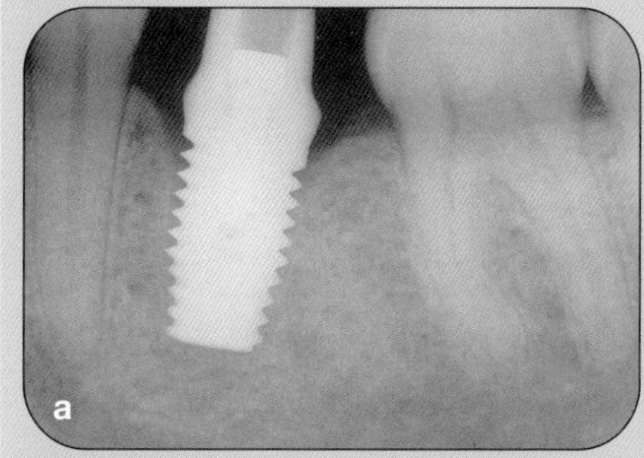

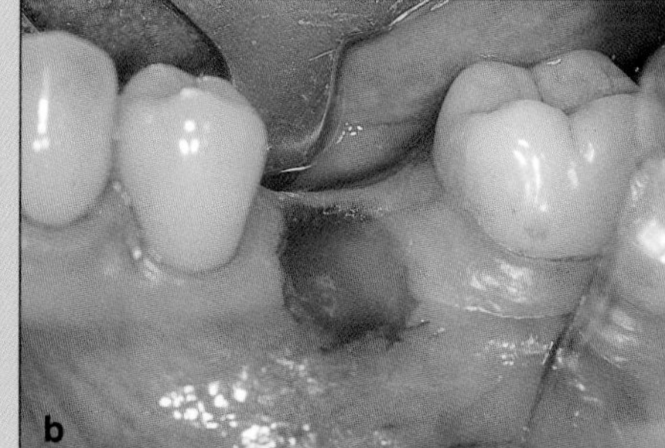

Fig 4-18a Preoperative radiograph demonstrating lack of osseointegration at this compromised mandibular first molar site.

Fig 4-18b Once the implant has been carefully removed, thorough curettage and perforation of the socket walls fails to stimulate bleeding. PRP solution will be used to ensure that a blood clot is present to initiate healing.

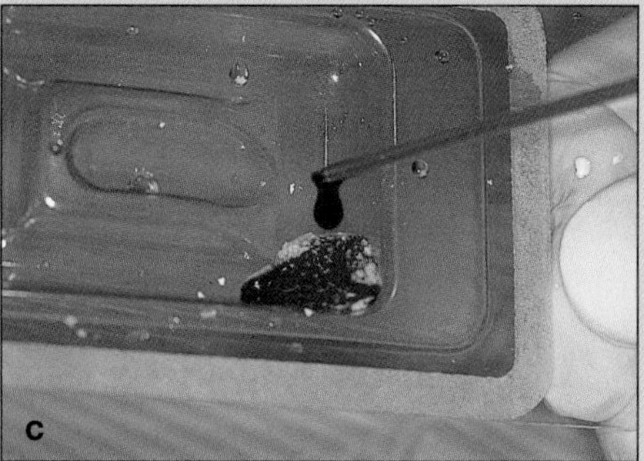

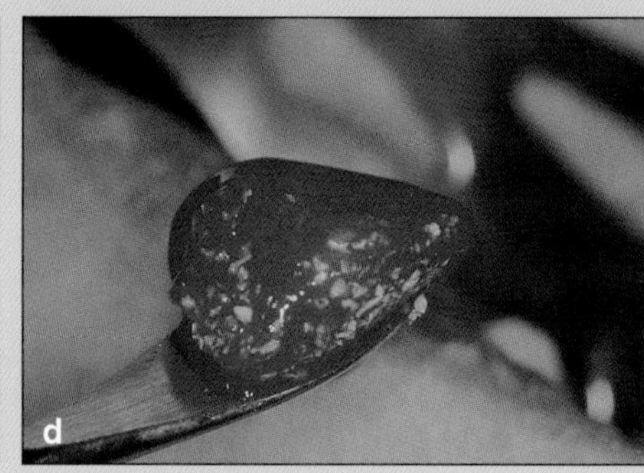

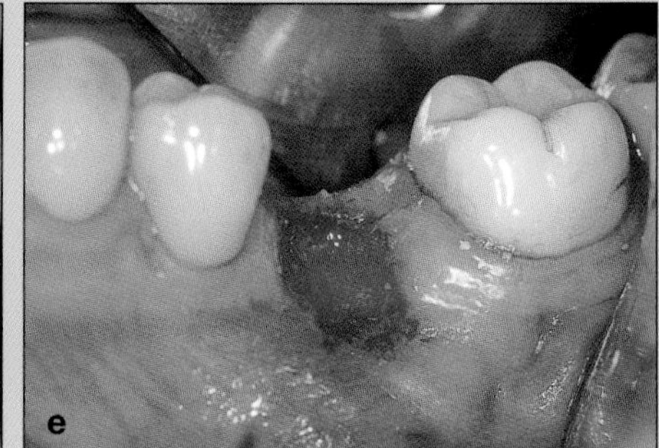

Figs 4-18c and 4-18d Mixing Bio-Oss with activated PRP solution results in a moldable graft that is conveniently delivered to the site. Autogenous bone was not used in this particular case.

Fig 4-18e The Bio-Oss-graft–PRP complex is immediately delivered and condensed into the socket. Additional PRP is injected into the grafted socket and left undisturbed before it is sealed with CollaPlug and Isodent tissue cement as previously described.

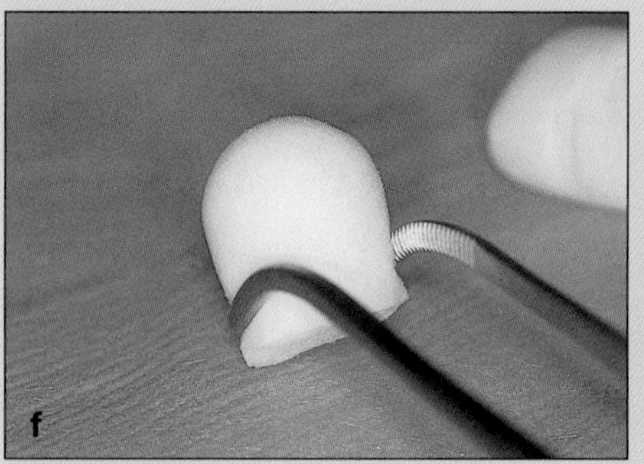

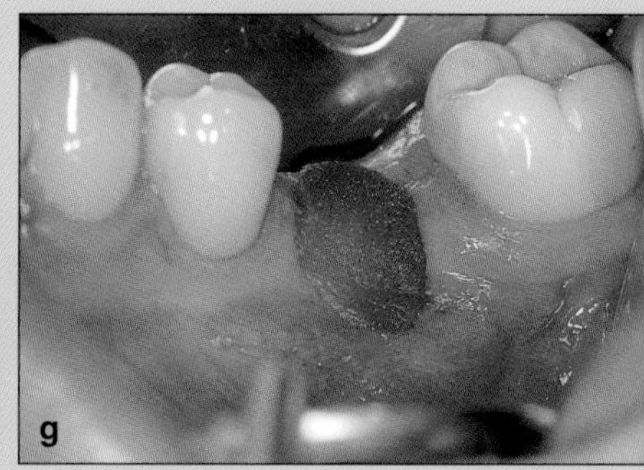

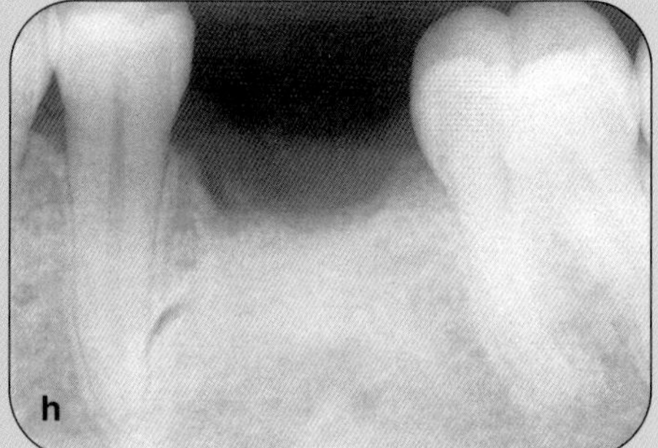

Figs 4-18f and 4-18g One half of a CollaPlug is prepared for delivery to the socket, where it is stabilized by absorbing the excess PRP solution. The site must be blotted with a dry sterile gauze before application of the tissue cement.

Fig 4-18h Postoperative radiographic view of the condensed Bio-Oss–PRP graft within the compromised socket.

site with a few drops of activated PRP and immediately delivering and condensing the graft at the site. After graft condensation is complete, the site is again moistened with a few drops of activated PRP solution and the CollaPlug material is immediately placed over the graft, where it becomes stabilized as it absorbs any excess PRP solution. Subsequently, the site is blotted with a dry sterile gauze, after which tissue cement is applied. For immediately placed implants, the author suggests injecting the activated PRP solution as the fixture is placed to its final sink depth. The PRP-graft mixture is delivered and condensed, and additional activated PRP mixture is injected as the fixture is delivered to full sink depth.

In summary, the author's 40-month experience indicates that the use of PRP may enhance wound healing and bone regeneration within extraction sockets in conjunction with immediate or delayed implant placement. The growth factors contained in PRP support the rationale for the inclusion of autogenous bone grafts mixed with Bio-Oss to take advantage of the theoretical benefits on these graft cells. Nevertheless, the au-

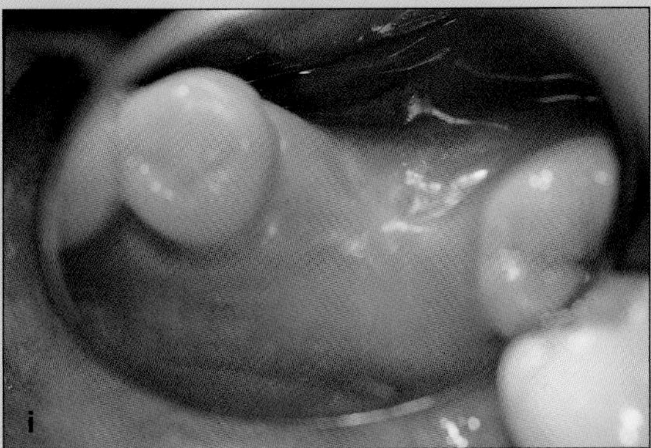

Fig 4-18i Excellent soft tissue healing 10 weeks after the procedure.

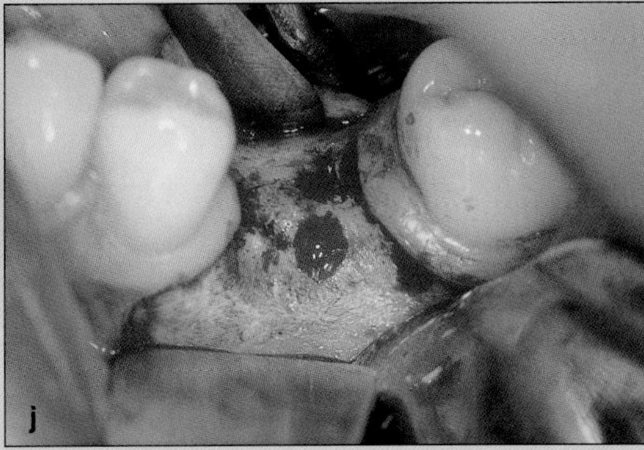

Fig 4-18j Upon site re-entry 3 months after the procedure, no Bio-Oss particles are discernible, indicating enhanced osseous healing. Newly formed cortex is also noted at previous defect site.

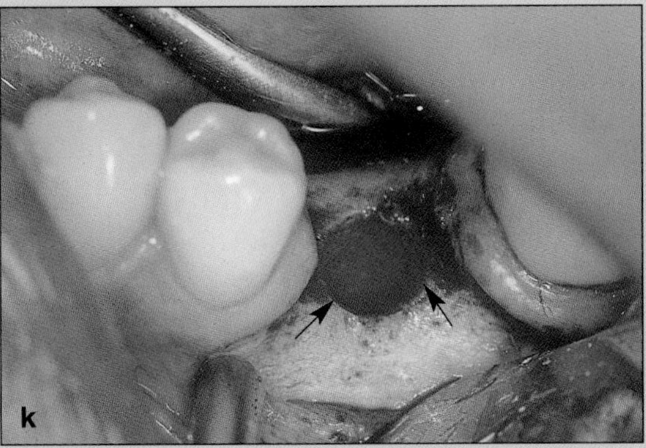

Fig 4-18k A core biopsy was performed prior to the osteotomy and implant placement. Although no Bio-Oss is visible, the buccal margin of the grafted socket *(arrows)* is discernable.

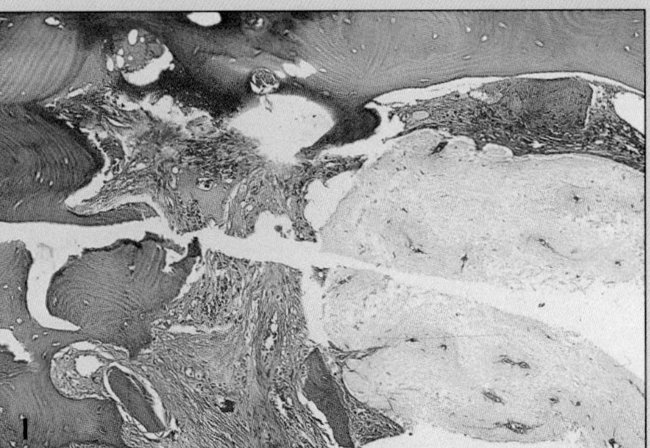

Fig 4-18l Histology of core biopsy demonstrates significant amounts of viable bone regenerated within the socket.

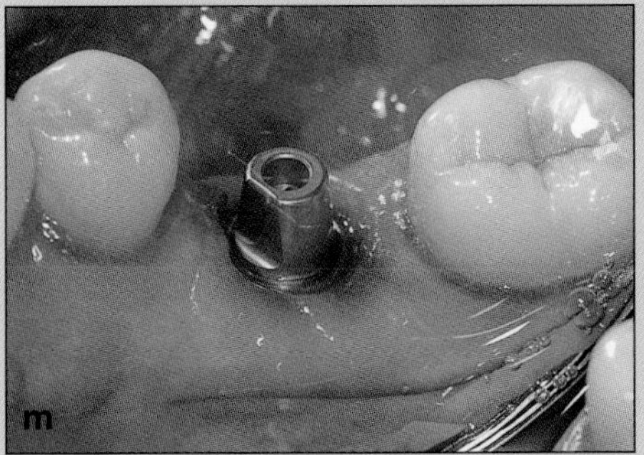

Fig 4-18m Three months after implant placement, the abutment is delivered. Note excellent soft tissue integration and prosthetic-friendly environment provided by one-piece nonsubmerged wide-neck implant.

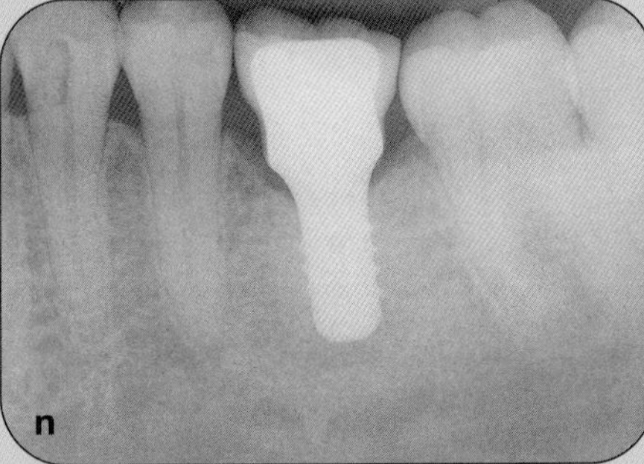

Fig 4-18n Radiographic view after delivery of final restoration demonstrating stable crestal bone and successful osseointegration of one-stage wide-neck implant (Straumann USA).

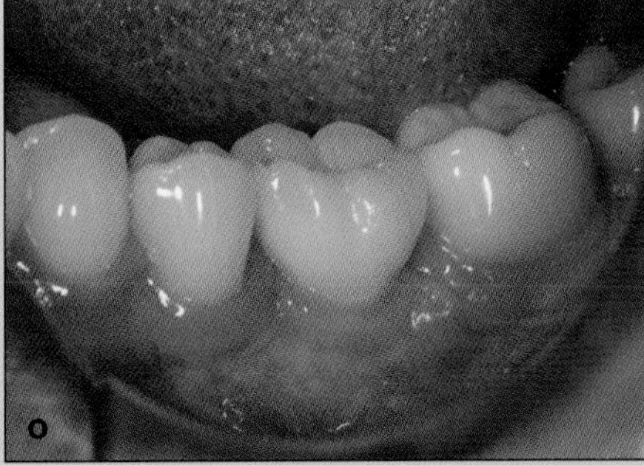

Fig 4-18o Final restoration has natural contours and a full occlusal table. Surrounding soft tissues are healthy. (Restoration by Dr Roy Greenberg, Miami, FL.)

thor has failed to observe any clinical advantages in including PRP in the treatment of intact healthy sockets with substantial osseous wall thickness (thick, flat periodontium). In the treatment of defect sockets or of sockets with inadequate wall thickness (thin, scalloped periodontium), where bone regeneration from within the graft may help bridge the gap across the defect, and in situations where guided bone regeneration is desired with particulate onlay bone grafts and resorbable barrier membranes are used, the author has observed that the use of a mixture of autogenous bone and Bio-Oss with PRP provides significant advantages.

Modified Bio-Col technique for full-arch immediate replacement of failing maxillary and mandibular dentition

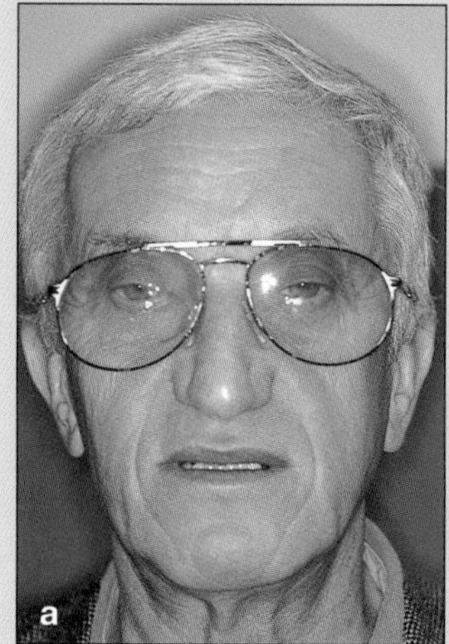

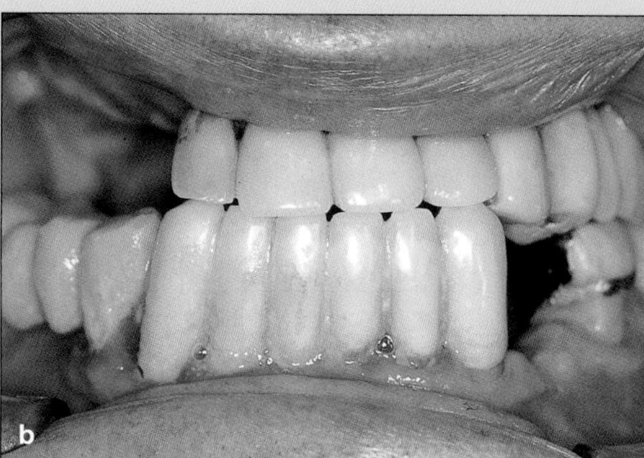

Fig 4-19a Preoperative view of a 64-year-old man with failing maxillary and mandibular dentition secondary to refractory periodontal disease.

Fig 4-19b Intraoral view demonstrating severity of periodontal destruction. A modified Bio-Col technique incorporating buccal flap elevation and repair of osseous defects with guided bone regeneration technique will be used in this case.

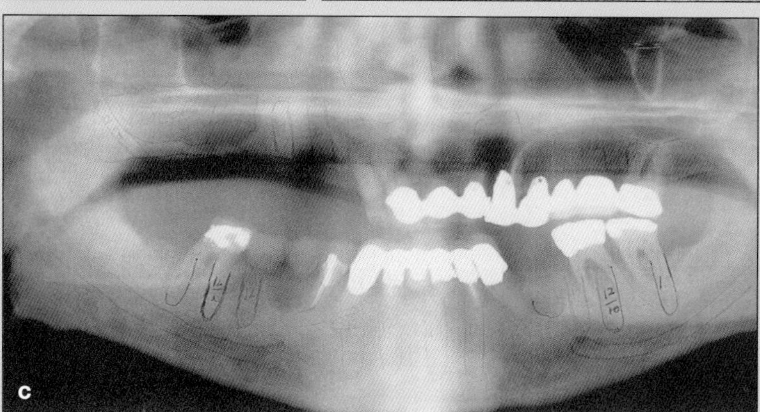

Fig 4-19c Pretreatment panoramic radiograph. Despite significant bone loss secondary to periodontal disease, adequate bone volume remains for placement of implants.

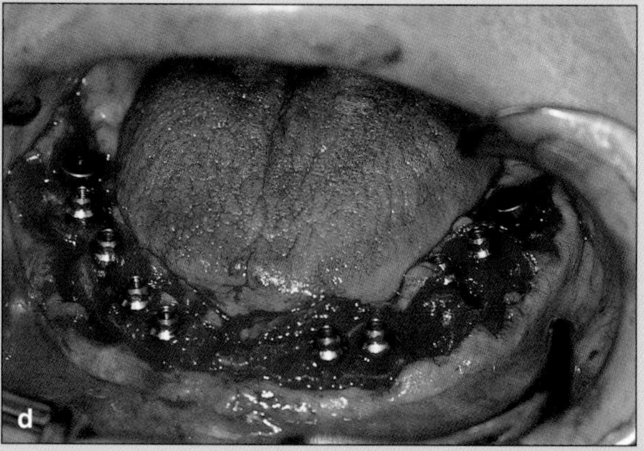

Fig 4-19d Remaining mandibular dentition has been removed, and 10 one-piece nonsubmerged implants have been placed in preparation for immediate loading.

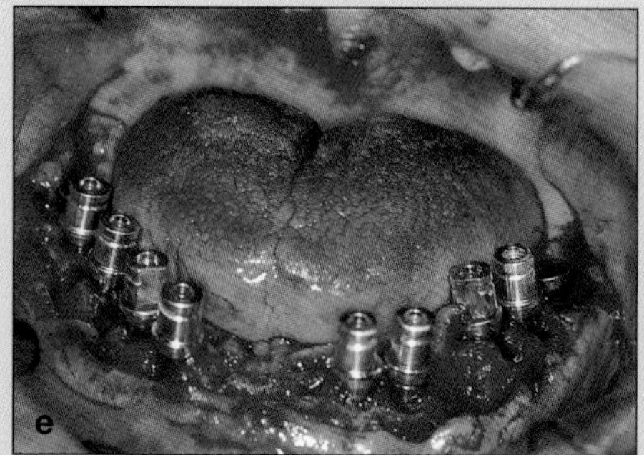

Fig 4-19e Repositionable impression copings have been secured to the implants.

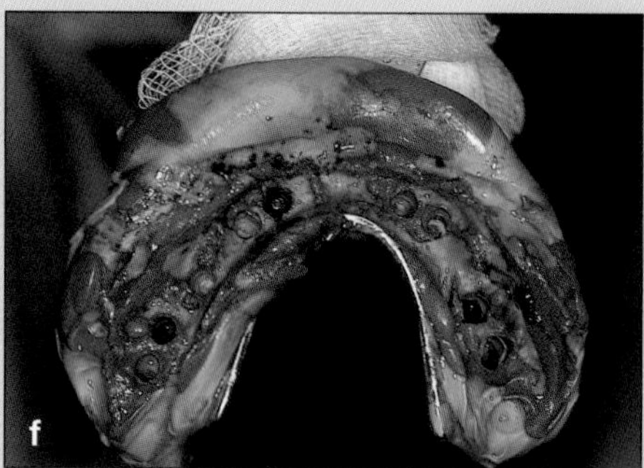

Fig 4-19f Mandibular full-arch impression registers the position of the immediately placed implants.

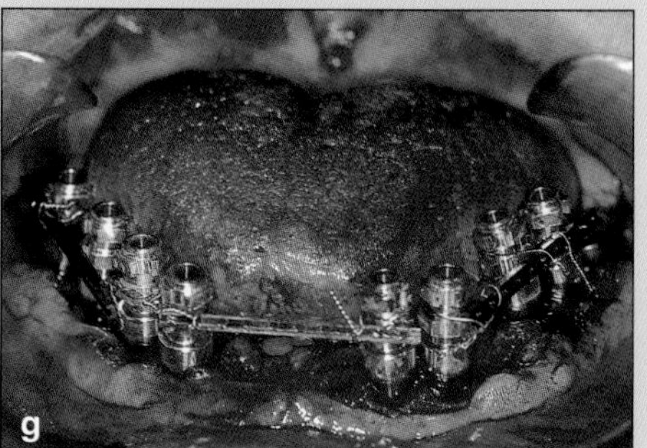

Fig 4-19g Nonrepositionable impression copings have been secured to the implants and connected with ligature wires and Zeza bar (Zeza, Miami, FL).

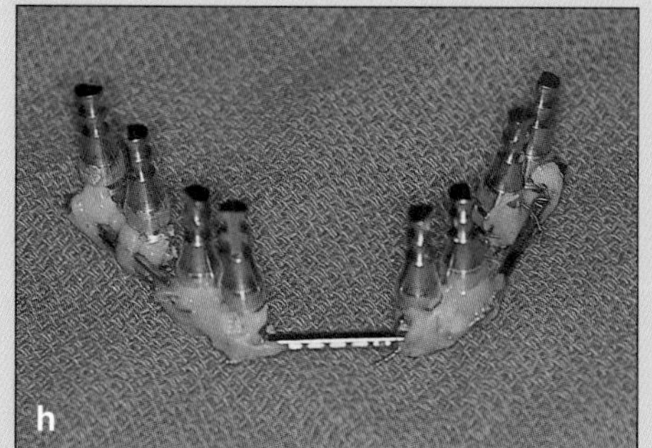

Fig 4-19h After further securing the Zeza bar with light-cured composite, the impression copings were removed as a single unit.

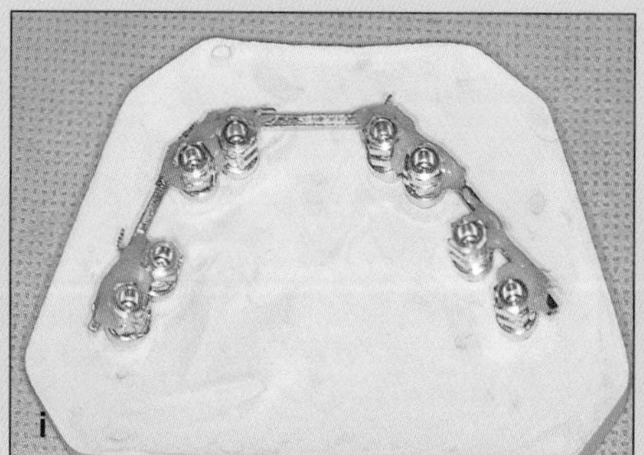

Fig 4-19i A master cast was fabricated using a fast-set zero-expansion stone. This provides a working model for the restorative dentist to fabricate the mandibular immediate-load, fixed prosthesis while the maxillary surgery is being performed.

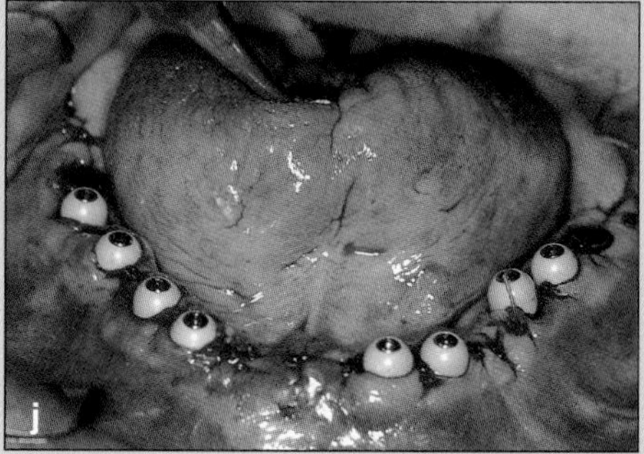

Fig 4-19j Osseous defects were grafted with a mixture of Bio-Oss, autogenous bone, and PRP. Bio-Gide membranes were then adapted over the grafts, and the buccal flaps were coapted to obtain circumferential adaptation around the Octa protective caps. Following wound closure, additional PRP solution was applied topically to gain a wound-sealing effect.

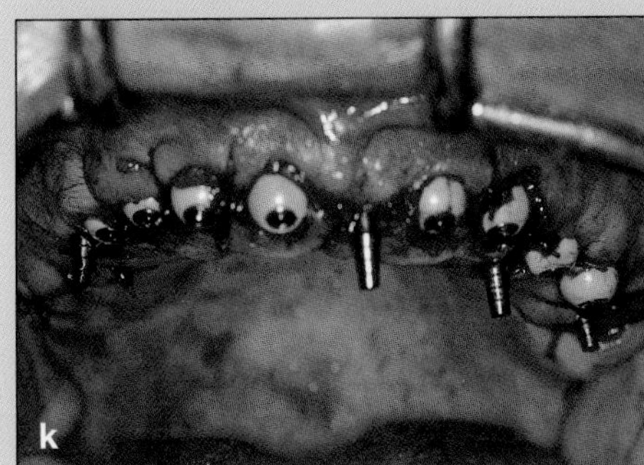

Fig 4-19k Remaining maxillary teeth have been removed, and 8 nonsubmerged implants (Straumann USA) have been placed using the Bio-Col technique. Because of poor bone quality, provisional implants were used to support the interim prosthesis and protect the implants from micromotion.

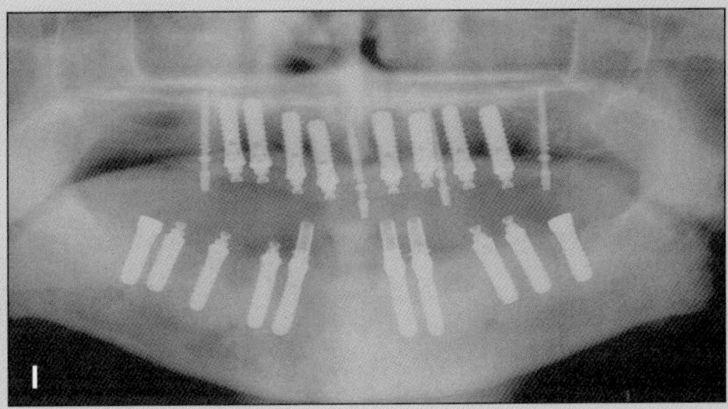

Fig 4-19l Panoramic radiograph taken after implant placement demonstrates good alignment and distribution of the implants.

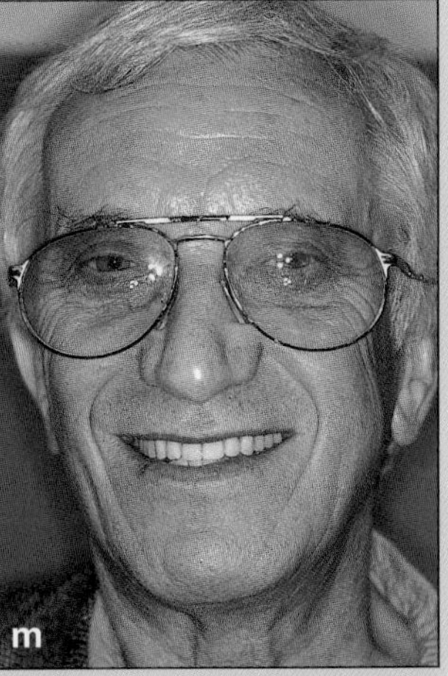

Fig 4-19m Post-treatment view of happy patient after delivery of maxillary and mandibular provisional restorations on the same day. Notice the immediate improvement in esthetics and lip support.

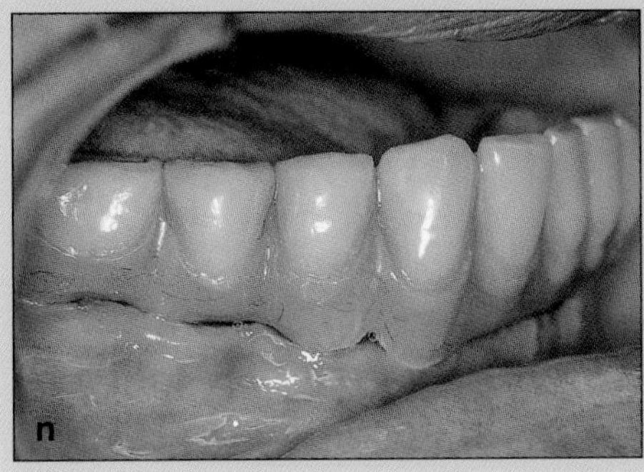

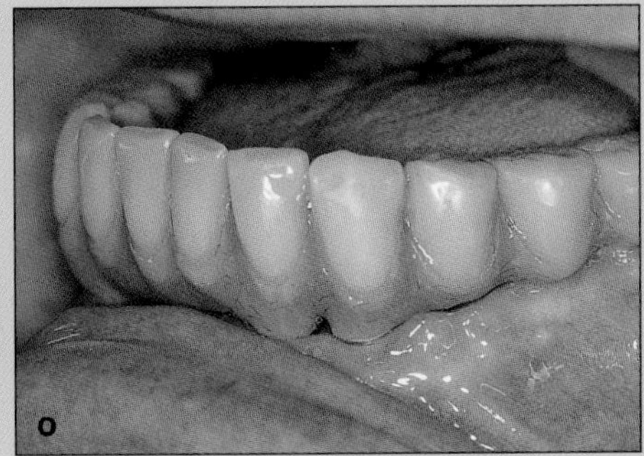

Figs 4-19n and 4-19o One year following delivery of mandibular fixed prosthesis. Stable, healthy peri-implant soft tissues are evident.

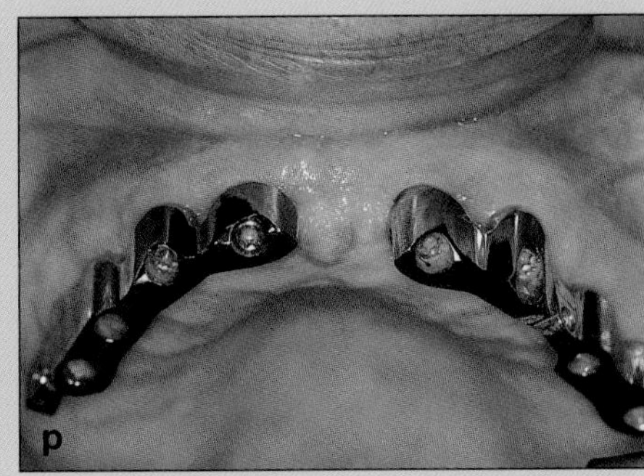

Fig 4-19p One year following delivery of precision maxillary fixed removable prosthesis. Healthy peri-implant soft tissues are evident.

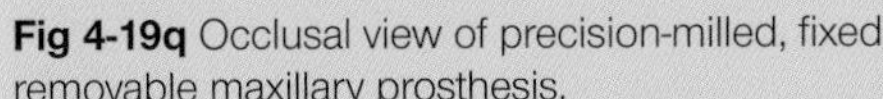

Fig 4-19q Occlusal view of precision-milled, fixed removable maxillary prosthesis.

Fig 4-19r Frontal view of final prosthesis 1 year after delivery. (Restoration by Dr Larry Grillo, Aventura, FL.)

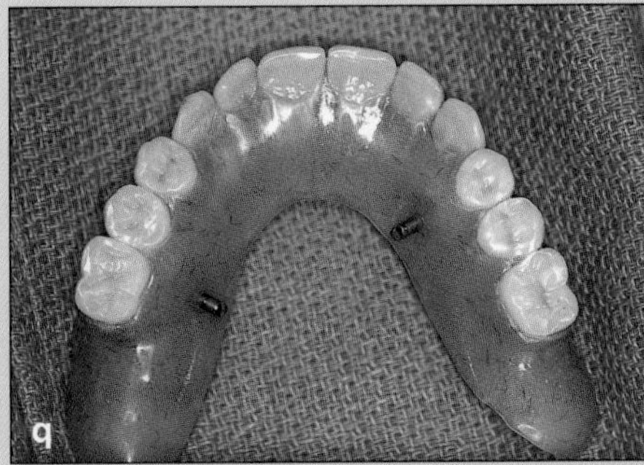

Fig 4-19s Panoramic radiograph 1 year after delivery of final restoration demonstrates stable osseous levels and integration of Bio-Oss grafts at all sites.

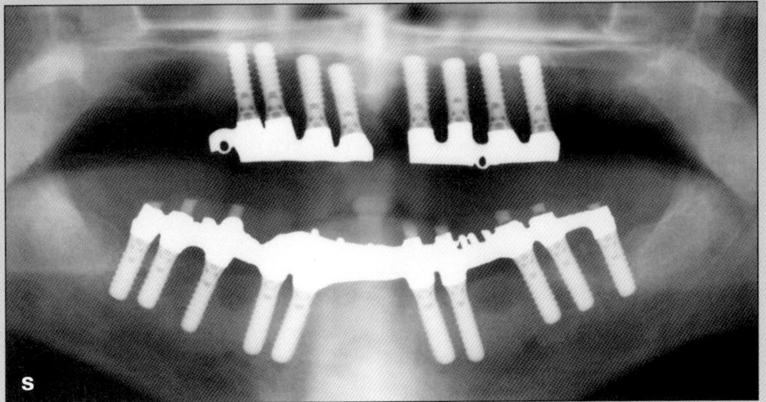

Summary

The Bio-Col technique is a straightforward and reproducible technique that has a biologic basis for success when used in conjunction with immediate implant placement or to potentiate sites for delayed implant placement. Nonetheless, it is important for the implant surgeon to recognize situations or conditions where the technique will not prevent the need for further site-development procedures. When a site is compromised by a history of trauma, infection, endodontic therapy, or previous surgeries, the surgeon should recognize that compromised circulation in the area might prevent adequate integration of the Bio-Oss graft material. Upon re-entry to such a site, the surgeon should not be surprised to find the material much as it was when it was placed. This may also occur at sites judged by history and clinical observation to have good regenerative potential when the details of the technique are not adhered to, when an incomplete technique without the prosthetic protocol is performed, or when micromotion is transmitted to the grafted site. This is consistent with our understanding of the important role that initial blood clot and/or graft stabilization and subsequent protection of a grafted site play in achieving guided bone regeneration. The need for additional site-development procedures should also be expected when tooth mobility, chronic irritation secondary to a violation of biologic width, or recurrent decay under an existing restoration is accompanied by edema of the soft tissues. These situations frequently lead to soft tissue recession that may also be accompanied by resorption of underlying alveolar bone. Similarly, whenever a tooth is removed in a patient with a thin, scalloped periodontium, there is significant risk of soft tissue recession and resorptive remodeling of the alveolus, which can result in early or late functional or esthetic compromises in implant therapy. Although the Bio-Col technique may not be able to completely prevent loss of hard and soft tissue volume and architecture in these instances, it minimizes the complexity of subsequent site-development procedures.

Finally, it is appropriate to address the question of whether the Bio-Col technique is always indicated to preserve hard and soft tissue alveolar ridge anatomy in preparation for delayed implant placement or in conjunction with immediate implant placement. Certainly, tooth extraction at healthy sites in patients with thick, flat periodontal phenotypes (abundant socket wall thickness) may escape significant resorptive remodeling changes that would compromise functional implant outcomes, but soft tissue collapse leading to an esthetic compromise is constant. Furthermore, since most patients fall somewhere in between the extremes of a thick, flat periodontium and the more vulnerable thin, flat periodontium, the author strongly suggests the use of the Bio-Col technique, especially in areas of high esthetic importance, whenever an implant replacement is planned following tooth removal. While success is certainly possible without the use of this technique, the functional and esthetic predictability realized in implant therapy is far greater when the implant surgeon routinely uses the Bio-Col technique, as summarized below.

1. Perform minimally traumatic tooth removal with preservation of hard and soft tissues in the area.
2. When bleeding is not abundant following curettage of the socket, perforate the socket walls to stimulate bleeding and enhance the invasion of osteoprogenitor cells into the socket.
3. Graft the bleeding socket with condensed Bio-Oss to provide an ideal osteoconductive scaffold that eventually will be replaced by vital mineralized bone through a slow resorptive process.
4. Perform immediate implant placement when indicated.
5. Isolate and seal the grafted socket or implant surgical site from the oral environment by condensing CollaPlug absorbable collagen material over the grafted area to the level of the free marginal tissues.
6. Secure the collagen material with a horizontal mattress suture in esthetic areas and with a continuous figure-eight suture in nonesthetic areas. Seal the surface of the collagen with Isodent tissue cement, avoiding overflow to the surrounding tissues.
7. Adapt and deliver an interim provisional restoration of ovate pontic design. The provisional restoration should replicate the contours of the natural tooth that was removed, support the surrounding soft tissues, and avoid loading of the underlying graft or immediately placed implant. Alternatively, use an anatomic healing abutment or a custom tooth-form healing abutment to provide immediate support of soft tissues when an implant is placed in a nonsubmerged fashion.

CHAPTER 5

Soft Tissue Grafting in Implant Therapy

The preceding chapters have established the critical role that the peri-implant soft tissues play in achieving and maintaining functional and esthetic success in implant therapy. When a clinical situation presents inadequate quality or quantity of soft tissue to provide a stable peri-implant environment, the implant surgeon must be equipped with the principles and techniques to reconstruct the missing soft tissue components. Moreover, when esthetics dictate that the implant be inconspicuous, the implant surgeon must be able to select the appropriate procedures necessary to restore natural soft tissue architecture. This chapter focuses on the principles of soft tissue grafting and the most common techniques and approaches used to enhance function and esthetics around dental implants.

Periodontal Plastic Surgery

In 1959, Friedman[1] coined the term *mucogingival surgery* and defined its scope to include the surgical management of shallow vestibules, aberrant frenula, and inadequate attached gingiva. In the early 1980s, a paradigm shift away from resective techniques and toward surgical procedures designed to reconstruct missing periodontal tissues in an esthetically pleasing manner occurred in surgical periodontal therapy. This shift in perspective came about as a result of increasing esthetic demands from patients and advances in surgical techniques and biotechnology. In 1988, Miller[2] introduced the term *periodontal plastic surgery* to include the broader scope of procedures that had evolved from traditional mucogingival surgery. According to Miller, the scope of periodontal plastic surgery includes surgical treatment for aberrant frenula, shallow vestibules, marginal tissue recession, deficient ridges, maintenance of ridge form after extraction of periodontally involved teeth, excessive gingival display ("gummy smile"), unerupted teeth requiring orthodontic movement, maintenance of interdental papillae, and mucogingival defects associated with dental implants.

In 1996,[3] periodontal plastic surgery was defined as "surgical procedures performed to prevent or correct anatomic, developmental, traumatic or disease-induced defects of the gingiva, alveolar mucosa or bone." Accordingly, periodontal plastic surgery for the implant patient includes the following procedures:

- Augmentation of attached tissues surrounding natural teeth and implant restorations
- Root and implant abutment coverage
- Correction of mucogingival defects around implants
- Edentulous ridge augmentation in preparation for prosthetic rehabilitation with conventional or implant prostheses
- Edentulous ridge preservation following tooth removal in preparation for prosthetic rehabilitation with conventional or implant prostheses
- Management of aberrant frenula
- Preservation or reconstruction of interdental or inter-implant papillae
- Surgical soft tissue sculpting procedures

Oral Soft Tissue Grafting with Dental Implants

Rationale for soft tissue grafting

The rationale for soft tissue augmentation around dental implants is similar to that around natural dentition. In general, experienced clinicians agree that an "adequate zone" of attached tissue around a natural tooth or implant prosthesis is desirable to better withstand the functional stresses resulting from mastication and oral hygiene efforts and to maintain predictable levels over time. In addition, most believe that an adequate zone of attached tissue is needed to withstand the potential mechanical and bacterial challenges presented by esthetic restorations—whether on natural teeth or dental implants—that extend below the free gingival margin. The initial potential mechanical challenges include tooth preparation, soft tissue retraction and impression procedures, cementation of provisional and permanent restorations, removal of implant healing abutments and their replacement with permanent abutments, implant-level impressions, and placement of provisional and permanent implant restorations. After final restoration, the intracrevicular esthetic restorative margins may continue to present a permanent inflammatory challenge to the surrounding soft tissue attachment apparatus. Some implant practitioners believe that the microgap at the site of abutment connection to two-piece implants may present a similar challenge.

Whether these challenges result in initial apical displacement of the marginal tissues or possibly even progressive loss of attachment depends on multiple factors, including the following:

- Patient age
- General health
- Host resistance factors
- Effect of systemic medications
- Periodontal phenotype
- Technique and effectiveness of oral hygiene
- Frequency and technique of professional oral hygiene care
- Operative technique
- Choice of restorative materials
- Initial location of restorative margin vis-à-vis circumferential biologic width requirements

- Prominence of implant position in alveolus
- Pre-existing bony dehiscence
- Design and surface characteristics of implant
- Depth of implant placement
- Thickness and apicocoronal dimension of attached tissue

Because multiple factors influence the health of the marginal tissues, prospective or retrospective experimental or clinical studies are difficult to design and conduct. Interpreting the results of these studies is even more difficult. Certainly, studies that consider primarily the apicocoronal dimension of attached tissue and its effect on marginal soft tissue health, without considering the other factors, are at best inconclusive. Therefore, the rationale for soft tissue augmentation around the natural dentition or the dental implant prosthesis should be based on clinical experience rather than on results from experimental or clinical studies.

Although clinicians agree that an adequate zone of gingiva is important for the maintenance of marginal tissue health, they do not agree on the precise gingival dimensions that constitute this adequate zone. Maynard and Wilson[4] state that an "adequate band" of keratinized tissue is fundamental to successful restorative dentistry when the margins of the restorations are extended under the free gingival margin. Although these authors recognize that many other factors, such as gingival thickness, also affect the adequacy of the gingival tissues, they define the dimensions of an adequate band of gingival tissue to be 5 mm. They further state that this band should be composed of 2 mm of free gingiva and 3 mm of attached gingiva. They point out that restorative procedures extending below the free gingival margin present a challenge to the periodontal attachment apparatus and may result in subsequent apical migration of marginal tissues. Therefore, they developed a rationale for fortifying the periodontal tissues via gingival augmentation prior to the restorative procedures when intracrevicular restorative margins are planned in areas consisting of alveolar mucosa or insufficient amounts of gingiva. The authors find that although restorations can be placed when less gingival tissue exists, success is far more predictable when the ideal dimensions are present.

Despite the many similarities between periodontal soft tissues and peri-implant soft tissues, they are not identical.[5] The lack of connective tissue attachment and the differences in the composition, vascularity, and orientation of the connective tissue surrounding a dental implant render the implant more susceptible to disease than its natural tooth counterpart. The soft tissue seal around a dental implant is formed by the junctional epithelium, which adheres to the abutment or implant body via a hemidesmosomal attachment. The implant surface does not have a functional connective tissue attachment analogous to the Sharpey's fiber insertion to the cementum of a natural tooth. Therefore, the biologic seal around an implant depends on the combination of the strength of the junctional epithelial attachment and the immobility of the peri-implant connective tissue. This immobility exists only when there is an adequate dimension of connective tissue in the peri-implant soft tissues. In addition, this connective tissue must be intimately adapted around the permucosal implant structures. The tonus of the circular connective tissue fibers that run around the implant and the attachment of connective tissue fibers extending from the alveolar crest to the free marginal gingiva provide the structural support and immobility needed to maintain the junctional epithelial seal.[6]

Although implant therapy can be successful in areas of alveolar mucosa, restorations are far more predictable when an adequate zone of attached tissue exists. When one considers that the periodontal attachment apparatus is mechanically superior to the protective soft tissue seal formed around an implant, it seems reasonable that the dimensions of gingival tissue surrounding an implant restoration should be equal to or greater than the 5 mm suggested by Maynard and Wilson.[4] At minimum, it seems logical to apply the same criteria where implant therapy is performed in areas of esthetic concern. When implant therapy is planned in nonesthetic areas, the author refers to the conclusions of Lang and Löe[7] that a zone of 2 mm of attached gingiva around the natural dentition is enough to maintain the health of the marginal tissues. Because of the tenuous nature of the peri-implant soft tissue seal, the author feels that this dimension is an absolute minimum and prefers a 3-mm zone of thick attached tissue around dental implants.

The author believes that the thickness of the attached tissue surrounding an implant restoration is as important as the apicocoronal dimension of the attached tissue. The clinician should realize that abutment connection and implant-level impressions are traumatic and may result in apical migration of the peri-implant soft tissues, with subsequent crestal alveolar bone loss. In addition, prosthetic attachments that allow apicocoronal movement of an implant-supported removable prosthesis continually challenge the tenuous peri-implant soft tissue seal. Therefore, even when supragingival implant restorations are fabricated in nonesthetic areas, there is a logical and biologic basis for fortifying the peri-implant tissues to withstand the trauma imposed by the necessary prosthetic procedures that extend below the level of the free gingival margin. In addition, the augmented peri-implant soft tissues will better resist future functional stresses imposed by mastica-

Table 5-1 Principles of oral soft tissue grafting

Preparation of recipient site	Management of donor tissue
• Ensure adequate vascularity to support the graft • Provide a means for rigid immobilization of the graft • Prepare uniform surface for intimate graft adaptation • Obtain hemostasis	• Harvest graft of adequate size to take advantage of peripheral circulation • Ensure a uniform graft surface for adaptation of recipient site • Ensure adequate thickness to obtain desired volume augmentation and for survival over avascular surfaces

tion, removal and replacement of removable prostheses, and oral hygiene efforts.

Goals of oral soft tissue grafting

The most obvious goal of oral soft tissue grafting in implant therapy is to create a stable peri-implant soft tissue environment by providing an adequate zone of attached nonmobile tissues with intimate adaptation to emerging implant structures. This results in the maintenance of the biologic soft tissue seal and a reduction in the incidence of peri-implantitis, which can jeopardize long-term success and patient satisfaction with implant restorations. An additional goal in esthetic implant therapy is inconspicuous reconstruction of natural soft tissue architecture to enable the emergence of harmonious implant restorations.

Surgical principles of oral soft tissue grafting

The principles that govern oral soft tissue grafting procedures are analogous to the basic principles of plastic and reconstructive surgery. It is useful to conceptually divide the surgical principles into those related to preparing the recipient site and those related to harvesting and securing the donor tissue at the graft site (Table 5-1).

The first principle of oral soft tissue grafting is that the recipient site must provide for graft vascularization. It is understood that free grafts initially survive by plasmatic diffusion and are subsequently vascularized as capillaries and arterioles form a vascular network providing the permanent circulation for the graft. When a recipient site is partially avascular (eg, a denuded root surface, exposed implant abutment, or area recently reconstructed with a block bone graft), it should be large enough to provide a peripheral source of circulation to support the free graft over the avascular or poorly vascularized areas. Although pedicle grafts and flaps have a contiguous blood supply, it is also good surgical practice to prepare a recipient site that can contribute circulation to ensure optimal results in the event of a reduction of circulation to a portion (most commonly, the margin) of the pedicle graft or flap.

The second principle of oral soft tissue grafting is that the recipient site must provide a means for rigid immobilization of the graft tissue. Initial graft survival requires that the graft be immobilized and intimately adapted to the recipient site. Mobility of the graft during initial healing can interfere with its early nourishment through plasmatic diffusion or can disrupt the newly forming circulatory supply to the graft, resulting in excessive shrinkage or sloughing of the graft.

The third principle is that adequate hemostasis must be obtained at the recipient site. Active hemorrhage at the site will prevent the intimate adaptation of the graft to the recipient site. Hemorrhage also will interfere with the maintenance of the thin layer of fibrin between the graft and recipient site, which serves to physically attach the graft to the recipient site and provides for the plasmatic diffusion that initially nourishes the graft before its vascularization. Preparation of a recipient site with a uniform surface enhances the intimate adaptation with the graft. Periosteum is generally considered to be an excellent recipient site for oral soft tissue grafts because it fulfills all of the requirements discussed above. In addition, decorticated alveolar bone can support and nourish a free soft tissue graft, although immobilizing the graft at the site is more troublesome.

The fourth principle of oral soft tissue grafting is that the donor tissue must be large enough to facilitate immobilization at the recipient site and to take advantage of peripheral circulation when root or abutment coverage is the goal. The graft also must be large enough to result in the desired volume augmentation after secondary contraction has occurred. In addition, the donor tissue harvest should ensure a uniform graft surface that facilitates intimate adaptation to the recipient site.

Finally, the surgeon should realize that graft thickness influences healing to some degree. When root coverage, abutment coverage, or soft tissue augmentation at implant sites is desired, grafts with a thickness greater than 1.25 mm are preferable. Although a higher percentage of success with thin and intermedi-

Maintainance of heterotopic specificity after transplantation of palatal connective tissue

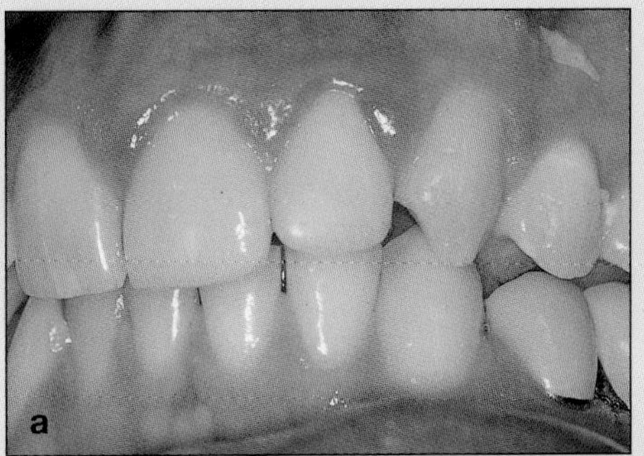

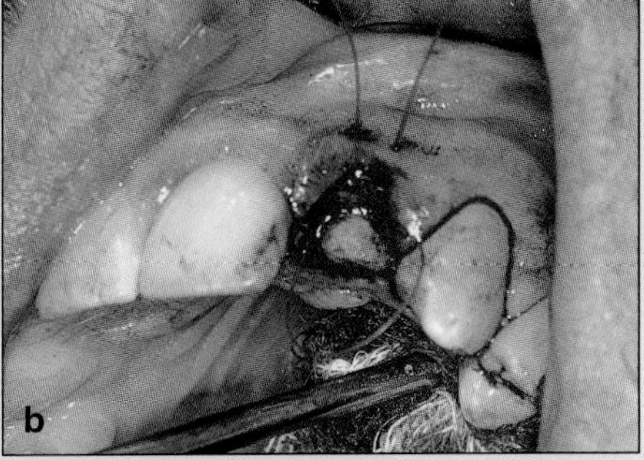

Fig 5-1a Presurgical view. Note Miller class I recession defect and poor-quality mucosal tissues surrounding fractured lateral incisor.

Fig 5-1b The tooth has been removed, and an immediate implant has been placed. After a split-thickness recipient site has been prepared, a subepithelial connective tissue graft is secured at the site.

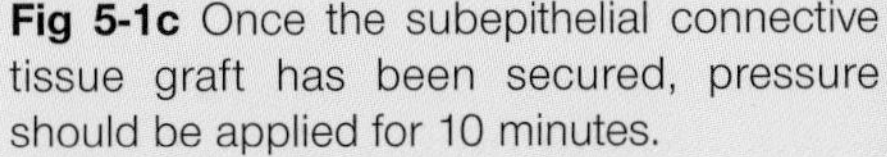

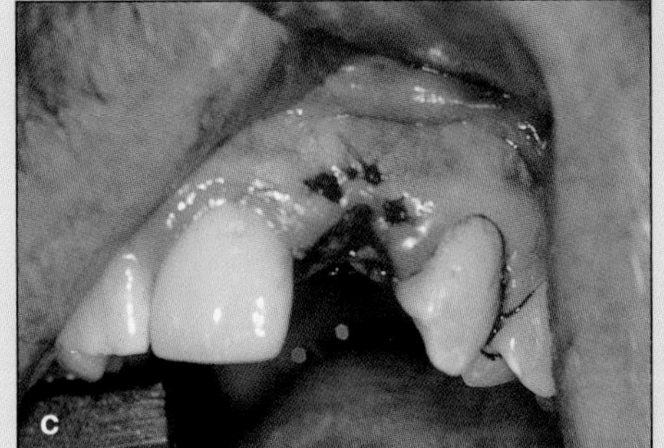

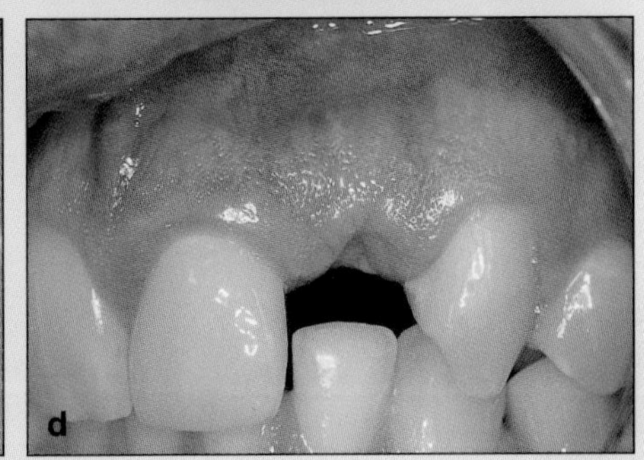

Fig 5-1c Once the subepithelial connective tissue graft has been secured, pressure should be applied for 10 minutes.

Fig 5-1d Patient initially lost to follow up returns 18 months later. Note the change in character of the soft tissues. Keratinization of the tissue is evident as a result of transplantation of palatal connective tissue.

ate split-thickness grafts (approximately 0.50 to 0.75 mm) has been reported, the use of thicker grafts as part of the contemporary surgical technique yields excellent results. Thicker grafts are especially useful for root and abutment coverage where graft healing over the central portion of the avascular surface is characterized by necrosis. The necrotic graft is gradually overtaken by granulation tissue from the periphery and ultimately forms a scar. The thicker grafts are better able to maintain their physical integrity during this process, which can take as long as 4 to 6 weeks. In contrast to skin grafts, oral soft tissue grafts undergo negligible primary contraction. Secondary contraction, which is rarely a problem for thick split-thickness grafts, is common when thin split-thickness grafts are used. In summary, harvesting a graft that is too small or too thin should be avoided by evaluating the donor site prior to surgery and applying the foregoing principles during recipient and donor site surgery.

Failure to adhere to these surgical principles will decrease volume yields of oral soft tissue grafting procedures. It also will increase complications such as inadequate volume yield, graft sloughing, wound breakdown, infection, and patient discomfort.

An important concept related to soft tissue grafting is the maintenance of heterotopic specificity after transplantation of palatal tissues.[8] This is an important consideration for the implant surgeon when performing subepithelial connective tissue grafts under alveolar mucosal recipient site tissue. In these instances, the underlying connective tissue will eventually determine the character of the overlying epithelium. In clinical practice, this phenomenon, known as "bleeding through" of keratinized tissue, is observed as progressive improvement in the color and character of the tissue over time (Fig 5-1). This understanding enables the surgeon to reassure patients that improvements in the appearance of soft tissue can be expected over time in these instances.

Modified Palatal Roll Technique for Dental Implants

In 1980, Abrams[9] first described the use of a connective tissue pedicle flap for augmentation of deficient edentulous ridges in preparation for fixed maxillary prostheses. He described a technique that involved rotating, or "rolling," a de-epithelialized connective tissue pedicle from the palate into a prepared labial pouch. The goal of the technique was to provide both buccal augmentation and vertical soft tissue augmentation at the edentulous site. The buccal augmentation re-created the appearance of a natural tooth root eminence. The vertical augmentation created a concave ridge form that provided an ideal prosthetic receptor site for convex pontic adaptation, ensuring both optimal esthetic emergence and cleansing ability. When successful, the technique allowed the restorative clinician to create a pontic restoration that was indistinguishable from the adjacent dentition.

In 1992, Scharf and Tarnow[10] described a modification of Abrams's original technique. They used a "trap door" approach by reflecting and preserving a partial-thickness flap overlying the area where the connective tissue pedicle would be subsequently harvested. After reflecting and rolling the connective tissue pedicle into position, the partial-thickness flap was used to cover the palatal donor site. This modified approach maximized the thickness of the connective tissue pedicle while minimizing the amount of exposed bone and, therefore, discomfort at the donor site. In 1995, Reikie[11] described the application of the trap door modification to enhance soft tissue contours around dental implant abutments.

The use of the palatal roll procedure can enhance the esthetic results of both conventional and implant-supported restorations by improving the soft tissue contours through which the restorations eventually emerge. This easy procedure provides the advantage of a single surgical site and a pedicled blood supply. Although originally described for use in the maxillary anterior area, the procedure often has limited use around dental implants in this area because the palatal anatomy may preclude the harvest of a connective tissue pedicle of sufficient thickness or length to gain significant soft tissue volume without increasing the risk of damage to adjacent neurovascular structures. An additional limitation is difficulty in adapting the rolled pedicle around an implant abutment or provisional restoration. This limitation becomes more obvious in the maxillary anterior area because of the complex cross-sectional anatomy of the incisors. Vertical releasing incisions on the facial aspect of the ridge often are required to allow proper adaptation of the pedicle around the implant components, resulting in an increased need for secondary gingivoplasty procedures.

The palatal roll procedure is usually performed in conjunction with second-stage surgery for submerged implants and simultaneously with nonsubmerged implant placement. The author feels that the palatal roll procedure is best suited for mild to moderate soft tissue augmentation around conventional or implant restorations located between the maxillary canine and the first molar, but the procedure continues to be useful for the correction of minor, very-small-volume soft tissue defects or surface irregularities around maxillary anterior implants. Nevertheless, the author prefers to correct most small-volume soft tissue deficiencies in the maxillary anterior area with interpositional subepithelial connective tissue grafts.

Modified roll technique for dental implants

The modified roll technique can be adapted for use around both submerged and nonsubmerged implants (Fig 5-2). The surgical procedure begins by outlining and dissecting a partial-thickness palatal flap overlying the area where the connective tissue pedicle will be subsequently harvested. A no. 15C scalpel is used to make two full-thickness vertical incisions extending from the crest of the alveolar ridge onto its palatal slope. These vertical incisions should spare the papilla and col area, and they should be long enough to allow the harvest of a connective tissue pedicle of sufficient length to reconstruct the site. The most favorable palatal anatomy is located between the canine and first molar, where the length and thickness of connective tissue that can be safely harvested is optimal. The length of the vertical incisions should correspond to the desired length of the connective tissue pedicle but may be limited by the depth of the palate at the proposed surgical site. Preoperative evaluation will determine if the palatal anatomy is favorable for the modified roll procedure or if another technique for soft tissue augmentation is indicated.

Next, a partial-thickness horizontal incision is made along the crest of the ridge to join the vertical incisions. Sharp dissection then creates a partial-thickness palatal flap (see Fig 5-2a). This dissection should be at least 1 mm deep to ensure that all of the epithelium and a thin layer of connective tissue are included with the palatal flap. Failure to do so can result in sloughing of the palatal flap and donor site exposure. In areas of prominent rugae, deeper dissection is recommended to avoid perforation of the cover flap.

After the split-thickness palatal flap has been reflected, the connective tissue pedicle is harvested. A no. 15C scalpel is used to make a horizontal incision through the connective tissue at the apical extent of the palatal dissection (see Fig 5-2b). This incision joins the previous full-thickness vertical incisions to outline the connective tissue pedicle. A Buser periosteal elevator is used to reflect the connective tissue pedicle starting apically at the horizontal incision and continuing coronally to the crest of the ridge (see Fig 5-2c). The Buser periosteal elevator or the paddle end of a membrane-placement instrument is used to create a subperiosteal tunnel starting at the buccal aspect of the ridge and extending just beyond the mucogingival junction (see Fig 5-2c). Alternatively, sharp dissection can be used to continue the pouch dissection beyond the buccal crest of the ridge in a supraperiosteal plane. This modification increases the elasticity of the cover pouch, facilitating the final positioning of the connective tissue pedicle and the adaptation of the rolled tissue around the emerging implant structures.

Modified palatal roll technique for dental implants

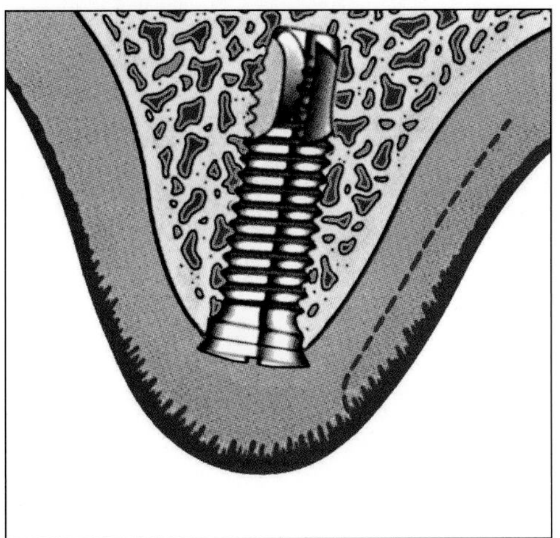

Fig 5-2a Cross section of maxillary alveolar ridge in the premolar region. A partial-thickness (approximately 1.0 mm) epithelial-connective tissue flap is outlined and elevated with sharp dissection.

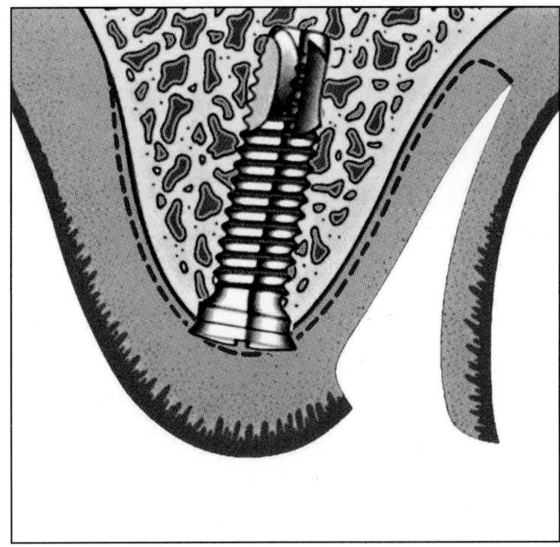

Fig 5-2b Full-thickness incisions outline the underlying connective tissue pedicle.

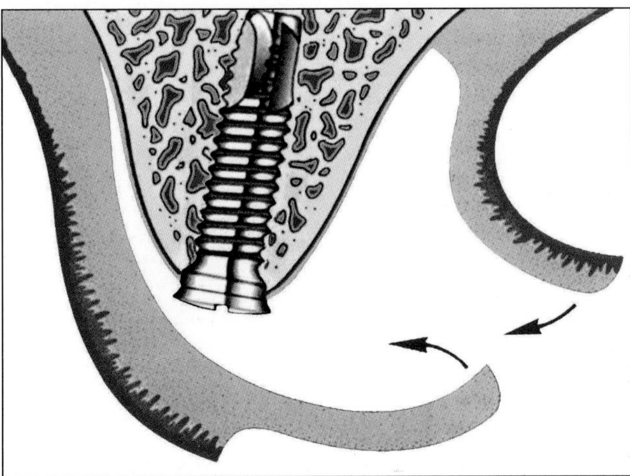

Fig 5-2c The connective tissue pedicle is elevated in a subperiosteal plane, and the dissection is extended onto the buccal aspect of the ridge. Alternatively, sharp dissection can be used for supraperiosteal dissection when tissue thickness is abundant.

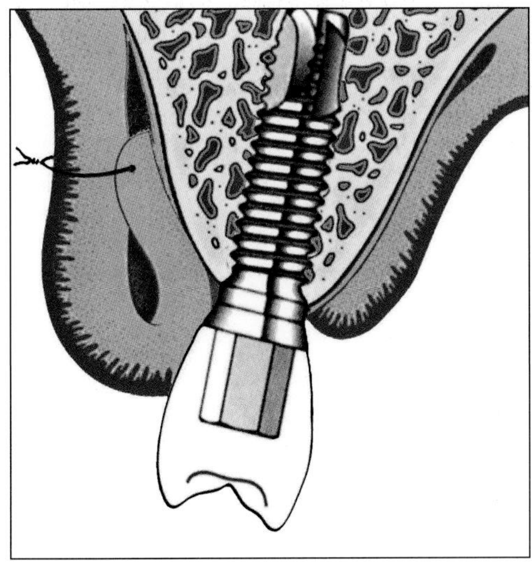

Fig 5-2d The connective tissue pedicle is rolled and secured in the resultant buccal pouch via a horizontal suture initiated and tied apically in the vestibule. Vertical releasing incisions are often required on the buccal aspect in order to adapt the tissue around an implant healing abutment or provisional restoration.

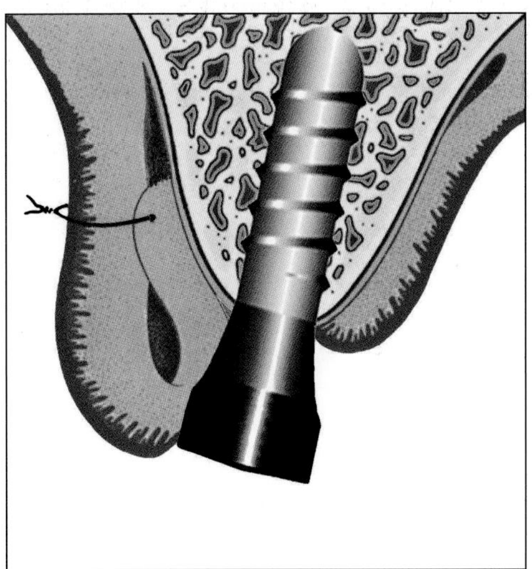

Fig 5-2e Modified palatal roll performed simultaneous with nonsubmerged implant placement.

Modified palatal roll technique performed at the time of implant exposure

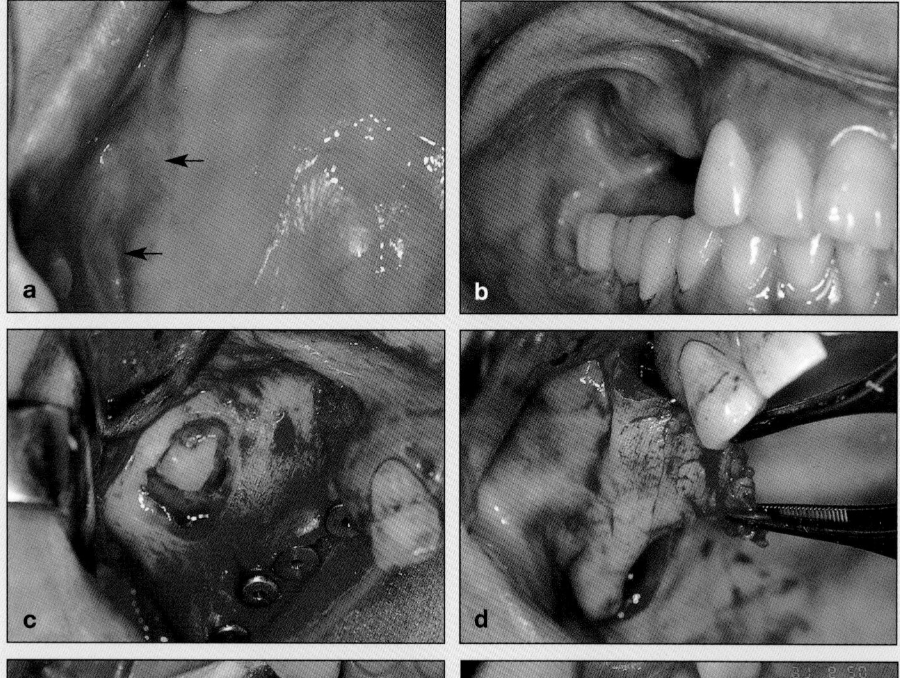

Figs 5-3a and 5-3b Presurgical occlusal and buccal views of edentulous maxillary quadrant. Note deficiency in buccal alveolar ridge contours and collapse of soft tissues in the buccal corridor *(arrows)*.

Fig 5-3c Placement of four submerged implants (3i, West Palm Beach, FL) performed simultaneously with a sinus lift bone graft procedure. Note the palatal crestal incision with a palatal bevel and a curvilinear-beveled releasing incision.

Fig 5-3d Subsequent to grafting, tension-free primary closure is obtained. A combination of horizontal mattress and simple interrupted sutures were used to close the crestal incision, and interrupted incisions were used to close the releasing incision. Four months later, a modified palatal roll dissection was performed at the time of implant exposure. Connective tissue pedicle is limited to the premolar–first molar area.

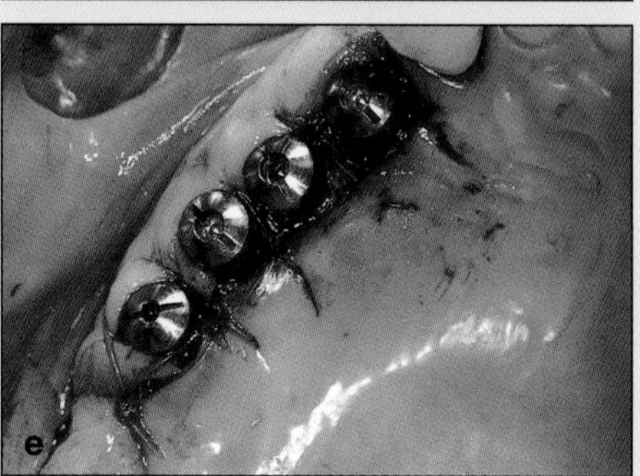

Fig 5-3e After abutment connection, the connective tissue pedicle is rolled and secured around the healing abutments on the buccal aspect. Vertical releasing incisions facilitate adaptation of the rolled pedicle around the implant abutments.

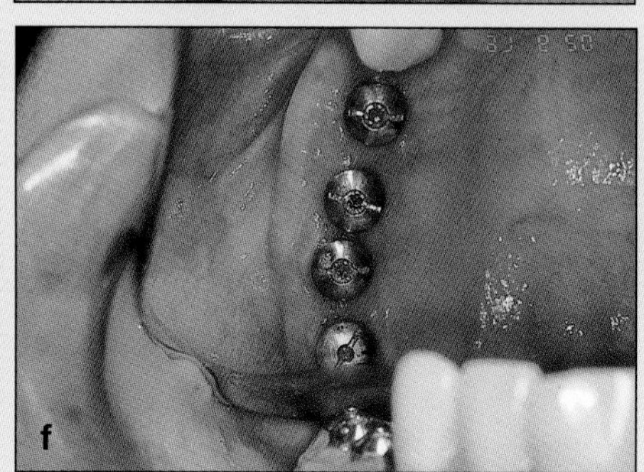

Fig 5-3f Six-week postoperative view. Excellent buccal soft tissue augmentation has been obtained.

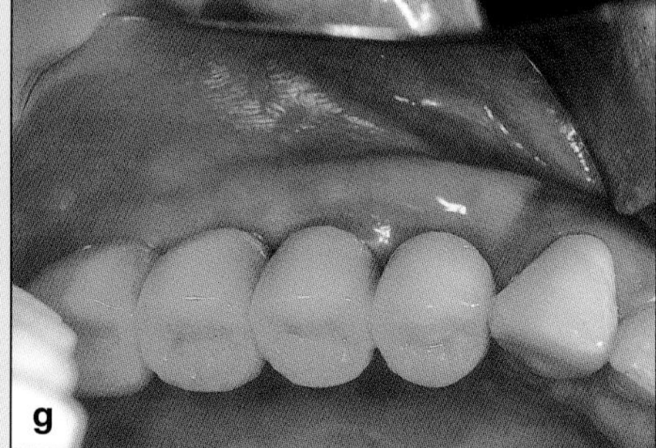

Fig 5-3g One year after delivery of the final restoration, successful reconstruction of deficient buccal soft tissue contours enhance the functional and esthetic result. Food impaction has been eliminated. (Restoration by Dr Larry Lesperance, South Miami, FL.)

In addition, the author often extends small vertical incisions buccally over the crest of the ridge to further facilitate the placement and positioning of the connective tissue pedicle in the buccal pouch by enlarging the entrance of the pouch (Fig 5-3). It is often necessary to extend these buccal vertical incisions beyond the mucogingival junction (Figs 5-4 and 5-5). This enables the precise vertical tissue repositioning often required to ensure the desired soft tissue augmentation around an emerging implant, as well as the realistic re-creation of the appearance of a root eminence at the implant site. This modification also allows the correction of distortions of the mucogingival junction resulting from previous site-preparation procedures. These considerations are especially important in areas of esthetic concern.

Once the buccal dissection has been completed, the connective tissue pedicle is rolled and positioned into the buccal pouch or under the buccal flap and secured with a mattress suture that originates through the buccal mucosa in the area of the mucogingival junction, passes into the buccal pouch, is passed through each corner of the apical end of the pedicle, and exits back through the buccal mucosa, where it is tied (see Figs 5-2d and 5-2e). When vertical incisions are extended buccally, additional sutures are used to re-adapt and secure the resulting buccal flap around the emerging implant. In both cases, secondary gingivoplasty is occasionally necessary to establish a harmonious gingival architecture that is free of surface irregularities. A diamond bur at high speed or a CO_2 laser may be used for this purpose.

Modified palatal roll technique synchronous with placement of a two-piece nonsubmerged implant at a lateral incisor implant site

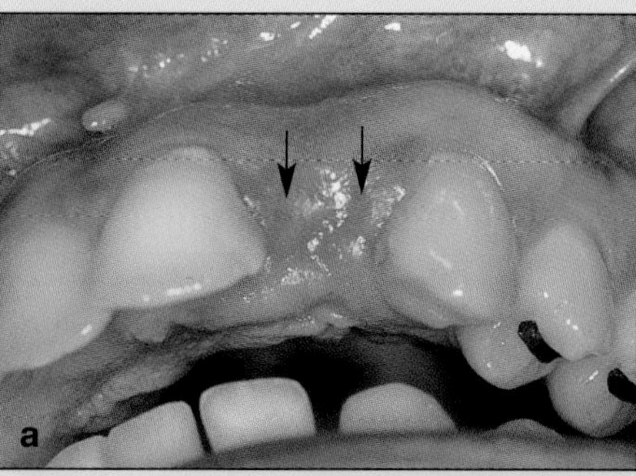

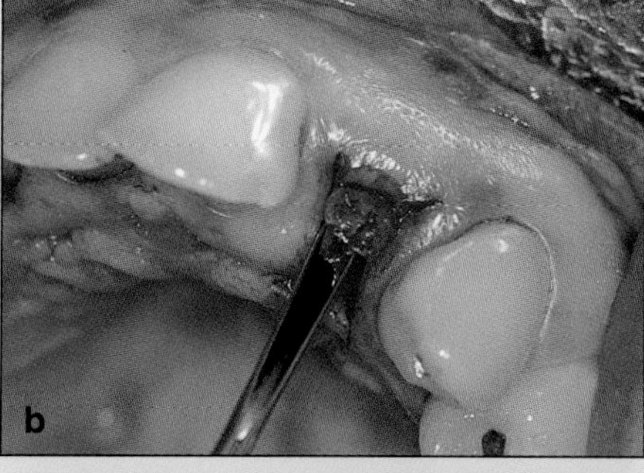

Fig 5-4a Presurgical occlusal view demonstrating a small-volume soft tissue defect in an area critical for esthetic restorative emergence *(arrows)*.

Fig 5-4b Following sharp dissection to elevate a split-thickness palatal flap, a connective tissue pedicle was outlined with sharp dissection and elevated with a membrane-placement instrument.

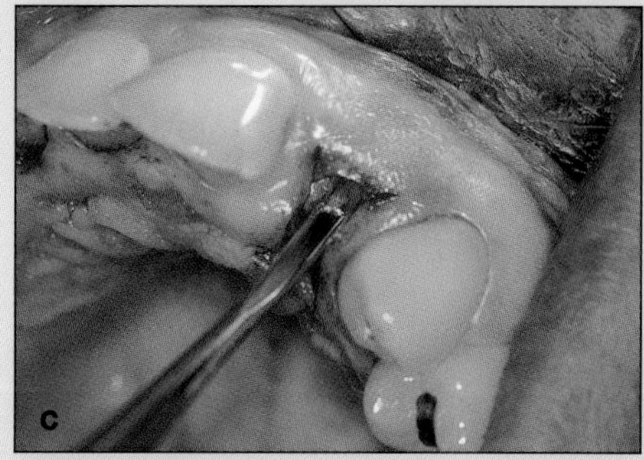

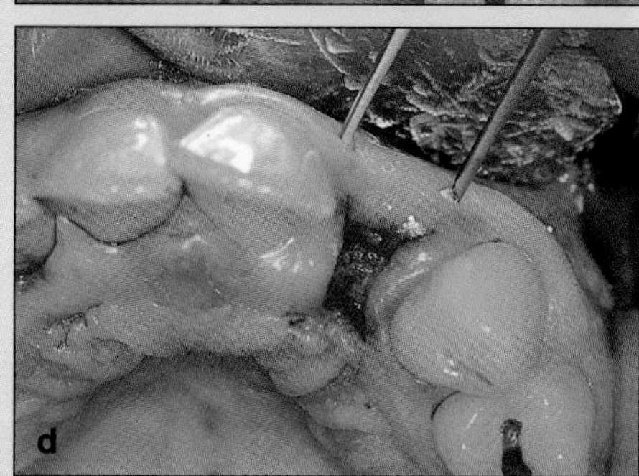

Fig 5-4c Subperiosteal dissection is continued to the facial to create a buccal pouch.

Fig 5-4d The small connective tissue pedicle has been rolled into the buccal pouch. Correction of the soft tissue defect is immediately realized.

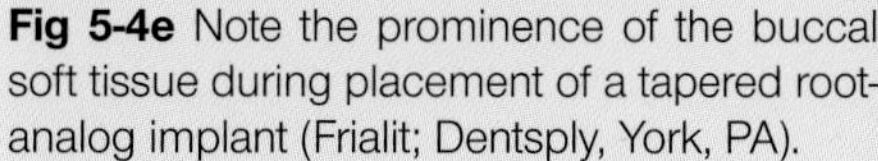

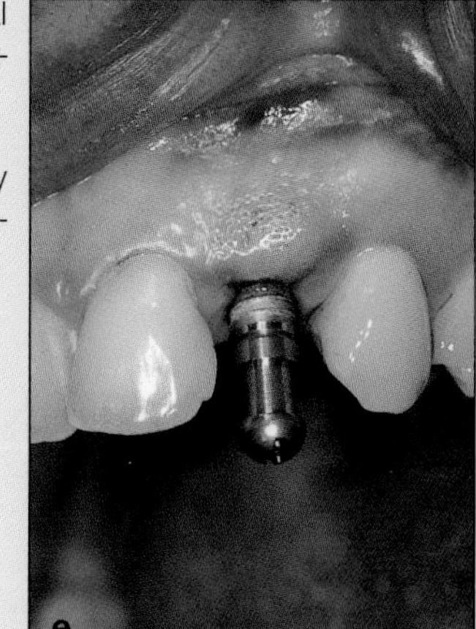

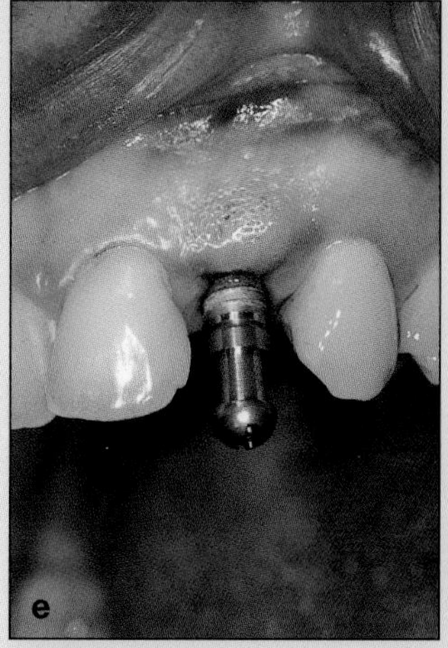

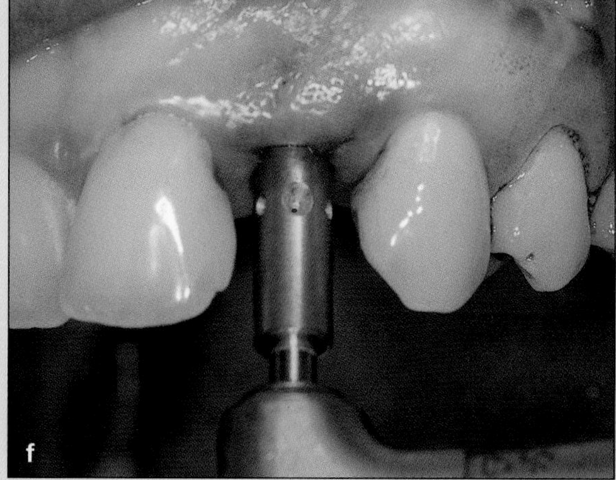

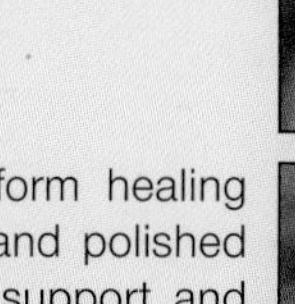

Fig 5-4e Note the prominence of the buccal soft tissue during placement of a tapered root-analog implant (Frialit; Dentsply, York, PA).

Fig 5-4f Sink depth of the fixture is carefully controlled to ensure an esthetic gingival pattern with the final restoration.

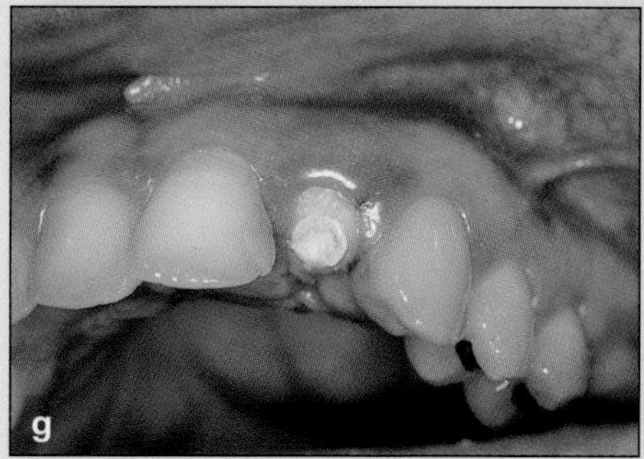

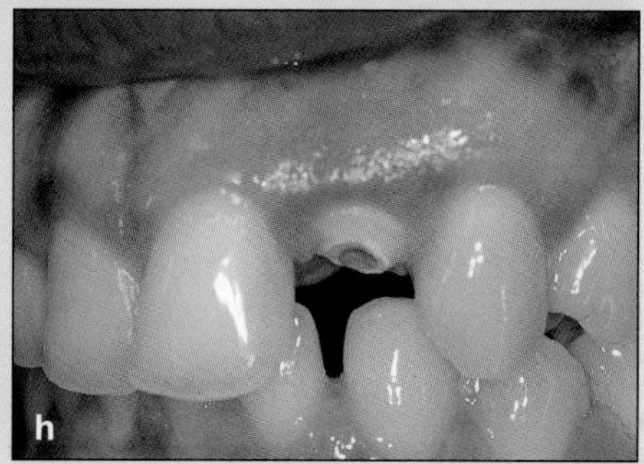

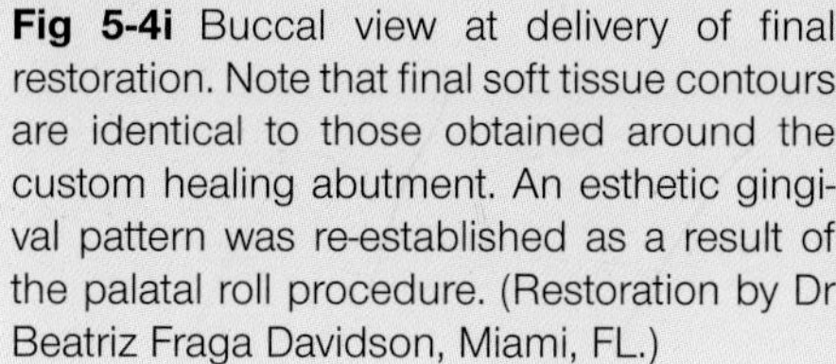

Fig 5-4g A customized tooth-form healing abutment, which was shaped and polished chairside prior to delivery, will support and guide the soft tissues during healing.

Fig 5-4h Buccal view 4 months after surgery showing the small-volume soft tissue defect successfully restored. Scalloped soft tissue architecture has been preserved, and tissues have been stabilized.

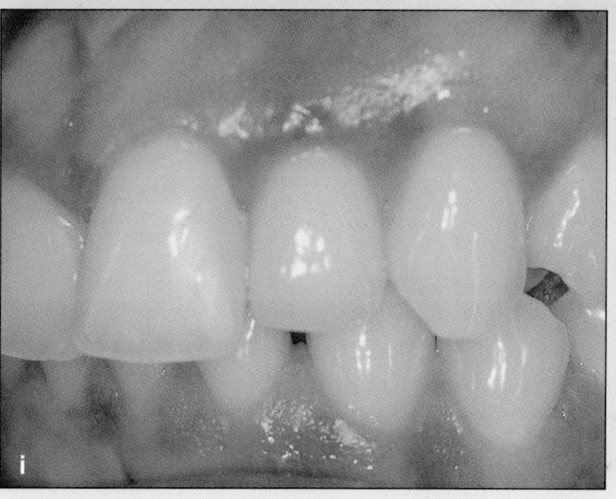

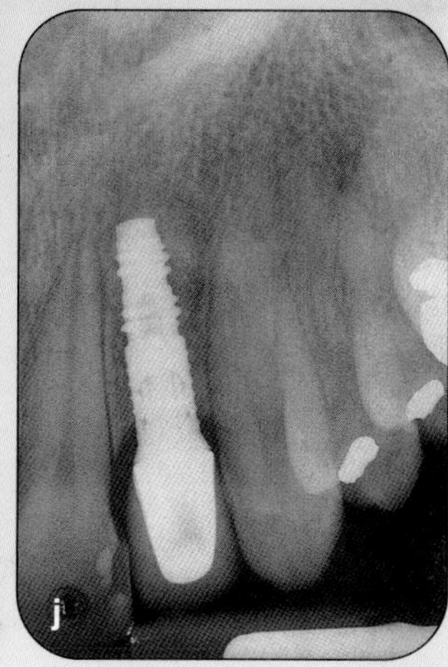

Fig 5-4i Buccal view at delivery of final restoration. Note that final soft tissue contours are identical to those obtained around the custom healing abutment. An esthetic gingival pattern was re-established as a result of the palatal roll procedure. (Restoration by Dr Beatriz Fraga Davidson, Miami, FL.)

Fig 5-4j Radiograph 1 year after delivery demonstrates stable bone levels and optimal fixture depth.

Modified palatal roll technique synchronous with placement of a one-piece nonsubmerged implant

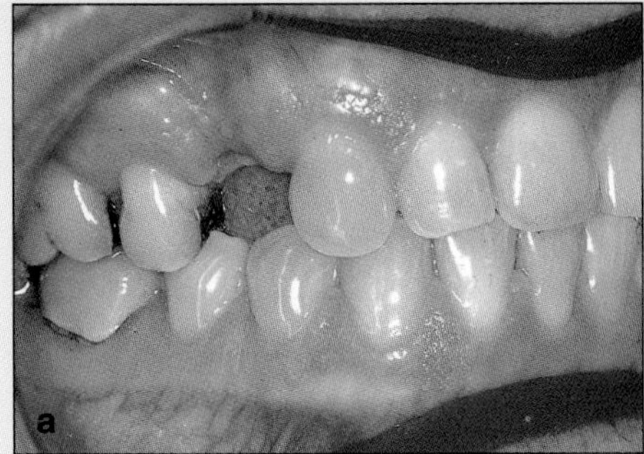

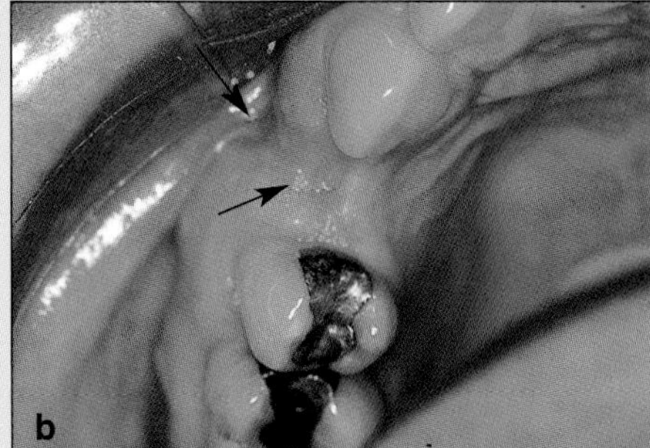

Figs 5-5a and 5-5b Presurgical views of premolar implant site with small-volume soft tissue defect. If left untreated, this defect will detract from smile esthetics. Note both the buccal and the vertical components of the defect *(arrows)*.

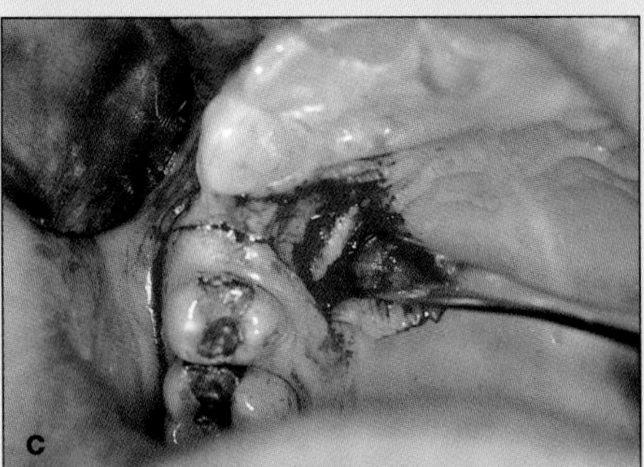

Fig 5-5c Outline and elevation of split-thickness palatal flap with sharp dissection.

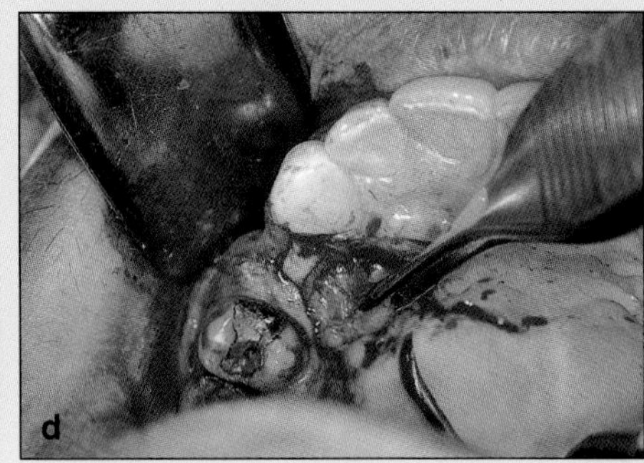

Fig 5-5d After outlining the connective tissue pedicle with sharp dissection, Adson tissue forceps stabilize the pedicle during subperiosteal elevation.

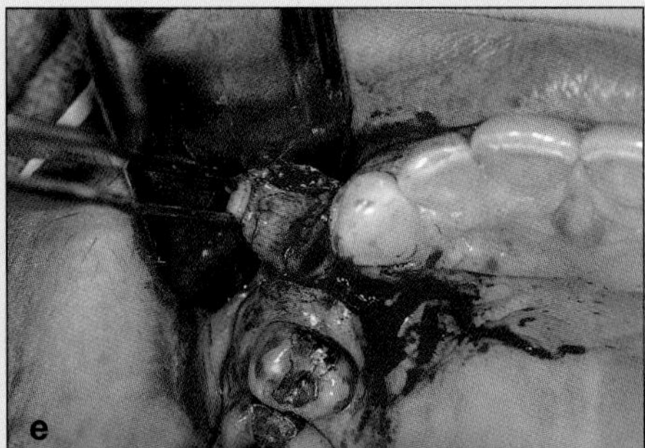

Fig 5-5e Subperiosteal dissection extended to create a buccal pouch. Because of the size of the pedicle, vertical releasing incisions were needed to be able to roll and subsequently adapt the tissue pedicle at the site.

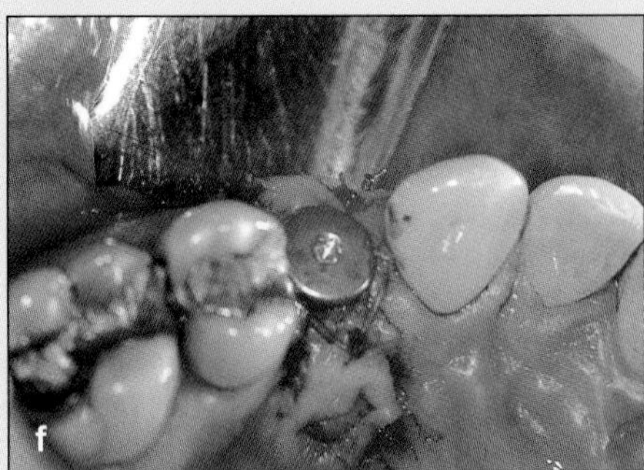

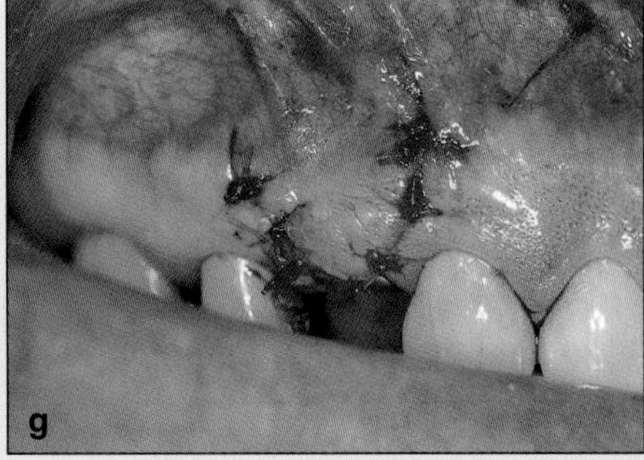

Figs 5-5f and 5-5g Following placement of a one-piece nonsubmerged implant (Straumann USA), the connective tissue pedicle was adapted and secured around the healing abutment.

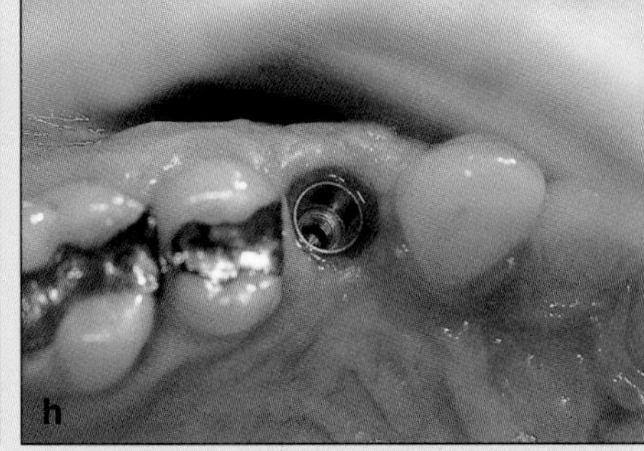

Fig 5-5h Occlusal view 3 months after the procedure. The soft tissue defect has been restored, and a prosthetic-friendly environment has been created for the restorative dentist.

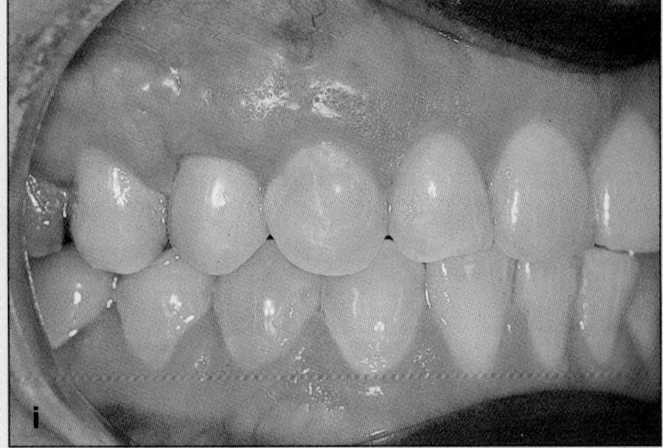

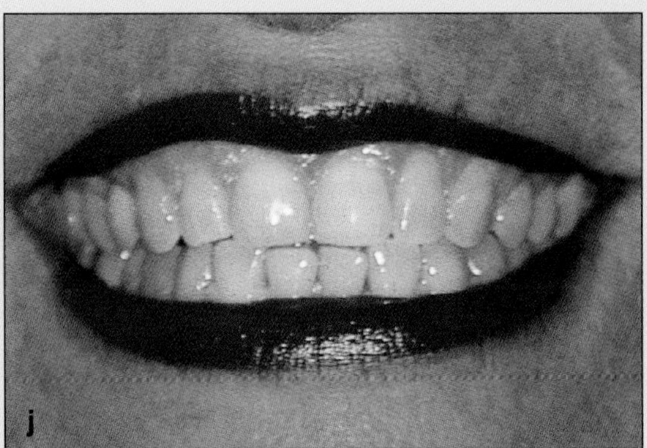

Figs 5-5i and 5-5j Final restoration has esthetic restorative emergence. Esthetic soft tissue contours have been restored and patient can smile freely. (Restoration by Dr Richard Mariani Sr, South Miami, FL.)

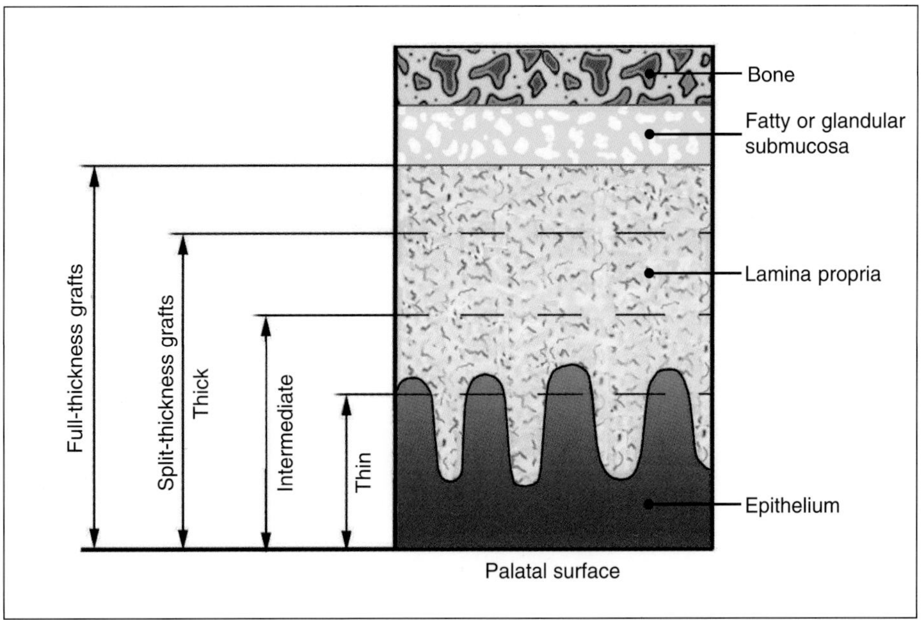

Fig 5-6 Classification of palatal mucosal graft thickness based on a cross section of the hard palate in the maxillary first molar position. Palatal mucosal grafts are classified as full thickness or split thickness. Full-thickness grafts include the epithelium and all of the lamina propria. Split-thickness grafts are further subclassified as thick, intermediate, and thin, depending on the amount of lamina propria included in the graft. Thick split-thickness and full-thickness grafts are typically used with the contemporary surgical technique. Harvesting of fatty or glandular tissue is undesirable.

Epithelialized Palatal Graft Technique for Dental Implants

The use of an epithelialized palatal graft for the treatment of a mucogingival defect has enjoyed a long history of predictable success. This versatile technique can be used not only to increase the dimensions of attached tissue around the natural dentition but also as a predictable method for covering denuded root surfaces. The term *free gingival graft* is a misnomer; it is commonly used to describe the transfer not of gingival tissue, which is seldom practical, but of epithelialized tissue harvested from the palate.

Early applications of gingival grafting involved placing grafted tissue below the existing mucogingival junction to increase the width of the attached tissue in the area. Excessive graft shrinkage, graft mobility, and conspicuous color mismatch with the adjacent tissues resulted. In their classic series of articles published in 1968, Sullivan, Atkins, and Gordon[12–14] described the surgical and biologic principles of successful free autogenous gingival grafting, an improved surgical technique, histologic observations of the graft site, and the treatment of gingival recession. Their application of plastic surgery principles to the treatment of mucogingival defects served as the basis for our understanding and development of a contemporary surgical technique for gingival grafting and modern periodontal plastic surgery procedures.

Sullivan et al[12–14] classified gingival grafts based on their thickness. They distinguished full-thickness grafts from split-thickness grafts and further subclassified the latter into thick, intermediate, and thin split-thickness grafts based on the thickness of connective tissue included in the harvest (Fig 5-6). They discussed in detail the influence of graft thickness on healing as well as characteristics of the grafted tissue after maturation.

When the purpose of the graft is to increase the zone of attached tissue, a thick split-thickness graft (0.75 to 1.25 mm thick) is preferred. When root or abutment coverage is desired, a split-thickness graft approaching full thickness, that is, 1.25 to 1.75 mm, is preferred. Early revascularization of full-thickness grafts is not as predictable as that of split-thickness grafts, but superior results are obtained with these grafts where root or abutment coverage is desired. However, the successful use of thicker gingival grafts is more technique sensitive, requiring absolute immobilization of the graft to a rigid recipient bed with meticulous suturing to ensure revascularization and to minimize primary and secondary contraction. In addition, coverage of an avascular area (denuded root or implant abutment) through the so-called bridging phenomenon as described by Sullivan et al[12–14] relies on collateral blood supply from the recipient site. Therefore, the recipient site and gingival graft must be large in relation to the area of root or abutment coverage desired. Once healed, thicker grafts resist the functional stresses of mastication, intracrevicular restorative procedures, and oral hygiene procedures better than thin grafts. Therefore, the author prefers to use full-thickness or thick split-thickness grafts and does not recommend the use of thin or intermediate split-thickness gingival grafts around dental implants or when root coverage is desired.

Indications and sequencing

The author primarily limits the use of the gingival graft to soft tissue augmentation in nonesthetic areas. The exception is the use of thick onlay gingival grafts for vertical augmentation of pontic or implant sites with large-volume soft tissue defects prior to implant placement or conventional restorations. In these situations, gingival grafting is staged with horizontal augmentation preceding vertical augmentation, which is performed secondarily. Usually, the gingival graft is indicated to extend the zone of attached tissue around the natural dentition or implant restorations. In addition, the gingival graft can be used to obtain root coverage or implant abutment coverage. However, when used for this purpose, the gingival graft is technique sensitive as compared to the use of a subepithelial connective tissue graft.

When there is an absence of attached gingival tissues at an edentulous implant site, the clinician should consider performing gingival grafting 8 to 12 weeks before implant placement. Doing so will improve the quality of tissue present at implant placement and during osseointegration. This will minimize complications such as wound dehiscence, cover screw exposure, or difficulty with interim removable restorations. These considerations are important when implants are planned in a severely atrophic maxilla or mandible that lacks attached tissue and buccal vestibular depth. They are also important in partially edentulous jaws where hard tissue augmentation is required before implant placement and the quality of the existing soft tissue provides an inadequate environment for coverage and vascularization of a bone graft. As a guideline, the author performs gingival grafting prior to implant placement when the width of remaining attached tissue is less than 3 mm and the height of the mandible or maxilla is less than 10 mm.

From a patient-management perspective, however, gingival grafting prior to implant placement can cause significant discomfort, which can discourage patients from completing the subsequent implant therapy out of fear that it will be even more painful. Therefore, if adequate gingival tissue (3 mm) exists at the implant site, gingival grafting can be performed at the second-stage surgery for submerged implants or simultaneously with nonsubmerged implant placement. In these cases, the existing attached tissues are preserved and repositioned to the lingual aspect of the implants, and the gingival graft is performed on the facial aspect. Additionally, gingival grafting can be performed 8 to 12 weeks after abutment connection or at any time after final restoration to correct any functional soft tissue deficiencies that develop. As discussed in chapter 3, the clinician should ensure that a minimum width of 3 mm of attached tissue is present lingual to emerging implants to avoid the difficulty of grafting soft tissue to gain adequate width of attached tissue lingually and the high incidence of peri-implantitis that occurs when mobile mucosal tissues are present.

Contemporary surgical technique

Recipient-site preparation

Beginning the surgical procedure with recipient-site preparation minimizes the time between graft harvest and transfer to the recipient bed. The first step is to outline the recipient site (Fig 5-7a). A no. 15C or similar scalpel blade is used to make a horizontal incision just coronal to the level of soft tissue augmentation desired; this incision should extend several millimeters beyond the area planned for augmentation. Vertical incisions should then be extended apically into the mucosa from the lateral aspects of the horizontal incision. These incisions should be made perpendicular to the surface of the existing gingival tissue to create a butt joint margin for subsequent graft adaptation. When working on natural teeth requiring root coverage, the horizontal incision extends through the interdental papilla coronal to the level of the cementoenamel junction of the involved dentition.

Sharp dissection is then performed in an apical direction to create a rigid periosteal recipient bed (Fig 5-7b). Vestibular extension is performed when the apicocoronal dimension of the recipient site is inadequate (less than 5 mm) for immobilization of an appropriately sized graft. Residual remnants of epithelium, connective tissue, or muscle attachments are removed with tissue nippers or sharp tissue scissors. The resultant flap is then usually excised to avoid possible displacement of the gingival graft after it is secured (Fig 5-7c). Alternatively, in certain instances (eg, severe alveolar atrophy), the resultant flap can be apically repositioned and secured at the base of the recipient site with sutures. A moist saline sponge is then placed over the prepared recipient site to obtain hemostasis.

Donor-site preparation

Donor-site evaluation is performed during the preoperative examination. Although the palatal mucosa is the most common donor source, edentulous ridge areas also can be used. Inflammation or hyperplasia of the

Epithelialized palatal grafting (gingival grafting): Contemporary surgical technique

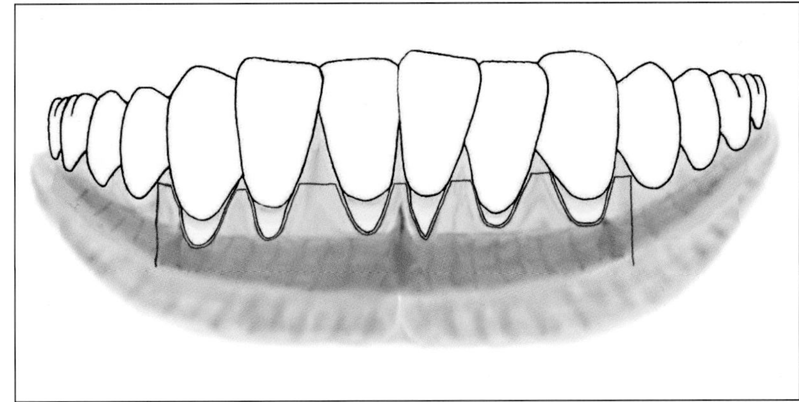

Fig 5-7a Miller class I and class II recession involving prominent mandibular anterior teeth with inadequate width of attached tissue and negligible vestibular depth. Prior to outlining the recipient site with partial-thickness incisions, hand or rotary instrumentation is used to mechanically reduce the convexity of the exposed roots. Afterward, they are chemically prepared with a supersaturated citric acid solution that is applied with a sterile cotton swab for 30 seconds. The horizontal incision is made at or just coronal to the level of root coverage desired. Vertical releasing incisions are carried inferiorly.

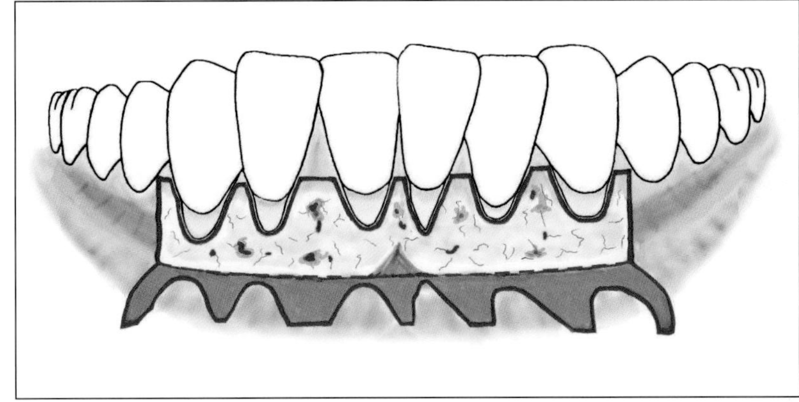

Fig 5-7b Sharp dissection is used to complete a supraperiosteal dissection. The resultant split-thickness flap is usually excised but may be retained and secured to the periosteum at the base of the dissection when significant alveolar ridge atrophy exists.

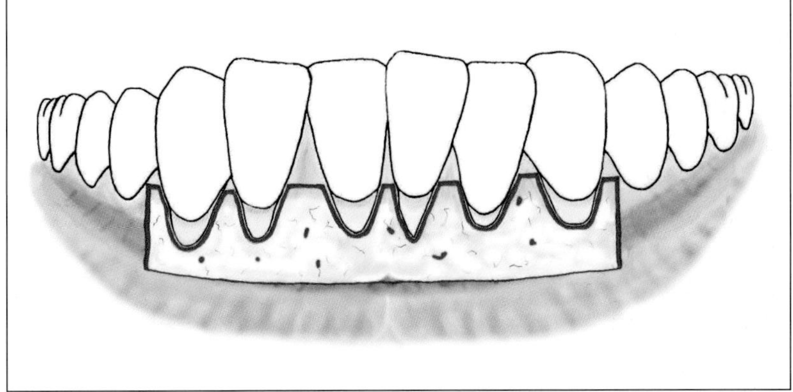

Fig 5-7c Residual elastic and muscular tissue are excised with tissue nippers or curved Iris tissue scissors. This results in a uniform recipient site, intimate adaptation, immobilization, and survival of the graft. Note that butt margins were created in the existing gingival tissues at the superior and lateral portions of the recipient site. Hemostasis is obtained, and moistened saline gauze is packed at the site.

donor site tissue should be resolved preoperatively. The smooth area of the palate in the premolar and molar region is the preferred area for harvest (Fig 5-7d). The dimensions of the donor site should exactly duplicate the dimensions of the recipient bed. A minimum of 5 mm in the apicocoronal dimension is desired for application around implants. A smaller graft will result in an inadequate band (less than 3 mm) of tissue should significant secondary graft contraction occur.

A periodontal probe or Castroviejo caliper is used to accurately transfer the recipient-site dimensions to the donor site. The donor tissue is outlined with partial-thickness incisions made in the palatal mucosa using a no. 15C blade on a round scalpel handle. Alternatively, a tinfoil template made on the recipient bed can be taken to the donor site and outlined with sharp dissection. A beveled vertical access incision at the anterior portion of the harvest outline allows the surgeon to visualize the plane of dissection and ensures that appropriate graft thickness is harvested. When this beveled access incision is made, sharp tissue scissors are then used to trim that portion of the graft to ensure subsequent butt joint marginal adaptation at the recipient bed (see Fig 5-7d).

Micro-Adson tissue forceps, a delicate skin hook, or a traction suture is used to apply gentle downward

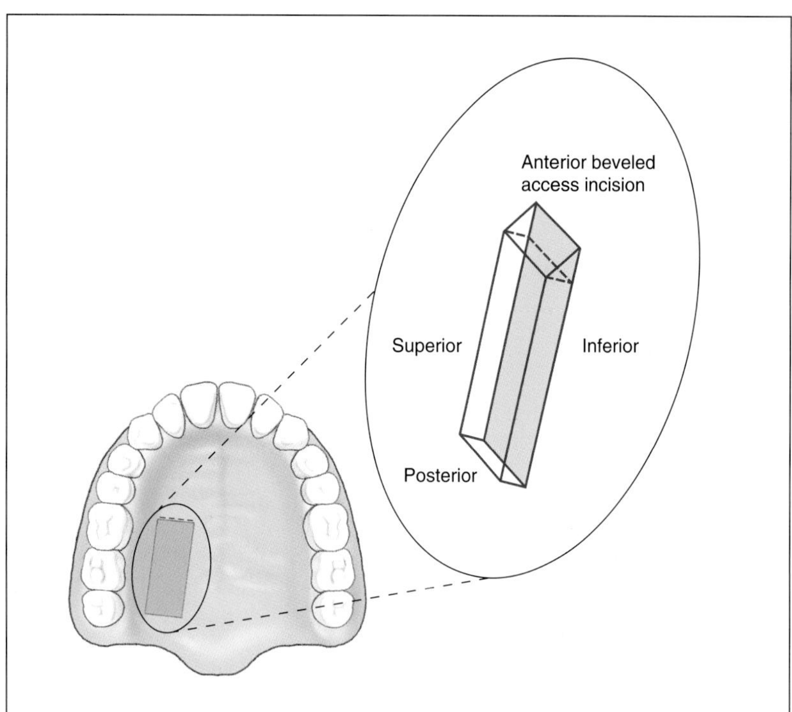

Fig 5-7d The donor tissue is sized to the recipient-site dimensions and outlined with partial-thickness horizontal and vertical incisions. The anterior vertical access incision is beveled to facilitate localization of the appropriate plane of dissection; the remaining incisions are made perpendicular to the surface. Adson tissue forceps are used to apply traction to the tissue at the access incision, and sharp dissection is used to harvest a uniform graft. Hemostasis is achieved with pressure or electrocautery. The donor site is then dressed with CollaCote (Centerpulse Dental, Carlsbad, CA) absorbable collagen dressing, and a palatal stent is provided to protect the site and improve patient comfort in the early postoperative period. The beveled portion of the graft is trimmed with a scalpel to prepare for butt joint marginal adaptation at the recipient site.

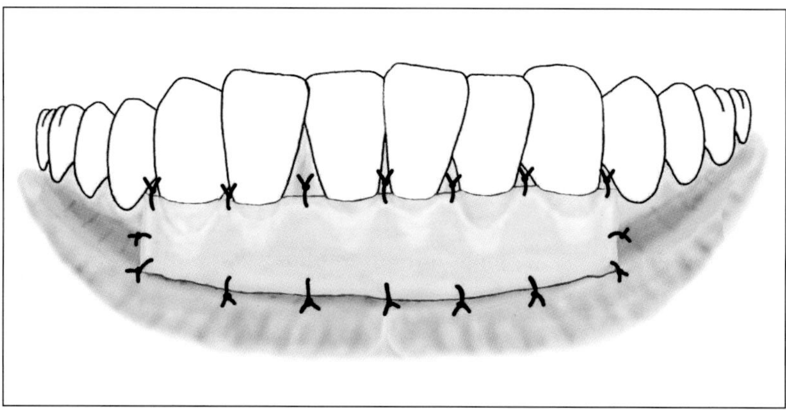

Fig 5-7e Immobilization of the graft at the recipient site begins with suture placement in each papillary area, working either from one side to the other or from the center laterally to ensure intimate adaptation and butt-joint marginal adaptation for survival of the graft over the exposed root surfaces. Sutures are then placed peripherally as needed to ensure graft immobilization, and pressure is applied for 10 minutes to promote the formation of a thin layer of fibrin that facilitates plasmatic circulation for early graft survival.

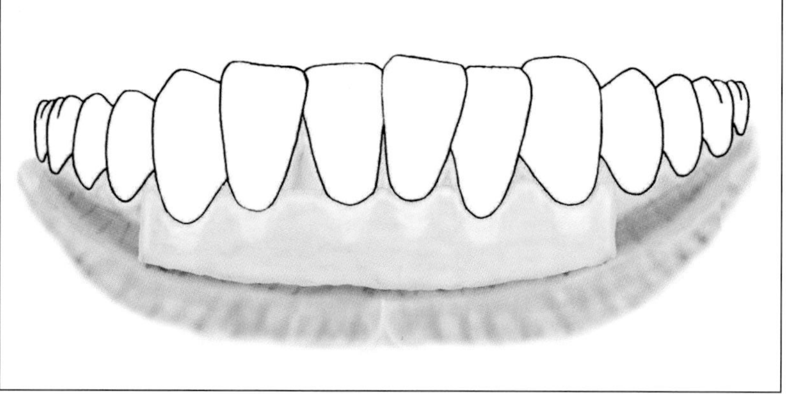

Fig 5-7f A successful outcome includes root coverage, increased width of attached tissue, and re-establishment of adequate vestibular depth. These are the goals of the contemporary surgical technique.

tension on the donor tissue during the dissection. The surgeon should take care during dissection to create a uniform graft surface, which will enhance the adaptation of the graft to the recipient site and thus facilitate subsequent graft revascularization. The graft is immediately taken to the previously prepared recipient site and sutured into place. Pressure is applied to the bleeding donor site with moistened saline gauze. An absorbable hemostatic dressing (CollaTape or Collacote; Centerpulse Dental) then is applied to the donor area and secured with Isodent tissue adhesive (Ellman International, Hewlett, NY). If the patient does not have a removable prosthetic appliance with palatal coverage, the use of a palatal stent will greatly diminish postoperative discomfort and is routinely used by the author.

Immobilization of the graft at the recipient site

Close adaptation of the gingival graft to the recipient site and rigid immobilization are critical for success with gingival grafting, especially when full-thickness grafts are used for root or abutment coverage. A uniform graft that is intimately adapted and secured to a properly prepared recipient site ensures excellent results. Intimate adaptation of the graft to the recipient site ensures initial nourishment of the graft via diffusion of nutrients from the host bed. This diffusion of nutrients is facilitated by a thin fibrin clot, which forms between the graft and the host bed. Subsequently, graft revascularization occurs as capillaries extend into the immobilized graft and form anastomosis with the graft's vasculature. An irregular graft or recipient-site surface allows pooling of blood between the host bed and the graft, thereby limiting both the early diffusion of nutrients to the graft and the subsequent extension of capillaries into it. Mobility of the graft essentially has the same deleterious effects.

Once the graft is harvested, it is immediately taken to the previously prepared, nonbleeding recipient site, where it is immobilized with sutures (Fig 5-7e). The contemporary surgical technique requires that the graft have an exact fit at the recipient site. The edges of the graft should form a butt joint with the periphery of the recipient bed to prevent sloughing of the margins of the graft and ensure smooth blending with the adjacent tissues. When root or abutment coverage is desired, sutures are placed in the periphery of the graft so as to stretch and adapt the graft to the recipient site. This process is initiated coronally by securing the graft at each papillary or interdental area. The author uses a P3 needle to place just enough 4-0 chromic gut sutures to rigidly immobilize the graft at the site.

Once the suturing has been completed, the thin fibrin clot is formed by applying pressure over the entire graft with a moistened saline sponge for a minimum of 10 minutes. Blood will be displaced from under the graft, and plasma will be converted to fibrin. The fibrin will further anchor the graft to the recipient bed and facilitate the diffusion of nutrients and metabolites until revascularization occurs. A periodontal dressing may then be applied over the graft; however, the author prefers not to dress the graft site to avoid the possible transmission of shearing forces from the dressing to the graft, which can prevent graft revascularization. This also allows visual inspection during postoperative examinations (Fig 5-7f). Although functional circulation exists 10 days after surgery, the graft continues to mature for 8 to 12 weeks, after which gingivoplasty can be performed (Fig 5-8).

The surgical technique for gingival grafting around dental implants is essentially the same. When gingival grafting is performed after implant abutment connection or delivery of the final restoration, a horizontal incision is made through the inter-implant papilla coronal to the desired final tissue position. This facilitates abutment coverage with the gingival graft. When gingival grafting is performed at second-stage surgery or simultaneous with nonsubmerged implant placement, the horizontal incision is made at the mucogingival junction, and any existing gingival tissues are repositioned to the lingual or palatal aspect of the implants (Fig 5-9a). This step is extremely important when implants are placed in the mandible because subsequent lingual soft tissue defects in this area are difficult to correct. A split-thickness dissection is then carried apically to create a uniform periosteal site. In the edentulous mandible, care must be taken to avoid damage to the mental nerve with vertical releasing incisions. In these instances, the author uses a midline vertical releasing incision and sharp dissection to create an adequate recipient site (greater than 5 mm apicocoronal dimension), as shown in Fig 5-9b. Subsequently, the mucosal flaps are excised and residual elastic or muscular tissue removed with tissue scissors or nippers (Fig 5-9c). When working in a severely atrophic mandible, the mucosal flaps are preserved and sutured to the periosteum at the base of the dissection. The technique for graft immoblization is also the same whether gingival grafting is performed around natural dentition, at second-stage surgery for submerged implants, or at the time of nonsubmerged implant placement. The graft is sutured to each papilla or inter-implant area coronally and then sutured to periosteum (Fig 5-9d) peripherally to rigidly immobilize the graft at the recipient site.

When grafting must be performed prior to implant placement (eg, in a severely atrophic maxilla or mandible less than 10 mm in height and with less than 3 mm of attached tissue), the author finds it useful to avoid significant dissection of the palatal or lingual tissues. Instead, a large recipient bed is created on the buccal aspect of the site extending far enough apically from midcrest to recreate the buccal vestibular fold. In these situations, the sutures should be placed approximately 5 mm apart to provide adequate immobilization of the graft while avoiding unnecessary trauma and hematoma formation at the periphery (Figs 5-10 to 5-17). A portion (3 mm or greater) of the mature grafted tissue is then repositioned lingually during subsequent implant surgery, providing good-quality gingival tissue for wound closure over submerged implants and circumferential adaptation of attached tissue around emerging implant abutments or one-piece nonsubmerged implants.

Gingival grafting for root coverage, increased width of attached tissue, and re-establishment of adequate vestibular depth around mandibular anterior teeth

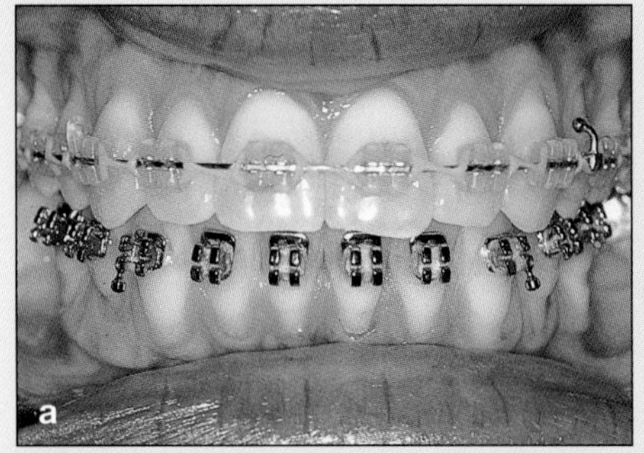

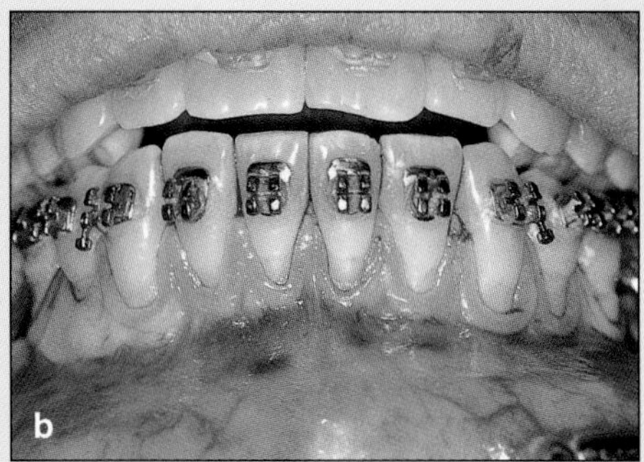

Figs 5-8a and 5-8b Presurgical view of Miller class I and class II recession around prominent mandibular anterior teeth in a patient with a thin, scalloped periodontium undergoing orthodontic therapy. The recession is progressive and the patient is experiencing sensitivity around the mandibular incisors.

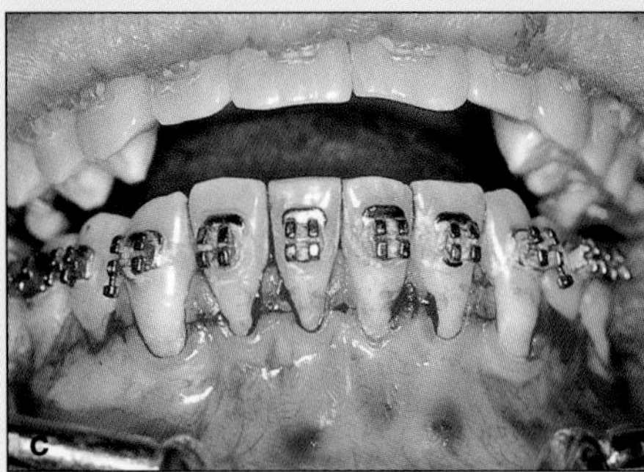

Fig 5-8c After mechanical preparation to reduce root prominence and chemical preparation to open dentinal tubules, partial-thickness horizontal and vertical incisions are made to outline the recipient site.

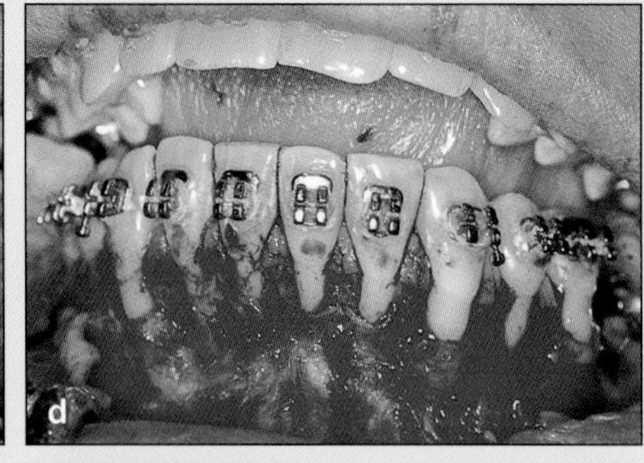

Fig 5-8d Sharp dissection is used to create a periosteal recipient site. Note the significant amount of root structure visible due to bony dehiscence. Mechanical and chemical preparation of nonexposed root surfaces is generally not indicated. The term *hidden recession* is commonly used to describe these dehisced root surfaces.

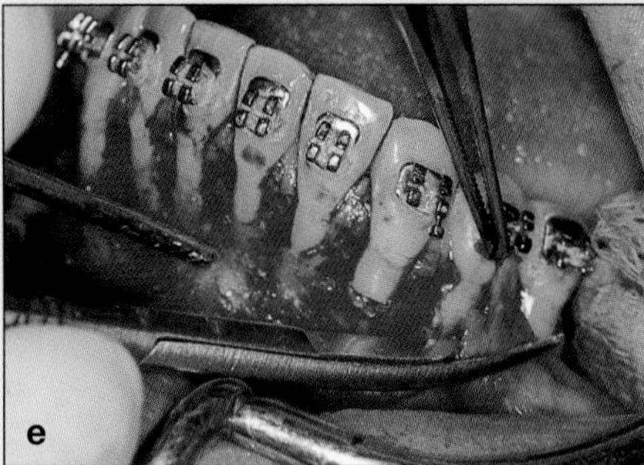

Fig 5-8e Curved Iris tissue scissors are used to excise the resultant flap, which consists of poor-quality mucosal tissues.

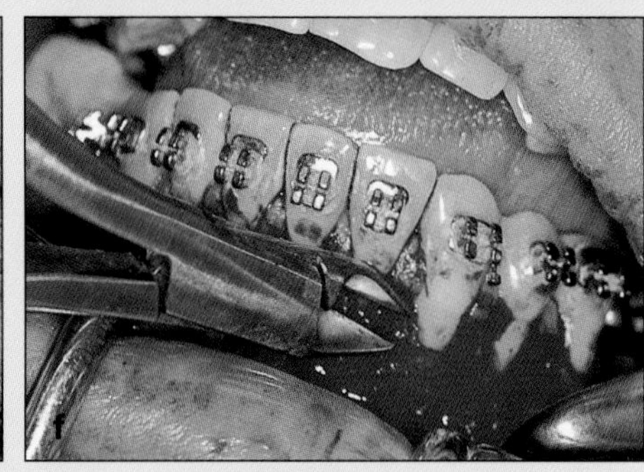

Fig 5-8f Tissue nippers are used to remove residual muscular and elastic tissue, resulting in a uniform recipient site that is rigidly immobile.

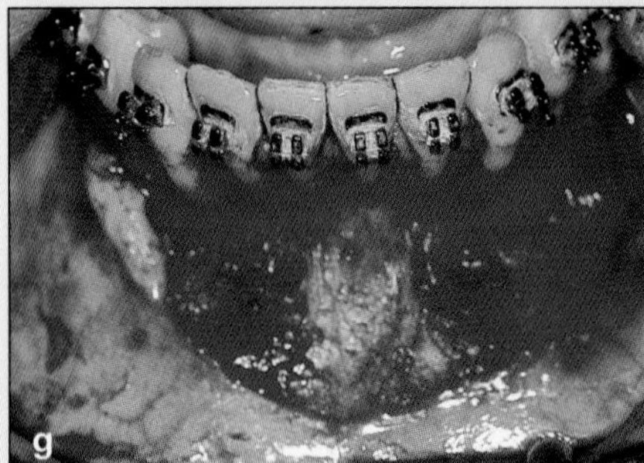

Fig 5-8g Hemostasis has been achieved via application of pressure at the site.

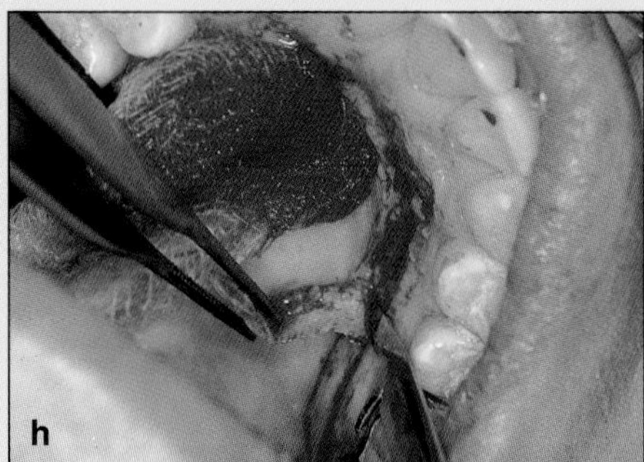

Fig 5-8h Donor-site surgery. After outlining the graft with partial-thickness incisions, a beveled access incision was made to establish a plane of dissection that includes all of the lamina dura (ie, full thickness).

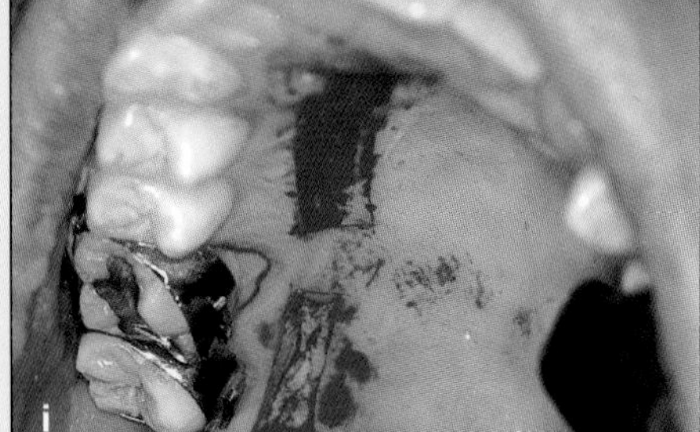

Fig 5-8i Donor-tissue harvest avoided a recession defect around the palatal root of the first molar.

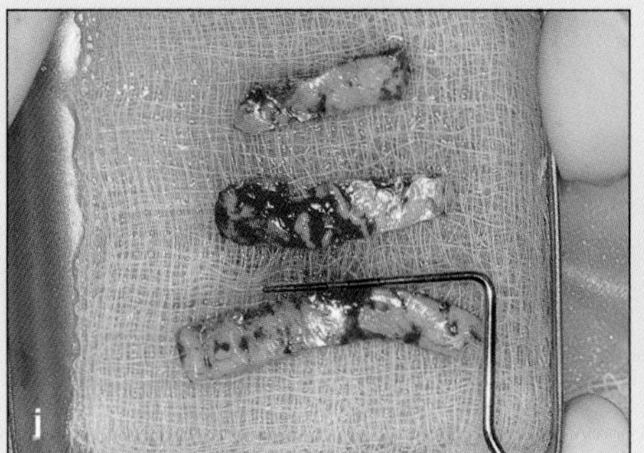

Fig 5-8j Three thick split-thickness grafts were harvested.

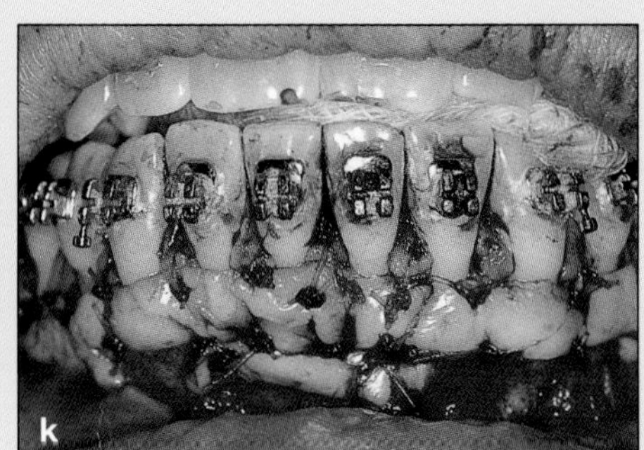

Fig 5-8k The grafts have been rigidly immobilized with meticulous suturing in each papilla area and peripherally. Butt-joint marginal adaptation at the horizontal incision in each papillary area is key to obtaining root coverage via the bridging phenomenon.

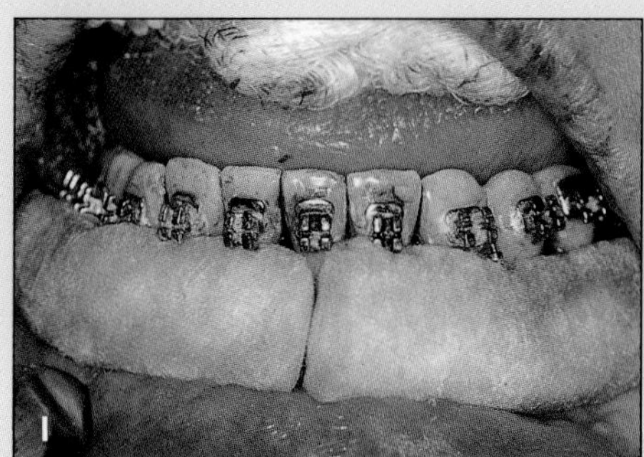

Fig 5-8l Pressure is applied with moistened saline gauze for 10 minutes to facilitate biologic immobilization via the formation of a thin fibrin layer intervening between the graft and the recipient site.

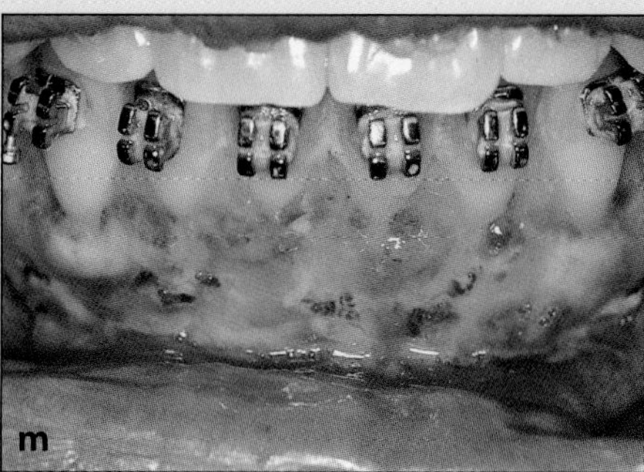

Fig 5-8m One-week postoperative view demonstrates superficial epithelial sloughing commonly seen with thick split-thickness grafts and early signs of a successful tissue transplantation.

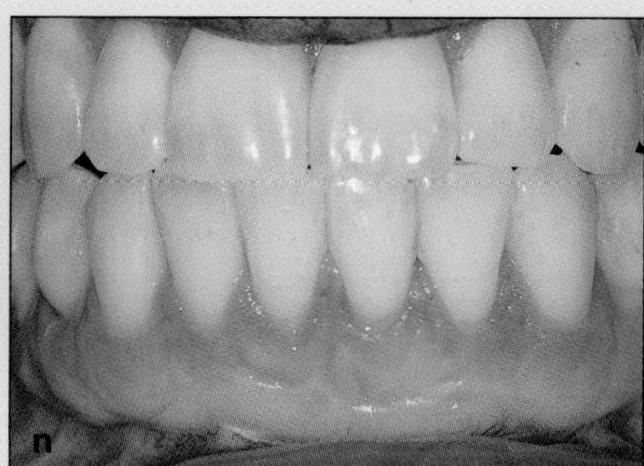

Fig 5-8n Final result 1 year after grafting procedure demonstrates successful root coverage, increased width of attached tissue, and re-establishment of adequate vestibular depth. Note improvement in soft tissue health compared with presurgical condition.

Gingival grafting to establish a stable peri-implant soft tissue environment in the edentulous mandible

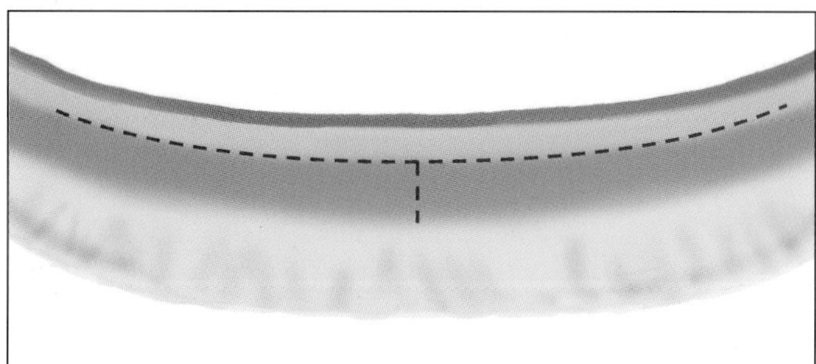

Fig 5-9a Edentulous mandible with a thin band (approximately 3 mm) of attached tissue on the ridge crest and inadequate vestibular depth, which will hinder the development of a stable peri-implant environment and limit access for patient oral hygiene following implant placement. Gingival grafting is planned simultaneous with nonsubmerged implant placement or at exposure of submerged implants. A full-thickness horizontal incision is made at the mucogingival junction and a partial-thickness vertical releasing incision is made at the midline.

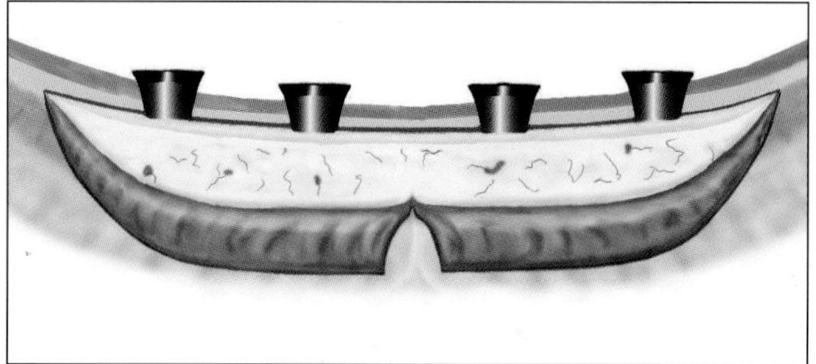

Fig 5-9b Subperiosteal reflection coronal to the horizontal incision is used to elevate and reposition the attached tissue to the lingual, thereby exposing the osseous ridge crest for implant placement. Split-thickness mucosal flaps are elevated with sharp dissection to create a periosteal recipient site. Nonsubmerged implants are placed or abutment connection is performed following a standard technique. In most cases, vertical releasing incisions are avoided laterally to minimize the possibility of damage to the adjacent mental nerve.

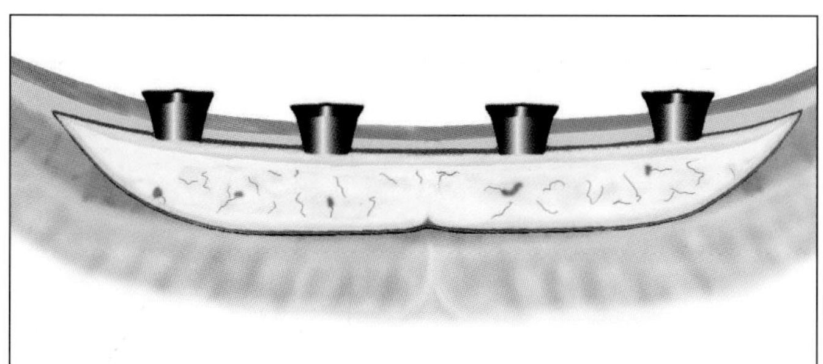

Fig 5-9c The resultant mucosal flaps are excised or repositioned and secured to the periosteum at the apical portion of the dissection when significant alveolar atrophy exists. Residual elastic and muscular tissues are excised with tissue nippers or curved Iris tissue scissors to create a uniform recipient site. Hemostasis is obtained prior to graft harvest.

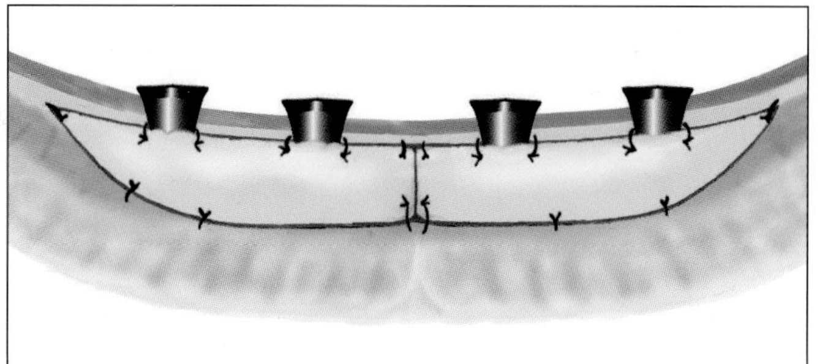

Fig 5-9d Palatal mucosal grafts are harvested to match the prepared recipient sites, and resective contouring is performed to allow intimate adaptation of the graft around the implants as well as to ensure butt-joint marginal adaptation of the graft with the lingual tissues. Immobilization of the graft begins with sutures placed in each inter-implant area superiorly and as needed peripherally. Pressure is applied with moistened saline gauze or cotton rolls for 10 minutes, after which graft immobilization is verified.

Gingival grafting at second-stage surgery in the edentulous mandible

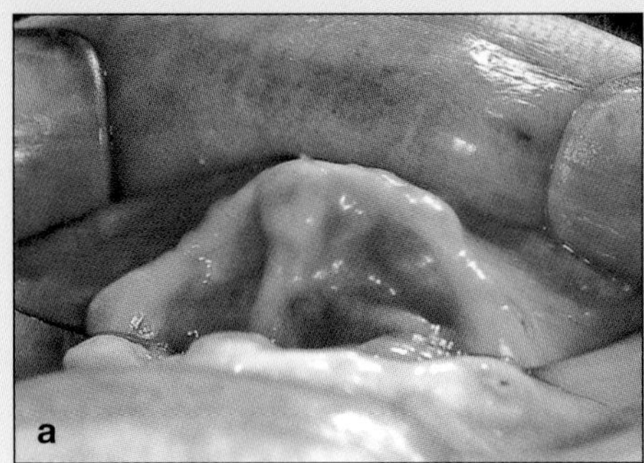

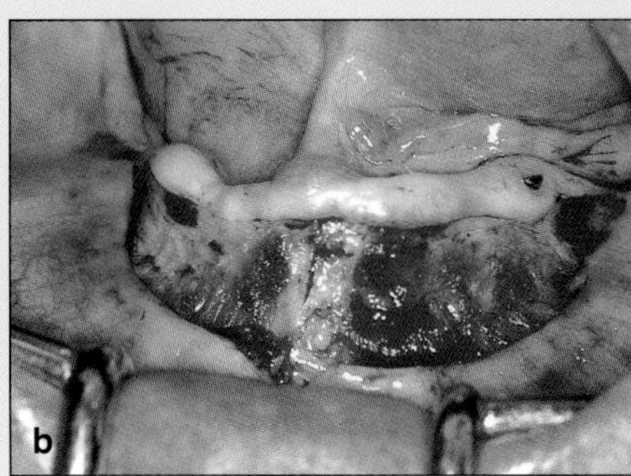

Fig 5-10a Four submerged mandibular implants (Nobel Biocare) are ready to be uncovered. The amount of attached tissue is inadequate to ensure a stable peri-implant soft tissue environment. The existing attached tissue should not be divided; instead the existing band should be preserved and repositioned to the lingual aspect of the emerging implants.

Fig 5-10b Horizontal incision made at the mucogingival junction is extended beyond the area of implantation. A uniform periosteal recipient site is created with sharp dissection.

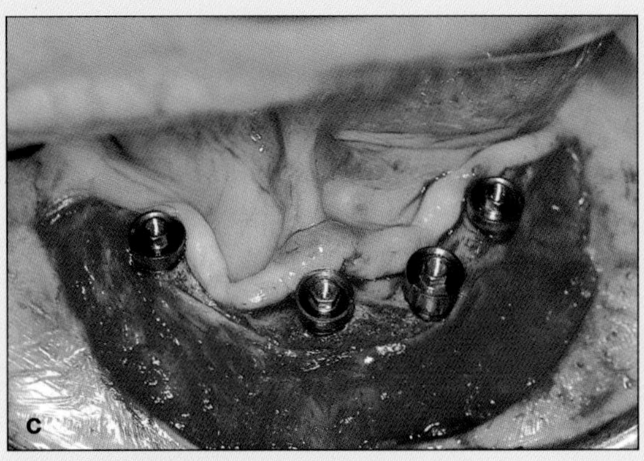

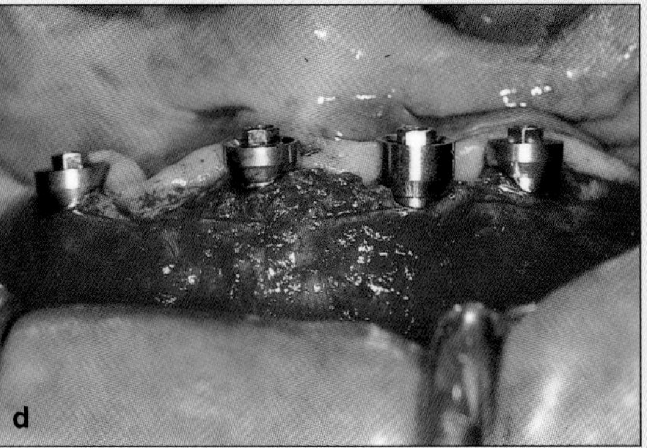

Figs 5-10c and 5-10d The thin band (approximately 3 mm) of attached tissue is repositioned to the lingual of the implants via subperiosteal elevation, and the abutments are secured. Excessive lingual reflection is minimized to avoid compromising circulation to the area.

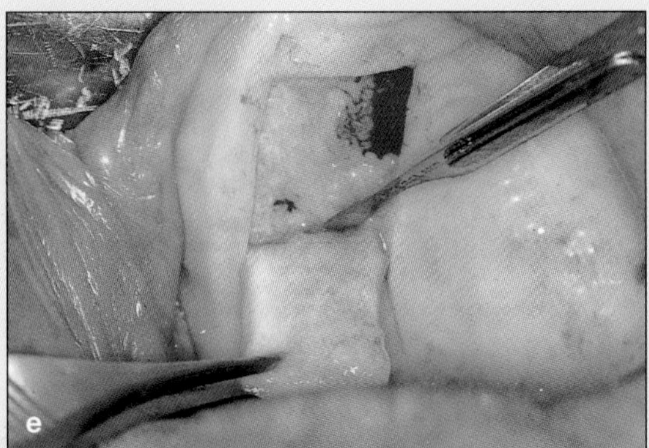

Fig 5-10e After the donor graft has been outlined with partial-thickness incisions, micro-Adson tissue forceps are used to apply gentle traction at the beveled access incision, and a uniform graft is harvested with sharp dissection.

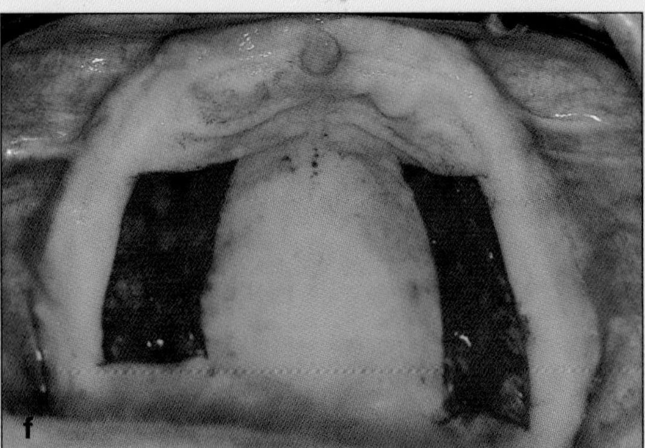

Fig 5-10f Hemostasis is obtained at bilateral donor sites with electrocautery and application of pressure with a moistened saline gauze. The donor sites will be dressed with CollaCote prior to protecting them with the patient's maxillary denture.

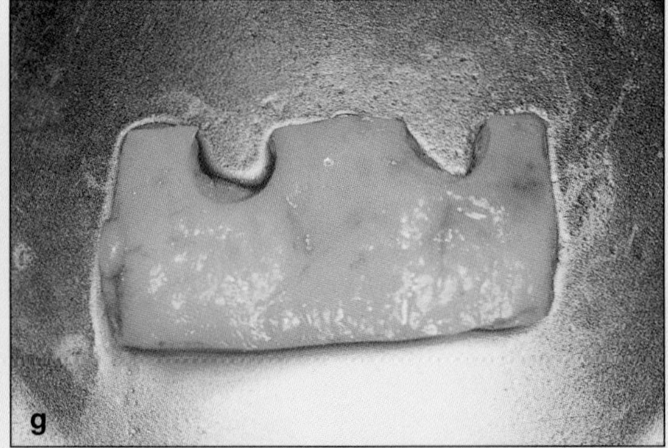

Fig 5-10g Each graft is marked, and resective contouring is performed with a fresh no. 15C scalpel to ensure intimate adaptation around the implant abutments and butt-joint marginal adaptation with the lingual tissues.

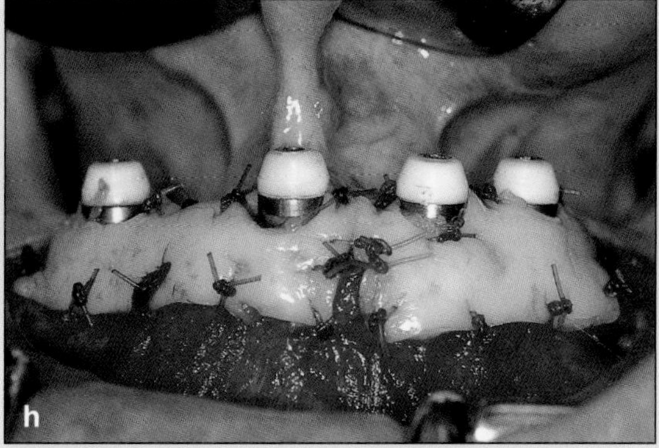

Fig 5-10h Gingival grafts have been adapted to and secured at the recipient site with meticulous suturing (4-0 chromic gut on a P3 needle). Initially, the grafts are secured to the repositioned lingual tissues with sutures in each inter-implant area.

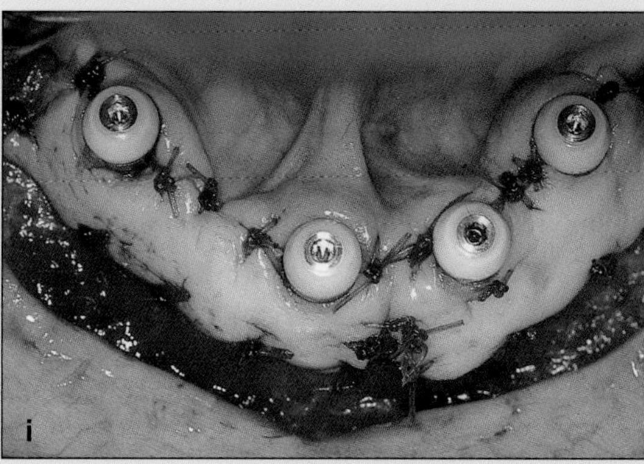

Fig 5-10i Sutures are also used to secure the grafts peripherally to periosteum. A buccal vestibular extension was performed to ensure absolute immobilization of the graft. Note that in this case the lingual frenum jeopardizes graft immobilization.

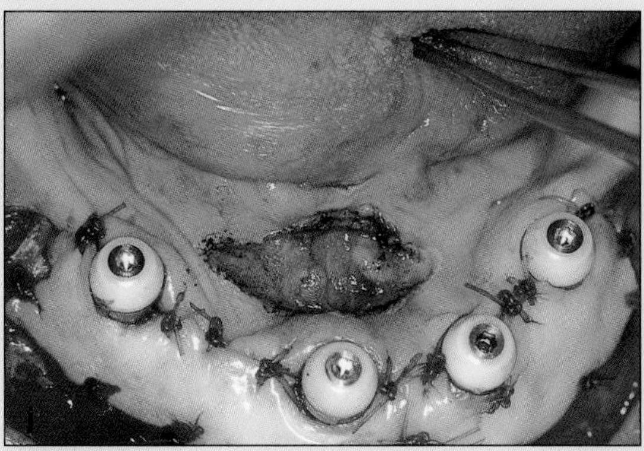

Fig 5-10j A CO_2 laser was used to release the aberrant lingual frenum, maintaining bi-pedicled circulation to the gingival tissue in that area.

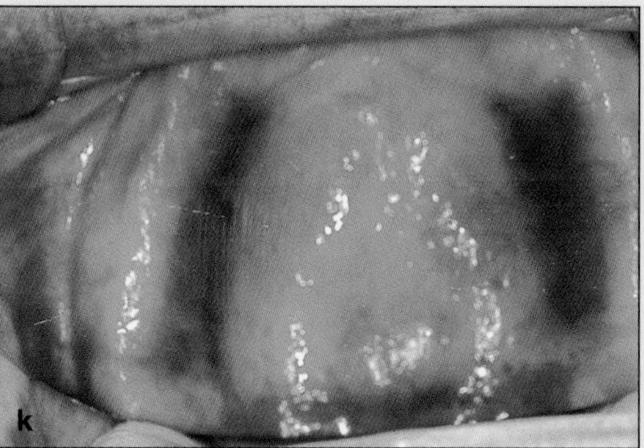

Fig 5-10k View of donor site 4 weeks after surgery.

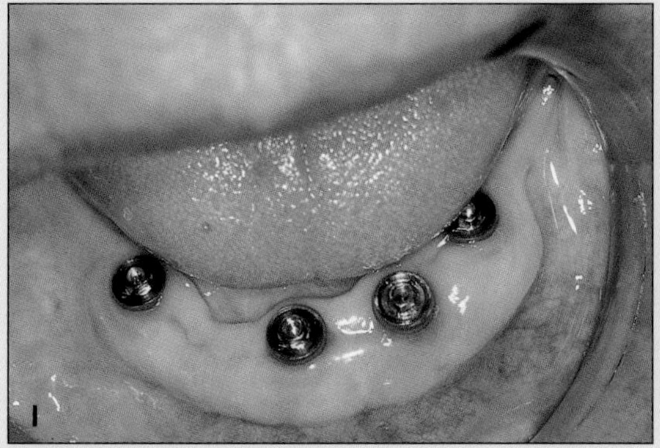

Fig 5-10l Four-week postoperative view of recipient site. Vestibular depth has been re-created, and an adequate band of attached gingival tissue now surrounds the abutments. The repositioned tissue has adapted well to the lingual aspect of the implants, and the lingual frenectomy was successful.

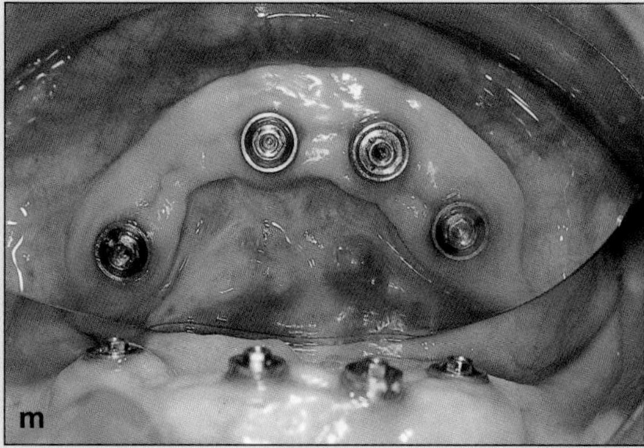

Fig 5-10m Eight-week postoperative view. The grafts have matured, and peri-implant inflammation is absent. Note the thickness of the healed grafts. This thick tissue will resist future functional stresses and facilitate restorative procedures.

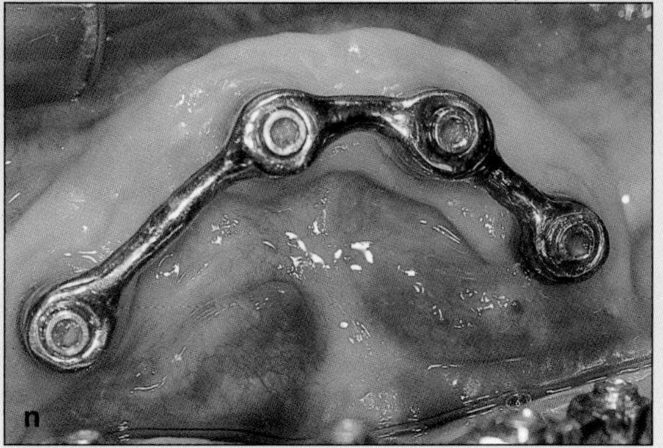

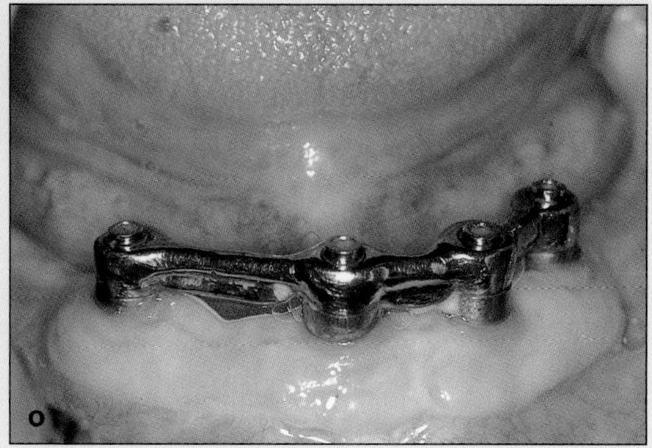

Figs 5-10n and 5-10o One-year post-restoration view demonstrating stability and health of attached peri-implant soft tissues. Maintenance of a lingual band of attached tissues and augmentation of buccal tissues has facilitated oral hygiene efforts for this patient with limited dexterity. (Restorative dentistry by Dr Faustino Garcia, Coral Gables, FL.)

Gingival grafting at second-stage surgery in the atrophic mandible

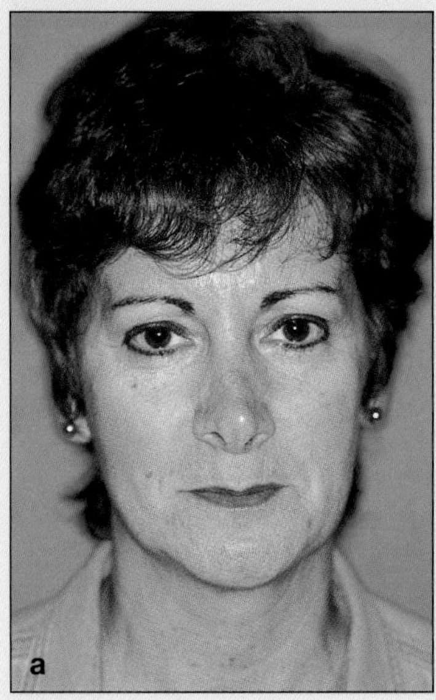

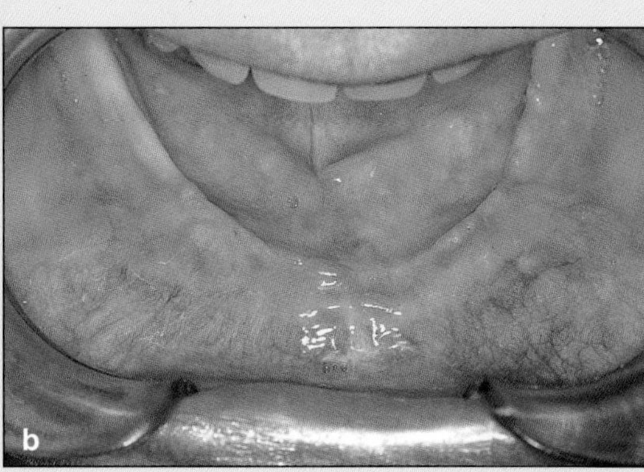

Fig 5-11a Frontal view of patient with atrophic mandible experiencing difficulty with unstable mandibular denture appliance. A fixed implant-supported appliance is planned to improve patient comfort and function.

Fig 5-11b Intraoral view of atrophic mandible with a thin band (approximately 3 mm) of attached tissue remaining. Mucosal tissues are bound down to the buccal aspect of the atrophic ridge. Gingival grafting is planned at the second-stage surgery. Use of a surgical guide indicated that the thin band of attached tissue at the ridge crest was located lingual to the proposed implant sites. Therefore, the attached tissues were not reflected to facilitate wound closure at first-stage surgery.

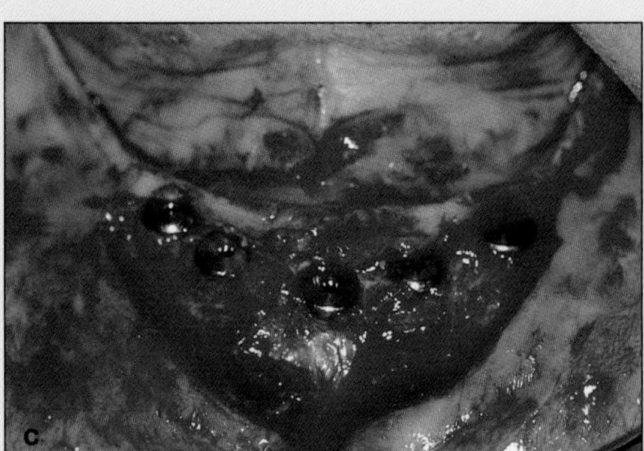

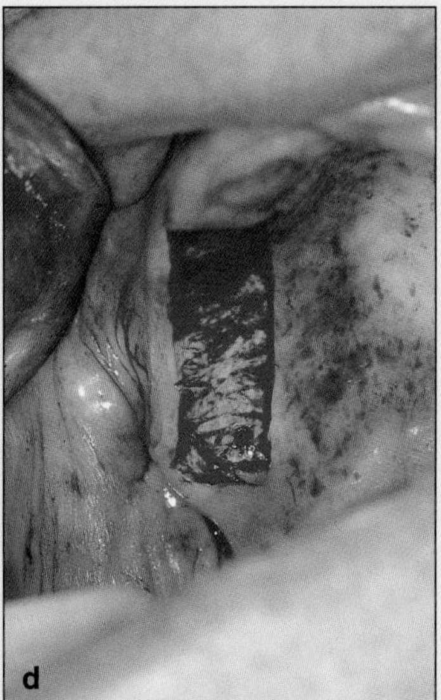

Fig 5-11c Second-stage surgery. Recipient-site preparation is initiated with a partial-thickness horizontal incision located at the mucogingival junction. Sharp dissection was performed over the implants and extended inferiorly to complete the supraperiosteal recipient site.

Fig 5-11d Thick split-thickness graft is harvested from a single donor site and divided to create two gingival strip grafts. In this case, the donor area included the alveolar ridge crest. Note that the plane of dissection at the ridge crest was inadvertently more superficial. This predisposes that portion of the graft to secondary contraction.

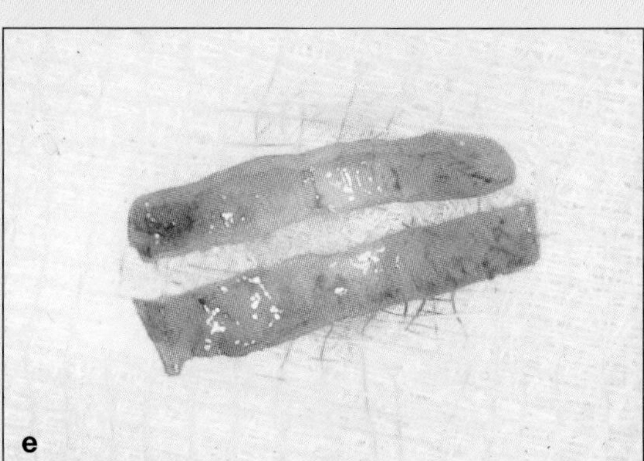

Fig 5-11e A fresh no. 15C scalpel was used to divide the graft into two 4-mm-wide gingival strip grafts. This eliminates the need for a second donor site.

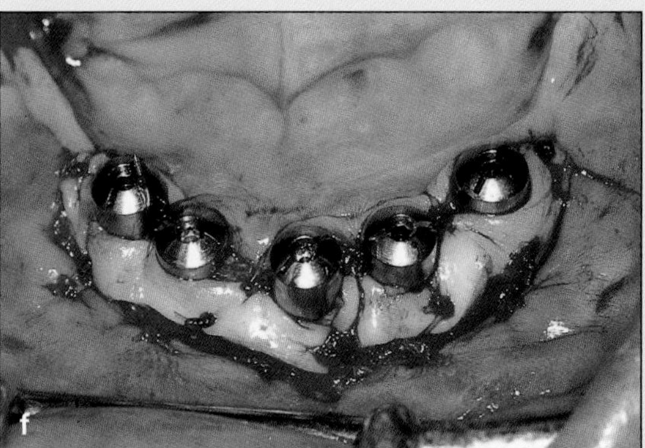

Fig 5-11f Temporary abutments have been placed, and gingival strip grafts have been contoured, adapted, and secured to the attached lingual tissues and the periosteum at the recipient site. Placement of permanent abutments at this time is preferred to avoid future disruption of the tenuous peri-implant soft tissue seal.

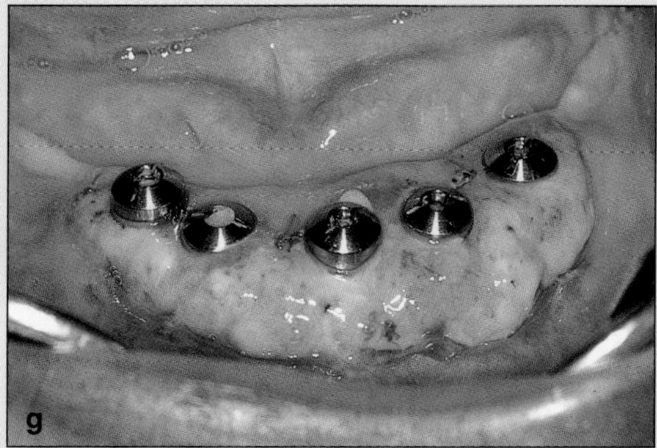

Fig 5-11g One-week postoperative view demonstrates initial revascularization of the graft. Superficial epithelial sloughing also is evident, as expected.

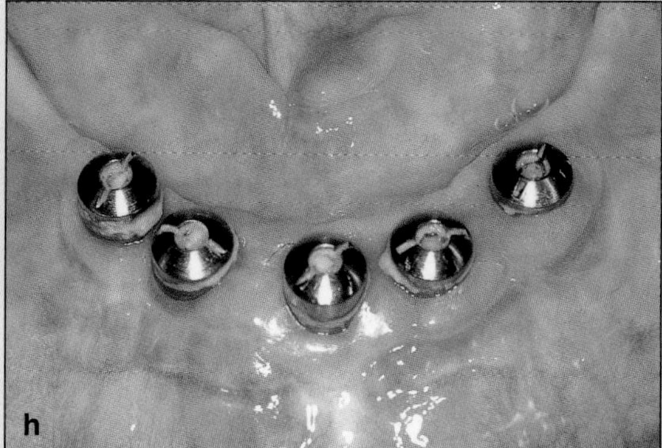

Fig 5-11h Four-week postoperative view. The gingival grafts have healed but are not completely matured.

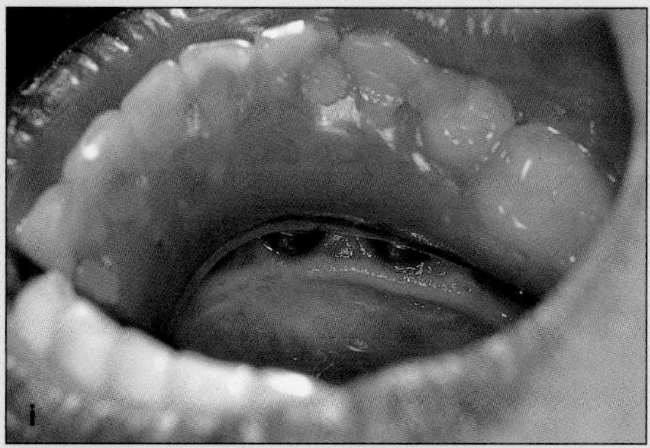

Fig 5-11i One-year postoperative lingual view. The original band of attached tissues was preserved on the lingual aspect of the emerging implants. Exceptional soft tissue health resulted from the preservation of the lingual attached tissues and reconstruction of the buccal attached tissues with gingival grafting. Oral hygiene has been facilitated by the presence of resilient attached tissues around the implants.

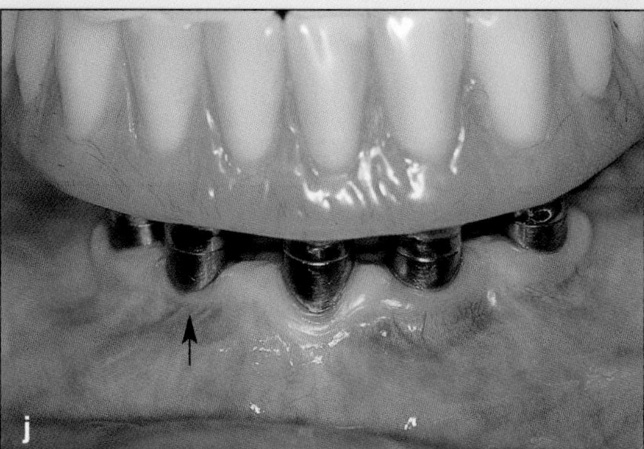

Fig 5-11j One-year postoperative view. The gingival strip grafts have undergone secondary contraction. Note that the thinner portion of the graft underwent greater secondary contraction *(arrow)*. The peri-implant soft tissues are healthy in appearance, nonmobile, and devoid of inflammation. A graft width of 5 mm or more generally eliminates problems encountered from secondary contraction but requires bilateral palatal harvest.

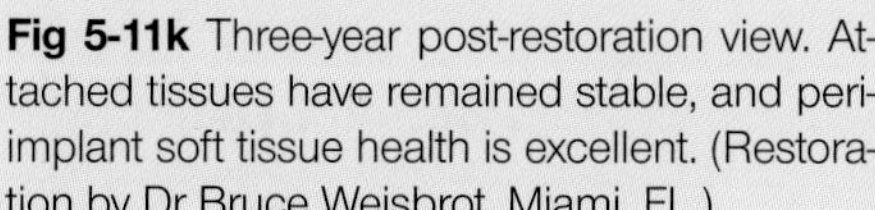

Fig 5-11k Three-year post-restoration view. Attached tissues have remained stable, and peri-implant soft tissue health is excellent. (Restoration by Dr Bruce Weisbrot, Miami, FL.)

Fig 5-11l Patient satisfaction is vastly improved by the treatment, which has facilitated oral hygiene procedures. Commonly encountered peri-implant soft tissue problems were avoided by the use of gingival grafting.

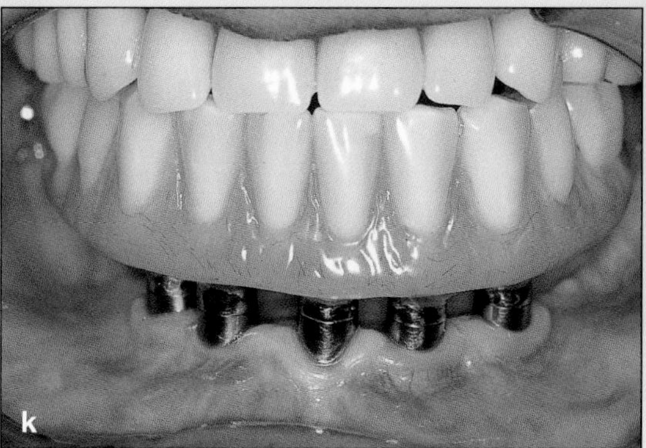

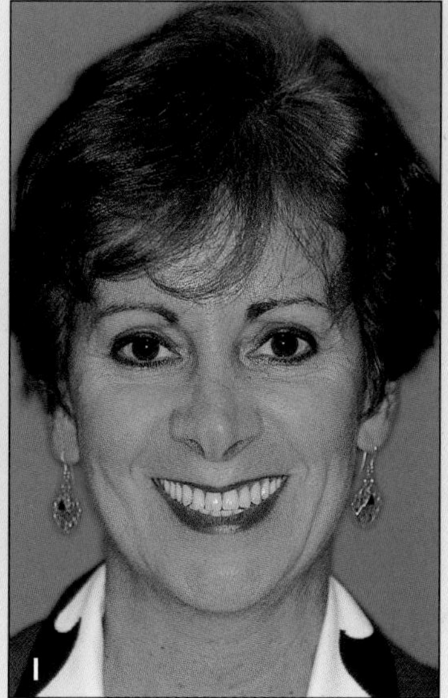

Gingival grafting performed simultaneously with nonsubmerged implant placement in the edentulous mandible

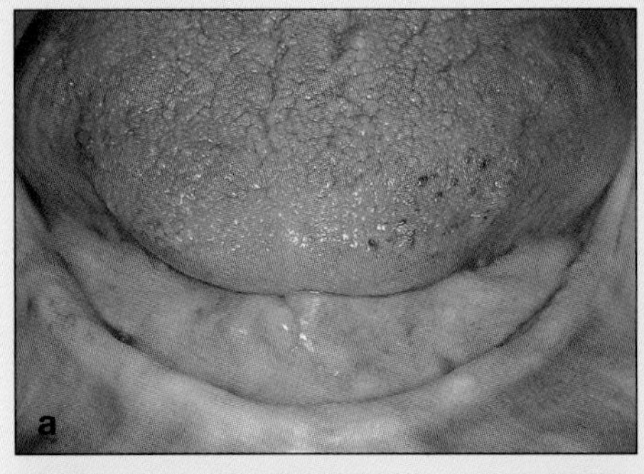

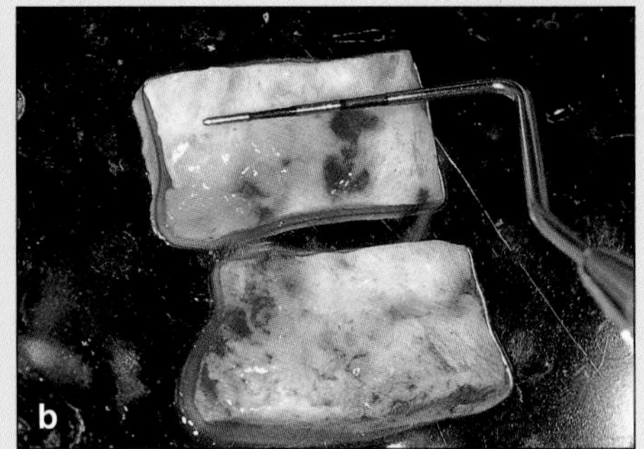

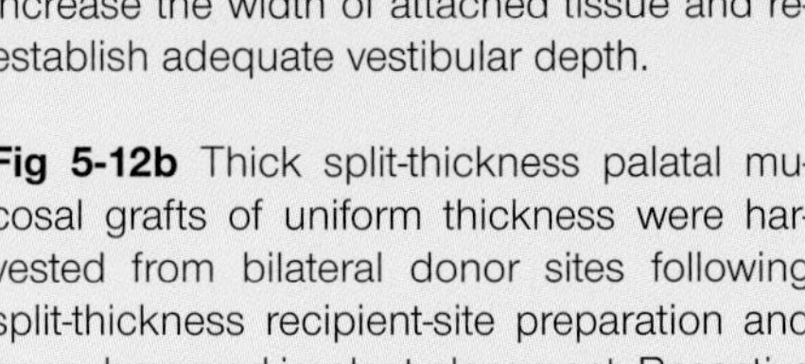

Fig 5-12a Preoperative view of edentulous mandible. Note the high muscle attachments and the thin band of attached tissue at the ridge crest. Gingival grafting is indicated to increase the width of attached tissue and re-establish adequate vestibular depth.

Fig 5-12b Thick split-thickness palatal mucosal grafts of uniform thickness were harvested from bilateral donor sites following split-thickness recipient-site preparation and nonsubmerged implant placement. Resective contouring is performed to allow close adaptation around nonsubmerged implant collars.

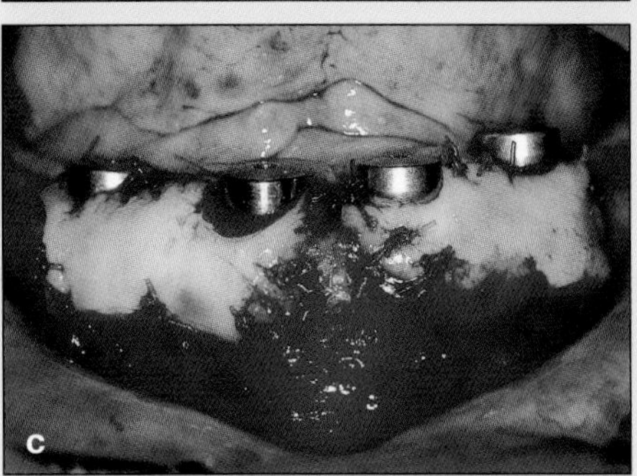

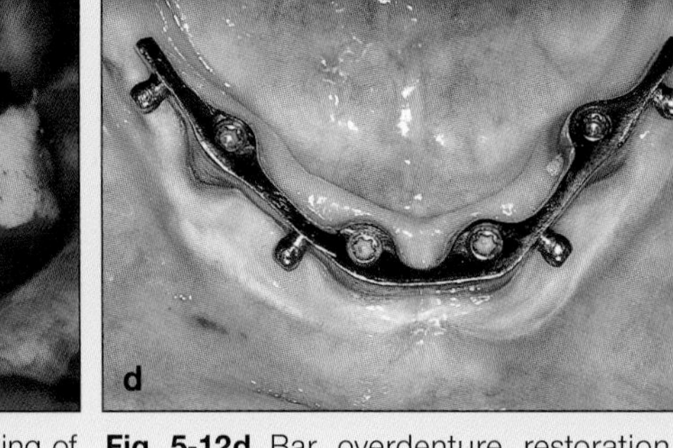

Fig 5-12c After reflection and repositioning of the thin band of attached tissues lingually to expose the ridge crest, sharp dissection was used to create a uniform periosteal recipient site. Subsequent to placement of four nonsubmerged implants (Straumann USA, Waltham, MA), gingival grafts were harvested, contoured, and rigidly immobilized at the recipient site.

Fig 5-12d Bar overdenture restoration in place. Adequate width of attached tissue and re-establishment of adequate vestibular depth has resulted in an optimal peri-implant soft tissue environment. Appropriate soft tissue management and grafting procedures performed in conjunction with nonsubmerged implant placement reduce treatment time and patient inconvenience. Final prosthesis includes extended flanges closely adapted to attached tissues to minimize the collection of food debris under the prosthesis. (Restorative dentistry by Dr Stephen Parr, Coconut Grove, FL.)

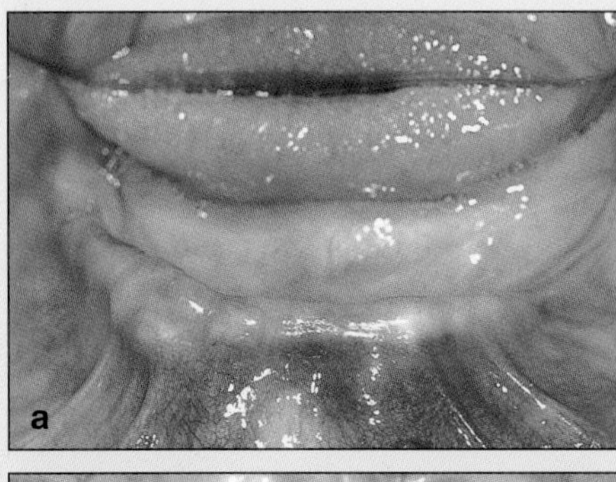

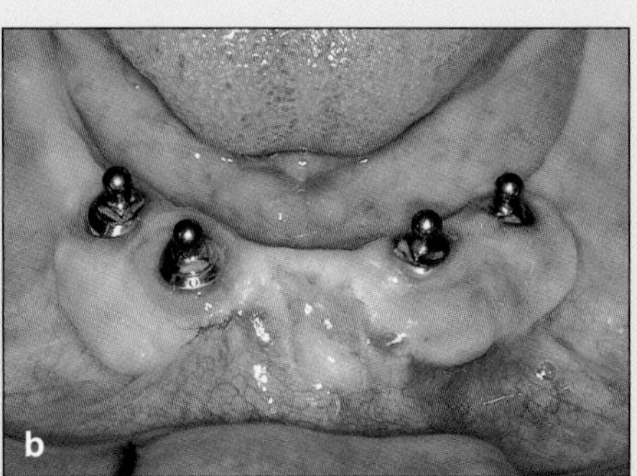

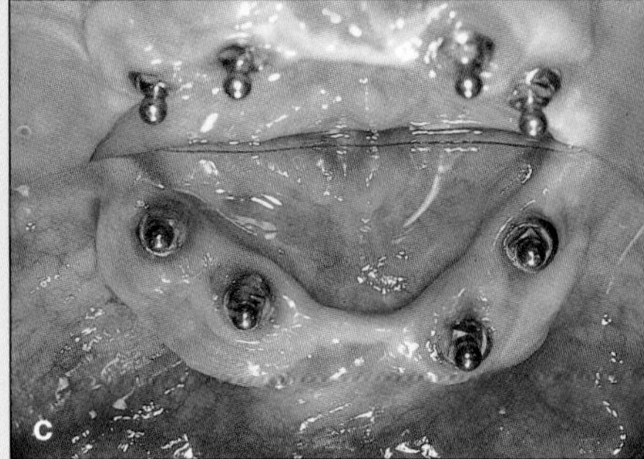

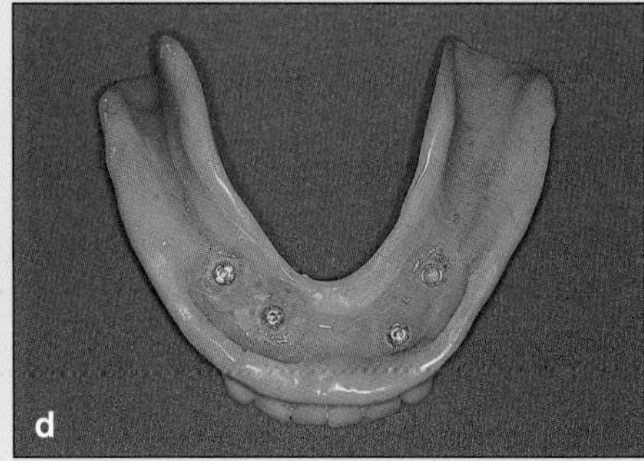

Fig 5-13a Presurgical view of another edentulous mandible with high muscle attachments, mobility of tissues at the ridge crest, and an inadequate width of attached tissue. An overdenture stabilized by four nonsubmerged implants with individual attachments was planned. Simultaneous gingival grafting was indicated.

Figs 5-13b and 5-13c At 3 months, the gingival grafts were fully matured and the peri-implant soft tissues were devoid of inflammation. The fortified peri-implant tissues are better able to withstand the repeated functional stresses created by the removable implant-supported prosthesis, virtually eliminating soft tissue problems. This is especially a consideration when resilient attachments are used to stabilize an overdenture.

Fig 5-13d Final prosthesis includes extended flanges that are intimately adapted to the grafted tissues in order to minimize collection of food debris under the flange. Grafting simultaneously with nonsubmerged implant placement reduced treatment time in this case. (Restorative dentistry by Dr Ralph Jacobson, Miami, FL.)

Gingival grafting at second-stage surgery to re-establish adequate vestibular depth

Fig 5-14a Presurgical view demonstrates high muscle attachments and inadequate vestibular depth *(arrow)* for oral hygiene maintenance of the proposed implant restoration.

Fig 5-14b At second-stage surgery, a split-thickness dissection created a labial recipient site. Subperiosteal dissection was used to elevate and lingually reposition the attached tissues at the ridge crest to allow for placement of permanent abutments (Nobel Biocare, Loma Linda, CA).

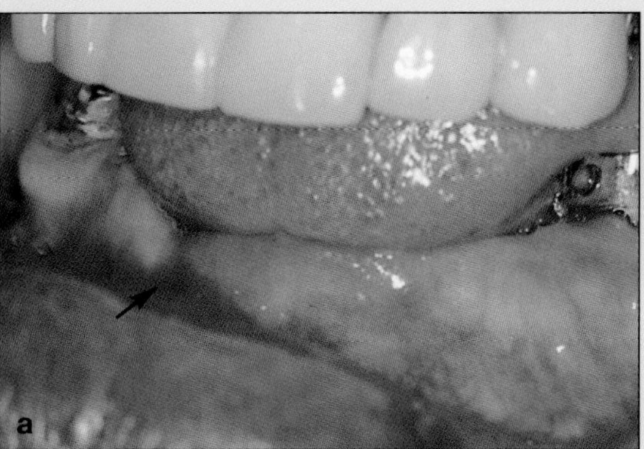

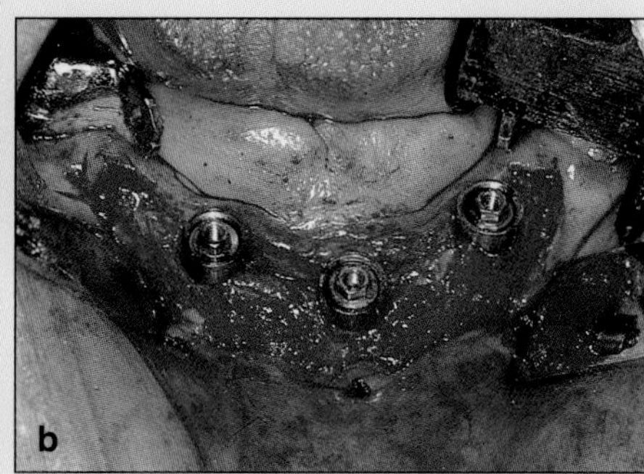

Fig 5-14c A large, thick split-thickness graft was harvested and divided into three individual grafts. Care was taken to maintain uniform thickness of the portion of the graft harvested over the ridge crest. The patient's partial denture served to protect the donor site during healing.

Fig 5-14d The grafts were secured to the repositioned lingual tissues and to the periosteum peripherally. Intimate adaptation of the grafts around the permanent abutments was obtained. No dressing was used at the recipient site.

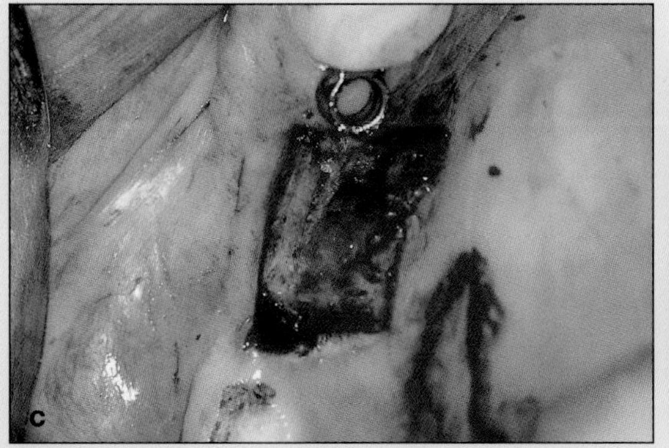

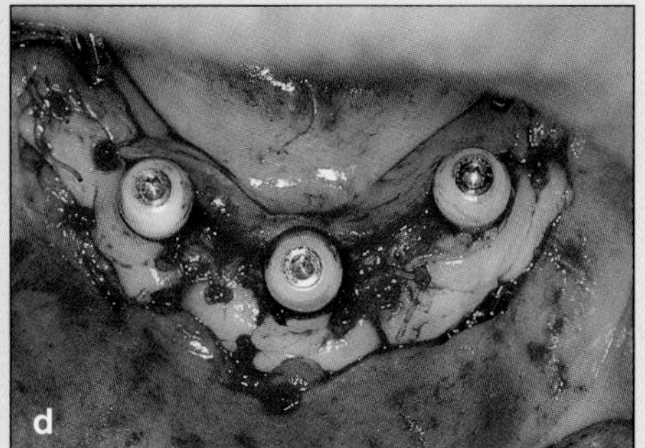

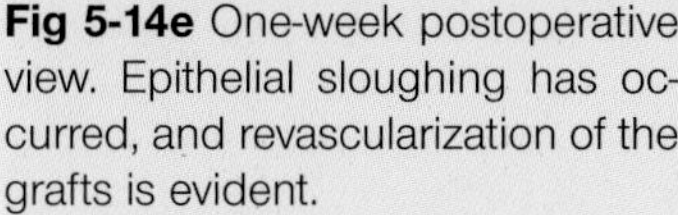

Fig 5-14e One-week postoperative view. Epithelial sloughing has occurred, and revascularization of the grafts is evident.

Fig 5-14f Occlusal view of restoration 1 year after delivery. Repositioning of the existing attached tissues to the lingual of the emerging abutments and gingival grafting on the labial aspect of the alveolar ridge has resulted in a healthy and stable peri-implant soft tissue environment.

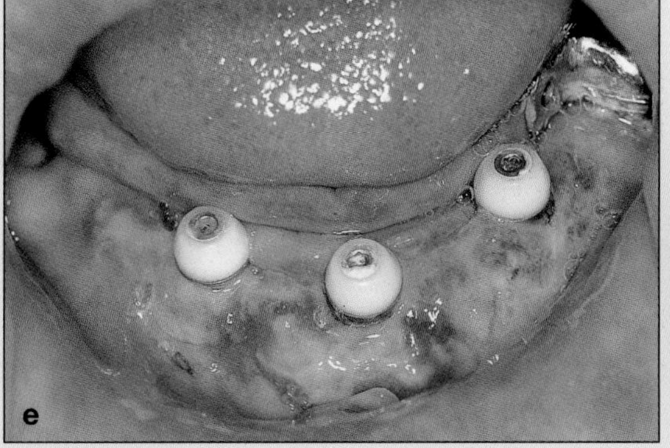

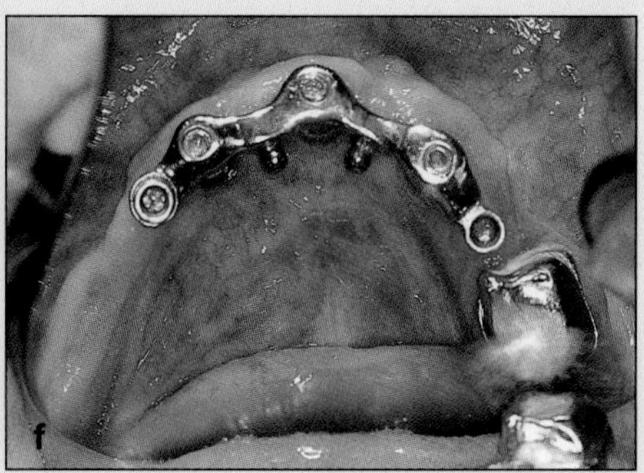

Figs 5-14g and 5-14h Frontal view of implant bar and healthy peri-implant soft tissues 1 year after delivery. Re-establishment of adequate vestibular depth *(arrow)* has facilitated the patient's oral hygiene efforts and allowed extension of the labial flange for both improved lip support and close adaptation of the removable restoration to the resilient grafted tissue, thereby minimizing collection of food debris. (Restorative dentistry by Dr Lea Kronacher, Miami, FL.)

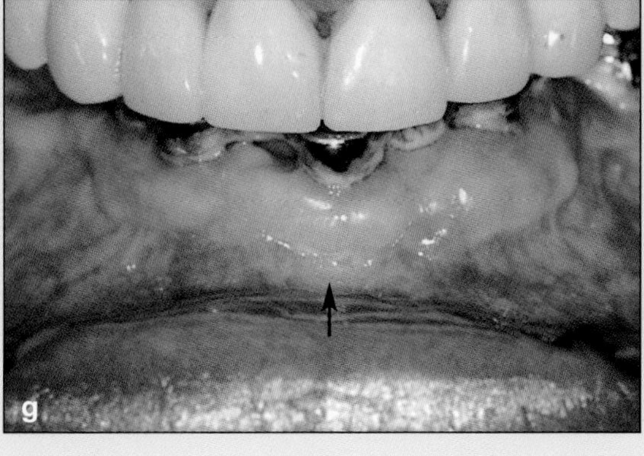

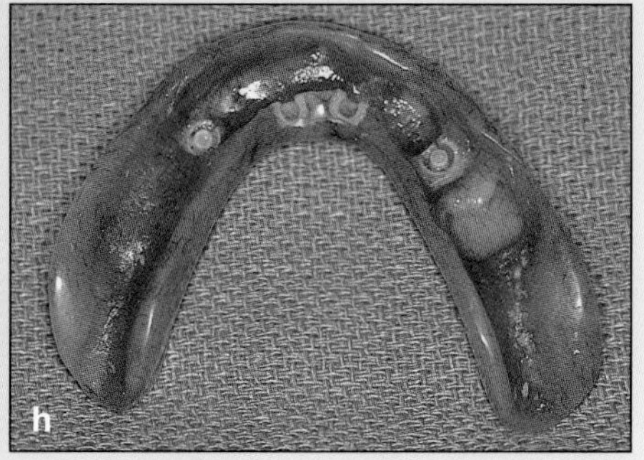

Gingival grafting in the edentulous maxilla to establish an adequate width of attached tissue

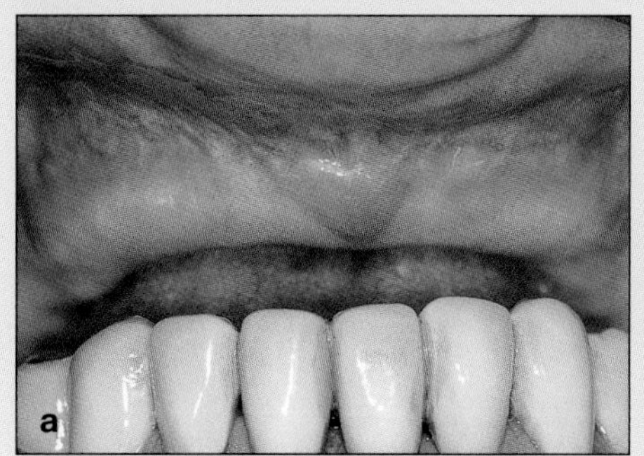

Fig 5-15a Presurgical view of edentulous maxilla following two iliac bone graft reconstructions. The first bone graft was performed via a Le Fort incision. However, the outcome of the bone graft did not allow for ideal implant positioning. Therefore, the author performed additional autogenous bone grafting simultaneous with implant placement through a peri-crestal approach.

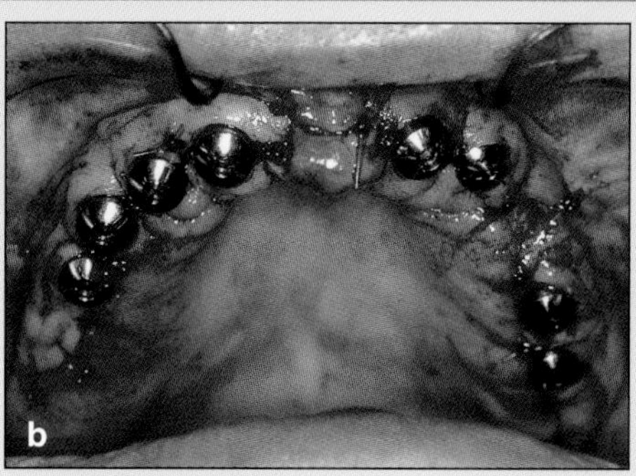

Fig 5-15b At second-stage surgery, a band of attached tissue was taken from the crest of the alveolar ridge and apically repositioned, contoured, and secured around the eight maxillary implants.

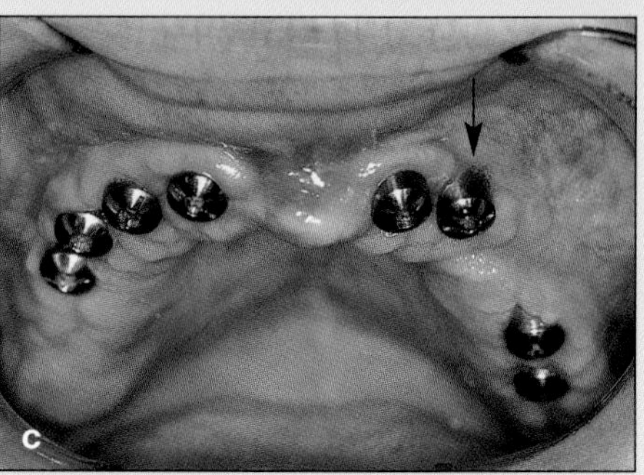

Fig 5-15c Soft tissue recession *(arrow)* is evident 8 weeks after second-stage surgery. This was attributed to compromised circulation to the flap margin as well as a poorly vascularized recipient site (recent block bone graft) for the apically repositioned pedicle flap used at the second-stage surgery. The result is an inadequate width of attached tissue and inadequate vestibular depth to ensure a stable peri-implant environment. Gingival grafting is indicated prior to restorative procedures, which could precipitate further recession and underlying bone loss.

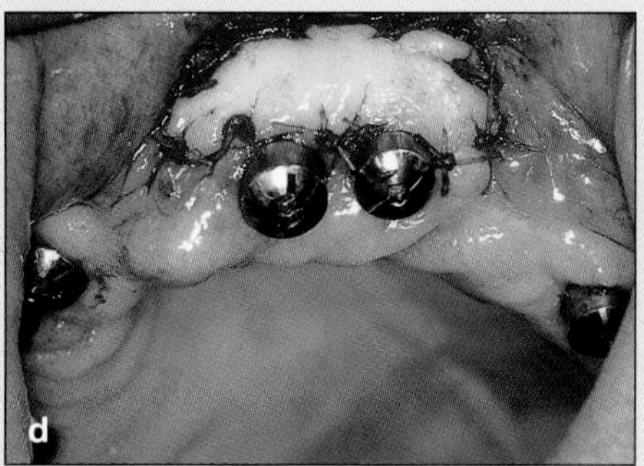

Fig 5-15d The recipient site and graft have been extended well beyond the area of recession to take advantage of peripheral circulation to nourish the graft and to compensate for the compromised circulation in the area previously bone grafted. Supraperiosteal dissection was performed to create a uniform recipient site with butt-joint marginal adaptation of the precisely sized palatal mucosal graft.

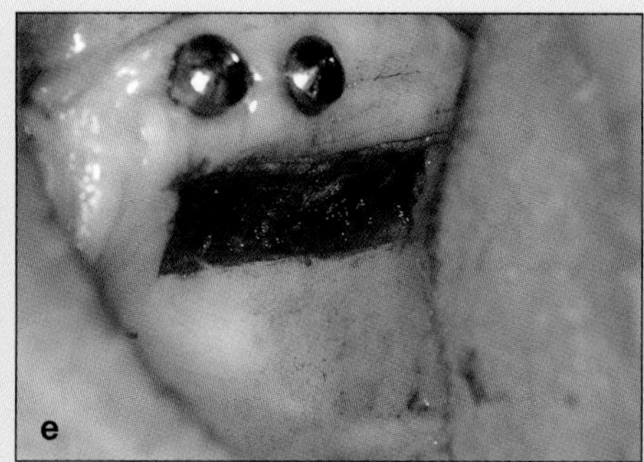

Fig 5-15e Hemostasis was obtained at the recipient site, which was subsequently dressed with CollaCote and protected with an interim complete denture.

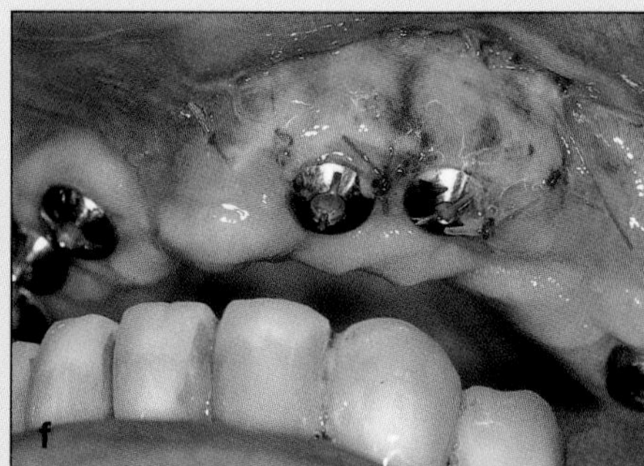

Fig 5-15f One-week postoperative view. The graft site is easily evaluated because a protective dressing was not used over the graft. Expected epithelial sloughing and early revascularization of the graft are evident.

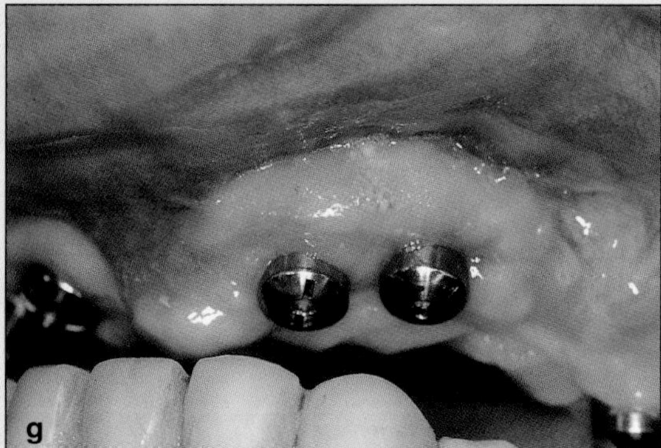

Fig 5-15g Six-week postoperative view. An adequate band of attached gingival tissue has been successfully reconstructed. Vestibular depth has been regained, providing access for oral hygiene and the necessary extension of the labial flange indicated for esthetic lip support. The grafted tissue will resist the trauma of the subsequent abutment connection or fixture-level prosthetic procedures and will facilitate future oral hygiene efforts.

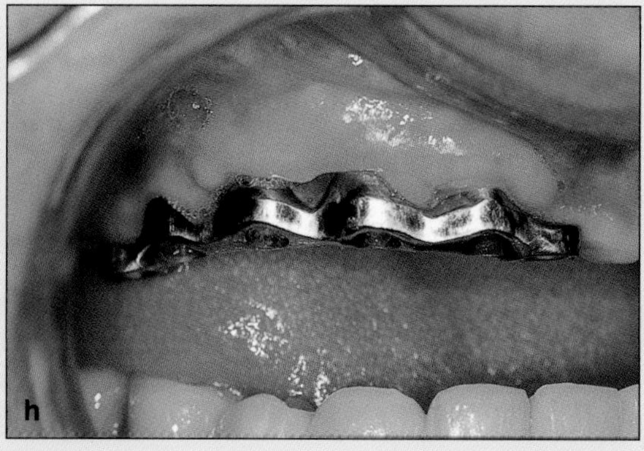

Fig 5-15h One year post-restoration. Excellent peri-implant soft tissue health and stability are evident. Prosthetic procedures and patient maintenance were facilitated as a result of the gingival graft. (Restorative dentistry by Dr Hank Baretto, Kendall, FL.)

Gingival grafting in the partially edentulous mandible performed simultaneously with nonsubmerged implant placement

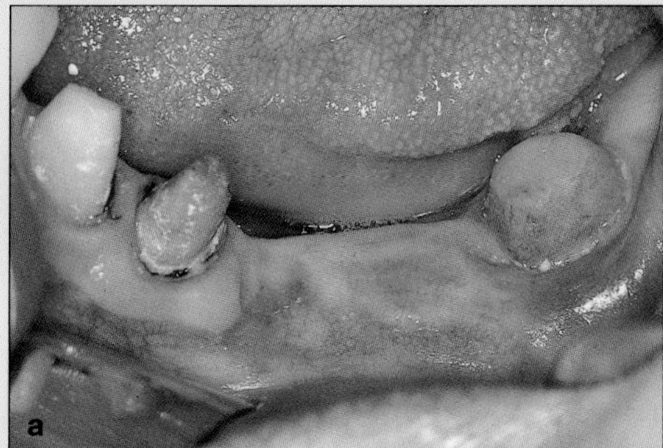

Fig 5-16a Preoperative view of partially edentulous site planned for nonsubmerged implant placement with simultaneous gingival grafting. Note the lack of attached gingival tissue extending distally adjacent to the natural tooth.

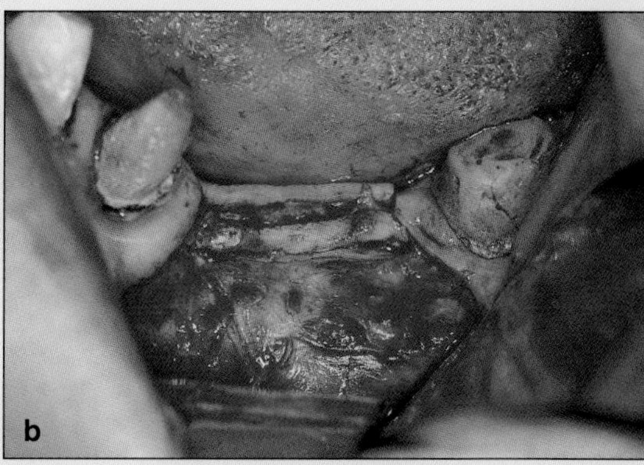

Fig 5-16b Because the horizontal incision was located at the mucogingival junction, reflection and lingual repositioning of the existing band of attached tissue were not necessary. A partial-thickness buccal flap was elevated and excised.

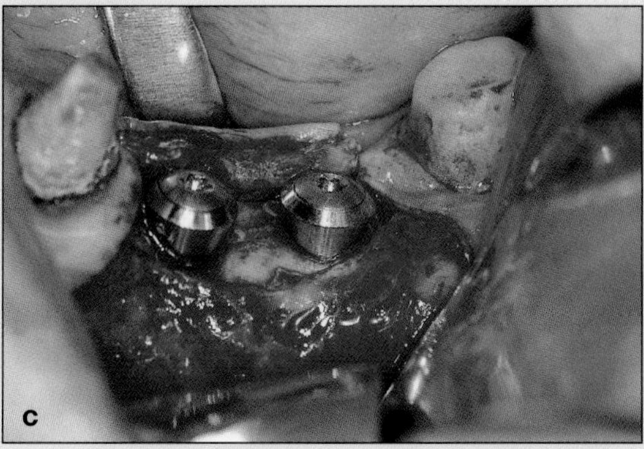

Fig 5-16c One-piece nonsubmerged implants (Straumann USA) were placed with low-profile closure screws to allow seating of the provisional fixed partial denture.

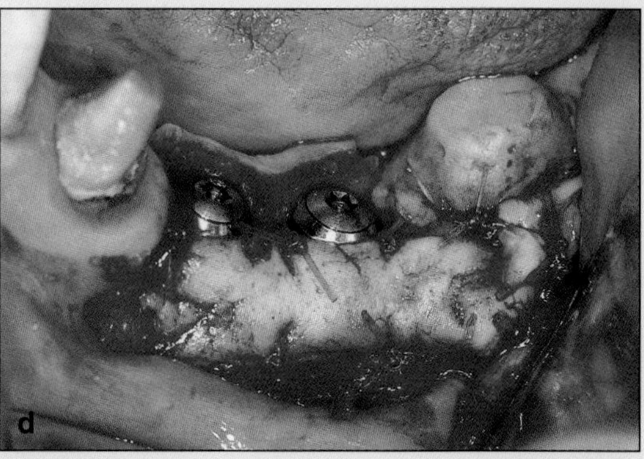

Fig 5-16d The gingival graft has been adapted around the permucosal portion of the implants and rigidly immobilized to the recipient bed with sutures.

Fig 5-16e Six-week postoperative view. The provisional prosthesis has been removed. The implants are osseointegrated and the gingival graft has matured. An adequate band of attached tissues has been reconstructed. The cervical portions of the implants have been successfully covered. This will allow esthetic emergence of the final restorations.

Fig 5-16f Six-week postoperative view. A tissue punch was used to remove excess gingival tissue from around the distal implant to facilitate prosthetics.

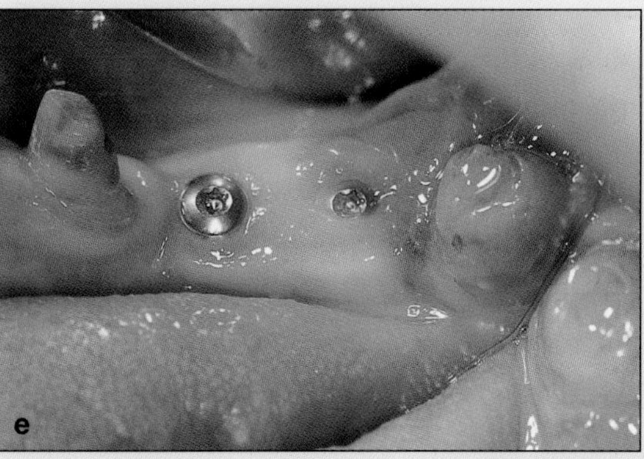

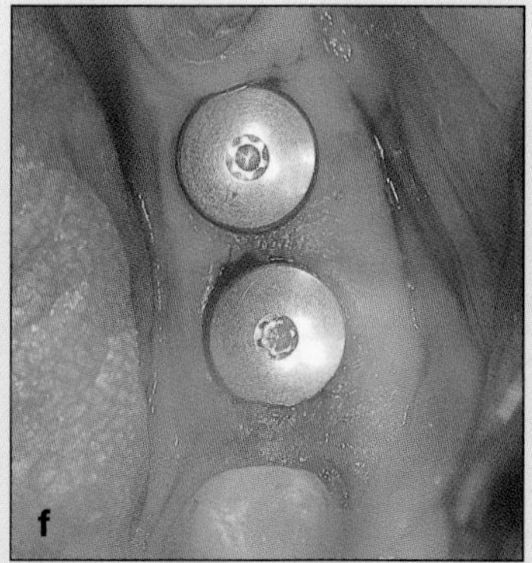

Fig 5-16g Final restoration was delivered 8 weeks following nonsubmerged implant placement with simultaneous gingival grafting, thereby reducing treatment time and enhancing patient satisfaction. Complete reconstruction of attached tissues is evident. (Restoration by Dr Jorge Blanco, Miami, FL.)

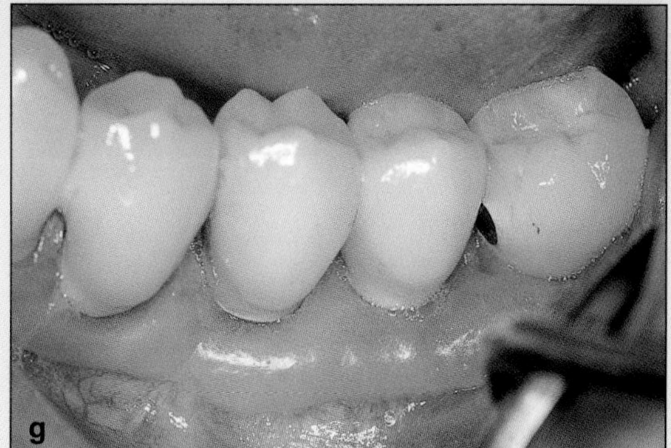

Gingival grafting in the partially edentulous mandible at second-stage surgery

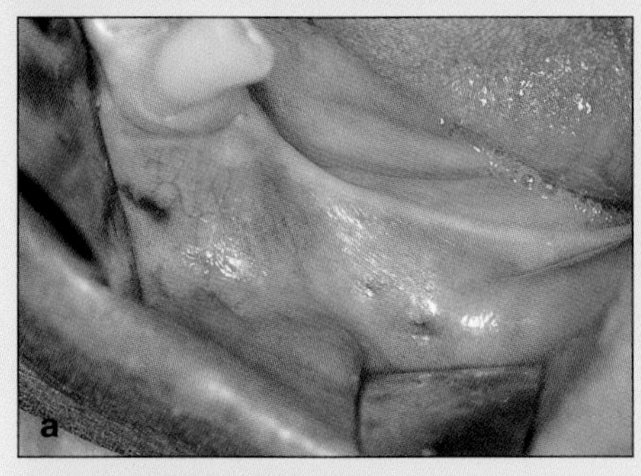

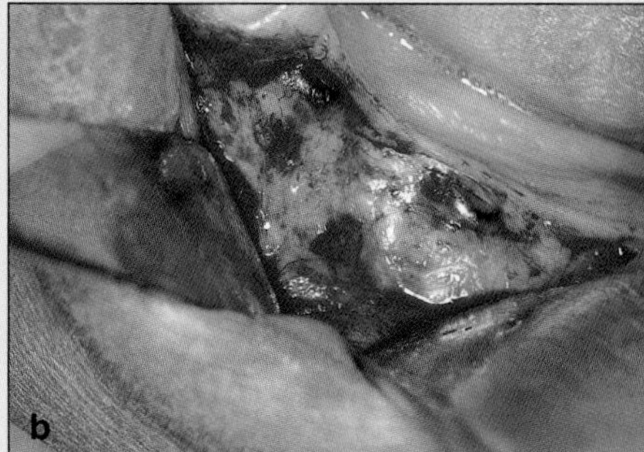

Fig 5-17a Preoperative view of the site. Note the thin band of attached tissue on the lingual crest of the ridge and the thin mucosal tissue through which implant cover screws can be visualized. A gingival graft is planned to provide an adequate band of attached tissue and reestablish vestibular depth.

Fig 5-17b A horizontal incision at the mucogingival junction initiates partial-thickness dissection to create a uniform recipient site.

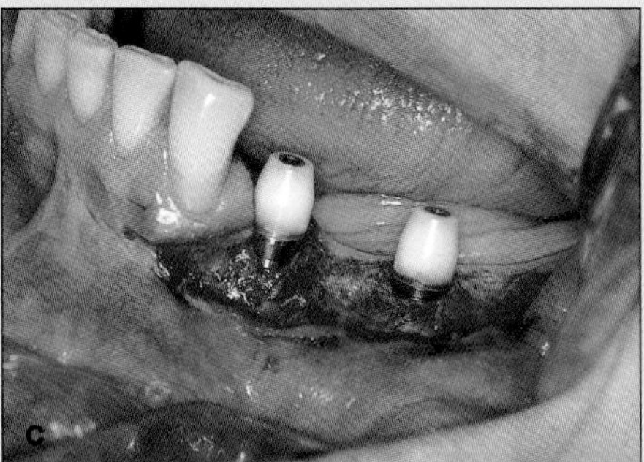

Fig 5-17c Permanent abutments with protective caps have been placed.

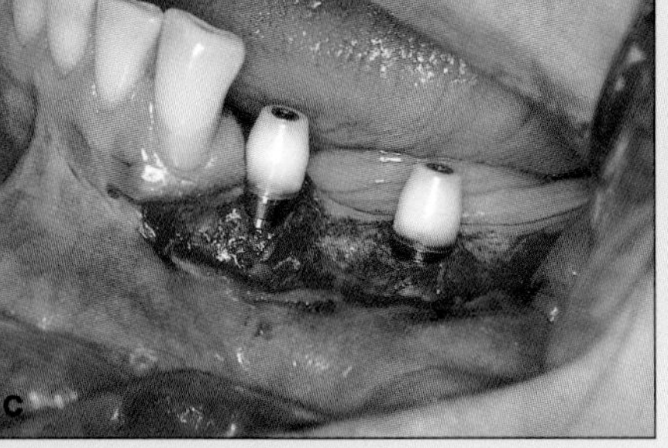

Fig 5-17d Graft immobilized with numerous 4-0 chromic gut sutures. Pressure was applied over the graft for 10 minutes.

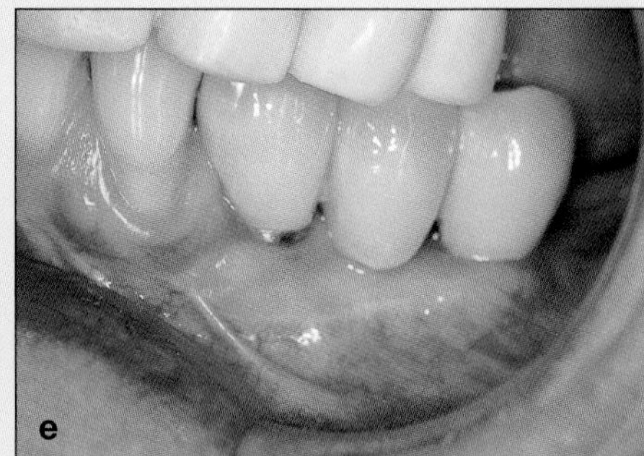

Fig 5-17e Adequate band of attached tissue and re-establishment of vestibular depth are evident. Note that extension of the recipient site and graft to include the papillary areas mesial and distal to the adjacent canine would have resulted in successful root and abutment coverage. (Restoration by Dr Richard Mariani Sr, Miami, FL.)

AlloDerm

AlloDerm (LifeCell, Branchburg, NJ) has been used as an alternative to harvesting autogenous epithelialized palatal grafts in periodontal surgery since 1996. AlloDerm grafts are composed of freeze-dried allograft skin processed to remove all immunogenic cellular components (epidermis and dermal cells), leaving a useful acellular dermal matrix for soft tissue augmentation. AlloDerm grafts can be used to increase the width of attached tissue around the natural dentition and implants, obtain root or abutment coverage, and correct small-volume soft tissue ridge defects.

The advantages of using AlloDerm include the elimination of donor site surgery for greater patient comfort, unlimited tissue supply, excellent handling characteristics, and decreased surgical time. Disadvantages include greater secondary shrinkage and slower healing at the recipient sites when used as an onlay graft or when complete coverage of an interpositional AlloDerm graft is not obtainable.

The surgical technique for using AlloDerm is essentially the same as for a gingival graft. The AlloDerm graft must be rehydrated for 10 minutes before use. Two distinct sides of the AlloDerm graft are identified by applying the patient's blood to each surface and rinsing with sterile saline. The connective tissue side will retain the red coloration while the basement membrane side will appear white in color. The connective tissue side contains pre-existing vascular channels that allow for cellular infiltration and revascularization. When used as an onlay graft to increase the width of attached tissues, the connective tissue side should be oriented toward and intimately adapted to the recipient site. The basement membrane side of the AlloDerm graft facilitates epithelial cell migration and attachment. When used for root or abutment coverage, the basement membrane side of the graft should be oriented toward the exposed root or abutment. Wherever possible, the author recommends preparing a larger recipient site (6 to 8 mm apicocoronal dimension) and immobilizing a larger AlloDerm graft compared to what is used when an autogenous gingival graft is performed. This will offset the additional shrinkage observed with AlloDerm onlay grafts (Fig 5-18).

In addition, the author has observed improvement in the rate of incorporation of AlloDerm onlay grafts when combined with platelet-rich plasma (PRP). In those instances, the AlloDerm graft is first soaked in nonactivated PRP solution prior to immobilization at the recipient site. Subsequently, activated PRP is used topically over the graft as a growth factor–enriched wound dressing (Fig 5-19).

AlloDerm used as an onlay graft at second-stage surgery to increase the width of attached tissue and establish adequate vestibular depth in the severely atrophic edentulous mandible

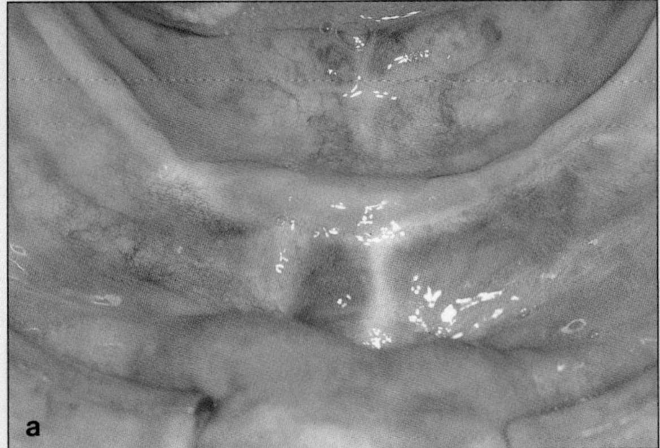

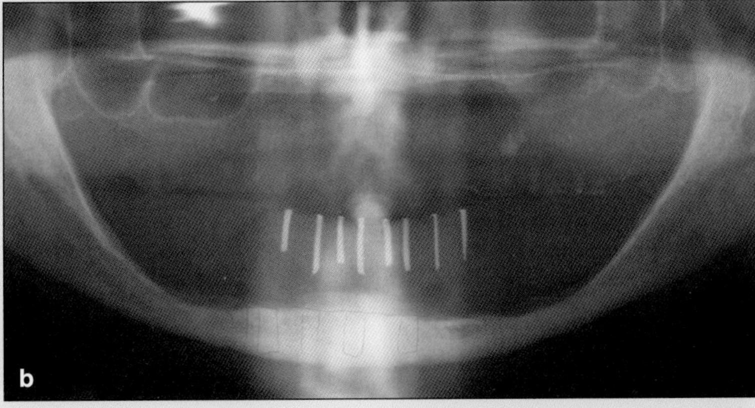

Figs 5-18a and 5-18b Preoperative and radiographic views of severely atrophic mandible prior to first-stage surgery. Note the thin band of attached tissue on the ridge, the high muscular attachments, and the inadequate vestibular depth. The surgical guide (denture duplicated in clear acrylic) was used to determine that the attached tissue was located lingual to the planned implant position.

Fig 5-18c Three months after placement of five submerged implants (Nobel Biocare), AlloDerm was used as an onlay graft. A horizontal incision located at the mucogingival junction and split-thickness recipient-site preparation initiates the second-stage surgery. Distal releasing incisions were not used to avoid damage to the mental nerve, and the resultant flaps were retained for subsequent apical repositioning.

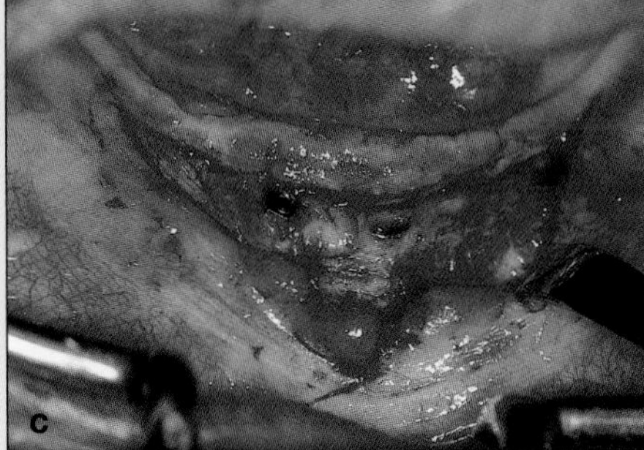

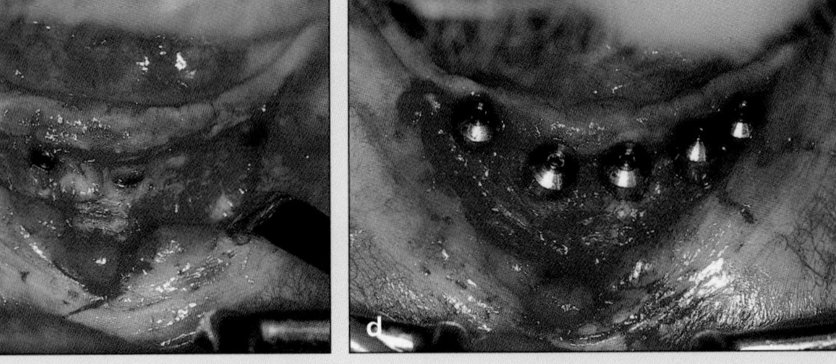

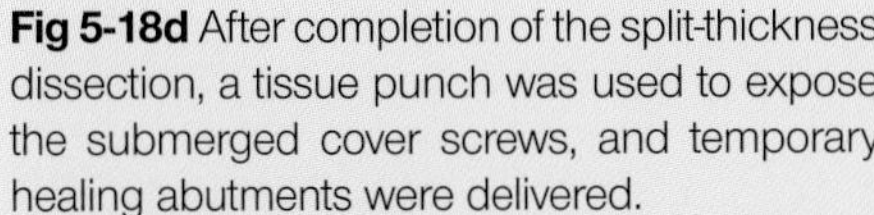

Fig 5-18d After completion of the split-thickness dissection, a tissue punch was used to expose the submerged cover screws, and temporary healing abutments were delivered.

Figs 5-18e and 5-18f After rehydration of the AlloDerm graft in sterile saline, blood from the surgical site is applied to both surfaces of the graft. The blood readily absorbs to the connective tissue surface, which retains a red color, but washes off the epithelial surface.

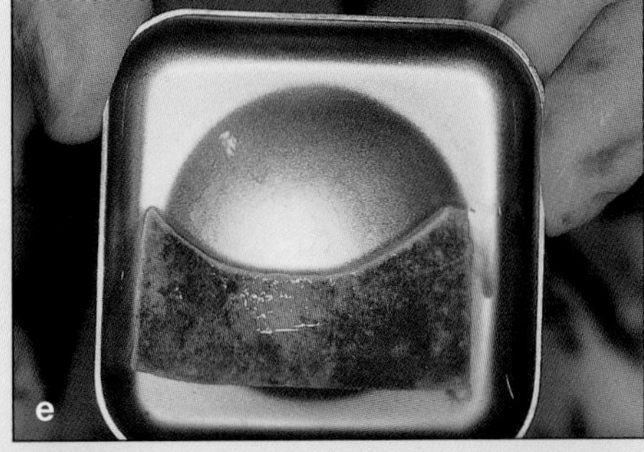

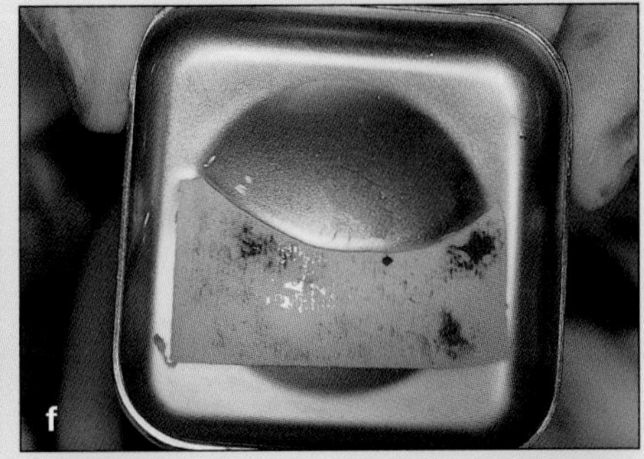

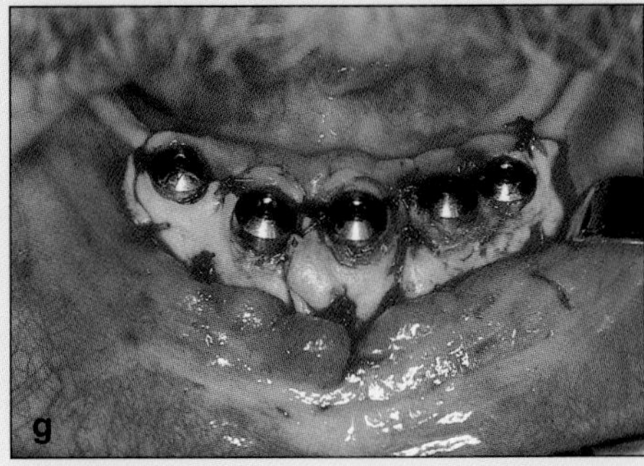

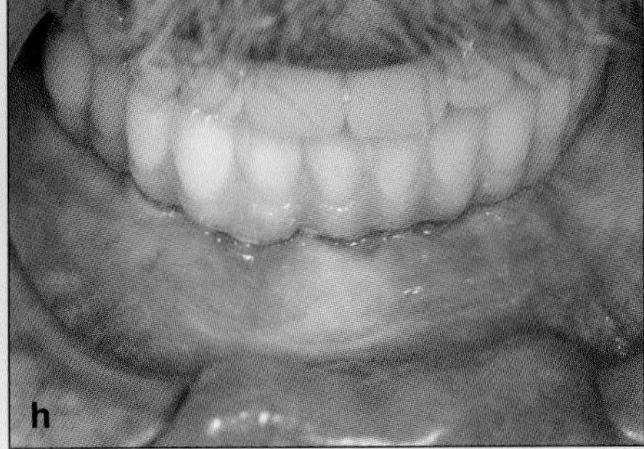

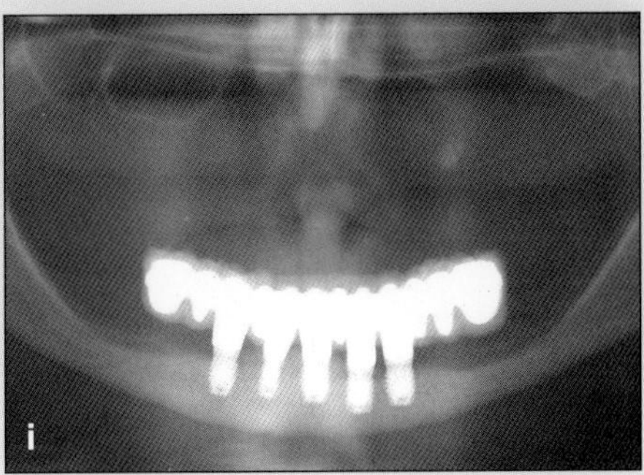

Fig 5-18g After apical repositioning and immobilization of the mucosal flaps to periosteum at the base of the recipient site, the AlloDerm graft was oriented with the connective tissue surface toward the recipient site and immobilized in the standard fashion by securing it first to the attached lingual tissues and then peripherally to periosteum with 4-0 chromic gut sutures.

Fig 5-18h Six months after delivery of the final restoration, it is clear that despite secondary contraction of the graft, a significant gain in vestibular depth was achieved, aberrant muscle attachments have been managed, and the buccal alveolar tissues are bound tightly around the emerging implant abutments. Oral hygiene has been facilitated and peri-implant soft tissue health is excellent.

Fig 5-18i Panoramic radiograph taken 6 months after delivery of the final restoration demonstrates stable osseous levels around all of the implants. Appropriate soft tissue management and use of AlloDerm as an onlay graft has enhanced the outcome of implant therapy in this challenging clinical situation. (Restoration by Dr Juan Diego Cardenas, Miami, FL.)

AlloDerm used as an onlay graft simultaneous with nonsubmerged implant placement in the edentulous mandible

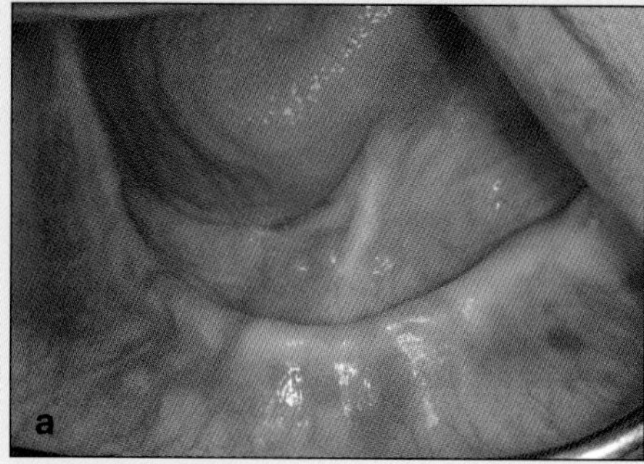

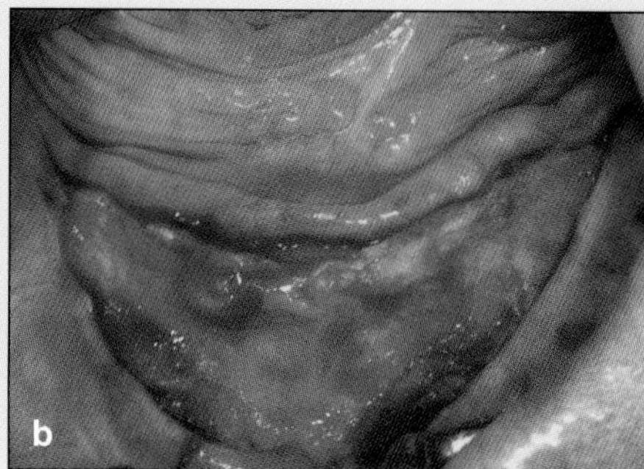

Fig 5-19a Presurgical view of edentulous mandible with a thin band of attached tissue, inadequate vestibular depth, and high muscle attachments.

Fig 5-19b A full-thickness horizontal incision made at the mucogingival junction initiated the procedure and provided access for nonsubmerged implant placement after subperiosteal reflection of the attached tissues to expose the ridge crest. Sharp dissection was used to create a uniform periosteal recipient site on the buccal aspect of the ridge. The resultant flaps were excised.

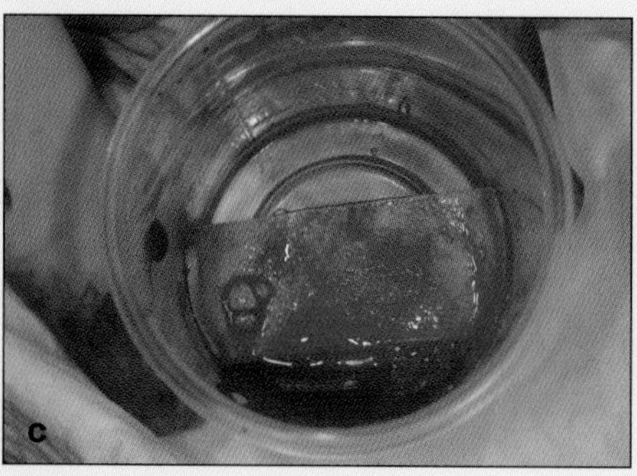

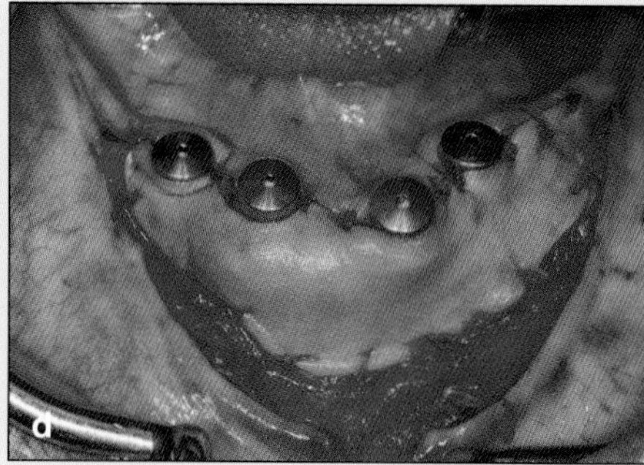

Fig 5-19c After initial rehydration in sterile saline, the AlloDerm graft was soaked in nonactivated (anticoagulated) PRP solution prior to being secured at the site.

Fig 5-19d After placement of four nonsubmerged TG implants (3i), the AlloDerm graft was placed with the connective tissue surface toward the periosteal recipient site and secured in the standard fashion with 4-0 chromic gut suture. Activated PRP solution should not be interposed between the graft and the recipient site because this would violate the principles of oral soft tissue grafting.

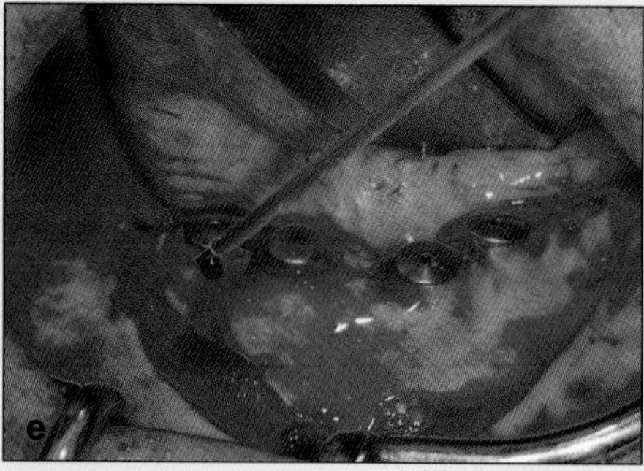

Fig 5-19e After applying pressure over the AlloDerm graft with moistened saline gauze for 10 minutes, activated PRP solution is placed over the surface of the surgical site and allowed to clot.

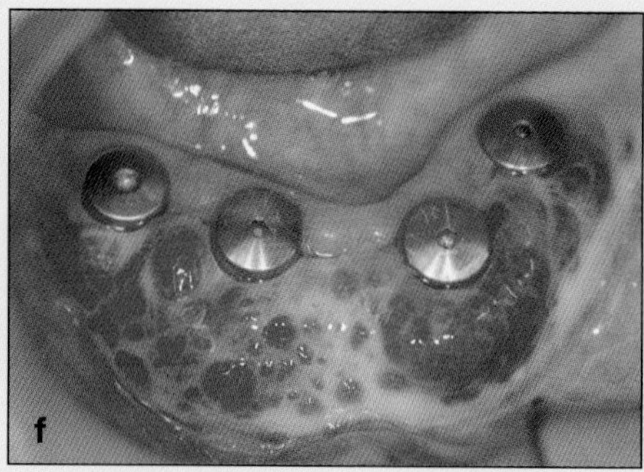

Fig 5-19f One-week postsurgical view. Rapid incorporation of the graft is evidenced by exhuberant replacement of the acellular dermal matrix with granulation tissue.

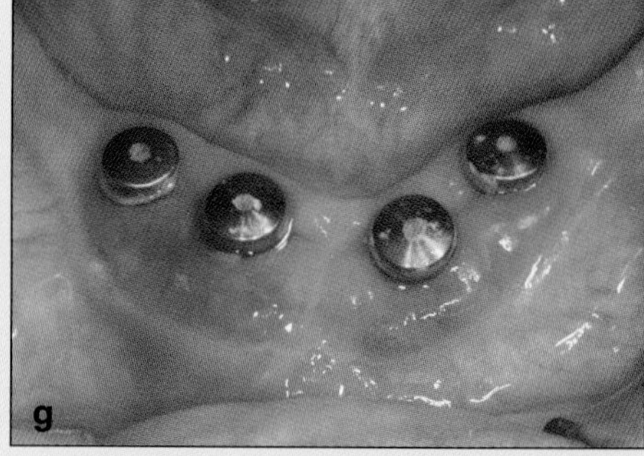

Fig 5-19g Two-week postsurgical view. The area where the AlloDerm graft was rapidly incorporated is easily discernable. Advanced rate of healing attributed to rigid immobilization of the graft to an oversized recipient site as well as the use of PRP.

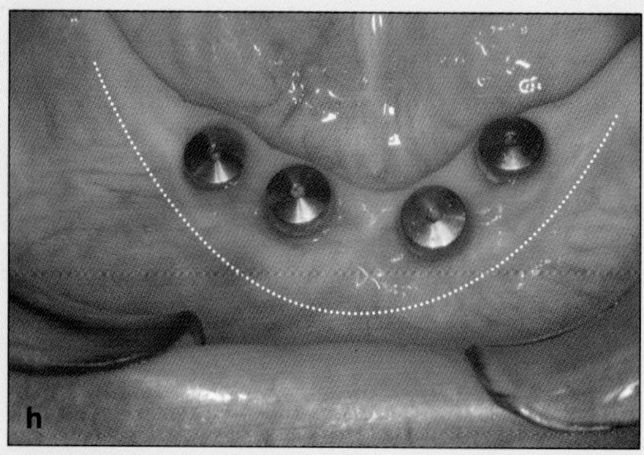

Fig 5-19h Eight-week postoperative view. The implants are integrated and the soft tissues are stable. Although secondary contraction of the AlloDerm grafted areas has occurred, a significant gain in vestibular depth and width of attached nonmobile tissues is evident on the buccal aspect of the nonsubmerged implants *(line)*. In addition, aberrant muscle attachments have been totally eliminated.

Subepithelial Connective Tissue Graft Technique for Dental Implants

In 1982, Langer and Calagna[15] introduced the subepithelial connective tissue graft as a new approach to anterior cosmetic enhancement. These authors described a technique for harvesting a subepithelial connective tissue graft from the palate and using it for localized ridge augmentation. They also discussed using the graft to obtain root coverage and correction of uneven gingival margins. The objective of using the connective tissue graft was to establish an esthetic gingival appearance that would allow prosthetic restoration of edentulous sites with fixed restorations of harmonious proportions.

The subepithelial connective tissue graft is an extremely versatile procedure to enhance soft tissue contours around the natural dentition and dental implants. The procedure combines the use of a free soft tissue autograft harvested from the palate that is interposed beneath a partial-thickness pedicle flap at the recipient site (ie, open approach). Alternatively, the graft can be secured in a split-thickness pouch prepared at the recipient site (ie, closed approach). An understanding of the anatomy of the palatal donor site allows the surgeon to predictably harvest the desired amount of connective tissue needed for soft tissue reconstruction without damaging adjacent neurovascular structures.

The graft is harvested internally from the palate, resulting in a partial-thickness donor site pouch, which allows for primary closure and thus a more comfortable palatal wound. Because the graft is positioned between the periosteum and a partial-thickness cover flap or pouch at the recipient site, it gains the advantage of a dual blood supply to support graft revascularization. As a result of the abundant blood supply available for healing, the connective tissue graft is less technique sensitive, easier to perform, and more predictable than the gingival graft. The connective tissue graft also results in superior color matching and esthetic blending at the recipient site.

Advantages of subepithelial connective tissue grafts

- Dual blood supply at recipient site
- Less invasive donor site wound
- Superior color matching
- Technically less demanding
- Not dependent on a smooth palatal surface for success
- Tremendously versatile

General considerations

Subepithelial connective tissue grafting is a versatile procedure. Because it yields exceptional color matching at the recipient site, it should be considered whenever soft tissue augmentation is required in an area of esthetic concern. The subepithelial connective tissue graft (ie, connective tissue graft) provides predictable soft tissue coverage of exposed root or abutment surfaces, and it can mask the gray metallic color that can penetrate the thin soft tissues surrounding an implant restoration. The graft can also be used to create the illusion of a root eminence and to enhance the esthetic results of either conventional or implant restorations by improving soft tissue contours. In addition to these esthetic enhancements, the connective tissue graft also improves the health of the peri-implant soft tissues by providing a zone of attached nonmobile soft tissue around permucosal implant structures.

Although the volume yield of a subepithelial connective tissue graft is dependent on the quality and quantity of the donor site tissue, a single graft usually is sufficient for reconstruction of small-volume soft tissue defects. Multiple grafts performed in a staged fashion are often necessary to reconstruct significant vertical soft tissue ridge deficiencies (large-volume soft tissue defects).

The initial harvest of a subepithelial connective tissue graft sometimes yields more fatty tissue than good-quality connective tissue, resulting in only partial reconstruction of deficient soft tissues at the recipient site. Because the quantity and quality of available tissues at individual donor sites varies, patients should be informed that a second graft might be needed if poor quality or inadequate volume of connective tissue is encountered at the initial harvest. In the author's experience, approximately 3 months of healing should be allowed prior to repeating the grafting. Harvesting a second connective tissue graft from the same donor site usually yields a tremendous increase (3 to 5 times) in good-quality connective tissue. This observation (the second-harvest effect) is not unexpected, as healing of the donor site is characterized by scar tissue formation. Use of an absorbable collagen material (CollaPlug; Centerpulse Dental) known to promote quick connective tissue ingrowth may contribute to the improvement in donor site tissue observed upon re-entry for a second harvest.

Subepithelial connective tissue grafting over a submerged implant

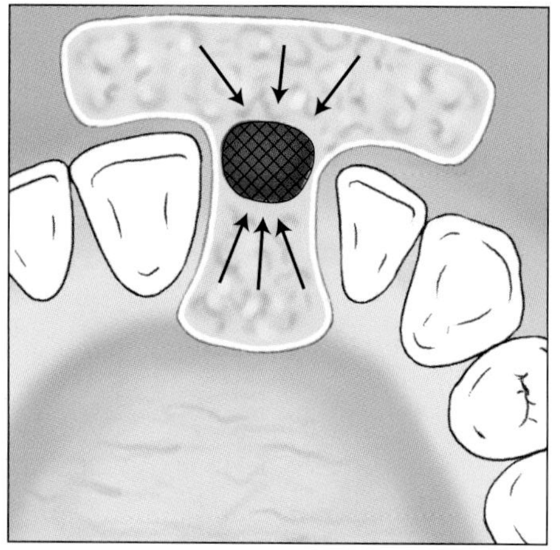

Fig 5-20a When a subepithelial connective tissue graft is performed prior to or synchronous with a submerged implant, the recipient site can be extended to the buccal and palatal aspects of the alveolar ridge to take advantage of peripheral circulation, thereby decreasing secondary contraction of the graft in the area critical for prosthetic emergence *(arrows)*. This is preferred whenever large-volume soft tissue defects will be reconstructed in stages prior to implant emergence.

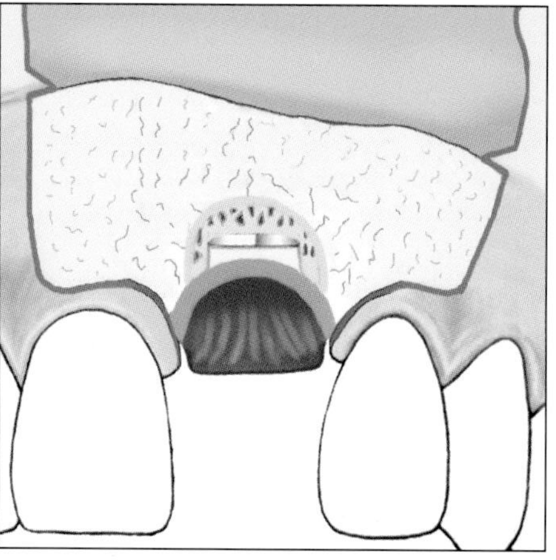

Fig 5-20b Modified dissection for simultaneous subepithelial connective tissue grafting with submerged implant placement. Note that full-thickness dissection is performed only in the area of osteotomy preparation, while partial-thickness (supraperiosteal) dissection is extended on the buccal and palatal aspects of the alveolar ridge and over the adjacent interdental bone.

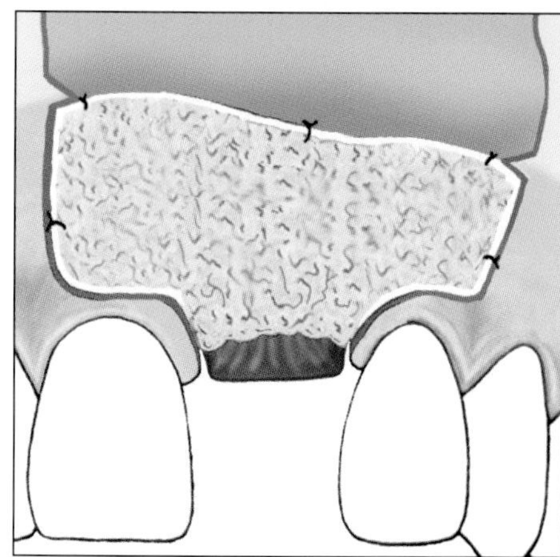

Fig 5-20c The subepithelial connective tissue graft is draped over the alveolar ridge and secured to the buccal and palatal aspects of the recipient site with 4-0 chromic gut suture. This technique is the same whether performed prior to implant placement, simultaneous with implant placement, or during the osseointegration period.

Indications and sequencing in implant therapy

The subepithelial connective tissue graft can be used to reconstruct missing soft tissue volume prior to implant placement, at the time of implant placement, during the osseointegration period, at abutment connection, and at any time during the recall period. When a small-volume defect in soft tissue contour is identified at an implant site, the author finds it most practical to perform subepithelial connective tissue grafting at the time of submerged implant placement or prior to nonsubmerged implant placement. Grafting prior to abutment connection or placement of a nonsubmerged implant facilitates reconstruction of missing soft tissue volume in the area critical for esthetic restorative emergence, because a large recipient site can be developed to include periosteal blood supply on both the buccal and palatal aspects of the alveolar ridge. This recipient-site design is ideal to support graft vascularization in the area critical for eventual prosthetic emergence (Fig 5-20).

Once an abutment is connected to a submerged implant or when a nonsubmerged implant is placed, the recipient bed can be developed only on the buccal aspect of the emerging implant, thus limiting the peripheral blood supply available to sustain the graft in the area critical for prosthetic emergence. Soft tissue contours certainly can be improved after the implant has emerged, but reconstruction of deficient contours in the area critical for esthetic restorative emergence may not be as predictable. Therefore, the author prefers to use a coronally advanced flap augmented by connective tissue when grafting at the same time as abutment connection or nonsubmerged implant placement (Fig 5-21). These situations necessitate adequate vestibular depth to allow the design of a flap of adequate elasticity to enable coronal positioning over the graft without a reduction of circulation to the margin of the flap. The use of an exaggerated curvilinear-beveled flap design, as described in chapter 3, facilitates passive coronal advancement in these situations. Preoperative evaluation of vestibular depth at the site will help the surgeon plan the most appropriate time to correct small-volume soft tissue contour defects.

When a large-volume defect in soft tissue contour is identified at an implant site, a staged approach using multiple subepithelial connective tissue grafts is recommended. When esthetic results are a concern, it is important to emphasize that the majority of the missing soft tissue volume should be reconstructed prior to implant emergence. After abutment connection or nonsubmerged implant placement, additional

Subepithelial connective tissue grafting technique at abutment connection or simultaneous with nonsubmerged implant placement

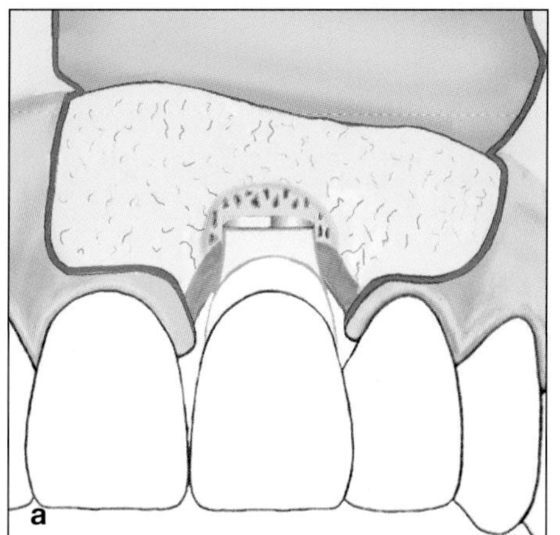

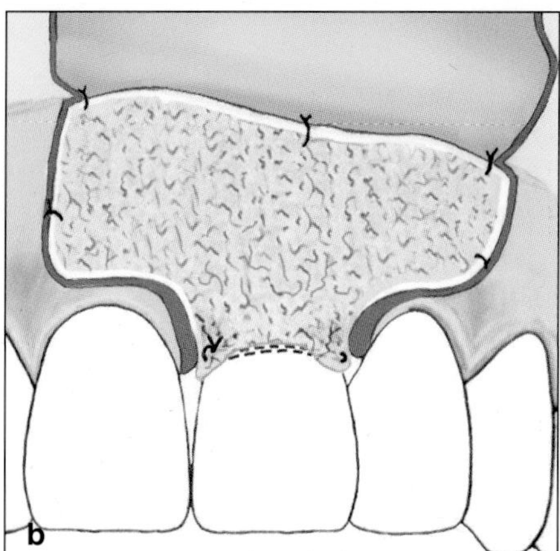

Fig 5-21a Recipient-site preparation for performing a subepithelial connective tissue graft in conjunction with implant exposure and delivery of custom abutment and provisional restoration. Partial-thickness incisions were used to outline a curvilinear-beveled flap. A uniform periosteal recipient site has been prepared on the facial aspect of the ridge.

Fig 5-21b Prior to graft immobilization, the adjacent attached tissues, including the papillary areas, have been de-epithelialized, thus facilitating immobilization of the graft around the periphery of the recipient site. A sling suture around the cervical aspect of the abutment improves graft immobilization.

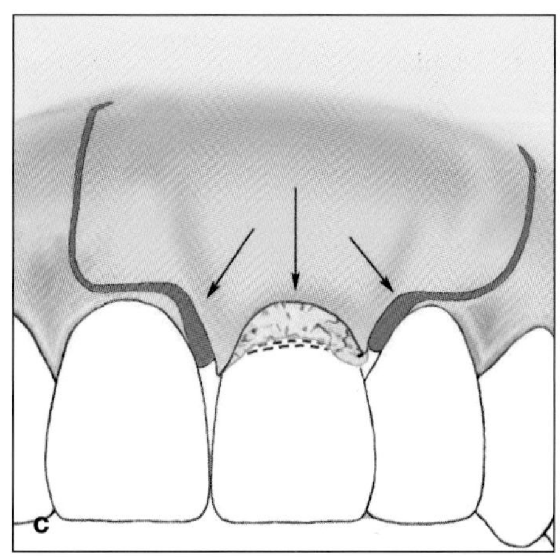

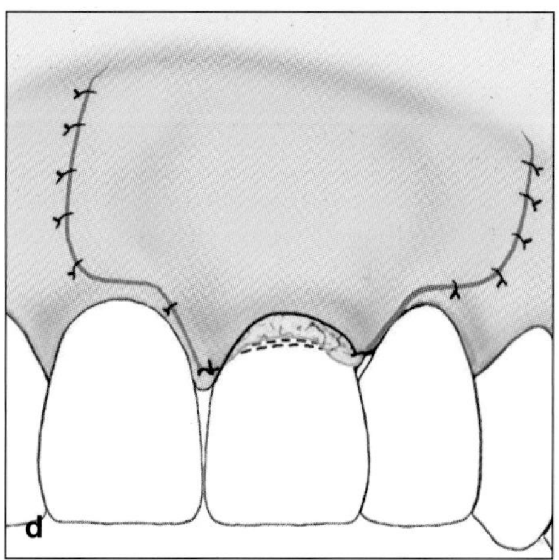

Fig 5-21c The cover flap is coronally advanced as it is coapted laterally to the extended wound margins created by the beveled incisions and de-epithelialized areas.

Fig 5-21d Sutures are placed in each papillary area or, alternatively, a single sling suture can be used to maintain desired coronal advancement of the cover flap prior to closing laterally. The sutures used to close the releasing incisions are then oriented to maintain coronal advancement.

subepithelial connective tissue grafts are reserved for the correction of residual small-volume soft tissue defects and fine-tuning of the soft tissue architecture around provisional restorations.

When a hard tissue defect is identified at an implant site, the surgeon must determine whether the quality of the soft tissue cover at the site is adequate to support the required hard tissue reconstruction. When preoperative evaluation reveals significant scarring from previous trauma, pathology, or multiple surgical procedures, the use of subepithelial connective tissue can improve the quality and quantity of the soft tissues prior to bone grafting. After a 3-month healing period, the hard tissue site development can be performed.

When a soft tissue defect develops shortly after implant placement or persists despite soft tissue grafting at the time of implant placement, subepithelial connective tissue grafting can be performed to reconstruct the defect during the osseointegration period. The surgeon should wait 8 to 12 weeks for initial osseointegration and soft tissue maturation before further soft tissue grafting. If a submerged implant was placed, the surgeon may have to decide whether to graft over the implant and delay abutment connection or perform the graft at the same time as abutment connection. In these situations, the author prefers to take advantage of the greater predictability of grafting over the implant and subsequently exposing the implant with a tissue punch or palatal peninsula flap, as described in chapter 3. Similarly, when soft tissue recession occurs after abutment connection or delivery of an implant-supported provisional restoration in an esthetic area, the surgeon must decide whether to resubmerge and graft over the implant or limit the recipient site to the buccal aspect of the ridge. This decision is primarily based on the available vestibular depth at the site, since predictable outcomes require coronal advancement of the cover flap.

Table 5-2 Recipient-site considerations

Open recipient site	Closed recipient site
• Easier to perform • Allows for direct visualization of dissection for uniform recipient site • Facilitates coronal advancement of cover flap • Use of releasing incisions sacrifices circulation • May require secondary gingivoplasty	• More difficult to prepare ("blind" technique) • Immobilization of graft is more technique sensitive • Limits coronal advancement • Contraindicated when vestibular depth is minimal • Preserves circulation to area • Allows for superior esthetics

Finally, connective tissue grafting can also be performed after prosthetic rehabilitation to treat soft tissue recession defects noted during the recall period. The cause of the recession should be determined and addressed. If overcontouring of the existing restoration is determined to be a contributing factor, the buccal contour should be reduced prior to grafting similar to the way in which prominent roots are mechanically reduced in preparation for root-coverage procedures. If implant malposition precludes coverage of an exposed abutment, a subepithelial graft can increase the width of attached tissue and thus prevent further recession.

Recipient-site considerations

As in gingival grafting, the subepithelial connective tissue graft procedure begins with preparation of the recipient site to minimize the time between graft harvest and transfer to the recipient bed. Beginning with this step also helps the surgeon to determine the precise dimensions of donor tissue needed for reconstruction and allows adequate time for hemostasis to be obtained at the recipient site.

The preparation of the recipient site involves either the elevation of a split-thickness flap through supraperiosteal dissection (open technique) or a supraperiosteal dissection, which avoids vertical releasing incisions to create an envelope or pouch (closed technique). The decision to use the open or closed technique at the recipient site when grafting around a natural tooth or an implant restoration depends on several factors (Table 5-2). The open technique for recipient-site preparation allows direct visualization during dissection, which ensures the preparation of a uniform recipient site. It also allows for significant coronal advancement when vertical soft tissue augmentation is needed over an exposed root or abutment surface. It is important to note that the vertical releasing incisions used in the open technique sacrifice some circulation to the flap and increase the need for secondary gingivoplasty. Although the use of a trapezoidal flap design has been advocated by some, the curvilinear-beveled flap design described in chapter 3 preserves circulation to the area, allows for significantly greater coronal flap advancement, and minimizes the need for secondary gingivoplasty. The incorporation of exaggerated curvilinear-beveled incisions effectively increases the size of the recipient site, thus increasing the peripheral blood supply available to sustain the graft. Passive coronal advancement of the cover flap and accommodation for buccal augmentation are achieved by extending the incisions well beyond the mucogingival junction and using apical cutback incisions rather than periosteal releasing incisions (see Figs 5-20 and 5-21). These modifications greatly reduce tension on the flap and minimize circulatory embarrassment to the flap margin, making this design especially useful for hard and soft tissue site development. In general, the author prefers the open technique for recipient-site preparation when the apicocoronal dimension of a recession defect exceeds 4 mm and the vascularity at the site will support a split-thickness dissection without significant risk of cover flap sloughing.

The closed technique avoids vertical incisions, thus preserving blood supply to the site and optimizing esthetic results. While the closed technique has advantages, it can be technically more demanding because it is a "blind" technique. Also, the closed technique does not allow for significant coronal advancement of the cover flap, possibly limiting vertical soft tissue augmentation. The closed technique is contraindicated whenever vestibular depth limits the preparation of an adequately sized recipient site. In general, the author prefers to use the closed technique when abutment or root exposure is less than 4 mm apicocoronally or when there is significant risk of sloughing of the cover flap because of poor vascularity at the site.

Recipient-site surgery

Closed approach

The technique for closed recipient-site preparation is identical whether performed around a natural tooth or an implant restoration. A horizontal incision is ex-

Subepithelial connective tissue grafting at a closed recipient site

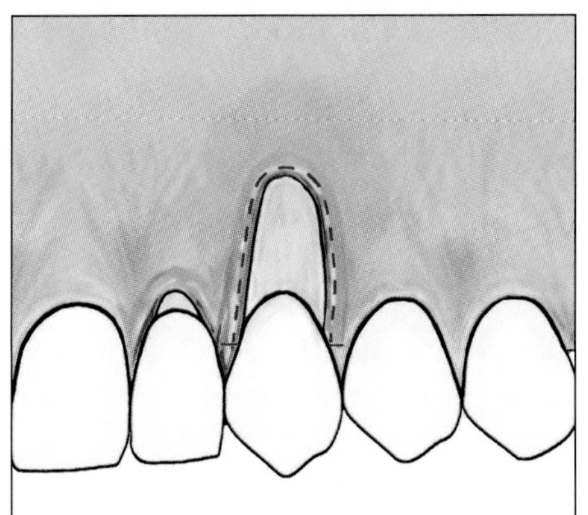

Fig 5-22a Gingival recession involving the maxillary canine and lateral incisor to be reconstructed in a staged approach. A partial-thickness horizontal incision is first extended mesial and distal to the recession defect just coronal to the level of root coverage desired. The scalpel is then oriented parallel to the tissue surface, and partial-thickness dissection is carefully performed, moving from each horizontal incision toward the center of the recession defect.

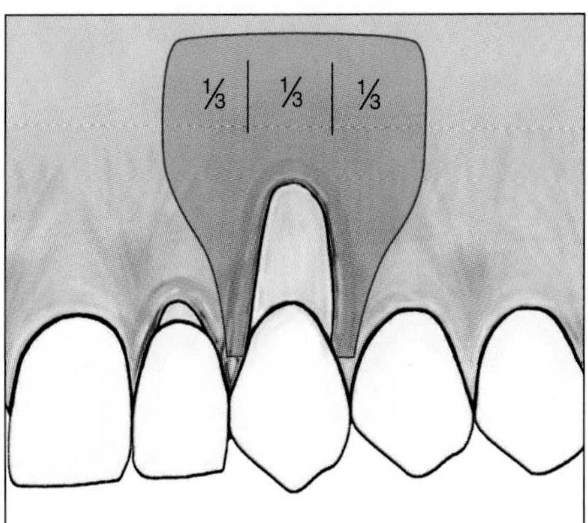

Fig 5-22b Outline of typical area for supraperiosteal dissection performed to develop an adequate closed recipient site for obtaining root coverage with a subepithelial connective tissue graft. As a general rule, the recipient site should be extended a sufficient distance mesial and distal so that the width of the recipient site is three times the width of the denuded root surface. This ensures enough peripheral circulation laterally to sustain the graft via the bridging phenomenon.

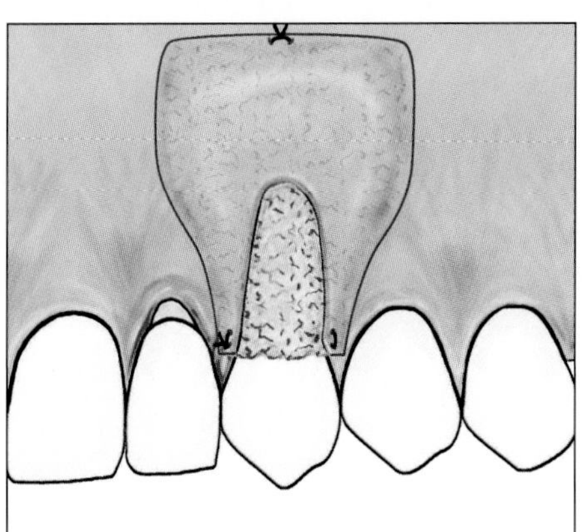

Fig 5-22c Passive seating and subsequent immobilization is accomplished by gently tugging on a horizontal mattress suture that is initiated from the depth of the vestibule, passes twice through the graft, and finally exits back into the vestibule several millimeters away from its entrance. A membrane placement instrument is used to help slide the graft slide into position. The suture is then secured to prevent coronal displacement of the graft. Next, a sling suture is passed around the cervical aspect of the tooth to immobilize the coronal aspect of the graft and the cover tissue is secured with interrupted sutures.

tended to the mesial and distal of the soft tissue defect just coronal to the level of root or abutment coverage desired (Fig 5-22a). Using a no. 15C scalpel, the surgeon makes this incision at a right angle to the epithelium at a depth of approximately 1 mm. The horizontal incisions not only mark the graft's final coronal position but also facilitate the pouch dissection and subsequent immobilization of the graft.

Next, the scalpel is oriented parallel to the tissue surface and the horizontal incisions are extended into the sulcus to create the entrance to the recipient site (Fig 5-22b). The split-thickness dissection is extended apically beyond the mucogingival junction at the mesial and distal aspect of the site before crossing the midline. To ensure that the recipient site can contribute adequate peripheral blood supply to sustain the graft, it is also important to extend the dissection well beyond the width of the soft tissue defect being corrected. As a general rule, the width of the recipient site should be three times that of the exposed root or abutment. This is accomplished by extending the defect to the mesial and distal (Fig 5-22b). The surgeon must take care to avoid perforating or tearing the overlying tissues with the scalpel; a meticulous technique is required to ensure a uniform recipient-site surface.

The blunt end of a membrane-placement instrument is then used to probe the resultant pouch and confirm that the dissection is complete. Occasionally, strands or webs of tissue extending from the overlying tissues to the periosteum will be detected in the apical extent of the dissection. If not released with sharp dissection, these tissue strands will prevent proper positioning and passive adaptation of the connective tissue graft within the pouch. A periodontal probe is then used to measure the dimensions of the recipient pouch and to guide the surgeon in the donor harvest, and pressure is applied with moistened saline gauze to obtain hemostasis.

Graft immobilization

When a closed recipient site is used, the dimensions of the donor connective tissue should closely match those of the recipient-site pouch. Curved Iris tissue scissors are used to size the graft prior to securing it in the pouch. The graft should always be oriented so that the periosteal side faces down at the recipient site.

A 4-0 chromic suture on a P3 or FS2 needle is used to place a horizontal mattress suture that enters the apical portion of the recipient pouch, engages the graft, and exits the pouch apically. This suture is used to gently "pull" the graft into the recipient pouch and secure the graft apically, thereby resisting subsequent coronal displacement.

First, the suture needle is passed through the vestibular mucosa into the recipient pouch and retrieved with forceps. The suture needle is then passed through the connective tissue side of the graft and back through the periosteal side of the graft. Next, the membrane-placement instrument is used to identify the apical extent of the recipient site, and the suture needle is passed back through the mucosal tissue to exit the pouch several millimeters laterally from where it entered. A fine hemostat is clamped across equal lengths of the suture material (approximately 3 inches), and suture scissors are used to cut away the remaining suture and needle.

The surgeon then uses the clamped suture material to slowly pull the graft into the recipient pouch, taking care not to tear the overlying tissue. The paddle end of the membrane-placement instrument is used like a shoehorn to guide the graft into the entrance of the recipient pouch. The flat portion of the instrument is moistened with saline and placed between the graft and the overlying tissue as the graft is gently pulled into the pouch. This technique prevents bunching of the graft at the entrance of the recipient pouch as well as excessive stretching of, and damage to, the overlying tissues. The spiked end of the membrane-placement instrument is then used to gently "push" the graft further into the pouch entrance while the clamped suture material is used to "pull" the graft apically. A triple tie secures the graft in the pouch. The graft is then secured coronally with interrupted sutures that pass through the graft and interproximal tissues (Fig 5-22c).

For close adaptation of the graft around an exposed root surface or implant restoration, the author uses a sling suture that passes around the tooth or implant restoration. This suture is passed through the coronal aspect of the graft and interproximal tissue on one side of the tooth or implant restoration, brought around the oral aspect of the tooth, passed back through the interproximal tissue and graft from the oral side, and then returned to its point of origin by passing it back through underneath the contact points, where it is secured with a triple tie.

After the graft is secured at the recipient site, the cover flap may be secured by interrupted sutures in the papillary area. These sutures are placed in the area of the horizontal incisions and passed through the papillary tissues without engaging the graft. Additionally, sutures can be placed to approximate the coronal margins of the pouch in an effort to cover more of the exposed graft. Because significant coronal advancement of the overlying tissues is not possible when a closed approach is used, a portion of the graft will remain uncovered. Whenever possible, it is recommended that two thirds or more of the graft be secured within the recipient site pouch. Gentle pressure is then applied over the graft site for a minimum of 10 minutes with moistened saline gauze.

Open approach

In the open approach to recipient-site preparation, the surgeon begins dissection by outlining the recipient site with partial-thickness horizontal and vertical incisions using a no. 15C scalpel blade on a round handle. The horizontal incision, which is performed first, extends mesial and distal to the soft tissue defect at a level just coronal to the final soft tissue position desired after augmentation. Exaggerated curvilinear-beveled incisions with tension-releasing cutback incisions, as described in chapter 3, are then initiated apically well beyond the mucogingival junction to outline the cover flap (Fig 5-23a). Next, sharp dissection is used to elevate a split-thickness flap. The dissection is initiated coronally with a no. 15C scalpel blade. Flap elevation is continued apically under direct vision with sharp dissection under tension, which the surgeon carefully maintains using micro-Adson tissue forceps. The goal is to maximize the thickness of the overlying tissue flap, leaving only a thin layer of immobile periosteum. When coronal advancement of the cover flap will be performed, the adjacent papillary areas are de-epithelialized with a fresh no. 15C scalpel. This further extends the wound margin, thereby reducing flap retraction and greatly enhancing incision line esthetics, and eliminates the possibility that the undersurface of the coronally advanced flap is coapted over an epithelial surface, thereby preventing initial wound healing and subsequently contributing to wound dehiscence in that area (Fig 5-23b). The dimensions of the recipient site are then measured with a periodontal probe, and hemostasis is obtained by applying gentle pressure with moistened saline gauze.

Graft immobilization

When an open recipient site is used, the dimensions of the donor connective tissue should closely match those of the recipient site. However, it is helpful if the donor tissue is trimmed to be slightly smaller than the open recipient site. This facilitates immobilization of the graft to the recipient site and suturing of the cover flap into position without unwanted engagement of the underlying graft, which can cause graft dislodgment secondary to swelling or retraction of the cover flap. Curved Iris tissue scissors are used to size the graft and remove any epithelial tissue that will be covered by coronal advancement of the cover flap.

When a graft will be placed around natural dentition or implant restoration(s), it is first adapted and secured coronally with sutures passed through the papillary area using a 4-0 chromic gut suture on a P3 needle (see Fig 5-21b). The first suture is passed through the graft and the mesial papillary tissue. The graft then is slightly stretched as sutures are placed in each successive papillary area, moving in a distal direction. Alternatively,

Subepithelial connective tissue grafting at an open recipient site

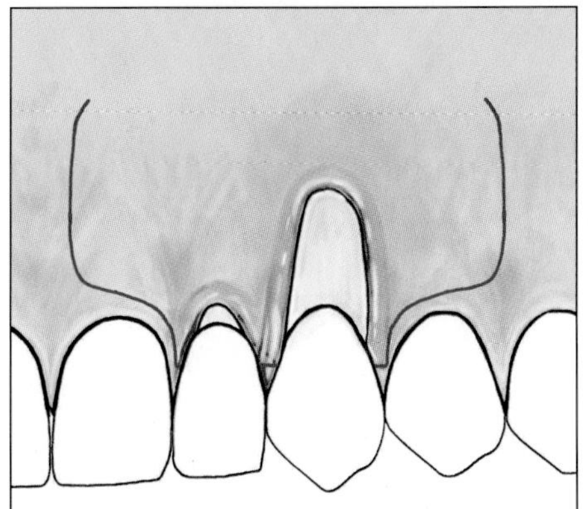

Fig 5-23a Typical outline for an open recipient site defined by partial-thickness curvilinear-beveled incisions and tension-releasing cutback incisions. This flap design facilitates coronal flap advancement and accommodation over a subepithelial connective tissue graft, improving the ability to gain vertical soft tissue reconstruction over denuded root or implant abutment surfaces.

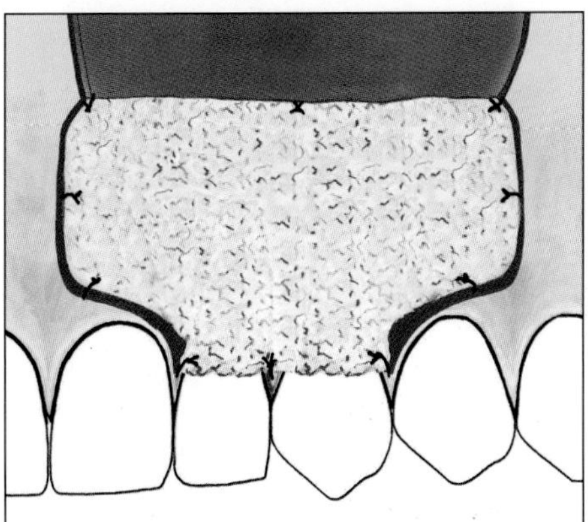

Fig 5-23b Prior to graft immobilization, the adjacent papillary areas are de-epithelialized with sharp dissection to create an exaggerated beveled wound margin. This facilitates securing of the subepithelial connective tissue graft to periosteum without distorting the tissues at the periphery of the site and subsequent closure of the cover flap without inadvertently engaging the immobilized graft. The graft is first secured coronally with interrupted sutures passing through the graft and each papillary area. Alternatively, sling sutures can be used for this purpose.

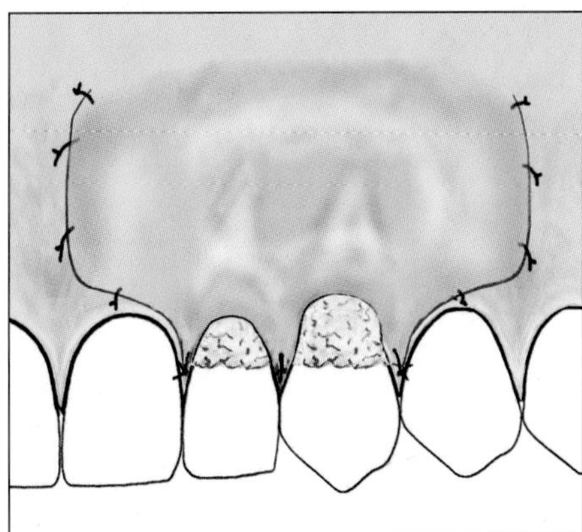

Fig 5-23c Passive flap coaptation is verified prior to closure of the cover flap. When adequate vestibular depth exists, the tension-releasing cutback incisions ensure passive coronal advancement of the flap. The cover flap is first secured with sling sutures that pass around the cervical aspects of the teeth. Subsequently, lateral wound margins are aligned and secured with sutures oriented to resist apical migration or displacement of the flap.

sling sutures can be used for this purpose. Next, the graft is secured laterally and apically to periosteum with additional sutures. Two passes—first through the graft, and second through the periosteum—are often needed to avoid tearing the underlying periosteum. The graft is stretched in a mesiodistal direction to improve its adaptation to the recipient site. Overstretching of the graft in an apical direction, however, could compromise the amount of coronal soft tissue augmentation achieved and thus should be avoided. The exaggerated curvilinear-beveled incision design not only extends the recipient site, providing additional circulation to sustain the graft, but also facilitates immobilization of the graft.

Next, the cover flap is secured coronally with interrupted sutures passing through the papillae. These sutures should pass through the facial flap, through the de-epithelialized papillary tissue, and return under the contact points, where they are tied facially (Fig 5-23c). Alternatively, a sling suture can also be used. In this case, the suture passes through the flap and the papillary tissue on the first pass; it then passes under the contact points as it returns to the facial aspect, where it is tied. Depending on the thickness of the cover flap tissue, 4-0 or 5-0 chromic gut suture on a P3 needle is used. Next, the cover flap is secured laterally. The curvilinear-beveled flap design facilitates alignment of the wound margins. The suture needle should be perpendicular to the beveled incision as it passes through the tissue. It also should be oriented in an apicocoronal direction as it is passed through the flap and adjacent tissue (see Fig 5-23c). A single pass is recommended to ensure precise positioning of the cover flap. The attached tissue contained in the flap is first precisely repositioned and secured with sutures placed laterally. The sutures then are placed apical to the mucogingival junction. Moistened saline gauze is used to apply gentle pressure at the site for 10 minutes; a periodontal dressing is not routinely used by the author.

Donor-site considerations

The dimensions of the connective tissue that can be safely harvested without damage to adjacent neurovascular structures depend on the size and shape of the patient's palate. The ideal location for harvesting connective tissue from the palate is in the premolar region, where the greatest tissue thickness is available for harvest without donor site morbidity. A graft with approximate dimensions of 14 mm in width and 12 mm in apicocoronal height can be safely harvested from the average palate. A graft of 14 mm in width and 17 mm in apicocoronal height can be obtained from a high-

Table 5-3 Dual- versus single-incision technique for harvesting subepithelial connective tissue

	Advantages	Disadvantages
Dual incision	• Easier to perform • Graft thickness defined by second incision	• Primary closure not always possible • Donor site pain more common • Dressing of donor site advisable
Single incision	• Allows for primary closure • Donor site pain uncommon • Dressing of donor rarely needed	• More technique sensitive • Uniform thickness not always obtained

arched palate. A shallow palate may limit the dimensions of safely available connective tissue to 14 mm in width and 7 mm in height and thus preclude the use of the graft to reconstruct some Miller class II or class III defects.[16]

Dual- and single-incision variations of the closed technique for harvesting connective tissue are commonly used (Table 5-3). Vertical incisions are avoided to preserve blood supply and minimize sloughing at the donor site. The dual-incision technique is easier to perform. Graft thickness is defined by the second partial-thickness incision, thereby ensuring a uniform thickness of donor tissue obtained. However, primary closure is not always possible, and donor site pain occurs with higher incidence when compared to the single-incision technique. Therefore, consideration should be given to the use of a protective palatal stent postoperatively. The single-incision technique is appropriate for the experienced surgeon. Primary closure is obtained and donor site pain is uncommon. Dressing of the donor site is rarely needed. However, this approach is more technique sensitive, and uniform graft thickness is more difficult to obtain.

The author prefers to harvest the underlying palatal periosteum with the connective tissue to improve the handling characteristics of the graft and to provide the periosteal vascular network for potential anastomotic connection during graft vascularization. The maxillary tuberosity is another potential donor site for subepithelial connective tissue grafts. Grafts procured from this area consist of very dense connective tissue, which provides the advantage of decreased tissue shrinkage after transfer but is more difficult to handle and secure at the recipient site.

Donor-site surgery

Dual-incision technique

Donor-site surgery begins with a full-thickness curvilinear incision made through the palatal tissues approximately 2 to 3 mm apical to the gingival margins of the premolars (Figs 5-24a and 5-24b). This incision can be made perpendicular to the surface of the palatal tissue, or it can be slightly beveled. When the first incision is made perpendicular to the palatal tissues, the thickness of the coronal portion of the graft is maximized; however, this usually eliminates the ability to obtain a passive primary closure. In contrast, beveling the first incision limits the thickness of the coronal portion of the graft but enables a passive primary closure in many cases. Next, a partial-thickness curvilinear incision is made approximately 2 mm apical to the first incision to complete an ellipse (Figs 5-24c and 5-24d). This incision defines the thickness of the subepithelial connective tissue graft to be harvested. The incision should be approximately 1 mm deep to ensure adequate thickness of the remaining cover tissue, thereby minimizing the incidence of sloughing at the donor site.

The scalpel then is oriented parallel to the surface of the palatal tissue, and sharp dissection is used to create a rectangular pouch (Figs 5-24e and 5-24f). The height of the palate determines the apical extent of the dissection. The mesiodistal extent of the dissection is determined by the length of the first and second incisions, which in turn are determined by the overall size of the palate and the width of the premolars. The scalpel blade is then used to complete the outline of the donor connective tissue graft with incisions that pass through the underlying connective tissue and periosteum just short of the mesial and distal extent of the pocket (Figs 5-24g and 5-24h). Doing so will avoid unnecessary trauma to the overlying palatal tissues when the scalpel is turned perpendicular to the surface of the donor tissue.

A Buser periosteal elevator and membrane-placement instrument are then used to carefully begin subperiosteal elevation of donor tissue at the coronal aspect of the dissection (Figs 5-24i and 5-24j). Once the coronal aspect of the graft has been elevated, it is carefully supported with tissue forceps, and the subperiosteal elevation is extended to the apical portion of the pouch. Next, gentle traction is placed on the elevated tissue with forceps, and a horizontal incision is

Subepithelial connective tissue grafting: Donor-site surgery, dual-incision technique

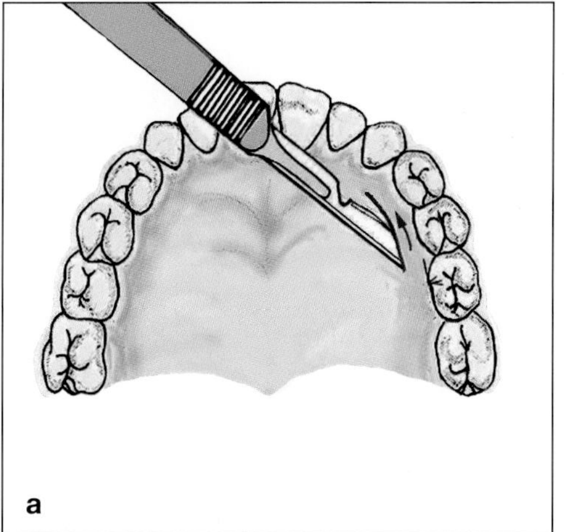

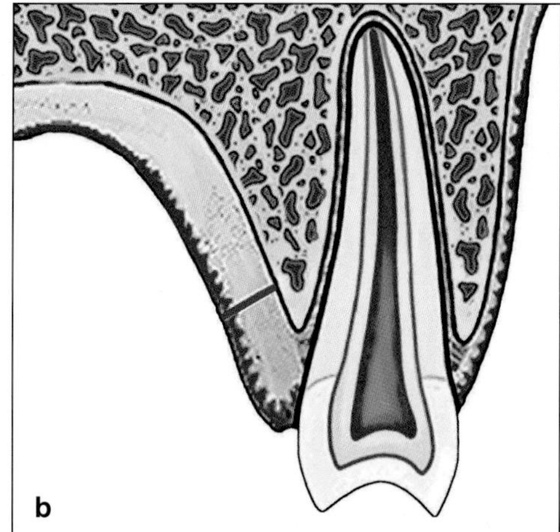

Figs 5-24a and 5-24b Occlusal and cross-sectional views of initial incision for harvesting a subepithelial connective tissue graft using a dual-incision technique. A no. 15C scalpel is used to make a full-thickness curvilinear incision approximately 3 mm apical to the adjacent premolars. Retracing the incision will ensure that the periosteum is completely incised. The incision should extend just mesial to the first premolar and just distal to the second premolar.

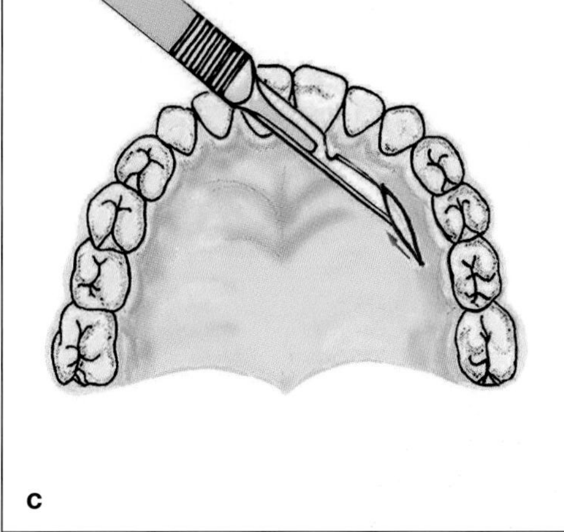

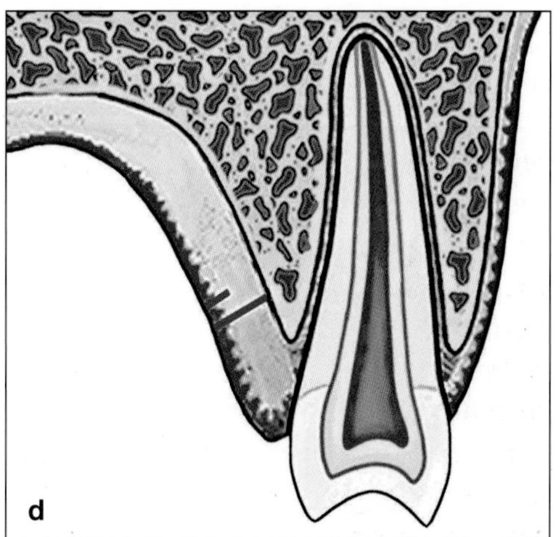

Figs 5-24c and 5-24d The second, partial-thickness incision is made with a fresh no. 15C scalpel blade and completes an ellipse. This incision should be made to the depth of the bevel of a no. 15C scalpel (approximately 1.0 mm). The depth of this incision defines the thickness of the donor tissue obtained.

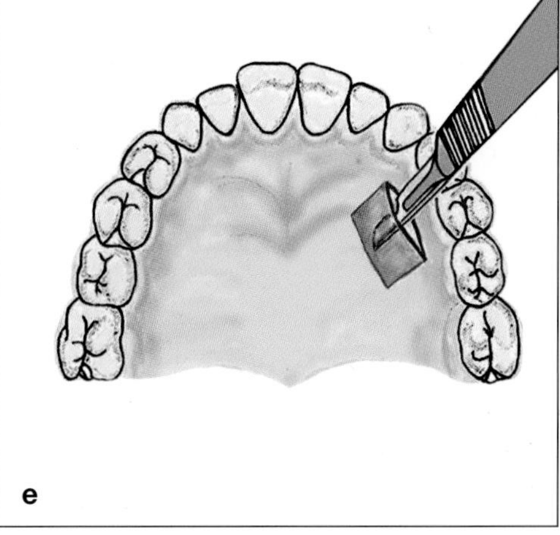

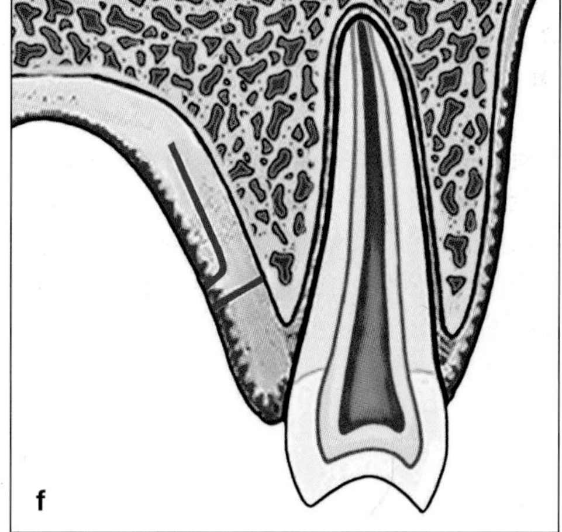

Figs 5-24e and 5-24f The tip of the scalpel is reoriented within the second incision to parallel the surface of the palatal tissues, and sharp dissection is used to create a subepithelial pouch. The apical extension of the dissection is determined by the size of the palate.

made through the apical aspect of the donor tissue from within the pouch. The harvested tissue is then transferred with tissue forceps to the recipient site or temporarily placed on a sterile gauze moistened with saline (Figs 5-24k and 5-24l).

The harvested tissue contains epithelium, connective tissue, and periosteum. Curved Iris tissue scissors are used to remove the epithelial tissue whenever it will be placed underneath the cover flap. The surgeon must avoid crushing or damaging the donor tissue as it is transferred to the recipient site or during removal of the unwanted epithelium.

Hemostasis is then obtained at the donor site by placing an absorbable collagen dressing (CollaPlug) and applying pressure with moistened saline gauze. The donor site is closed using 4-0 chromic gut suture on a P3 needle. Interrupted sutures are secured in the interproximal area (Figs 5-24m to 5-24n).

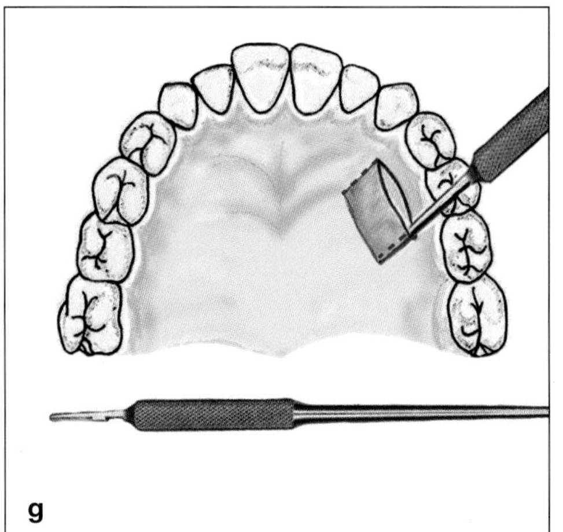

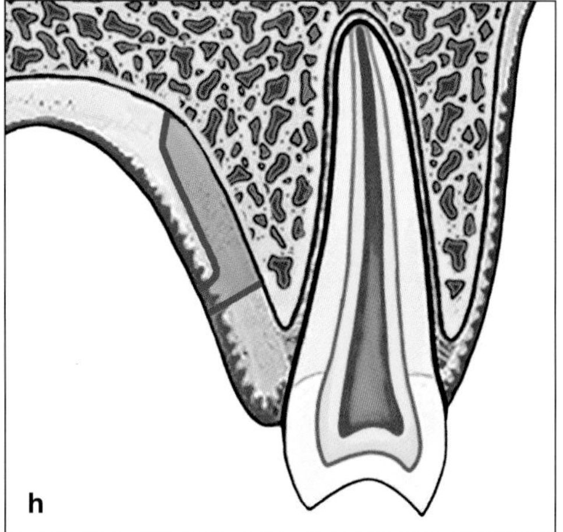

Figs 5-24g and 5-24h Next, from within the pouch vertical incisions are made with a no. 15C scalpel through the connective tissue and periosteum to define the width of the donor tissue. To avoid tearing the overlying tissues, these incisions are located just short of the mesial and distal extent of the pouch dissection, allowing reorientation of the scalpel blade perpendicular to the surface of the palatal tissues. The low profile of the round handle scalpel facilitates this maneuver.

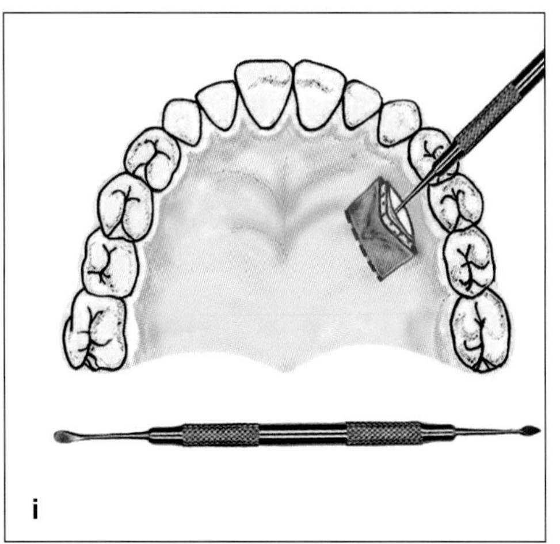

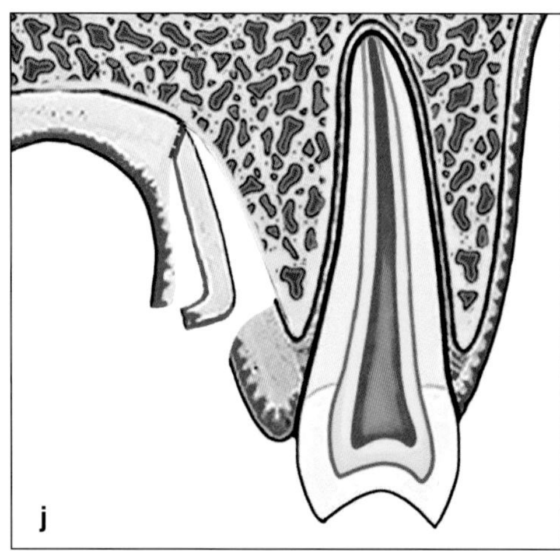

Figs 5-24i and 5-24j Subperiosteal dissection is then performed using the paddle end of a Buser periosteal elevator or a membrane-placement instrument (Hu-Friedy, Chicago, IL). The coronal portion of the donor tissue is stabilized with Adson tissue forceps while the subperiosteal dissection is completed. A horizontal incision made at the apical extent of the dissection under gentle traction completes the donor tissue harvest.

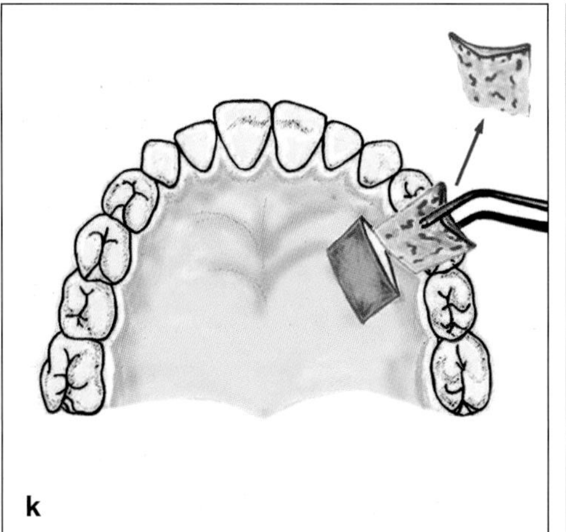

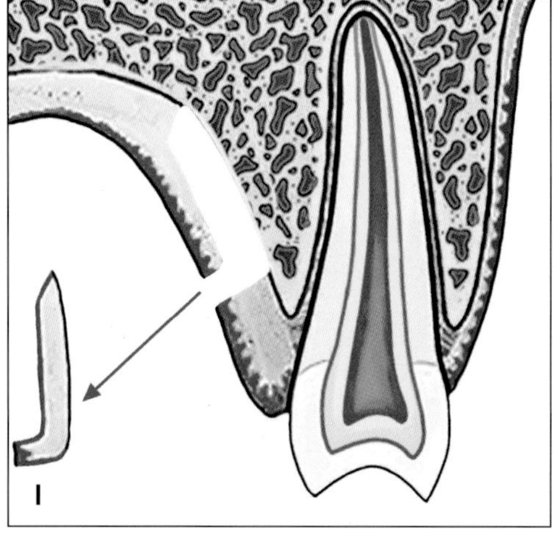

Figs 5-24k and 5-24l The donor tissue, consisting of epithelium, connective tissue, fat, and periosteum, is then immediately taken to the recipient site, where it is adapted and immobilized. The epithelial strip included with the graft should be excised with sharp tissue scissors whenever that portion of the graft will be submerged under a cover flap or pouch at the recipient site.

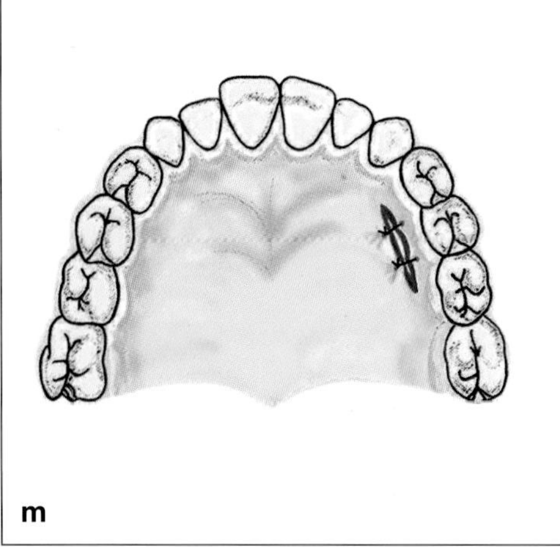

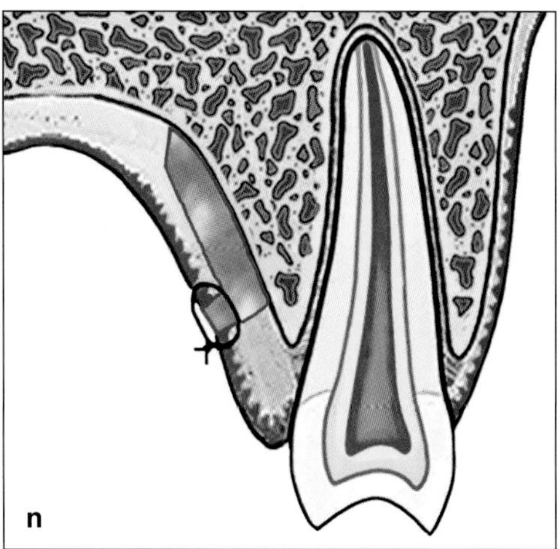

Figs 5-24m and 5-24n CollaPlug absorbable collagen dressing is used to aid in hemostasis and to fill the considerable dead space that results from the donor tissue harvest. Chromic gut suture (4-0) on a P3 needle is used for closure of the donor-site wound. Sutures are conveniently passed through the area of the gingival embrasures of the adjacent premolars. In most instances the wound will heal by secondary intention.

Subepithelial connective tissue grafting: Donor-site surgery, single-incision technique

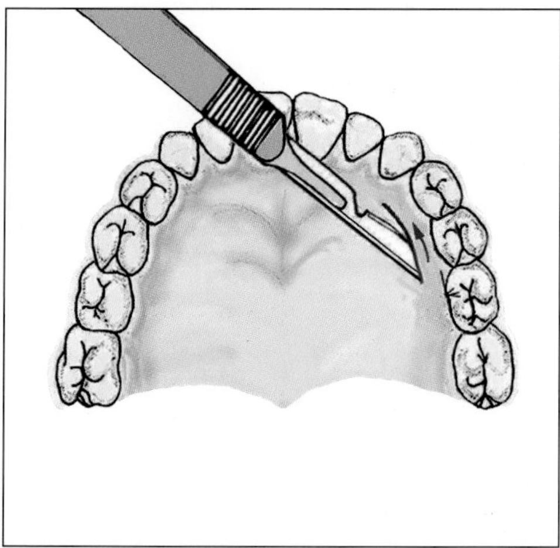

Fig 5-25a A no. 15C scalpel is used to make a full-thickness curvilinear incision approximately 2 to 3 mm apical to the adjacent premolars. The incision is slightly beveled in an apical direction to extend the wound margin and facilitate primary closure of the donor site. Retracing the incision will ensure that the periosteum is completely incised. The incision should extend just mesial to the first premolar and just distal to the second premolar.

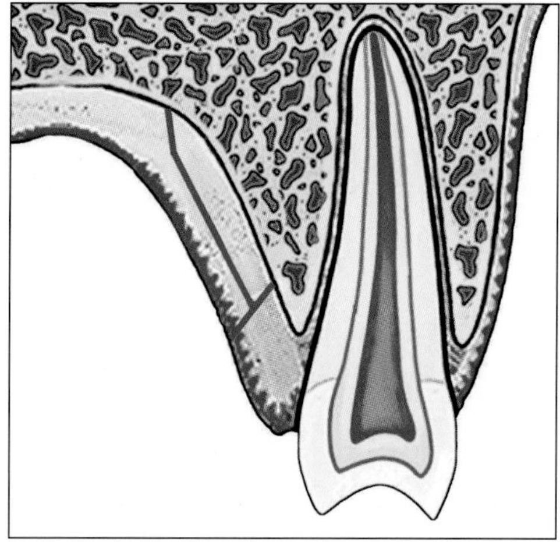

Fig 5-25b A fresh no. 15C scalpel blade is reoriented within the first incision to parallel the surface of the palatal tissues. The tip of the scalpel blade is placed within the first incision, and lateral pressure is used to ensure that adequate cover tissue thickness remains. The remainder of the donor-tissue surgery is identical to that described for the dual-incision technique with the exception that primary closure is usually obtained.

Single-incision technique

The single-incision technique uses only one incision to establish access to both subperiosteal and subepithelial planes of dissection. The technique begins with a full-thickness curvilinear incision through the palatal tissues approximately 2 to 3 mm apical to the gingival margins of the premolars. The incision should be slightly beveled. Next, the scalpel is reoriented within the incision until it is parallel to the surface of the palatal tissue. A subepithelial incision parallel to the external surface of the palatal tissue is then made and extended to create a rectangular pouch. After making the first incision, the surgeon may find it useful to perform subperiosteal elevation coronally. This will improve visualization of available soft tissue thickness before defining the subepithelial plane of dissection (Fig 5-25; see also Fig 5-24b), thereby aiding the surgeon in establishing the appropriate subepithelial plane of dissection. The remainder of the surgical procedure is identical to the procedure described for the dual-incision technique (see Figs 5-24g to 5-24n).

When thin palatal tissues are present, donor-site harvest can be facilitated by the use of local anesthetic or sterile saline solution injected in the subepithelial plane to create a ballooning effect. This common plastic surgery technique decreases the technical difficulty of establishing a subepithelial plane of dissection via the single- or dual-incision approach. The result is the harvest of a uniform graft. When local anesthetic solution is used for this purpose, the author prefers to limit the concentration of vasoconstrictor (0.25% bupivacaine with 1:200,000 epinephrine) to avoid postoperative donor-site complications such as sloughing of the cover palatal tissues. This approach greatly facilitates the surgeon's ability to obtain a uniform graft of adequate thickness even when this anatomic limitation is present.

Sequential subepithelial connective tissue grafts for root coverage of maxillary canine and lateral incisor

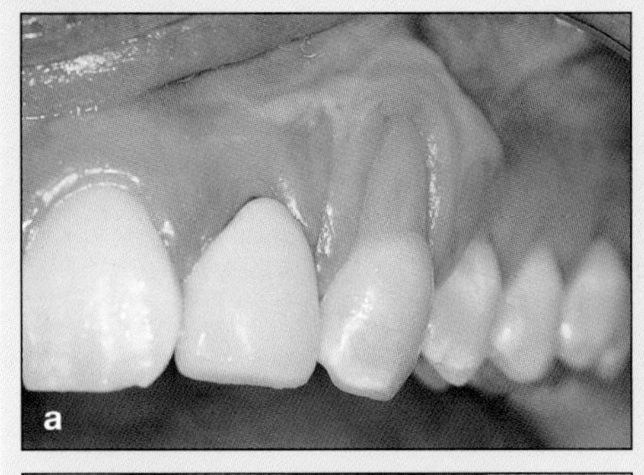

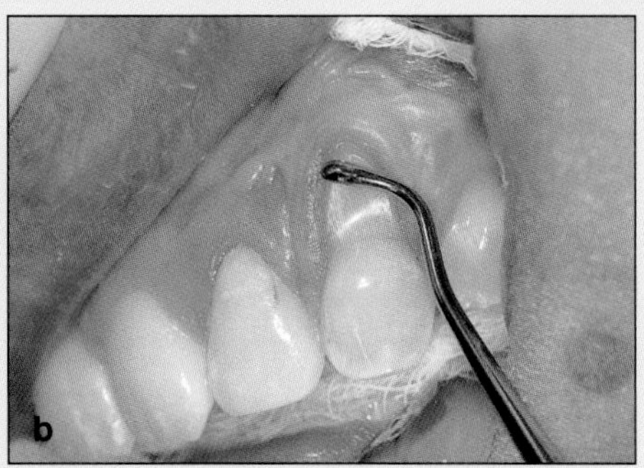

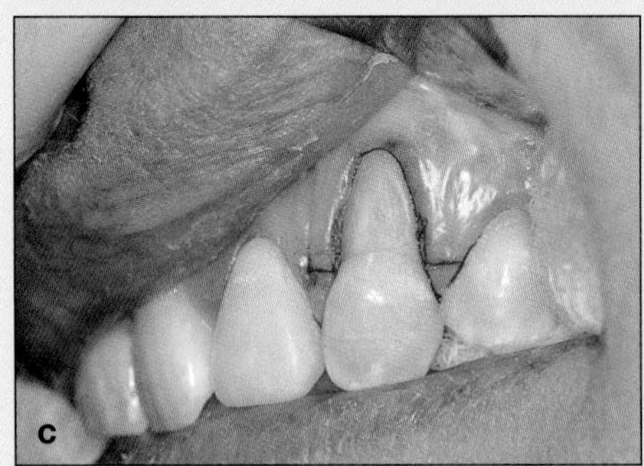

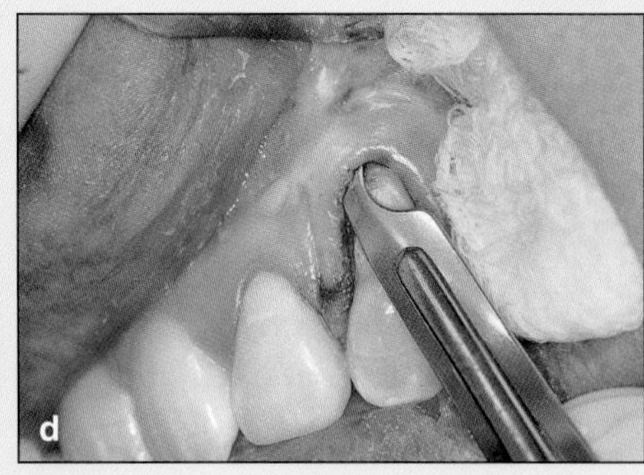

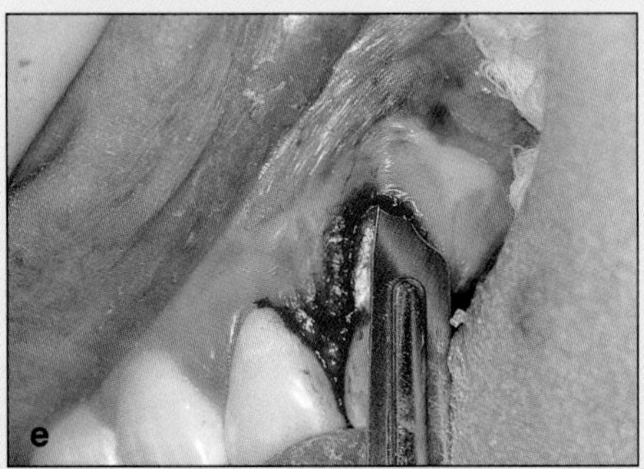

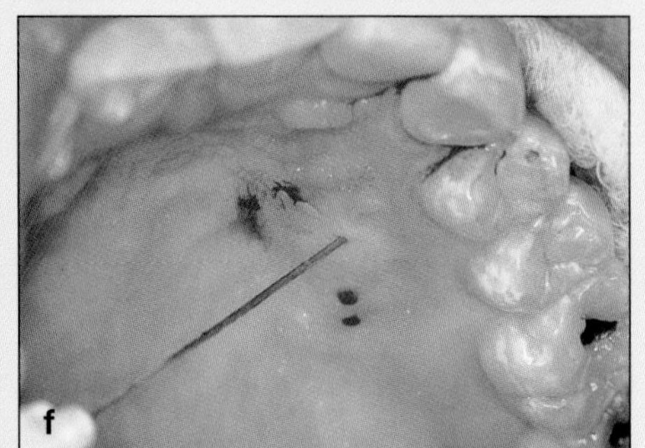

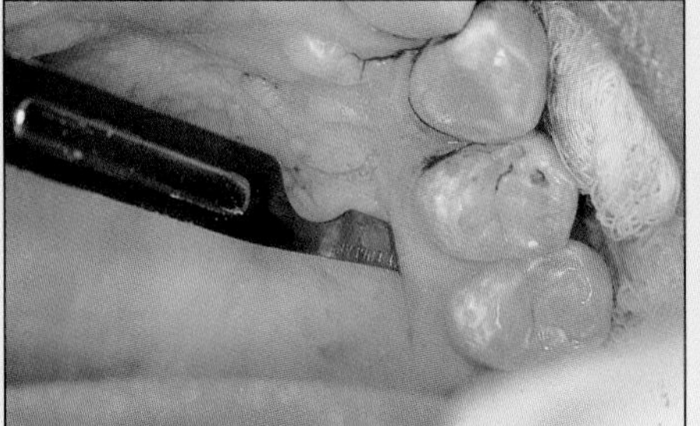

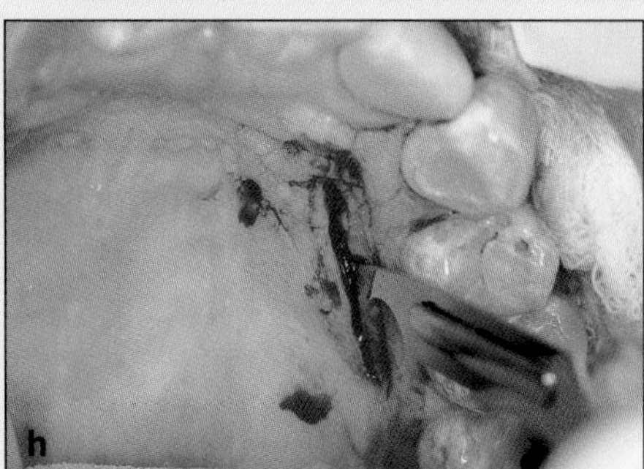

Fig 5-26a Presurgical view of maxillary canine with Miller class III recession defect and Miller class I recession on the lateral incisor. Scarring is a result of two previous gingival grafts, which failed to achieve root coverage. There is no interdental bone or soft tissue loss. A closed approach was selected for the first procedure to preserve circulation and avoid the predisposition for cover flap sloughing. An open approach was selected for the second procedure to obtain 100% root coverage.

Fig 5-26b Mechanical preparation converted the Miller class III defect to a Miller class II defect amenable to complete correction.

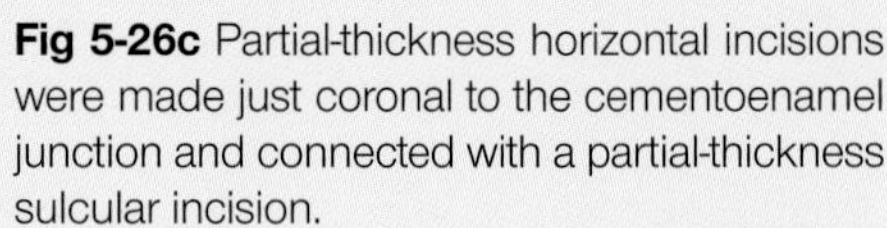

Fig 5-26c Partial-thickness horizontal incisions were made just coronal to the cementoenamel junction and connected with a partial-thickness sulcular incision.

Fig 5-26d Sharp dissection begins at the mesial horizontal incision and moves toward the center of the defect. The dissection then proceeds from the distal horizontal incision and moves toward the center of the defect to complete the entrance to the pouch.

Fig 5-26e Sharp dissection is now extended to the full depth of a no. 15C scalpel blade. The blunt end of a membrane-placement instrument is used to confirm that no webs of tissue remain to hinder passive positioning of the graft.

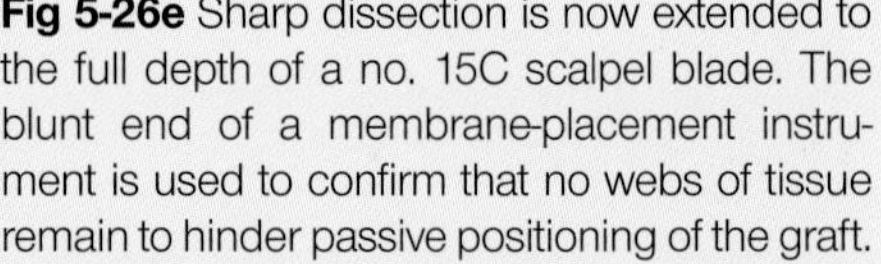

Fig 5-26f The local anesthetic needle is used to estimate the thickness of available tissue in the area.

Fig 5-26g A full-thickness curvilinear incision is made 2 to 3 mm apical to adjacent premolars and extended just beyond the area of the premolars. Next, a partial-thickness incision is made to complete a small ellipse for defining the thickness of the donor tissue.

Fig 5-26h The scalpel is reoriented to parallel the surface of the palatal tissues, and apical dissection is performed through the second incision. Vertical incisions through the donor connective tissue and periosteum are made just short of the mesial and distal extent of the dissection.

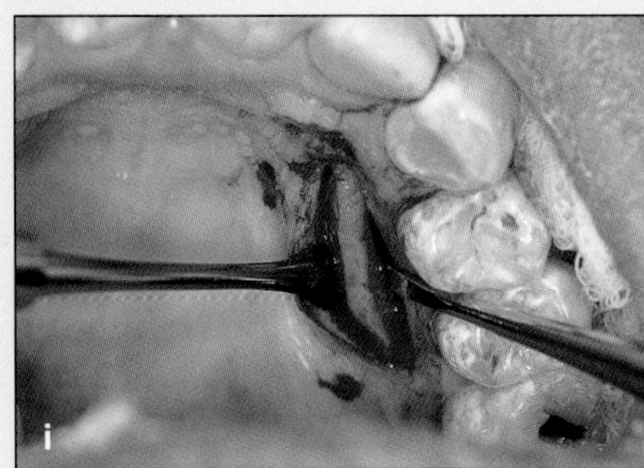

Fig 5-26i The paddle ends of the Buser periosteal elevator and membrane placement instrument are used to carefully complete subperiosteal elevation within the pouch.

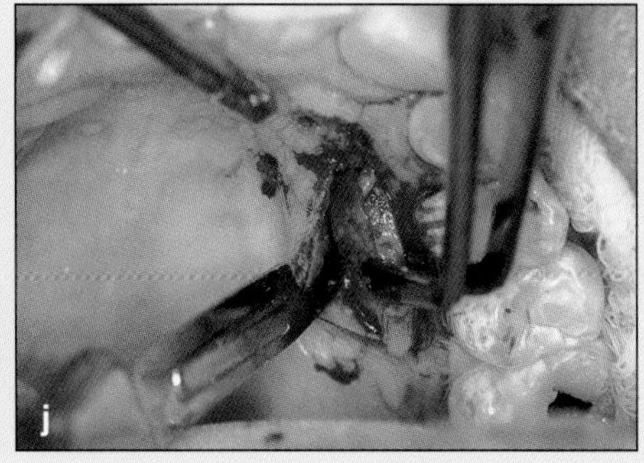

Fig 5-26j A horizontal incision made at the apical extent of the dissection through connective tissue and periosteum completes the donor tissue harvest.

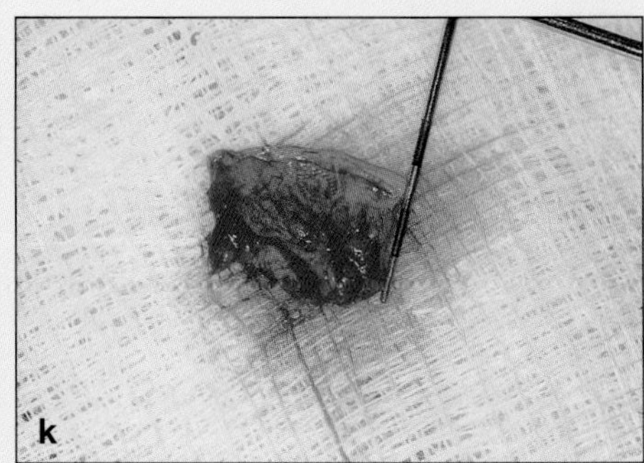

Fig 5-26k The donor tissue is uniform in shape and includes epithelium, connective tissue, fatty tissue, and periosteum.

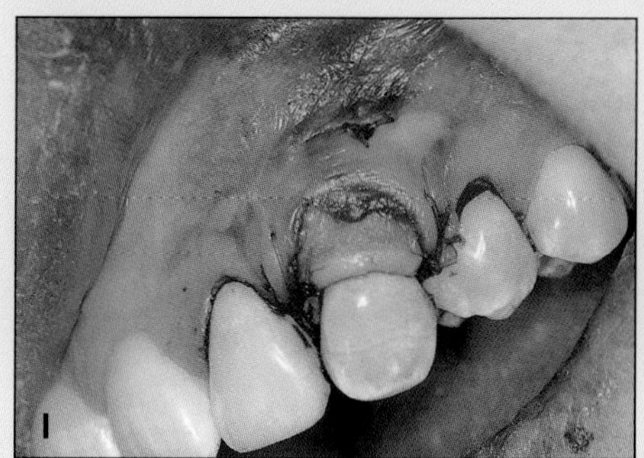

Fig 5-26l The graft is passively positioned using a horizontal mattress suture. A sling suture secures the graft coronally around the cervical area of the tooth.

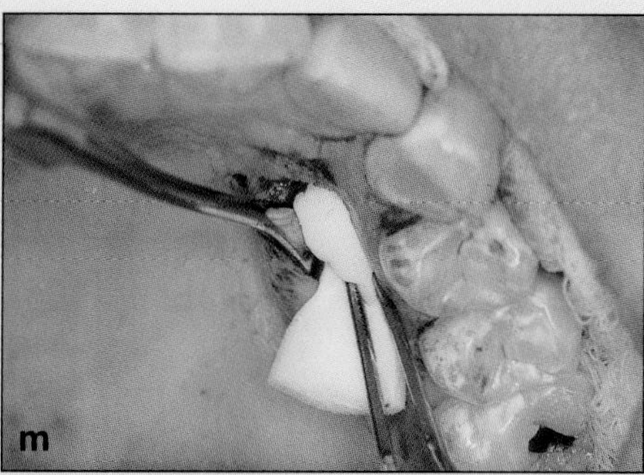

Fig 5-26m CollaPlug absorbable collagen dressing is used to obliterate the dead space, aid in hemostasis, and promote quick connective tissue ingrowth at the donor site.

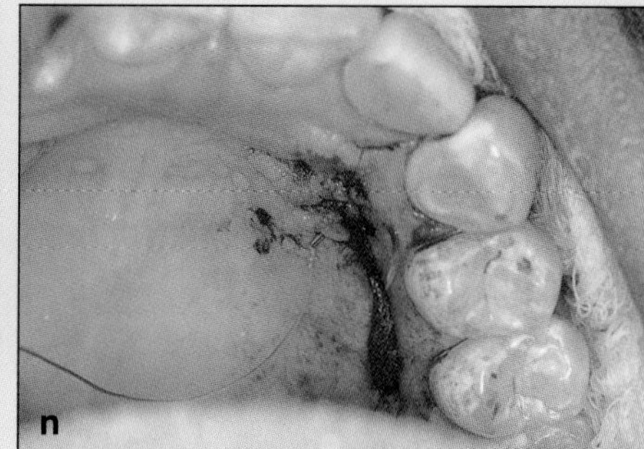

Fig 5-26n A 4-0 chromic suture on a P3 needle is used to close the donor site. The needle is conveniently passed through the area of the gingival embrasure.

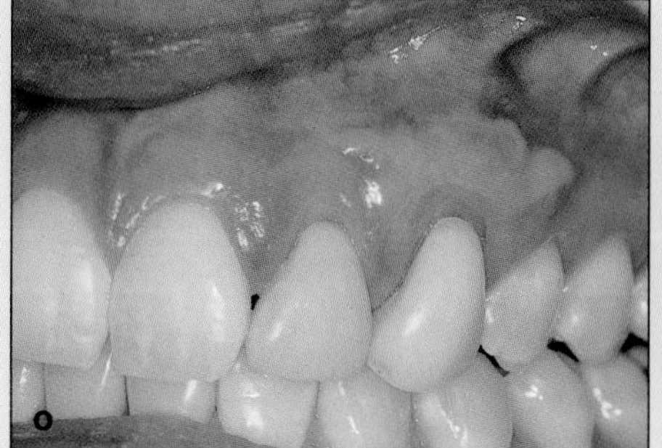

Fig 5-26o Three-month postoperative view. Provisional restorations define the final tissue levels needed to re-create an esthetic gingival appearance.

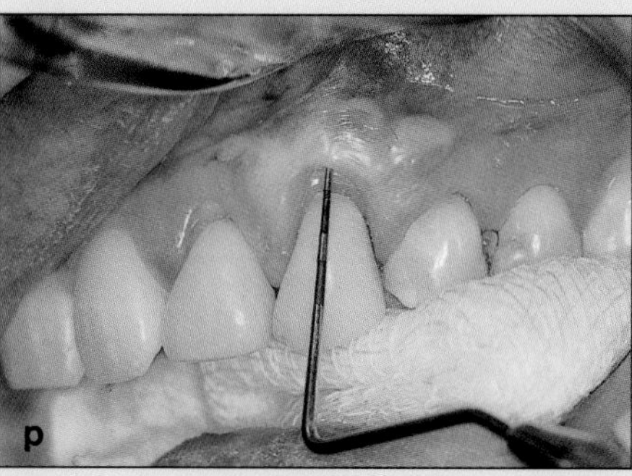

Fig 5-26p Moderate probing pressure measures a sulcus depth of 1.0 mm at the center of the defect. Partial root coverage was obtained.

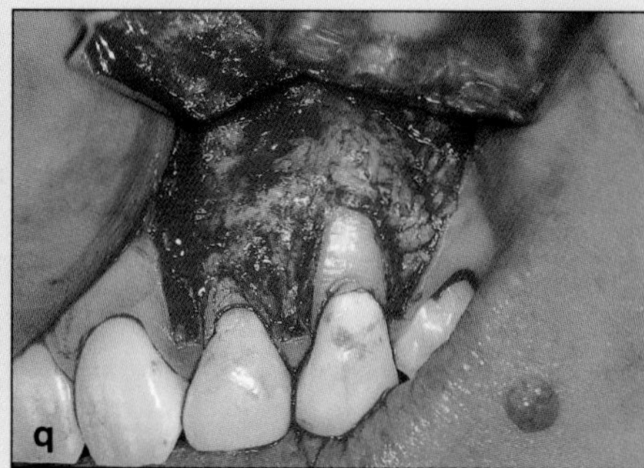

Fig 5-26q Following mechanical and chemical preparation of the exposed root surfaces of the lateral incisor and canine teeth, a partial-thickness open flap has been elevated.

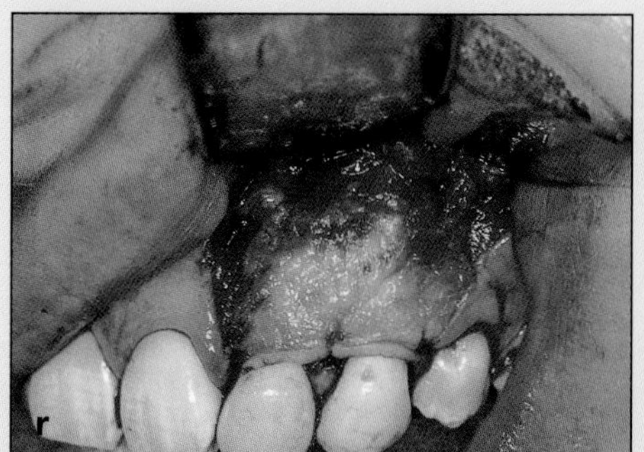

Fig 5-26r The epithelial strip that results from the dual-incision approach is trimmed away with a scalpel and the graft is intimately adapted and secured at the recipient site. The coronal portion of the graft is initially secured at each papilla. Sutures immobilize the graft to periosteum at the periphery of the recipient site.

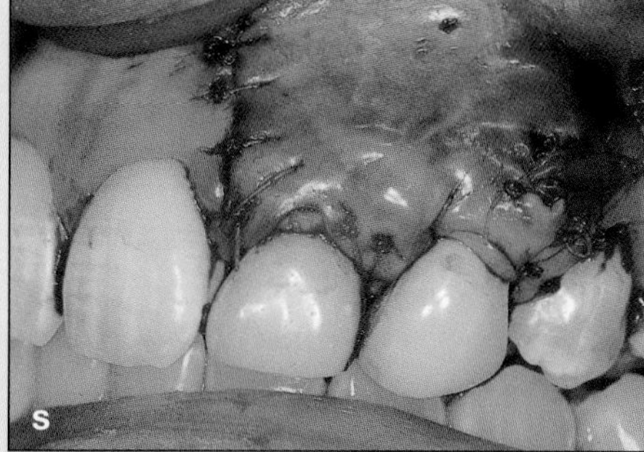

Fig 5-26s The cover flap is coronally repositioned and secured with cervical sling sutures and interrupted sutures along the lateral wound margins. Care is taken to avoid passing the suture through the underlying connective tissue graft.

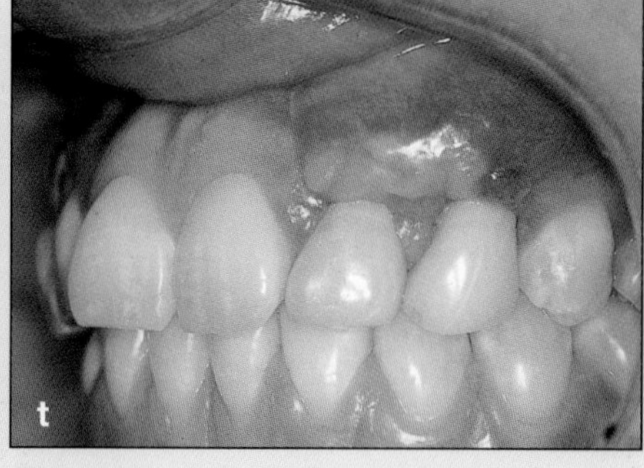

Fig 5-26t One-month postoperative view. Generally, the center portion of the graft becomes necrotic and is slowly replaced by granulation tissue, which subsequently undergoes cicatrix formation.

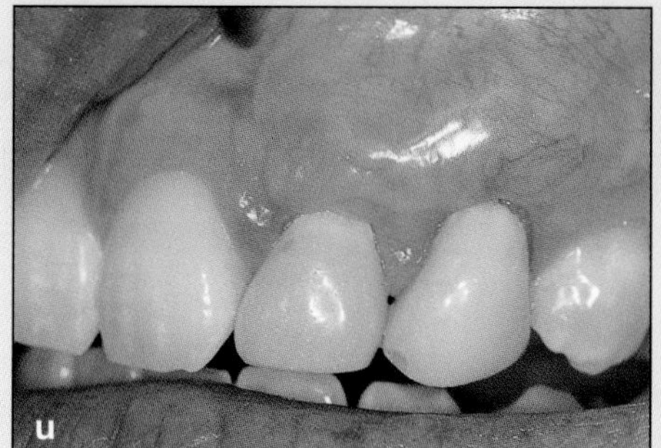

Fig 5-26u Three-month postoperative view. Esthetic soft tissue resurfacing was performed to blend the contours between the graft and adjacent papillary areas.

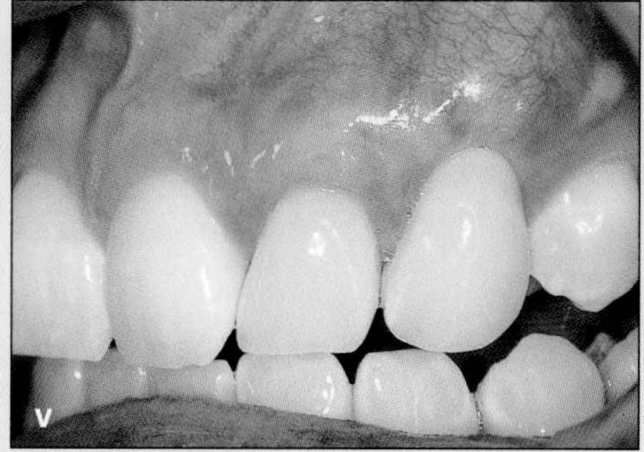

Fig 5-26v Six-month postoperative view demonstrates complete root coverage and reestablishment of an esthetic gingival appearance.

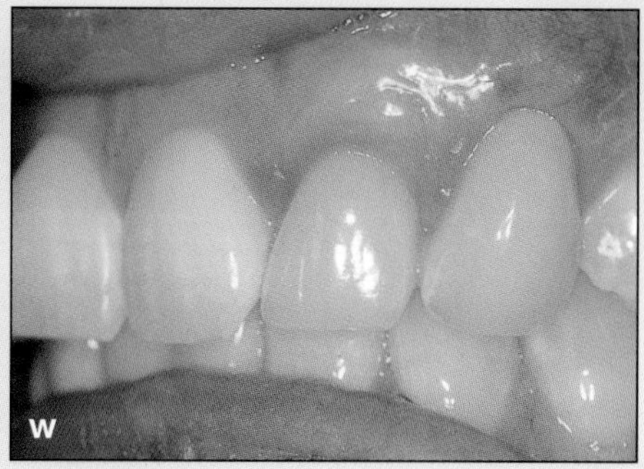

Fig 5-26w Two-year postoperative view. Soft tissues at grafted areas are healthy and stable. (Restoration by Dr Larry Grillo, Aventura, FL.)

Subepithelial connective tissue graft for root coverage of Miller class I and II defects

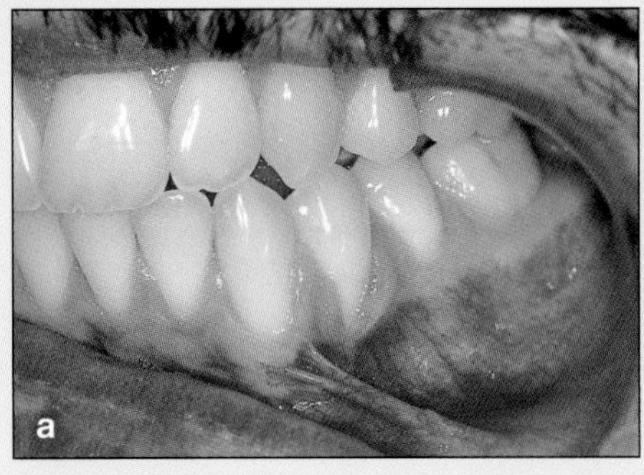

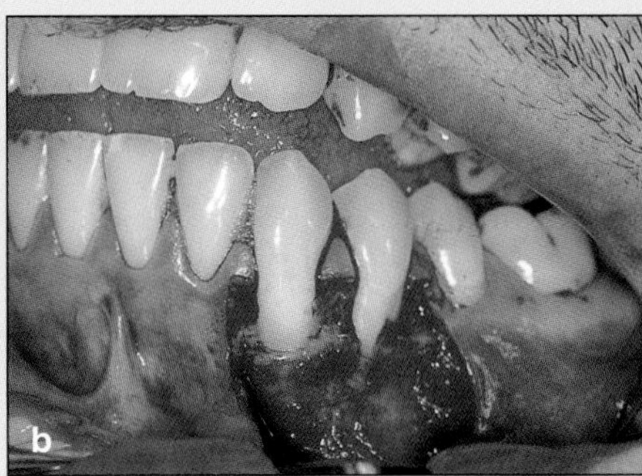

Fig 5-27a Presurgical view of mandibular canine (Miller class I recession) and premolar (Miller class II recession). An open flap approach is indicated to fully release the aberrant frenum under direct visualization with minimal risk to the adjacent mental nerve.

Fig 5-27b Following mechanical reduction and chemical preparation of the excessively prominent roots, sharp dissection is used to create a partial-thickness periosteal recipient site. A significant amount of root dehiscence or "hidden recession" is evident.

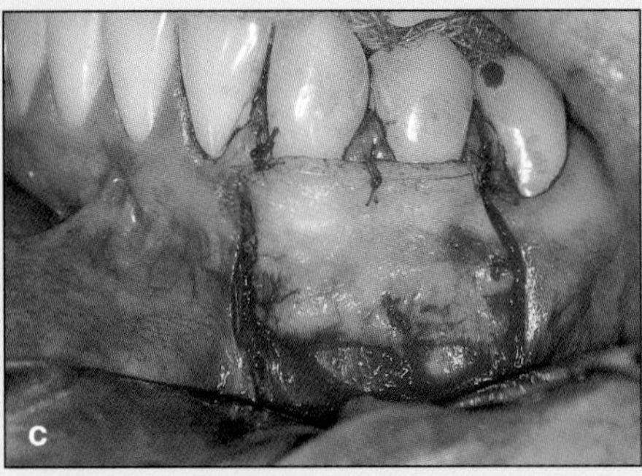

Fig 5-27c A subepithelial connective tissue graft was harvested via a dual-incision approach, after which the epithelium was excised from the graft. The graft was adapted with the periosteal surface facing toward the periosteal recipient site.

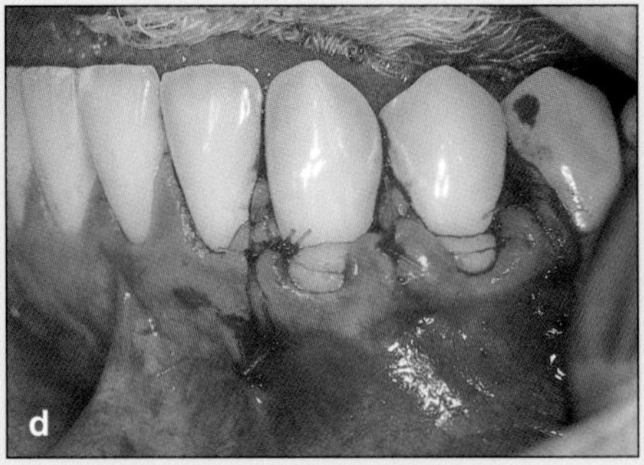

Fig 5-27d The flap was apically repositioned and secured with sling sutures. Note that the apical repositioning of the cover flap eliminated the aberrant frenum but resulted in exposure of some of the connective tissue graft.

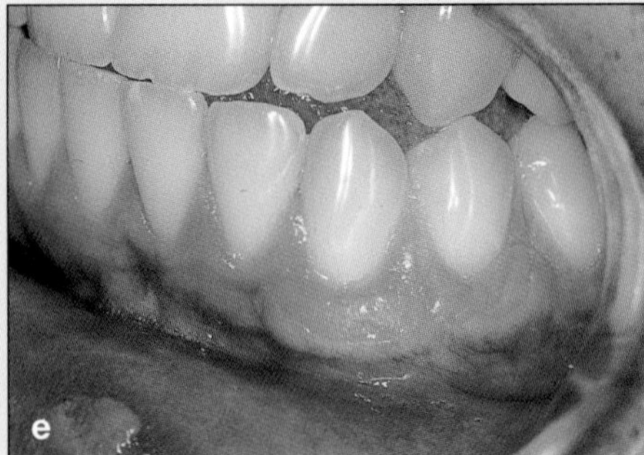

Fig 5-27e One-year postoperative view demonstrates complete root coverage, increased width of attached tissue, and elimination of the aberrant frenum.

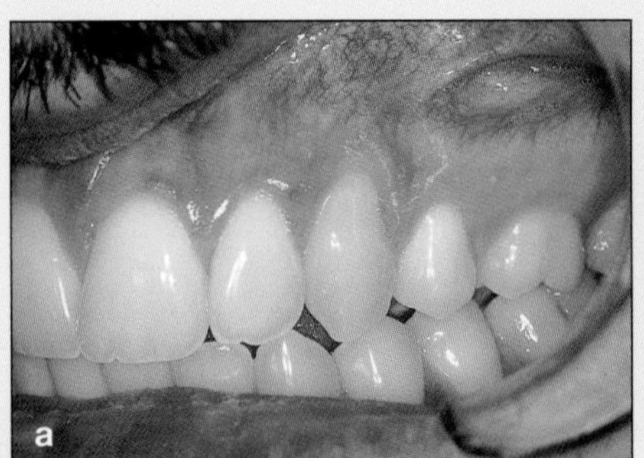

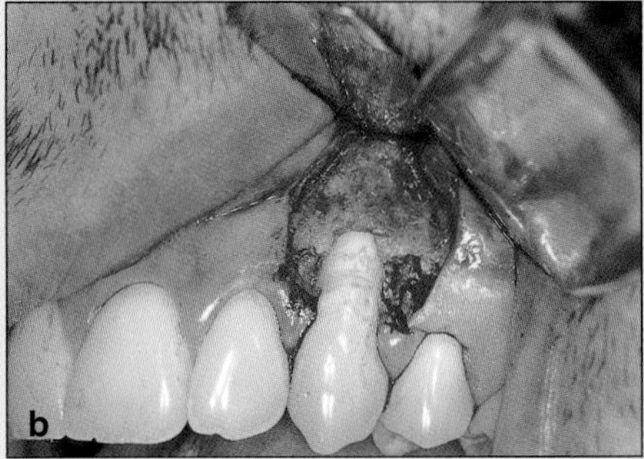

Fig 5-28a Preoperative view of another Miller class I recession defect on a maxillary canine in a patient with a thin, scalloped periodontium. An open approach provides the technical advantage of direct visualization, minimizes soft tissue trauma during graft immobilization, and facilitates subsequent coronal repositioning of the cover flap for greater vertical soft tissue augmentation.

Fig 5-28b Following root planing and chemical preparation, sharp dissection is used to create a partial-thickness periosteal recipient site. A significant amount of "hidden recession" is common in patients with a thin, scalloped periodontium.

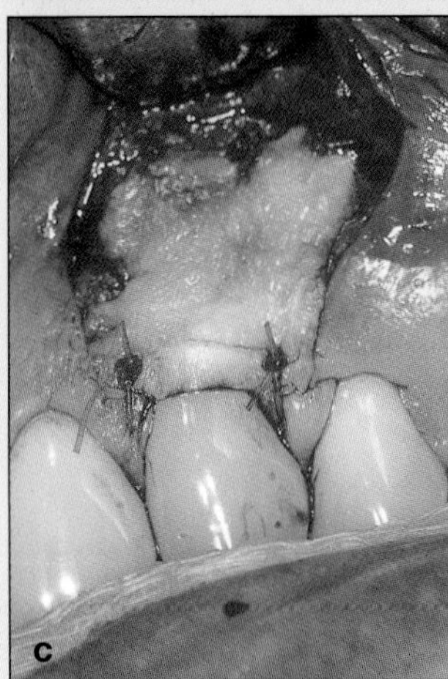

Fig 5-28c A connective tissue graft was harvested via a dual-incision approach. The graft is adapted and secured with the periosteal surface facing down using chromic gut suture on a P3 needle.

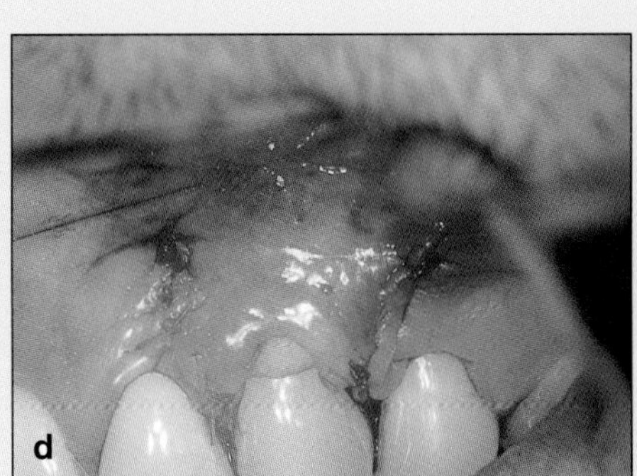

Fig 5-28d A fresh no. 15C scalpel was used to de-epithelialize the attached tissue adjacent to the recipient site, including a portion of the papilla. The flap was coronally advanced and secured with cervical sling sutures and interrupted sutures placed along releasing incisions.

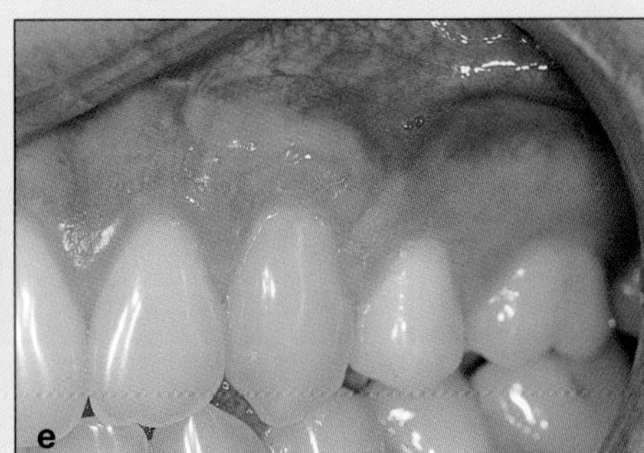

Fig 5-28e Six-month postoperative view demonstrates complete root coverage, increased width of attached tissue, and acceptable gingival esthetics. The patient declined esthetic soft tissue resurfacing.

Subepithelial connective tissue grafting for partial root coverage of mandibular canines via a closed approach

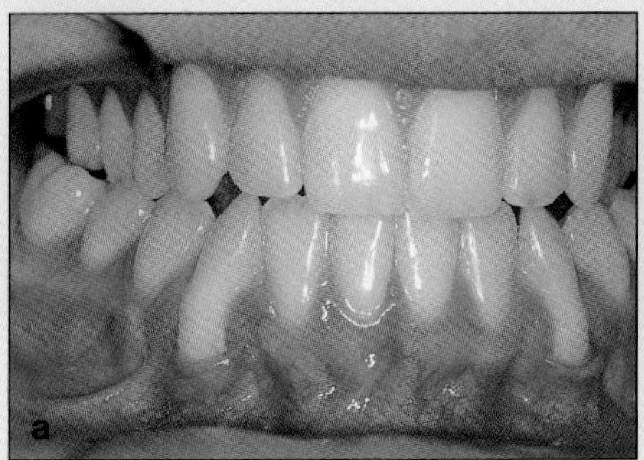
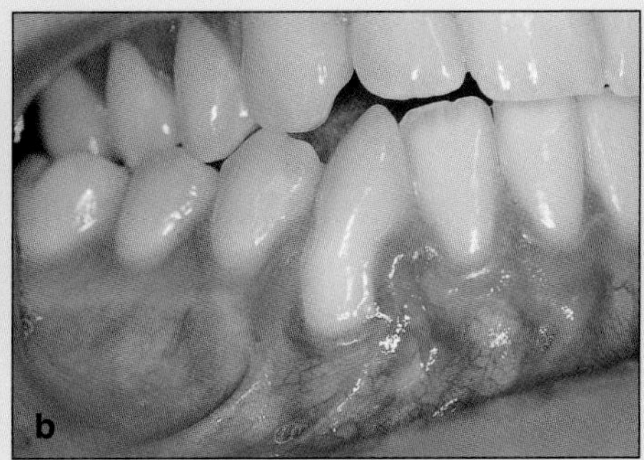
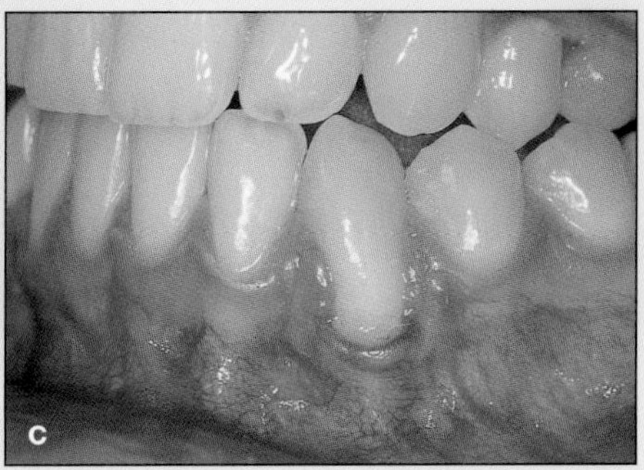

Figs 5-29a to 5-29c Presurgical view of malposed mandibular canines with Miller class III recession. Trauma from masticatory forces and food collection caused chronic tissue inflammation and progression of tissue recession. Subepithelial connective tissue grafts were planned via a closed approach in order to obtain partial root coverage and to increase the width of attached tissue so as to resist future mechanical trauma and halt the progression of recession.

Figs 5-29d and 5-29e Presurgical radiographs demonstrate adequate interdental bone height for successful root coverage if not for the excessive root prominence.

Fig 5-29f Mechanical and chemical preparation of the exposed roots was performed to reduce their prominence. Connective tissue grafts were harvested from bilateral palatal donor sites via a single-incision approach and immobilized in the closed recipient sites. The recipient sites were modified by extending the coronal horizontal incisions and de-epithelializing the mesial aspect of the adjacent papilla.

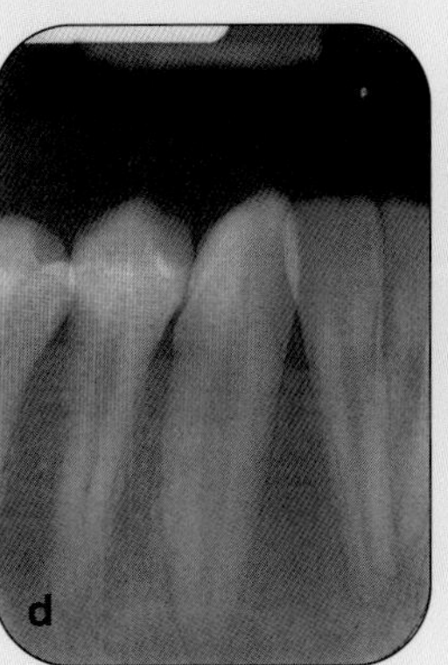
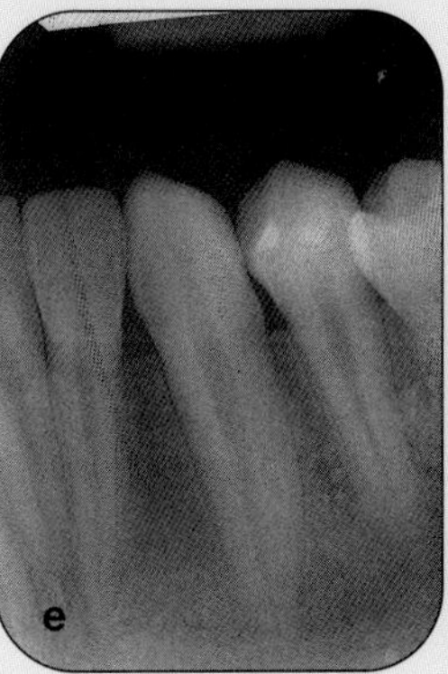
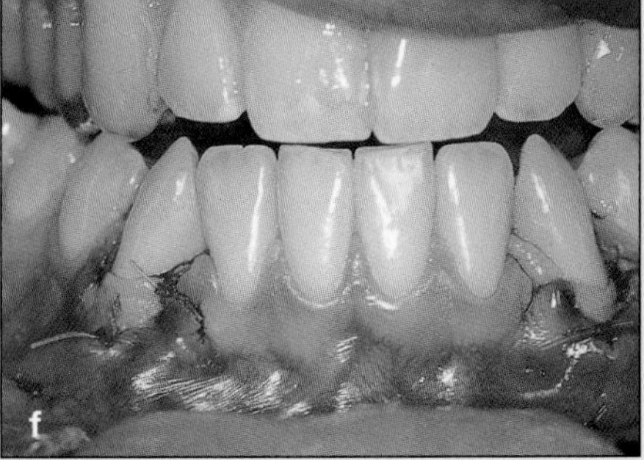

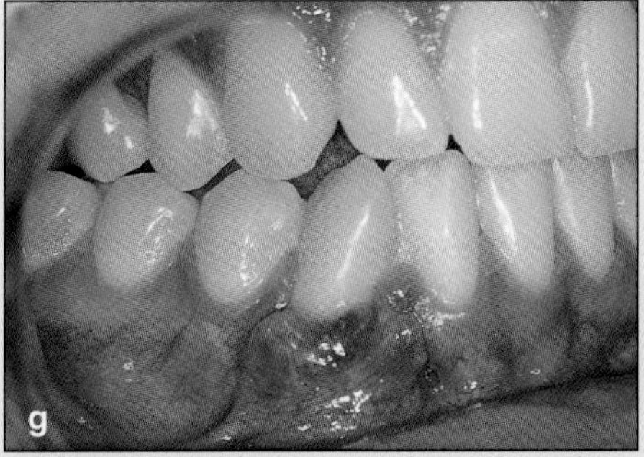
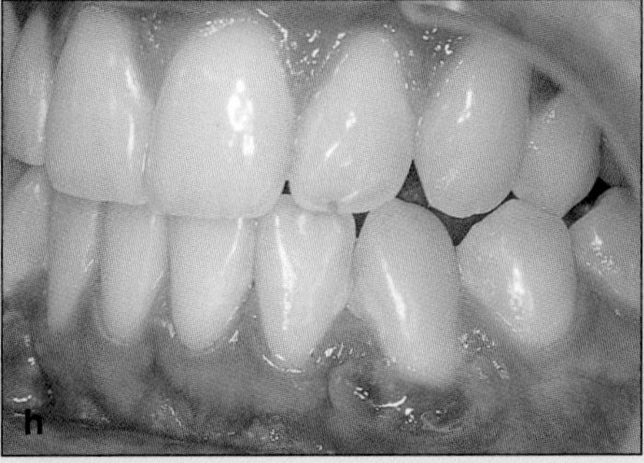

Figs 5-29g and 5-29h Two-week postoperative view. Granulation tissue is replacing those portions of the donor graft overlying the central portions of the denuded root surfaces, which had initially become necrotic.

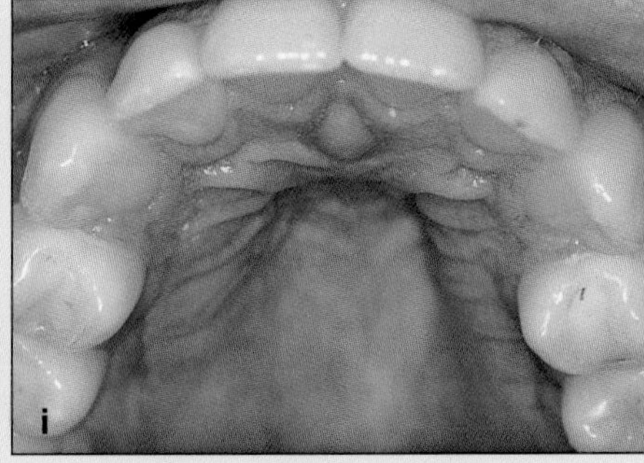

Fig 5-29i Two-week postoperative view of donor sites. Healing by primary intention is evident.

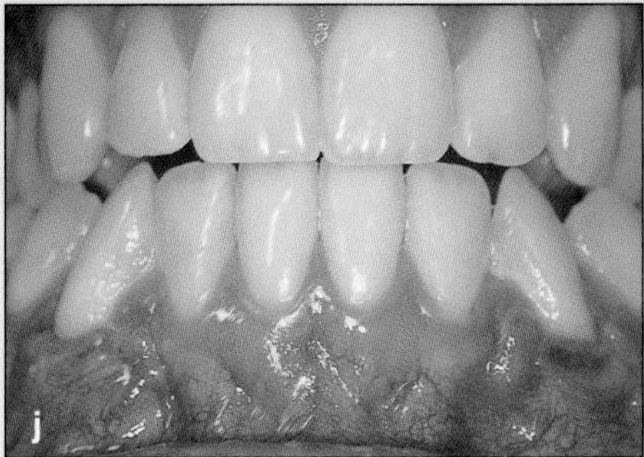

Fig 5-29j Four-week postoperative view. Re-epithelialization of the grafted tissues at the right canine site indicates complete incorporation of the graft. Incomplete incorporation of the grafted tissue is still evident at the left canine site.

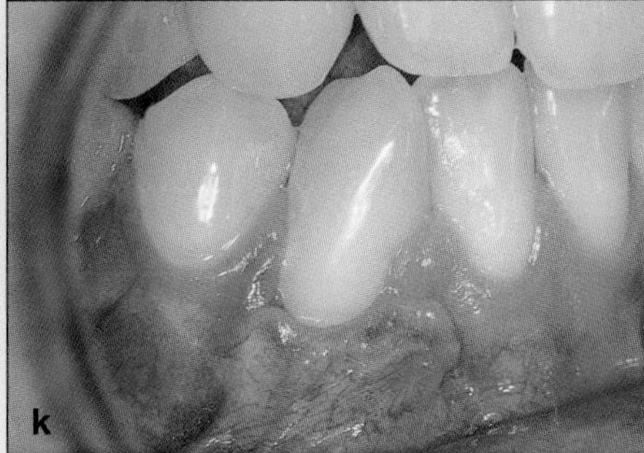
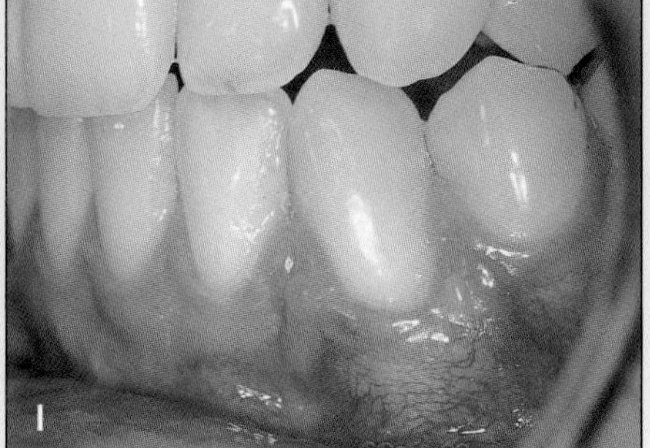

Figs 5-29k and 5-29l One-year postoperative view. Scarring from modifications to the closed recipient sites is evident. The tissues are bound down, but the bleeding through of keratinized tissues that follows the transfer of subepithelial connective tissue is still incomplete. Successful root coverage, estimated at 80%, was attributed to both the reduction of root prominence and modification of the recipient site to take advantage of the abundant circulation provided by the adjacent papillae, which were unusually large.

Subepithelial connective tissue grafting performed simultaneously with implant placement via an open approach

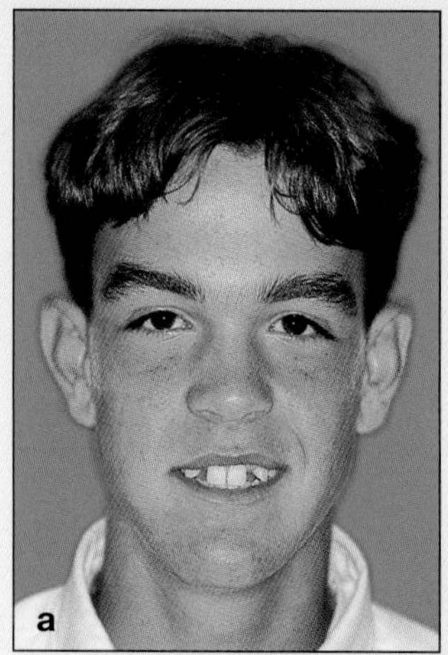

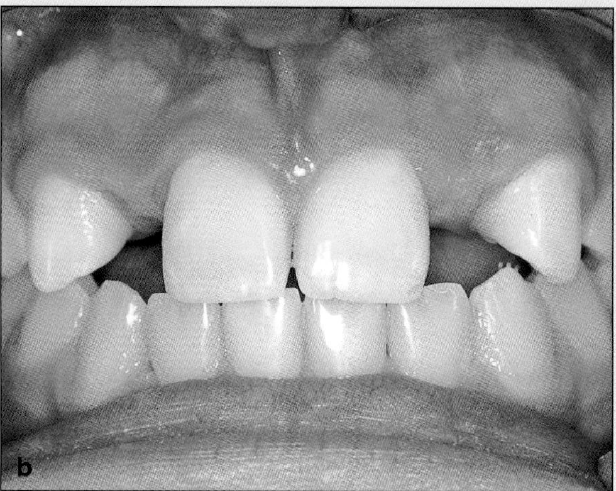

Fig 5-30a Preoperative view of 16-year-old male patient with congenitally missing lateral incisors. Note generous tooth exposure when lips are at rest.

Fig 5-30b Small-volume combination defects are evident at the lateral incisor sites. Connective tissue grafts will be performed simultaneously with implant placement. The abundant vestibular depth will facilitate the expansion of the soft tissue envelope at the sites via coronal advancement of cover flaps, thereby camouflaging the defects.

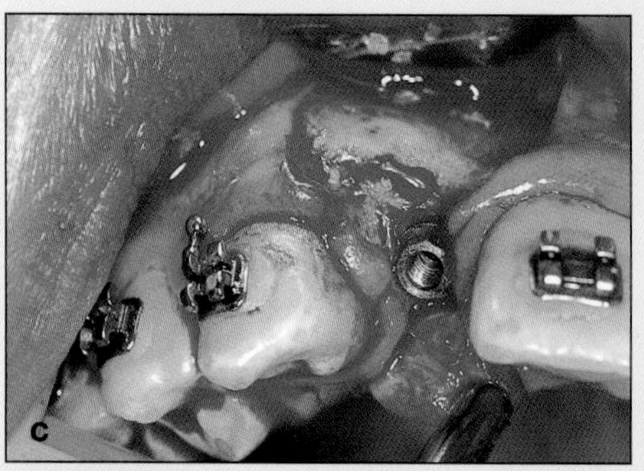

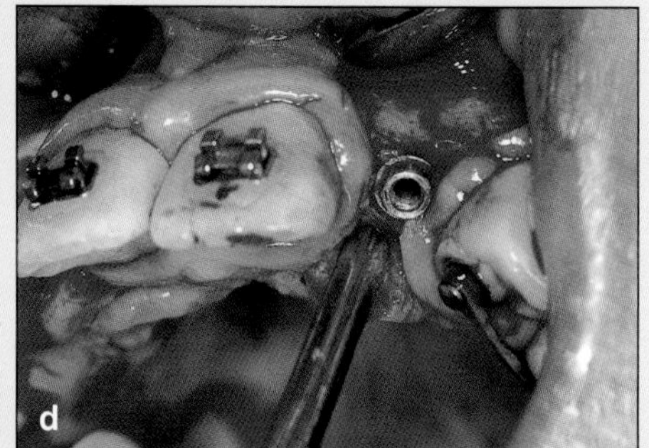

Figs 5-30c and 5-30d A curvilinear-beveled flap was used with full-thickness dissection at the alveolar crest and partial-thickness dissection over the buccal and palatal aspects of the alveolar ridge. In addition, tension-releasing cutback incisions were used. Nonsubmerged narrow-neck implants (Straumann USA) were placed as recommended with the transmucosal portion of the implant located supracrestally.

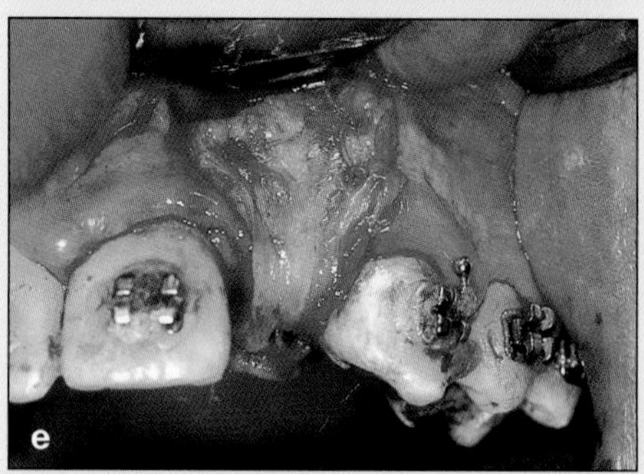

Fig 5-30e A subepithelial connective tissue graft was adapted over the nonsubmerged implants and secured to facial and palatal periosteum. Subsequently, the cover flaps were coronally advanced, and tension-free closure was obtained over the implant neck and connective tissue graft, thereby expanding the soft tissue envelope.

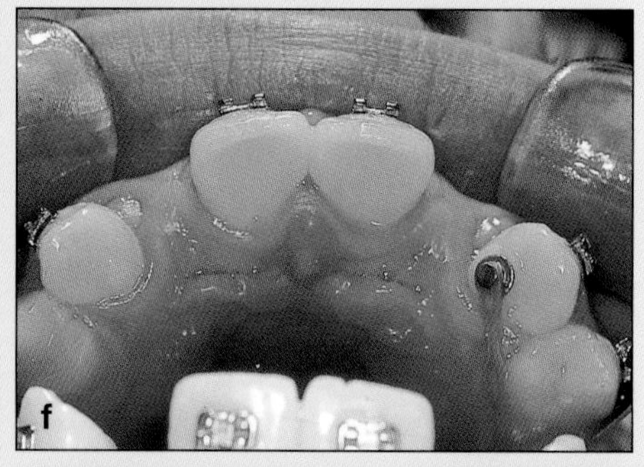

Fig 5-30f Three-month postoperative view. Tissue-punch exposure is planned to preserve soft tissue ridge augmentation.

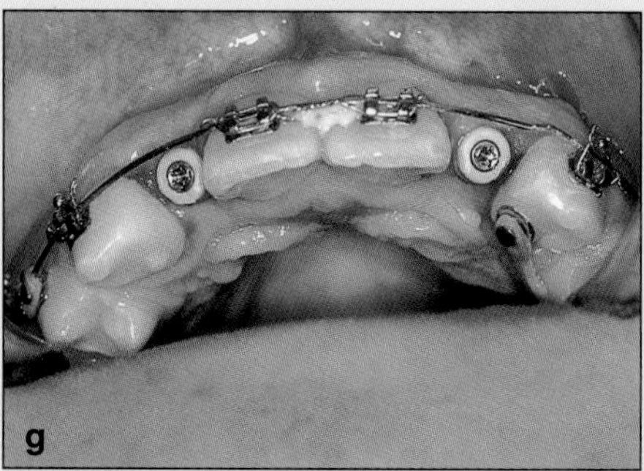

Fig 5-30g One week following tissue-punch exposure and placement of healing abutments. Note that significant vertical and buccal soft tissue augmentation have been achieved, thereby camouflaging the small-volume combination defects at the sites.

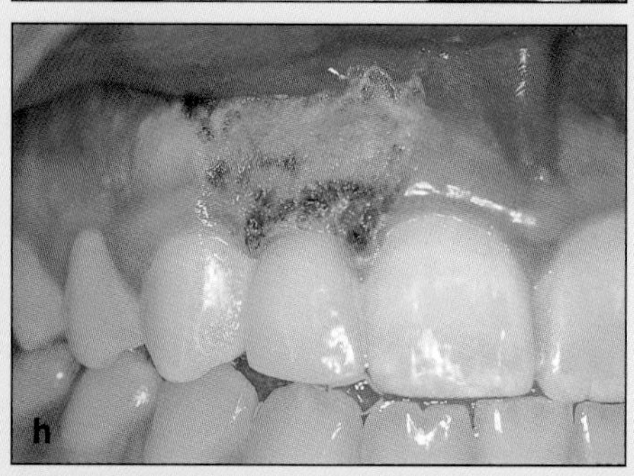

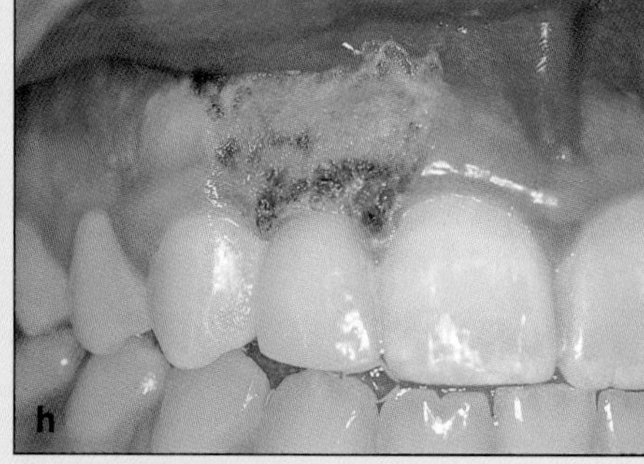

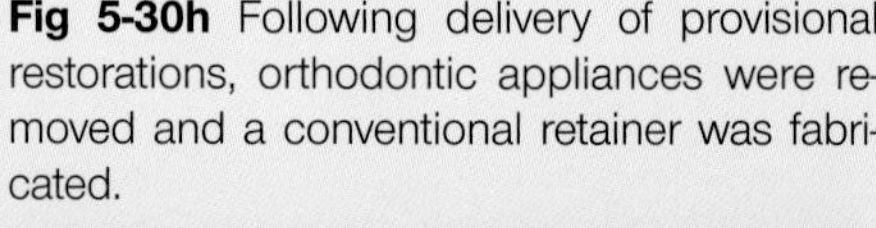

Fig 5-30h Following delivery of provisional restorations, orthodontic appliances were removed and a conventional retainer was fabricated.

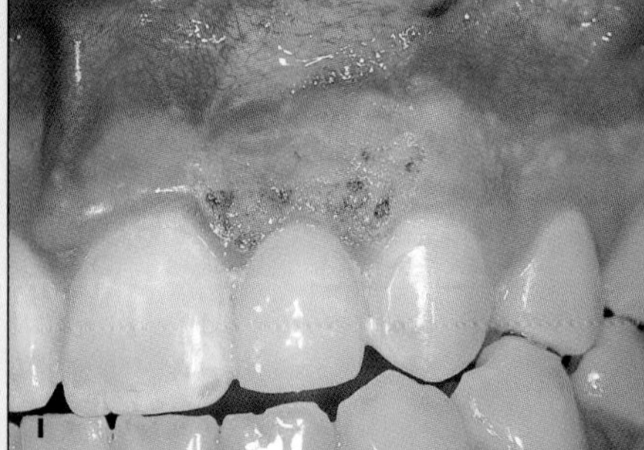

Fig 5-30i Esthetic laser soft tissue resurfacing was performed to remove surface tissue irregularities, thereby enhancing esthetics.

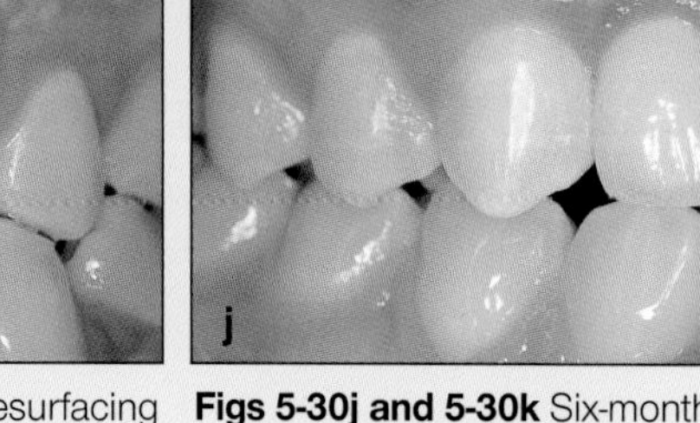

Figs 5-30j and 5-30k Six-month post-restoration view. A slight red discoloration of the marginal tissues persists around the right lateral incisor restoration but has completely faded at the left lateral incisor site. This discoloration is a normal finding at sites where soft tissue grafting and laser resurfacing have been performed and may persist up to 18 months afterward.

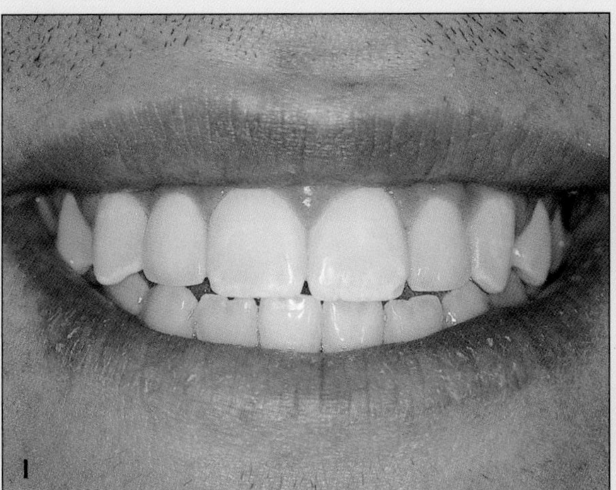

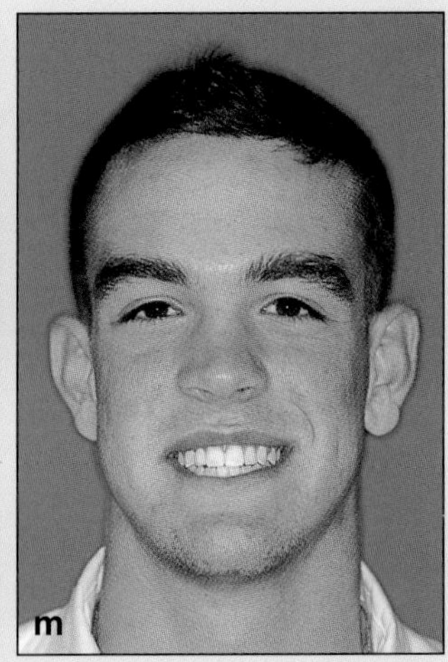

Figs 5-30l and 5-30m One-year post-restoration view. The soft tissue augmentation in conjunction with implant replacement was critical for esthetic success in this case. Good color match is now evident. A straight gingival pattern was obtained on the right side and a sinuous pattern on the left side. Total treatment time, including presurgical orthodontic therapy and growth monitoring, was 30 months; 7 months elapsed from implant placement until delivery of final restorations. (Orthodontics by Dr Richard Mariani Jr, South Miami, FL; restoration by Dr Richard Mariani Sr, South Miami, FL.)

Fig 5-31a Preoperative view of edentulous maxillary left central incisor site with small-volume soft tissue esthetic ridge defect located in the area critical for esthetic restorative emergence.

Fig 5-31b Modified curvilinear-beveled flap for simultaneous implant placement and subepithelial connective tissue grafting includes full-thickness (ridge crest) and partial-thickness dissection (buccal and palatal alveolar ridge). Surgical indexing was performed.

Fig 5-31c Donor subepithelial connective tissue graft has been adapted over the implant cover screw and alveolar ridge and secured with 4-0 chromic gut suture on a P3 needle.

Fig 5-31d Cover flap was passively re-adapted and secured with 4-0 chromic gut sutures. Note that primary closure was not obtained over that portion of the graft at the buccal ridge crest and that the flap was modified in this case to simultaneously manage an aberrant midline frenum.

Fig 5-31e Two-week postoperative view demonstrates complete epithelialization of exposed donor connective tissue located at the buccal ridge crest and apparent correction of small-volume soft tissue defect.

Fig 5-31f Five-month postoperative view demonstrates successful correction of small-volume soft tissue esthetic ridge defect. The site is ready for abutment connection.

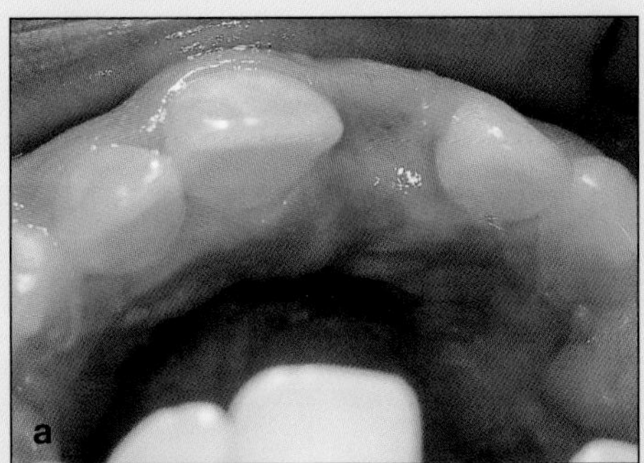

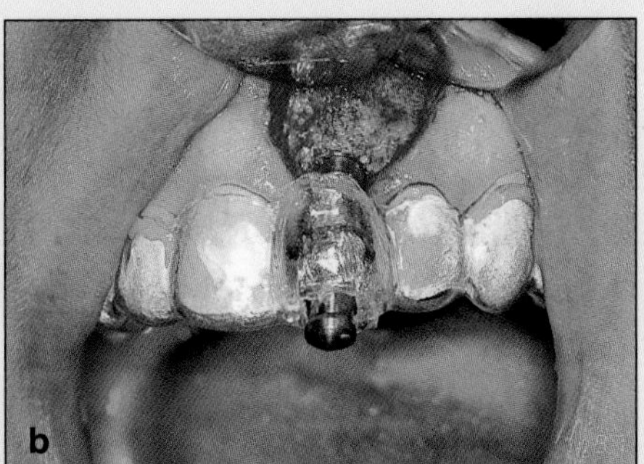

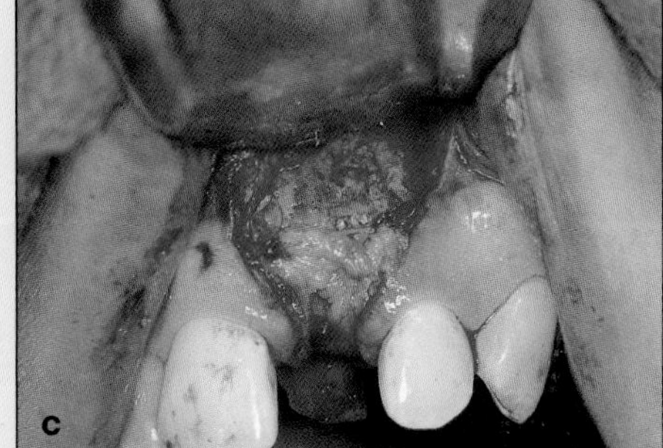

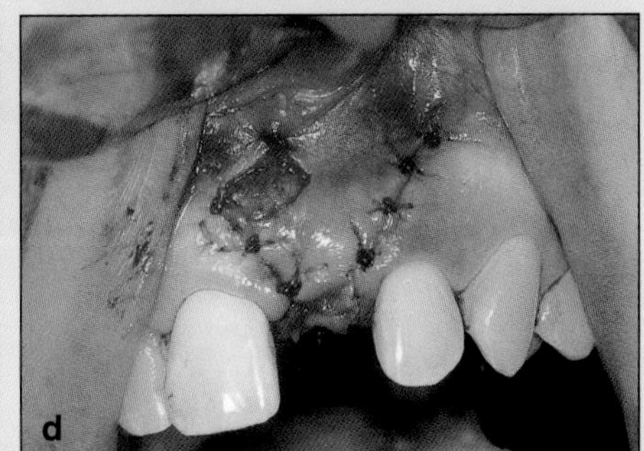

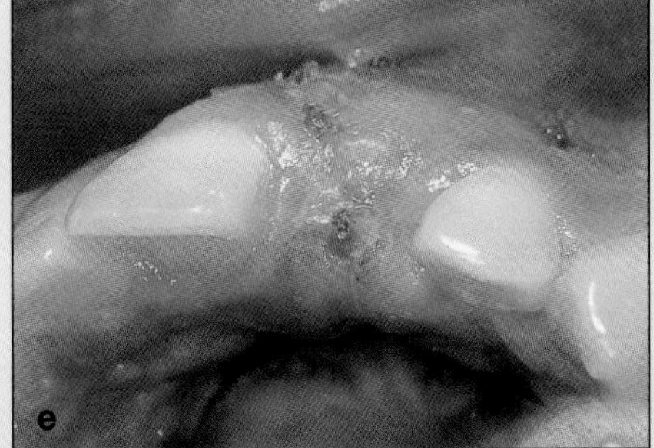

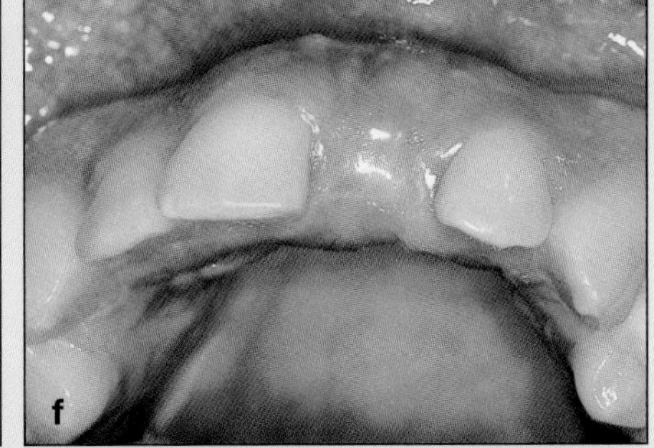

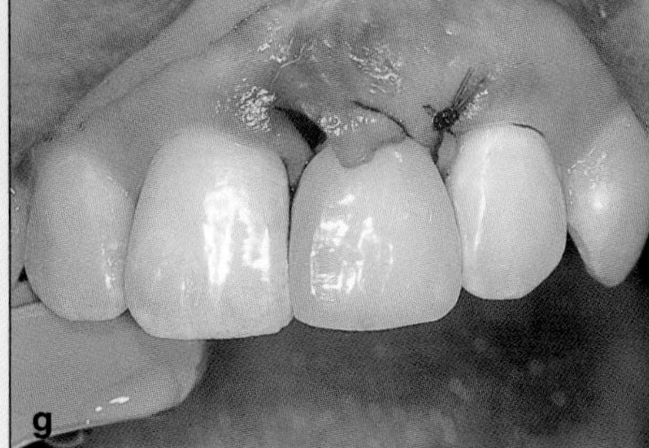

Fig 5-31g After de-epithelializing the adjacent midline papillae, a small cutback incision was made to define a pedicle that would be passively rotated and secured around the provisional restoration.

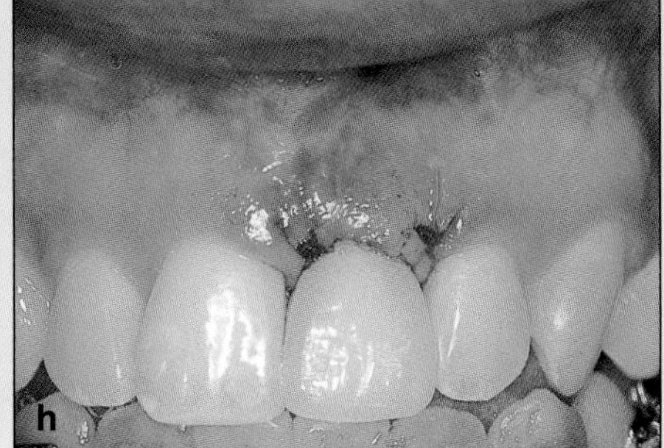

Fig 5-31h Chromic gut suture (5-0) on a P3 needle was used to secure the resultant flap and pedicle. Symmetrical gingival height was maintained between the central incisors.

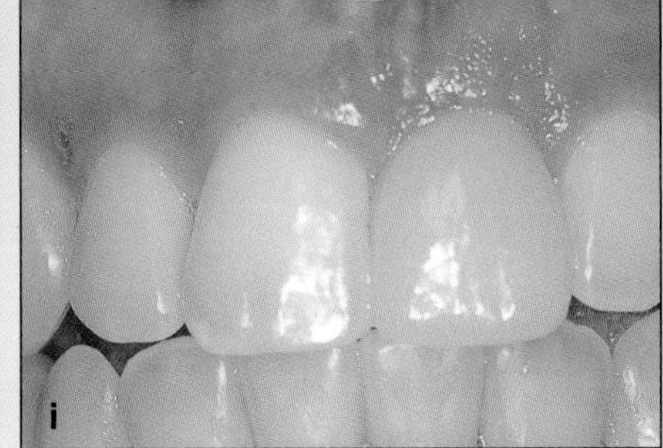

Fig 5-31i Final restoration 6 months after delivery. The small-volume esthetic ridge defect was successfully reconstructed. (Restoration by Dr Jorge Hernandez, Miami, FL.)

Subepithelial connective tissue grafting performed simultaneously with implant placement via an open approach

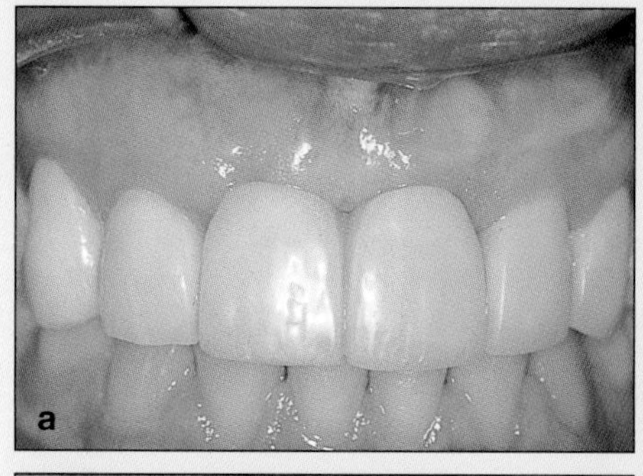

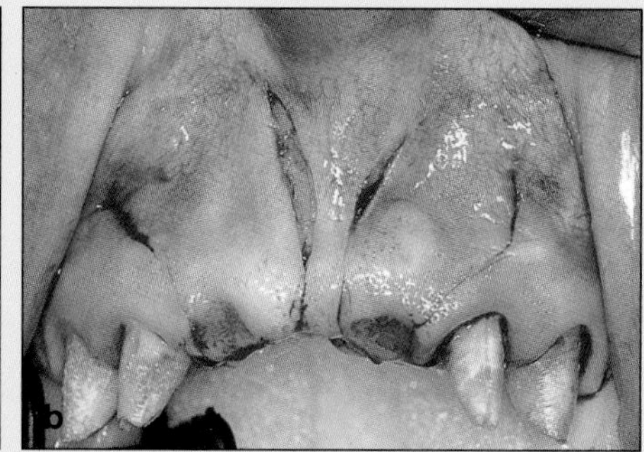

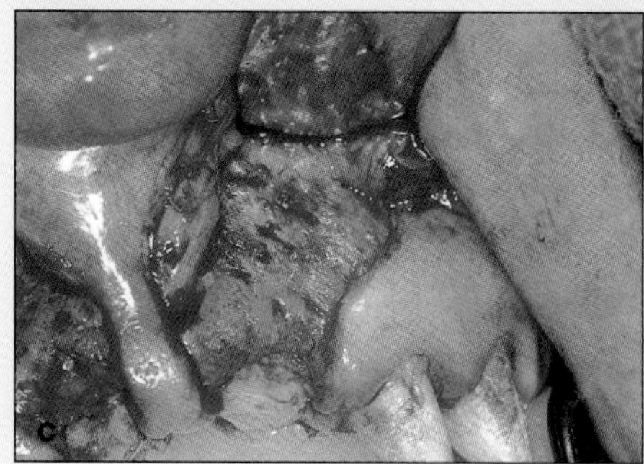

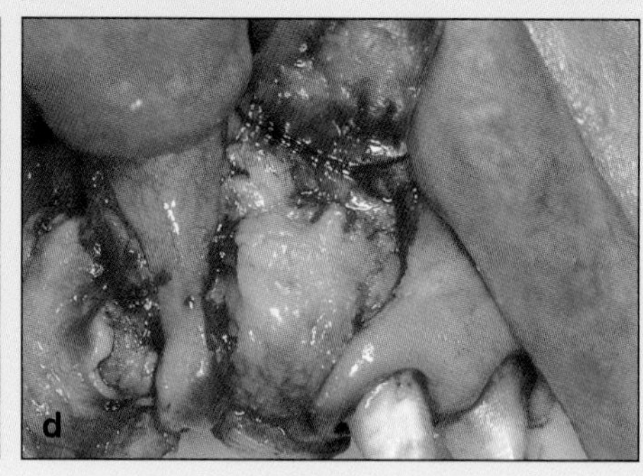

Fig 5-32a Preoperative view of edentulous maxillary central incisor sites with small-volume soft tissue esthetic ridge defects. Horizontal and vertical augmentation will be necessary to achieve implant restorations with natural emergence. The position of the midline papillary tissue was slightly compromised.

Fig 5-32b Curvilinear-beveled flaps have been outlined with partial-thickness incisions. Elevation of the midline papillary tissue was avoided to preserve tissue height. The tissues in the ridge lap pontic site are extremely thin and circulation is probably compromised.

Fig 5-32c To avoid compromising circulation to the flap margins, full-thickness dissection was performed to expose the ridge crest. Partial-thickness dissection was performed on the buccal aspect of the alveolar ridge.

Fig 5-32d The grafts were adapted over the implant cover screw and alveolar ridge with the periosteum facing down.

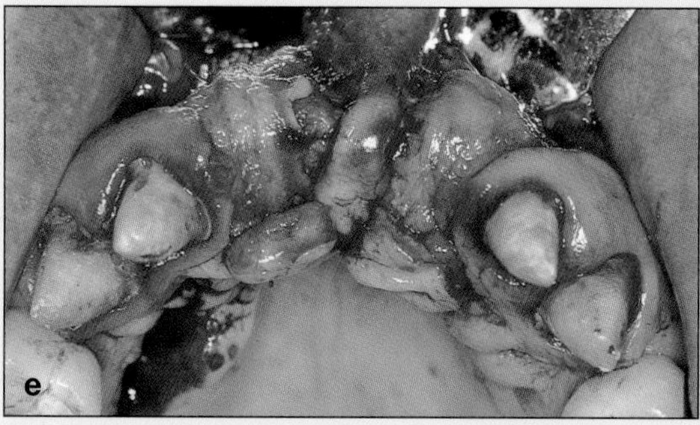

Fig 5-32e Occlusal view prior to coronal advancement and securing of cover flaps. The highest-quality connective tissue was centered at the buccal ridge crest (ie, the area critical for prosthetic emergence). The grafts were immobilized with careful suturing.

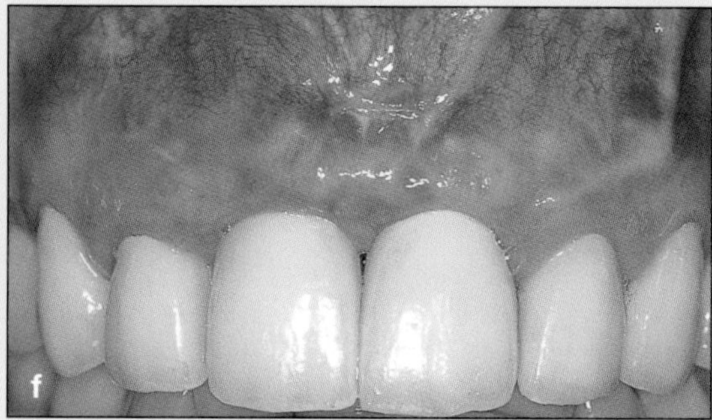

Fig 5-32f One year after delivery of the final restoration. The central midline papilla was preserved, adequate width and thickness of attached tissue were restored, and peri-implant soft tissue health is excellent. Failure to perform soft tissue augmentation would have resulted in a functional and esthetic compromise for this patient. (Restoration by Dr Marshall Brothers, Miami Beach, FL.)

Subepithelial connective tissue grafting performed during the osseointegration period via a closed approach

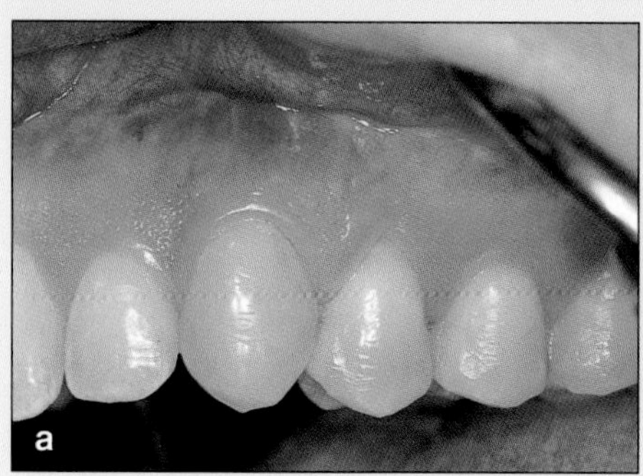

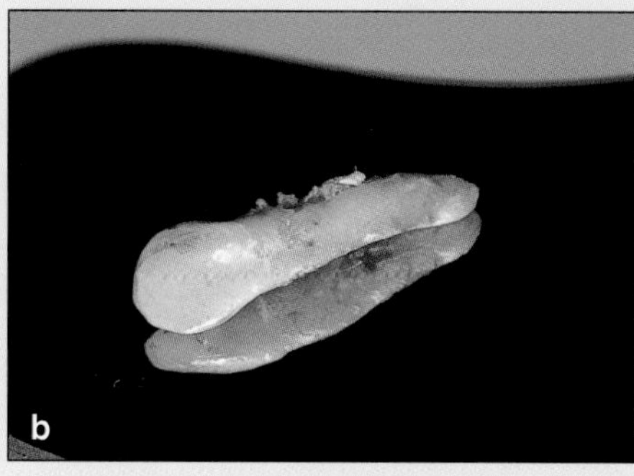

Fig 5-33a Presurgical view of failing maxillary canine at site where circulation has been compromised by previous orthognathic and endodontic surgery. Note extremely thin tissue and thin, scalloped periodontium. It is predictable that soft tissue recession will occur despite use of alveolar ridge preservation technique in conjunction with tooth removal and immediate implant placement.

Fig 5-33b Tooth was removed with minimal trauma using periotomes. Note the compromise that resulted from previous efforts to salvage the tooth.

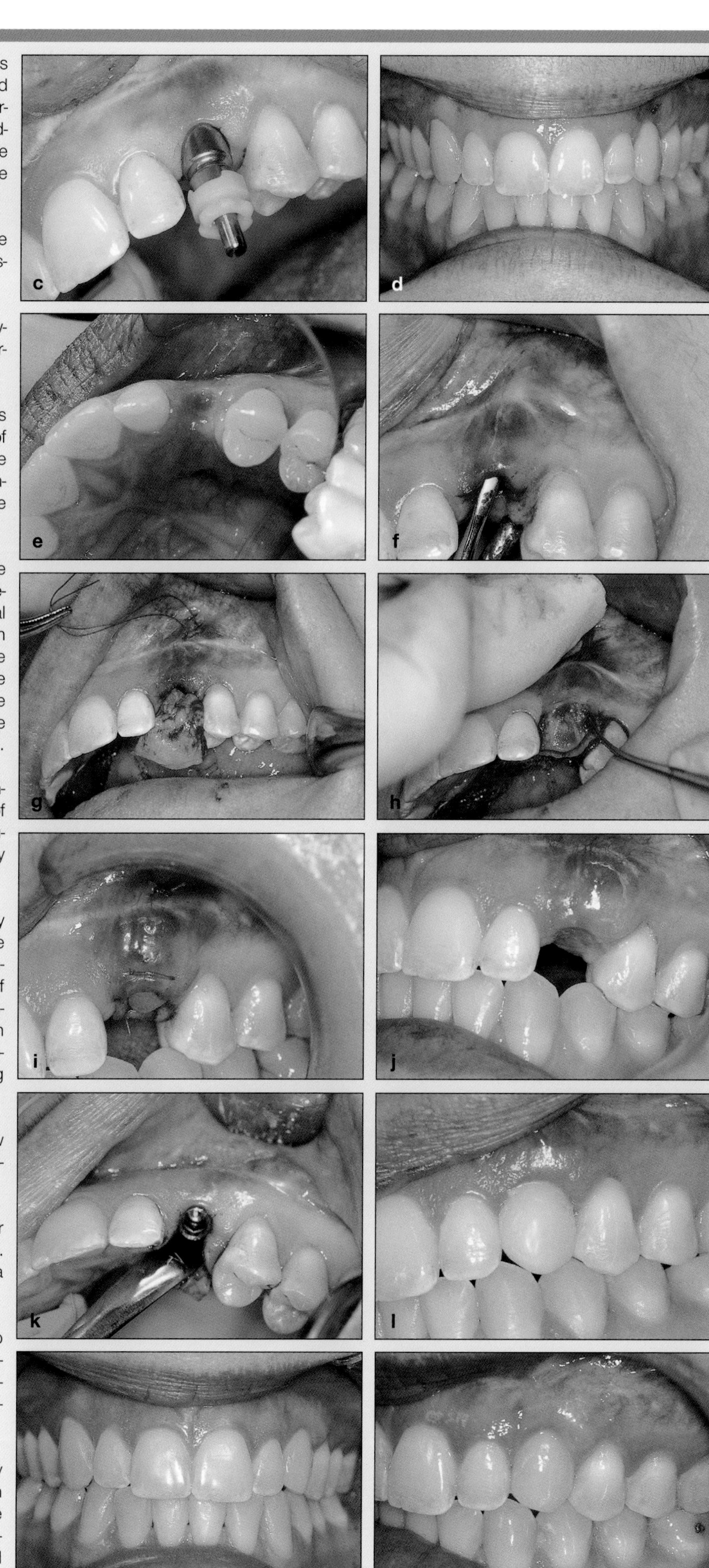

Fig 5-33c A palatal peninsula approach was used to gain access for implant placement and surgical indexing. This approach conserves circulation to the buccal soft tissues while providing access and direct visualization of fixture depth relative to the palatal and crestal ridge crests during implant placement.

Fig 5-33d Two-week postoperative view. Note lack of canine eminence secondary to soft tissue shrinkage.

Fig 5-33e Two-month postoperative view showing that the morphology of the defect is primarily in the horizontal plane.

Fig 5-33f Partial-thickness horizontal incisions were made just coronal to the desired level of augmentation required for esthetic restorative emergence. These incisions define the entrance or "mouth" of the closed recipient site and facilitate subsequent graft immobilization.

Fig 5-33g The subepithelial connective tissue graft is immediately transported to the prepared site, where it is attached to a horizontal mattress suture. This suture is initiated through the vestibule just apical to the depth of the recipient-site preparation and retrieved from the entrance of the recipient site, passed twice through the graft, and passed back out into the vestibule adjacent to the area where it entered.

Fig 5-33h Gentle apical tugging on the horizontal mattress suture is combined with the use of the blunt end of a membrane-placement instrument moistened with sterile saline to gently guide the graft into the site.

Fig 5-33i The apical horizontal suture is loosely secured to prevent coronal displacement of the graft by tissue edema. Similarly interrupted sutures are used to secure the coronal portion of the graft. The cover tissues demonstrate compromised circulation as anticipated based on previous history of the site. The closed approach provides the advantage of preserving circulation by avoiding releasing incisions.

Fig 5-33j Three-month postoperative view demonstrates complete restoration of small-volume soft tissue ridge defect.

Fig 5-33k Exposure of implant 5 months after placement via a palatal peninsula approach. Custom Protec abutments (Dentsply) and a provisional restoration were delivered.

Fig 5-33l The U-shaped palatal peninsula flap provided access for delivery of a custom temporary abutment and cementation of the provisional restoration while avoiding buccal releasing incisions.

Figs 5-33m and 5-33n One year after delivery of the final restoration. The closed approach preserved much-needed circulation at this site and avoided any additional soft tissue scarring. (Restoration by Dr Fred Witkoff, Coral Gables, FL.)

Subepithelial connective tissue graft performed in the recall period via a closed approach

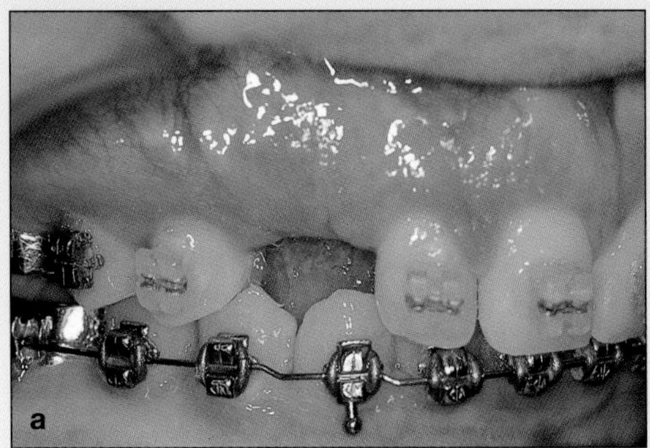

Fig 5-34a View of implant site prior to second-stage surgery. A palatal peninsula approach was used for placement and surgical indexing of a submerged implant.

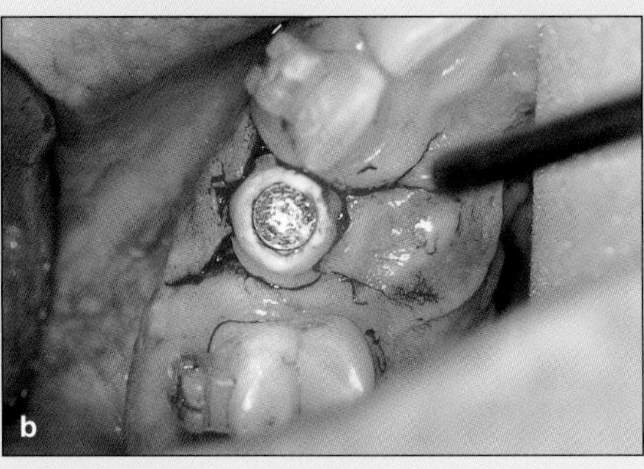

Fig 5-34b Occlusal view of second-stage surgery with delivery of custom ceramic abutment. Small beveled incisions through the buccal tissues were necessary to fully seat and secure the ceramic abutment on the 5.0-mm-diameter external hex implant (Nobel Biocare).

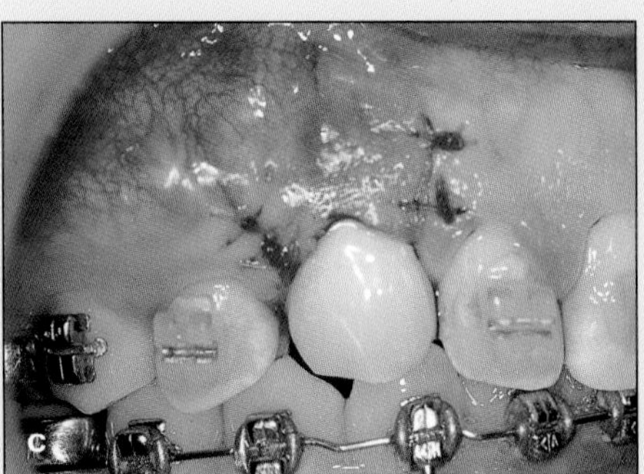

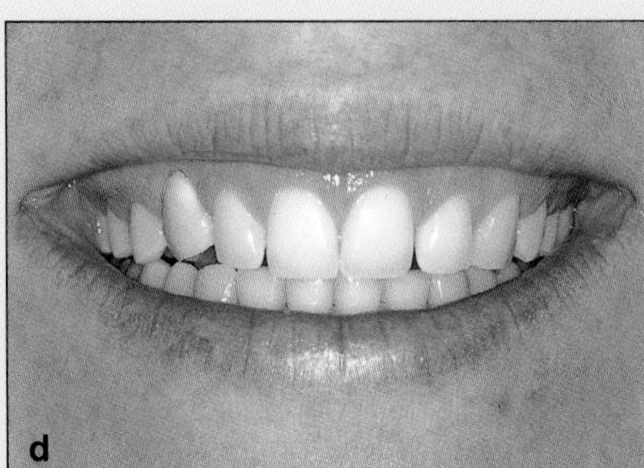

Fig 5-34c Primary closure of the abbreviated beveled incisions was accomplished after cementation of the provisional restoration with 4-0 chromic gut suture on a P3 needle.

Fig 5-34d Six months after delivery of the final restoration, a Miller class II recession defect and metal showthrough with tissue discoloration were evident at the implant site. Several factors contributed to the loss of soft tissue volume. The most significant factor was the placement of a large-diameter implant with slightly excessive buccal inclination. This was compounded by the use of a ceramic abutment, which caused excessive prominence of the implant restoration and led to soft tissue recession.

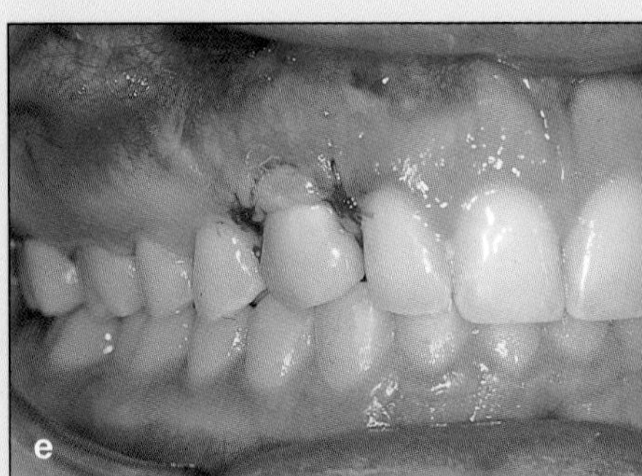

Fig 5-34e After mechanical reduction of the ceramic restoration, a subepithelial connective tissue graft was harvested, passively positioned, and immobilized within the closed recipient site.

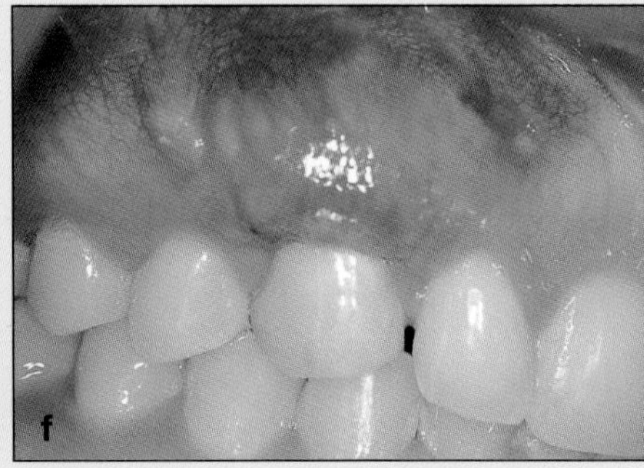

Figs 5-34f and 5-34g Two-week postoperative view demonstrates partial re-epithelialization of previously exposed donor tissue and apparent complete abutment coverage.

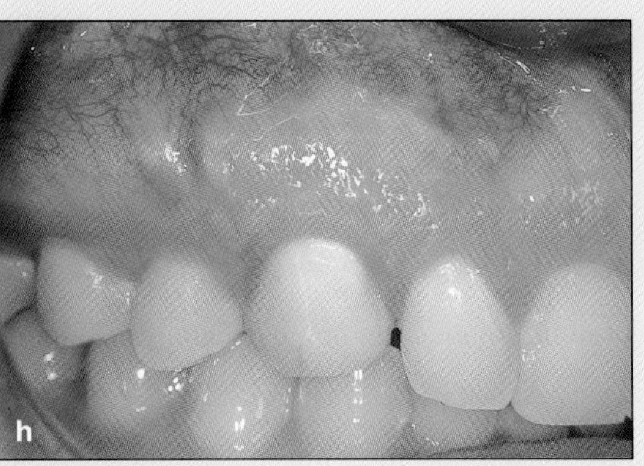

Fig 5-34h One-year postoperative view demonstrates complete abutment coverage and elimination of metal showthrough. Natural gingival esthetics have been restored and peri-implant soft tissue health is excellent. (Restoration by Dr Jose Rodriguez-Cepero, Miami, FL.)

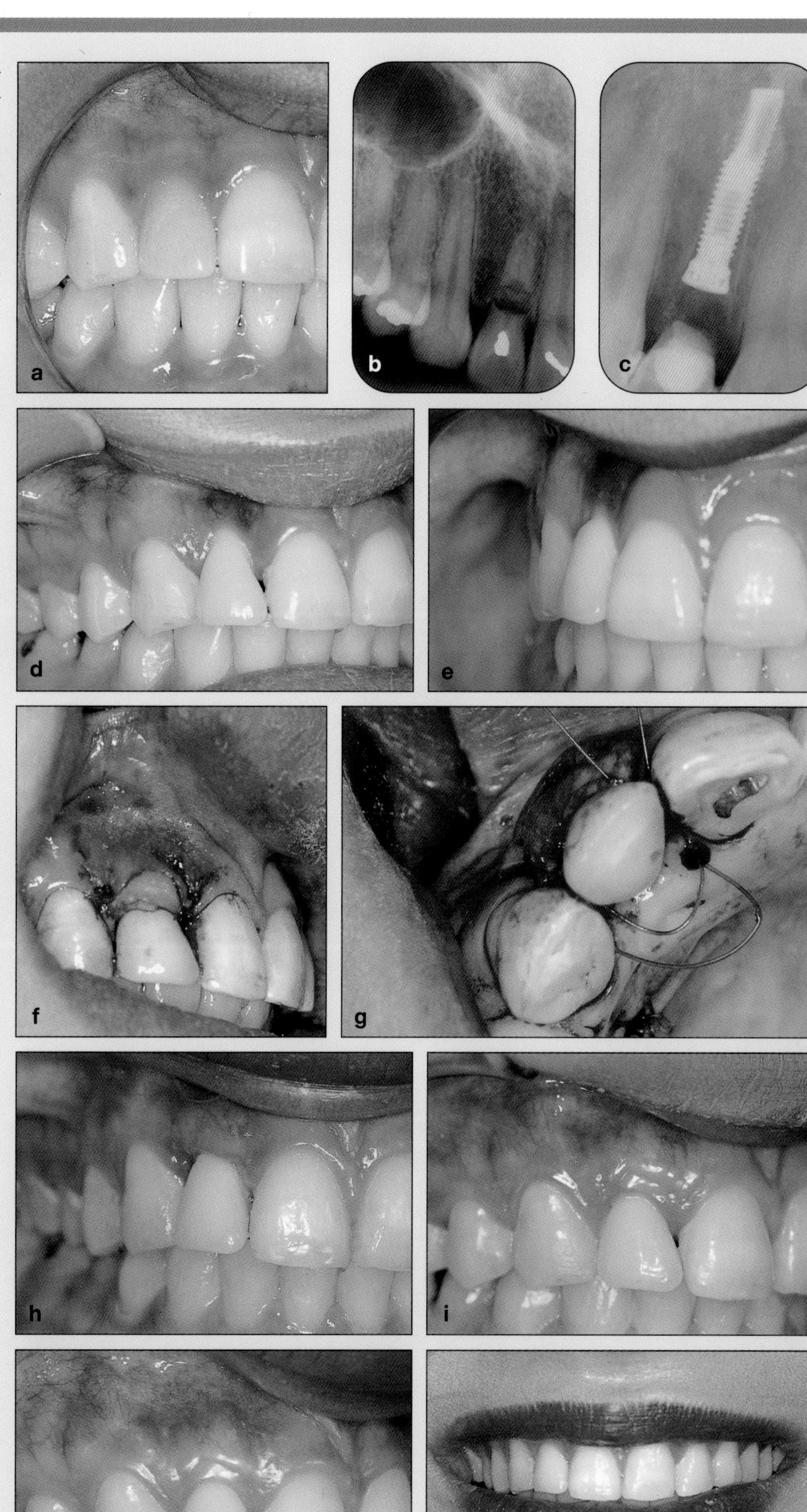

Fig 5-35a Preoperative view of failing right lateral incisor secondary to post-traumatic resorption in a patient with an extremely thin, scalloped periodontium. The surgical plan was to remove the tooth and perform immediate implant replacement with the Bio-Col alveolar ridge preservation technique. The patient opted not to proceed with recommended soft tissue grafting and accepted the risks, including possible implant failure and a nonrestorable esthetic defect.

Fig 5-35b Preoperative radiograph of failing lateral incisor. The small volume of interdental bone on the mesial contributes to blunting of the interdental papillae.

Fig 5-35c Postoperative radiograph. The axial inclination of the implant was adjusted to avoid further compromise to the interdental bone on the distal of the adjacent central incisor. The crown of the natural lateral incisor was modified into an ovate pontic and used to create a resin-bonded temporary Maryland fixed partial denture to optimally preserve soft tissue architecture and prevent transmission of micromotion during the osseointegration period.

Figs 5-35d and 5-35e One year after delivery of the final restoration, progressive soft tissue recession has occurred and peri-implant tissues are inflamed and in jeopardy of complete dehiscence. Surgical plan for correction was to perform abutment coverage procedure with subepithelial connective tissue graft via a closed approach.

Figs 5-35f and 5-35g Intraoperative views of abutment-coverage procedure. A subepithelial connective tissue graft was passively positioned in a closed recipient site and secured with an apical horizontal mattress suture and a cervical sling suture.

Fig 5-35h One-month postoperative view demonstrates complete epithelialization of previously exposed donor graft. Adequate soft tissue thickness has been restored and complete abutment coverage is evident.

Fig 5-35i One-year postoperative view demonstrates excellent peri-implant soft tissue esthetics and health. Papillae are still blunted.

Figs 5-35j and 5-35k Three-year postoperative view demonstrates regeneration of previously blunted mesial papilla. Excellent color match is evident and the tissue transformation and keratinization are complete. Reconstruction of this small-volume soft tissue defect was critical in this area of high esthetic importance, as evidenced by exposure in the relaxed smile position. (Restoration by Dr Ricardo Gonzales, Miami, FL.)

Postoperative period

During the first 24 to 48 hours following oral soft tissue surgery, the graft is nourished through diffusion from the recipient bed. Capillary proliferation begins within 24 hours, but an adequate blood supply is not established until the 7th or 8th postoperative day. Although fibrous attachment to the recipient site is complete by the 10th postoperative day, gingivoplasty should be delayed for 2 to 3 months. Intracrevicular implant prosthetic procedures should be delayed for 3 months or more to allow sufficient time for the development of a stable sulcus. Proceeding prior to this can result in soft tissue recession. Postoperative instructions include routine measures such as gentle pressure over the site for 4 to 6 hours after surgery; application of ice externally for 24 hours; and a liquid diet for 24 hours, followed by a puree diet for an additional week. In addition, patients should be told to limit themselves to light physical activity for 7 to 10 days following surgery.

Patients should be instructed that if postoperative bleeding occurs, they should apply gentle pressure with moistened gauze at the donor or recipient site. When root- or abutment-coverage procedures are performed, spontaneous bleeding may occur as late as 14 to 21 days following surgery as capillaries proliferate into the portion of the graft that covered the avascular root or abutment. Patients should be instructed to expect significant swelling at the recipient sites and to use donor site protective stents continuously for the first week, removing them only for oral hygiene maintenance.

If root or abutment coverage was performed, the patient is instructed to avoid brushing in the area. Initially, a cotton swab can be used to cleanse the area for the first 7 to 10 days. Subsequently, the author recommends the use of a Biotene Ultra Soft toothbrush (ICP Medical, St Louis, MO) to maintain oral hygiene for the following 4 to 6 weeks. The patient also should be instructed to avoid chewing hard foods in the surgical areas for 4 to 6 weeks after root- or abutment-coverage procedures.

Summary

This chapter provides the basis for the successful application of oral soft tissue grafting in implant therapy and a clear explanation of the indications, advantages, expected outcomes, and limitations of the most commonly used soft tissue grafting techniques. The modified palatal roll procedure is generally used to correct very-small-volume soft tissue defects simultaneously with abutment connection or nonsubmerged implant placement. This procedure is limited by the thickness and length of the pedicle that can be harvested from the palate in a specific area. The gingival graft technique has broad applicability in nonesthetic areas, where it rapidly provides keratinized tissue necessary to establish a stable peri-implant environment in edentulous and partially edentulous cases. For avulsive injuries that involve the alveolar ridge, use of sequential gingival grafts provides both the quantity and quality of tissue necessary for subsequent bone grafting procedures. The contemporary surgical technique for gingival grafting allows for success even when such injuries occur in esthetic areas. Because it is extremely versatile, the subepithelial connective tissue graft is the most commonly used oral soft tissue graft in areas of esthetic importance. Its greatest drawback is the need for several procedures to reconstruct large-volume defects at implant sites. Finally, the principles of oral soft tissue grafting presented in this chapter were the basis for the development of the VIP-CT flap, which is the subject of the next chapter.

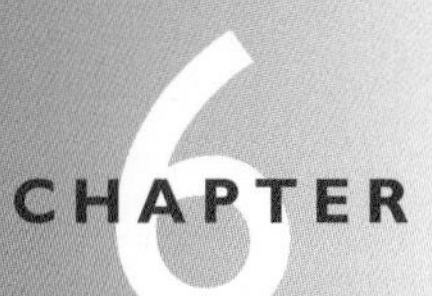

CHAPTER 6

Vascularized Interpositional Periosteal–Connective Tissue (VIP-CT) Flap

This chapter presents the rationale, biologic basis, and detailed surgical technique for the VIP-CT flap. The impetus for the development of this innovative soft tissue site-development technique was twofold. The author recognized the need for a technique that would allow successful reconstruction of large-volume soft tissue esthetic ridge defects with a single procedure. By maintaining a contiguous blood supply, use of a pedicled flap allows the transfer of a greater volume of soft tissue when compared to free soft tissue grafts, which undergo significant secondary soft tissue contraction. Furthermore, the author recognized the many advantages that a pedicle flap would provide when simultaneous hard and soft tissue esthetic implant site development was desired.

Although an axial-pattern palatal flap was preferable, the course of neurovascular structures through the palate from the greater palatine to incisive foramina precluded the development of such a flap with sufficient length for use in the anterior maxillary area. Instead, taking advantage of the abundant perfusion pressure available from the connective tissue–periosteal vascular plexus located adjacent to the incisive foramen, the author designed a random-pattern periosteal–connective tissue flap that would allow rotation of a vascularized pedicle to the anterior maxillary area, including the midline papillary area. Refinements in the initial flap design and surgical technique improved the ability to provide esthetic implant replacements at compromised anterior maxillary sites with large-volume combination ridge defects with a level of predictability not achieved through existing techniques and site-development protocols.

Rationale and Biologic Basis

Chapter 5 described several surgical techniques for enhancing soft tissue contours at edentulous sites in preparation for implant or conventional restoration; however, each technique has its own limitations. The modified palatal roll technique is limited by the thickness and length of the pedicle that can be harvested without damage to adjacent neurovascular structures or risk of sloughing of the cover flap. Thus, unfavorable palatal anatomy often excludes the use of this technique for significant soft tissue enhancement at implant sites in the maxillary anterior area. The poor color match that results at the recipient site often limits use of the gingival graft in esthetic areas. Although extremely versatile, the subepithelial connective tissue graft often requires several procedures to reconstruct large-volume soft tissue defects.The survival of free soft tissue grafts depends completely on the circulation at the recipient site; therefore, these grafts lack the biologic basis for predictable simultaneous hard and soft tissue reconstruction.

Currently accepted protocols for esthetic implant site development commonly involve staged reconstruction of hard and soft tissue ridge defects. In most instances, hard tissue grafting precedes soft tissue grafting, followed by implant placement. Large-volume hard tissue defects are first reconstructed with a combination of autogenous corticocancellous block bone grafts surrounded by a particulate mixture of autogenous cancellous bone and a xenograft bone mineral (Bio-Oss; Osteohealth, Shirley, NY) used as an osteoconductive volume expander. To achieve guided tissue regeneration, these composite grafts are usually covered with a bioabsorbable collagen membrane. After bone graft maturation (4 to 6 months), soft tissue grafting is performed either prior to, simultaneous with, or following implant placement. When the soft tissues at a particular recipient site are extremely thin or scarred, soft tissue augmentation prior to hard tissue grafting is indicated. This prepares the soft tissue envelope at the site by providing viable mesenchymal cells to contribute to bone graft healing. This also improves the structural integrity of the soft tissue and hence the handling characteristics during the bone graft surgery. In these instances, a minimum of 3 months is required for maturation of the soft tissue graft prior to proceeding with the bone graft procedure. Based on these existing protocols, site development typically involves two or three surgical procedures performed over a period of 9 to 12 months. Subsequently, an additional 4 to 6 months are needed for osseointegration and fine-tuning of soft tissue esthetics with provisional restorations and soft tissue "touch-up" procedures. Therefore, total treatment time with previously described techniques and protocols typically ranges from 13 to 18 months.

To overcome the limitations of the previously described techniques and protocols and to fulfill the need for predictable simultaneous hard and soft tissue site development in the maxillary anterior area, the author developed the vascularized interpositional periosteal–connective tissue (VIP-CT) flap. This innovative technique involves the development of a random-pattern periosteal–connective tissue flap from within the palatal soft tissues that is rotated into the recipient site and interpositioned beneath the recipient-site flap. The design of the donor- and recipient-site flaps allows tension-free closure of the cover flaps; the result is a true interpositional flap and a donor site that heals by primary intention. The flap, which consists of periosteum and connective tissue, depends for its survival on the connective tissue-periosteal vascular plexus supplied by the adjacent greater palatine artery as it approaches the incisive foramen.

Once developed, as described below, the flap is flexible enough to allow augmentation of edentulous sites between the ipsilateral premolar and central incisor areas. In addition, the flap has proven successful for vertical augmentation of the midline maxillary interdental papilla, allowing the re-creation of positive gingival architecture around central incisor implant replacements to serve as the focal point of the smile. Augmentation of the papilla between the central incisors or the midline papillary area can require a flap length-to-width ratio of 4:1 or greater. Because of close proximity to the greater palatine vessels, the flap has sufficient perfusion pressure from the subepithelial-periosteal vascular plexus to easily sustain flaps rotated to these areas. This should not be surprising because the abundant vascular supply in the oral and facial areas commonly allows the use of random-pattern flaps with length-to-width ratios of 5:1 for the reconstruction of oral and facial defects. Nevertheless, during the development phase of this procedure, the author used Doppler flow measurements taken before flap elevation and after flap rotation and immobilization to verify maintenance of an intact circulation (Figs 6-1a and 6-1b). Initially, an abbreviated tension-releasing cutback incision made in the base of the flap at the pivot point (point of maximum tension) was required in a significant number of cases for passive rotation to the desired recipient site. Again, the perfusion pressure to the flap is generous enough to prevent vascular embarassment in these circumstances, as long as the length-to-width ratio of the flap falls within the pa-

Rationale and biologic basis for VIP-CT flap

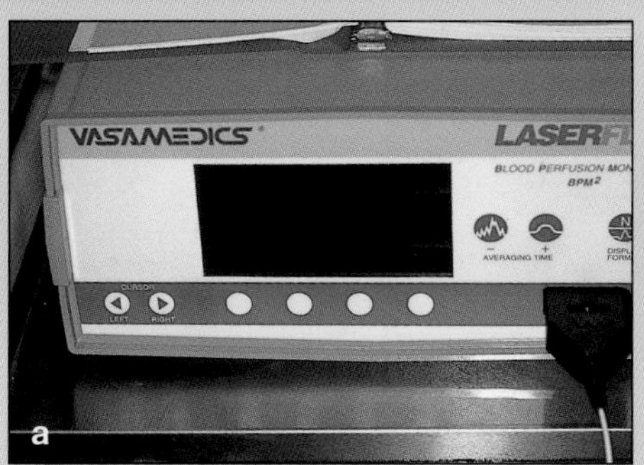

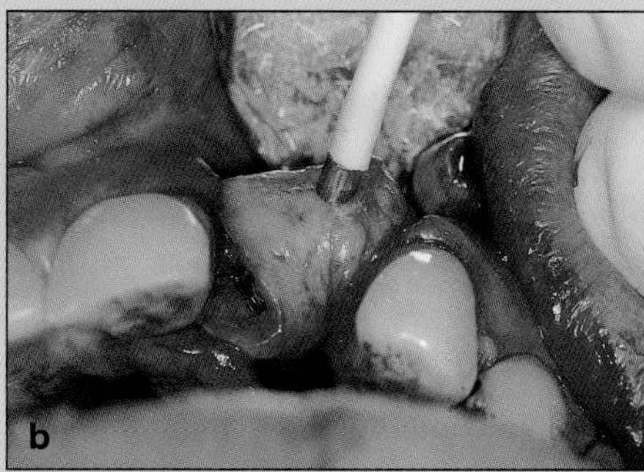

Figs 6-1a and 6-1b *(a)* During the development phase of the VIP-CT flap, Doppler flow measurements (Laserflo BPM[2]; Vasamedics, Eden Prairie, MN) were used to verify the maintenance of intact circulation to the flaps once they were passively rotated into their recipient sites. In addition, measurements were recorded in order to compare the relative effects that tension-releasing cutback incisions versus subperiosteal elevation and undermining techniques had on flap circulation. The trends that were observed indicated that subperiosteal undermining preserved flap circulation and facilitated tension-free rotation. Therefore, tension-releasing cutback incisions, which in some cases diminished circulation, especially in shallow palates, were subsequently avoided whenever possible. In addition, measurements verified maintenance of intact circulation for flap length-to-width ratios approaching 5:1, allowing for augmentation of the midline central papilla. *(b)* Laser Doppler probe verifies circulation to connective tissue margin of the VIP-CT flap after passive rotation to an anterior maxillary site.

rameters discussed above. Nevertheless, subsequent refinement of the surgical technique to include subperiosteal undermining of the base of the flap across the midline of the palate made virtually obsolete the use of tension-releasing cutback incisions. This modification also greatly simplified the surgical procedure.

The advantages of the VIP-CT flap technique in esthetic implant therapy include the ability to perform large-volume soft tissue augmentation at esthetic sites with a single procedure, maintenance of an intact vascular supply, excellent esthetic blending at the recipient site, minimal postsurgical shrinkage, and a minimally invasive donor-site wound. Of greatest significance, the pedicled blood supply, derived from the connective tissue–periosteal vascular plexus, provides a biologic basis for predictable simultaneous hard and soft tissue esthetic implant site development even at compromised sites. Thus, treatment time and patient inconvenience are dramatically reduced. Furthermore, there is clinical evidence that when the VIP-CT flap is used to enhance the soft tissue cover prior to or simultaneous with bone grafting, bone graft maturation is enhanced (Fig 6-2). This is consistent with our understanding of the two-phase theory of osteogenesis and our experience in maxillofacial reconstruction.

Advantages of the VIP-CT flap:

- Allows large-volume soft tissue augmentation at esthetic sites with a single procedure
- Maintains an intact vascular supply (random pattern)
- Provides excellent esthetic blending at the recipient site
- Minimizes postsurgical shrinkage
- Allows for primary closure of the donor site
- Dramatically reduces treatment time
- Dramatically reduces patient inconvenience
- Enhances bone graft maturation
- Provides a biologic basis for predictable simultaneous hard and soft tissue esthetic implant site development

Simultaneous hard and soft tissue implant site development

Simultaneous hard and soft tissue grafting with a free soft tissue autograft draped over a block or particulate bone graft lacks any biologic basis for predictable success and ignores two basic principles of oral soft tissue grafting: *(1)* the recipient bed (composite bone graft and membrane) does not easily allow for rigid immobilization of the soft tissue graft, and *(2)* the majority of the recipient bed is unable to vascularize the graft. Therefore, decreased volume yields from the soft tissue graft and possible compromise of the underlying bone graft are to be expected. Although it has been theorized that a free soft tissue graft immediately adapted over a bone graft will function as a biologic membrane barrier, providing guided bone regeneration, one must consider that revascularization of the soft tissue graft in these situations is, for the most part, dependent on the cover flap. Because revascularization of the soft tissue graft gradually occurs over the first 7 to 10 postoperative days, phase-two bone graft healing, which begins between 10 and 14 days postoperatively, is subject to a compromise due to lack of vascular and cellular contributions normally provided by the surrounding soft tissues. Furthermore, when an edentulous site is re-entered for implant placement 4 to 6 months after hard tissue augmentation, as described above, vascularization of the composite bone graft system is seldom suffi-

Enhanced bone graft outcomes via simultaneous rotation of a vascularized periosteal-connective tissue flap

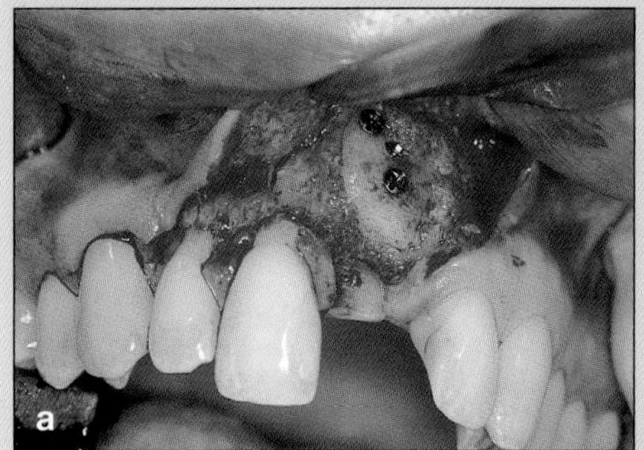

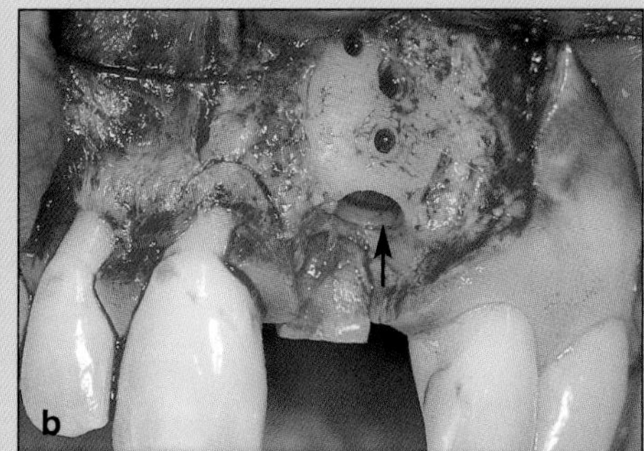

Fig 6-2a Re-entry to site 4 months after simultaneous hard and soft tissue site development for implant placement and esthetic crown lengthening of adjacent dentition. A corticocancellous block bone graft was secured at the prepared recipient site with three Mincro rigid fixation screws (Osteomed, Addison, TX). Autogenous particulate bone and Bio-Oss mixture in a 1:1 ratio was condensed around the periphery of the block. The VIP-CT flap was large enough to completely cover the bone graft with intact periosteum, thereby eliminating the need for a barrier membrane in this case.

Fig 6-2b Clinical evidence of advanced integration of both corticocancellous block and particulate bone grafts. It is difficult to discern where the edges of the block graft were initially located. Bleeding from the surface of the grafts demonstrates revascularization. The palatal wall of the osteotomy is within the recently grafted block bone graft *(arrow)*. The cancellous portion of the block graft will contribute to osseointegration of the implant.

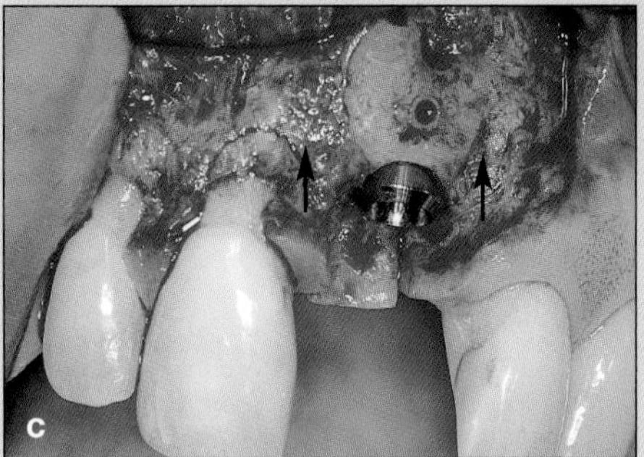

Fig 6-2c One-piece nonsubmerged implant (Straumann USA) has been placed according to a surgical guide, which was also used to guide crown extension of adjacent teeth. Note advanced integration of Bio-Oss particles within the surrounding particulate graft *(arrows)*.

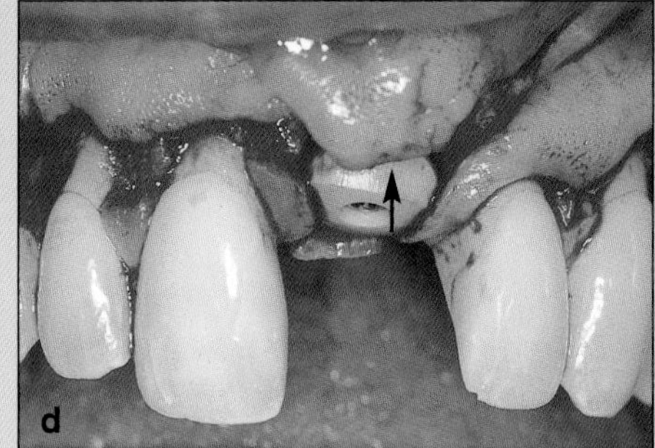

Fig 6-2d Upon reapproximation of the cover flap, the thickness of the soft tissue in the area where the VIP-CT flap was rotated into the site is notably increased *(arrow)* compared to that found in the adjacent areas. Minimal postoperative soft tissue shrinkage occurs following use of the VIP-CT flap compared to that normally observed following free soft tissue grafting techniques.

cient to nourish free soft tissue grafts performed at that time. Although a supraperiosteal dissection and a modified flap design (chapter 3) are used to maximize the available blood supply at the recipient site, at best the site provides a partially vascular recipient bed. This often results in some degree of shrinkage of the free soft tissue autograft placed at these partially avascular recipient sites, thus requiring additional procedures to gain sufficient soft tissue augmentation to ensure esthetic restorative emergence. In summary, when free soft tissue grafts are used as part of simultaneous hard and soft tissue implant site development, a successful outcome is dependent on selecting a case where all clinical parameters related to achieving the desired hard and soft tissue augmentation are favorable. Such factors include favorable history leading to tooth loss, favorable osseous defect morphology, use of autogenous bone, the presence of good-quality soft tissues at the site, and the absence of recognized anatomic limitations, as discussed in chapter 2. In clinical practice, this ideal set of circumstances rarely presents itself. Instead, patients with large-volume hard and soft tissue esthetic ridge defects as well as those presenting with large-volume combination esthetic ridge defects usually have significant history resulting in tooth loss that compromised the area and led to the ridge defects with unfavorable morphologies, to compromised soft tissues, and in a significant percentage of cases, to one or more anatomic limitations that further hinder successful site-development efforts.

Conversely, it is well recognized based on our experience in maxillofacial reconstruction that the addition of vascularized soft tissue flaps improves the potential volume yields of autogenous bone grafts by providing additional circulation and a source of healing-capable mesenchymal cells derived from connective tissue to support osteogenesis, as described in the two-phase theory of osteogenesis.[1] The additional vascularity and cellularity provided by use of a pedicled flap in simultaneous hard and soft tissue implant site development improves the predictability of the result obtained and expands the indications of this simultaneous approach to include the compromised sites most often encountered in clinical practice.

When simultaneous hard and soft tissue reconstruction is performed with the VIP-CT flap, site development is completed in 4 months. Soft tissue refinement or touch-up procedures are then performed at the time of implant placement. Average treatment time is thus reduced from 13 to 18 months to just 8 to 10 months for large-volume hard and soft tissue combination defects (see chapter 2).

Provisional restoration following use of the VIP-CT flap for large-volume hard and soft tissue reconstruction

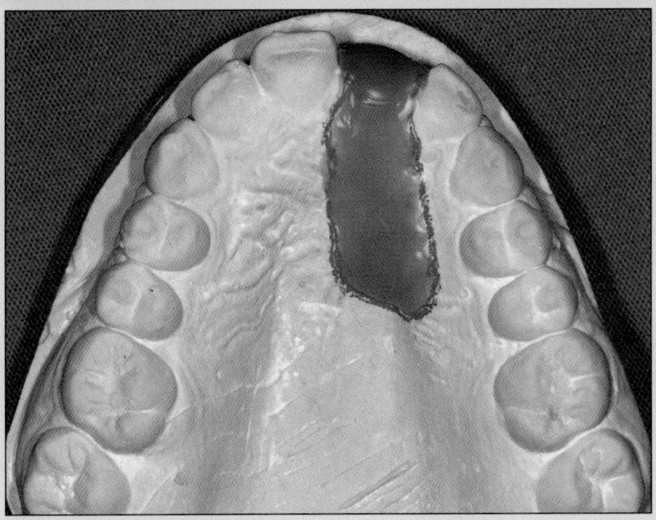

Fig 6-3a Diagnostic cast altered by wax relief of donor and recipient sites for VIP-CT flap. There is a large-volume combination defect involving the left central incisor site. Simultaneous hard and soft tissue reconstruction is planned with the VIP-CT flap. A pontic tooth is adapted on the ridge after the wax relief of the grafted area has been added. Next, using this altered cast, an Essex provisional restoration will be fabricated.

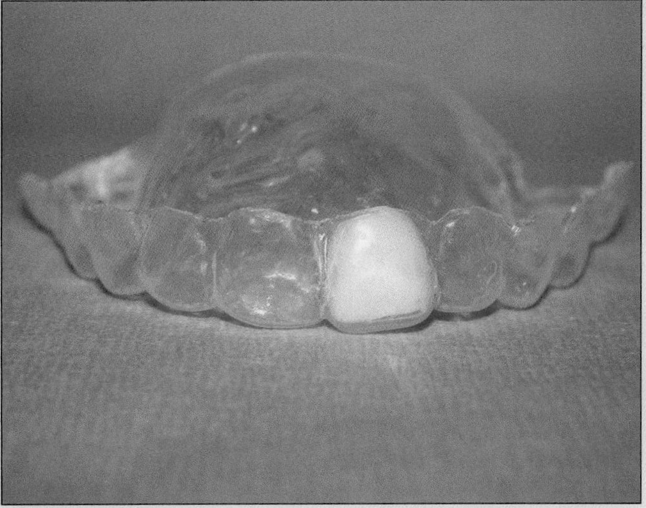

Fig 6-3b Essex-type provisional restoration fabricated by surgical team using 0.08 mm Visacryl material and the MiniSTAR device. The edges of the provisional are polished and disinfected for immediate delivery following the surgical procedure and typically are used to provide an interim provisional restoration that protects the palatal donor sites and avoids impingement and transmission of micromotion to the bone and soft tissue recipient site during the first 10 to 14 days following surgery, after which a more definitive interim provisional restoration is delivered by the restorative dentist.

General Considerations

As in subepithelial connective tissue grafting, the size and shape of the donor palate may limit the use of the VIP-CT flap technique. For instance, in a shallow palate, the flap width obtainable may be as small as 5 mm, limiting the ability to rotate the flap beyond the first premolar or canine area. Therefore, preoperative assessment of the donor site is critical. In addition, use of the VIP-CT technique results in excess tissue bulk in the anterior palate, which prohibits the use of a removable provisional prosthesis in the initial postoperative period. Use of a removable provisional prosthesis not only jeopardizes the circulation to the flap secondary to compression but also may interfere with healing of the cover flaps secondary to the introduction of micromotion. Furthermore, the increased soft tissue bulk in the palate may prohibit the possibility of using a pre-existing removable prosthesis, even with significant modifications.

In the author's experience, provisionalization is best accomplished initially with an Essex retainer modified to house a pontic tooth or teeth at the graft site and provide full palatal coverage. This type of provisional restoration protects the surgical site and provides an esthetic solution for the patient during the initial healing period of 10 to 14 days. Prior to surgery, a diagnostic cast of the maxillary arch is obtained. The cast is altered by adding wax at the deficient site to simulate the proposed hard and/or soft tissue augmentation. In addition, wax relief of the cast is applied to simulate the increased palatal soft tissue bulk that results from the rotated interpositional flap (Fig 6-3a). Subsequently, one or more selected pontic teeth are secured at the edentulous site and 0.08 mm Visacryl material is used in the MiniSTAR device (Great Lakes Orthodontics, Tonawanda, NY). The edges of the Essex provisional restoration are polished using an assortment of polishing burs and stones and disinfected for delivery at the time of surgery (Fig 6-3b).

After initial healing (10 to 14 days), a provisional composite resin-bonded fixed restoration is then recommended to support and sculpt the soft tissue architecture at the site and can be used until the subsequent implants are ready to be restored. Alternatively, an Essex provisional restoration without palatal coverage can be used. The resultant excess palatal tissue provides an additional source of connective tissue should soft tissue touch-up procedures be indicated following implant placement or abutment connection. It should be noted, however, that even in severe ridge defects the presence of this excessive soft tissue bulk palatal to the emerging implant restorations often camouflages blunted papillary tissues and should be maintained unless it is uncomfortable for the patient or interferes with phonetics.

As discussed above, the VIP-CT flap technique involves the development of an interpositional periosteal–connective tissue flap from within the palatal soft tissues, which is passively rotated anteriorly for reconstruction of soft tissue deficiencies existing in the ipsilateral maxillary premolar, canine, and incisor regions. The flap design is identical whether the procedure is performed prior to implant placement, at the time of implant placement, or during the osseointegration period. When the procedure is performed prior to implant placement, a split-thickness recipient site is recommended. When the technique is performed at the time of implant placement, the recipient-site flap should be full thickness in the area of osteotomy preparation and modified to partial thickness apically, again providing a means of immobilizing the flap to a partially vascularized recipient site (as discussed in chapter 5). When the procedure is performed in conjunction with hard tissue grafting, the surgical site is extended peripherally beyond the bone graft area with split-thickness dissection, thus providing a means of immobilizing the flap to a partially vascularized recipient site. In addition, the attached buccal tissues and papillary areas adjacent to the site can be de-epithelialized, providing another vascularized area for flap immobilization. Despite the pedicled blood supply to the VIP-CT flap, such maneuvers are consistent with good surgical principles. Alternatively, the flap can be secured directly to a block bone graft using sutures passed through transosseous perforations made with a small wire-passing bur.

Careful subperiosteal elevation during flap development will yield an intact periosteum, which aids in the ability to rigidly immobilize the flap at the periphery of the exaggerated recipient site or directly to the block bone graft. Any portion of the bone graft not covered by the VIP-CT flap should be covered by an absorbable collagen membrane. In order to predetermine this, the author suggests that the VIP-CT flap be developed immediately following the rigid fixation of the block bone graft in the area. Next, passive rotation of the VIP-CT flap over the secured bone graft will demonstrate the amount of coverage obtainable. The surgeon should keep in mind that stretching the flap to obtain more coverage of the bone graft is contraindicated, as this will compromise circulation to the flap margin. Subsequently, particulate graft material is packed around the periphery of the block graft, and the absorbable collagen membrane is appropriately sized and adapted over those portions of the bone graft that will not be covered by the VIP-CT flap. Following this procedural sequence will facilitate completion of the surgery and ensure guided bone regeneration for the entire hard tissue graft at the site.

Potential Complications

Complications experienced by the author during the development phase of this technique were limited to donor-site sloughing and dehiscence of recipient-site incisions. Donor-site sloughing occurs when the subepithelial plane of dissection results in a thin palatal soft tissue cover flap with compromised circulation. In addition, when deep palatal rugae are present, the surgeon may inadvertently "buttonhole" the palatal cover flap, resulting in exposure of denuded palatal bone at the site. When this occurs, it is extremely painful for the patient. Use of a palatal stent or interim provisional restoration fabricated on a master cast that has been altered by wax relief in the areas mentioned above minimizes the negative impact on the patient when one of these technical errors occurs during surgery. On several occasions, dehiscence was experienced at the recipient-site incisions following a VIP-CT flap procedure. Two distinct causes were attributed to the observation of problematic wound healing in these areas. Initially, the author used a dual-incision approach for development of the VIP-CT flap. In two cases, the epithelium harvested with the flap was incompletely excised before the pedicled flap was interposed beneath the recipient-site flap, resulting in persistent swelling of the mesial releasing incision. Subsequent exploration of the wound, excision of wound margins, and re-closure resolved the problem without compromise to the final result. In addition, the author noted that when large-volume hard and soft tissue combination defects were simultaneously reconstructed with autogenous corticocancellous block grafts and the VIP-CT flap, the large amount of coronal advancement of the exaggerated curvilinear recipient-site flaps routinely resulted in coaptation of the undersurface of the flap over the epithelial surfaces of the attached tissue at the buccal ridge crest as well as the papilla and col adjacent to the site. Problematic wound healing was subsequently avoided by using a single-incision approach for the dissection and by routinely de-epithelializing the col, papillary areas, and buccal gingival surfaces around the adjacent dentition. In fact, significant improvements in wound healing and incision-line esthetics were observed after incorporating these modifications into the procedure. Unexpectedly, the author also observed improvement in height and volume of the interdental papilla treated in this manner, presumably due to survival of the vascularized pedicle flap interposed between the de-epithelialized col and papilla and the coronally advanced recipient-site flap.

Another observation commonly noted as a result of correction of large-volume hard and soft tissue defects with the VIP-CT flap was temporary loss of vestibular depth at the sites due to the dramatic coronal advancement of the recipient flap obtained through the use of exaggerated curvilinear-beveled incisions. Most often this is easily managed with the use of a CO_2 laser to plasty the mucosal tissues in the area. In some cases, apical repositioning of the recipient flap was necessary to realign the mucogingival junction, thereby improving esthetics at the site.

Surgical Procedure

The surgeon begins by first outlining and preparing the recipient site and then proceeds to donor-site preparation. An exaggerated curvilinear-beveled flap design is used at the recipient site, as described in chapters 3 and 5. Abbreviated vertical releasing incisions are made on the palate at the mesial and distal aspect of the recipient site. This allows full exposure of the ridge crest for hard tissue grafting or implant placement. The palatal incision at the distal aspect of the recipient site parallels the gingival margin on the oral aspect of the adjacent tooth (Fig 6-4a). After recipient-site preparation, donor-site preparation begins by extending this incision horizontally to the distal aspect of the second premolar. To facilitate subsequent closure of the donor site, the orientation of this incision should be slightly beveled and follow a path approximately 2 mm apical to the free gingival margins of the canine and premolar teeth (see Fig 6-4a). As in the single-incision technique for harvesting a free subepithelial connective tissue graft (see chapter 5), sharp dissection is then used internally to create a split-thickness palatal flap in the premolar area. The subepithelial dissection is carried anteriorly toward the distal aspect of the canine. The surgeon should be careful to maintain adequate thickness of the palatal cover flap to avoid sloughing. In most cases, the dissection will have to be deeper in the area of the palatal rugae to avoid perforating the cover flap (Fig 6-4b).

Next, a vertical incision is made internally through the connective tissue and periosteum at the distal extent of the subepithelial dissection, as far apically as possible without damaging the greater palatine neurovascular structures. Using a Buser periosteal elevator and a membrane-placement instrument, the surgeon then carefully elevates the resultant periosteal–connective tissue layer, beginning in the second premolar area and working toward the anterior extent of the dissection (see Fig 6-4b). In most cases, this careful subperiosteal dissection will yield intact periosteum on the undersurface of the pedicle, which will aid in subsequent rigid immobilization of the graft. Furthermore, intact periosteum potentially provides osteoblastic activity if applied over a bone graft when simultaneous hard and soft tissue site development is performed. If difficulty is encountered in maintaining the integrity of the periosteum when subperiosteal elevation is performed, the author finds it useful to perform subperiosteal elevation alternately at the mesial and distal extents of the donor site until the dissections converge. A second incision is then initiated under tension internally at the apical extent of the previous vertical incision and extended horizontally anterior to the distal aspect of the canine. The outline of the periosteal–connective tissue pedicle is now complete. Limiting the incisions to the anatomic landmarks given ensures that the margin of the pedicle is safely harvested from the palatal area where the thickest amount of connective tissue is available without risk of damage to adjacent neurovascular structures. Next, a Buser periosteal elevator is used to carefully elevate the periosteal–connective tissue pedicle and undermine the full thickness of palatal mucosa and periosteum at the base of the pedicle to or beyond the midline of the palate (Fig 6-4c). This subperiosteal elevation or undermining begins at the distal aspect of the dissection in the area of the second premolar and is carried anteriorly toward but short of the incisive foramen so as to avoid compromise to the neurovascular structures in this area. Doing so provides additional elasticity at the base of the pedicle to allow passive rotation to the recipient site without the need for a tension-releasing cutback incision. Thus, the two distinct planes of dissection performed have defined an interpositional periosteal–connective tissue pedicle flap without disrupting its circulation. The subepithelial plane is superficial to the greater palatine vessels but deep enough to avoid sloughing of the palatal cover flap. The subperiosteal plane is deep to the greater palatine vessels and limited anteriorly and posteriorly to avoid damage to the neurovascular structures as they course through the palate.

Tension-releasing cutback incisions extended into the base of the pedicle flap in order to allow passive ro-

Surgical technique for the VIP-CT flap

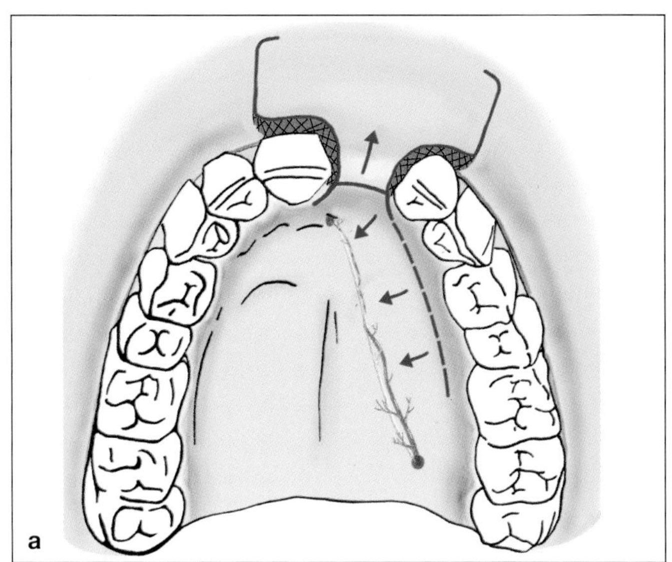

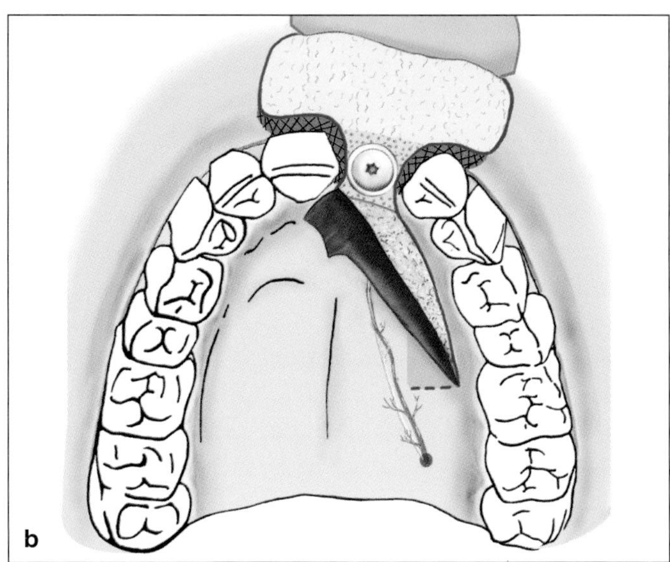

Figs 6-4a and 6-4b Exaggerated curvilinear-beveled incisions with tension-releasing cutback incisions outline the recipient-site flap when the VIP-CT flap is used as part of implant site development. When used for correction of large-volume soft tissue defects prior to implant placement, partial-thickness curvilinear-beveled incisions are initiated in the vestibule and sharp dissection is used to prepare a periosteal recipient site. When the VIP-CT flap is performed simultaneously with implant placement, partial-thickness incisions are also initiated in the vestibular area on the buccal aspect of the alveolar ridge but are continued as full-thickness incisions over the ridge crest. Full-thickness periosteal elevation is then limited to the area of implant placement (palatal and buccal ridge crest), and partial-thickness dissection is performed apically to create a periosteal recipient site on the buccal aspect of the ridge.

The abbreviated palatal crestal incisions located at the mesial and distal extent of the recipient site are always full thickness. Subperiosteal reflection is always performed to expose the palatal aspect of the ridge crest and to identify the location of the incisive foramen. This ensures that the base of the flap will be full thickness in this area, thereby preserving circulation and minimizing damage to the neurovascular structures. When simultaneous hard and soft tissue reconstruction is performed, all incisions that outline the recipient site are full thickness, and subperiosteal reflection is used to expose the bone graft recipient site. In cases where a high vaulted palate provides for the development of a VIP-CT flap with enough length to completely cover the bone graft and extend beyond the bone graft area, partial-thickness dissection can be extended peripherally to aid in subsequent immobilization of the periosteal–connective tissue flap over the bone graft with sutures. Once the recipient-site flap has been elevated, a fresh no. 15C scalpel is used to de-epithelialize the adjacent attached tissues on the buccal aspect of the ridge as well as the papilla and col adjacent to the site *(cross-hatched areas).* Doing so allows for overlap of the cover flap as it is coronally advanced to accommodate the increased contours from the hard tissue graft and/or the VIP-CT flap, thereby preventing wound-healing problems at the incision lines.

Subsequent to recipient-site preparation, the donor-site surgery begins. The full-thickness palatal incision located at the distal aspect of the recipient site is extended to parallel the gingival margin of the adjacent canine and premolar teeth *(dotted line).* This incision should be located 2 to 3 mm apical to the gingival margins and incorporate a slight apical bevel similar to the incision used when a free subepithelial connective tissue graft is harvested via the single-incision technique. Within this incision, a fresh no. 15C scalpel is reoriented parallel to the surface of the palatal tissues, and sharp dissection is used to define the subepithelial plane of dissection beginning at the distal end of the beveled incision (ie, distal of the second premolar, mesial of the first molar), working mesially to the distal aspect of the canine. As in the harvest of a free subepithelial connective tissue graft, the apical extension of the subepithelial dissection is determined by the size and shape of the palate *(shaded area).* Similarly, the plane of dissection should be deep enough to maintain adequate palatal cover tissue thickness to minimize unwanted postoperative sloughing. Returning to the distal extent of the subepithelial dissection, a vertical incision is made through the underlying connective tissue–periosteal layer. This incision defines the distal margin of the periosteal–connective tissue flap.

tation to the midline are rarely necessary when subperiosteal undermining is performed. When unavoidable, these relaxing incisions are initiated at the pivot point of flap rotation along the line of greatest tension. Although the line of greatest tension is the radius of the rotation arc created by the apical horizontal incision, the pivot point may not coincide with the termination of that incision. This is because the periosteal undermining causes a favorable displacement of the flap's pivot point and in most cases allows for tension-free rotation of the flap into the maxillary anterior area without the need for a tension-releasing cutback inci-

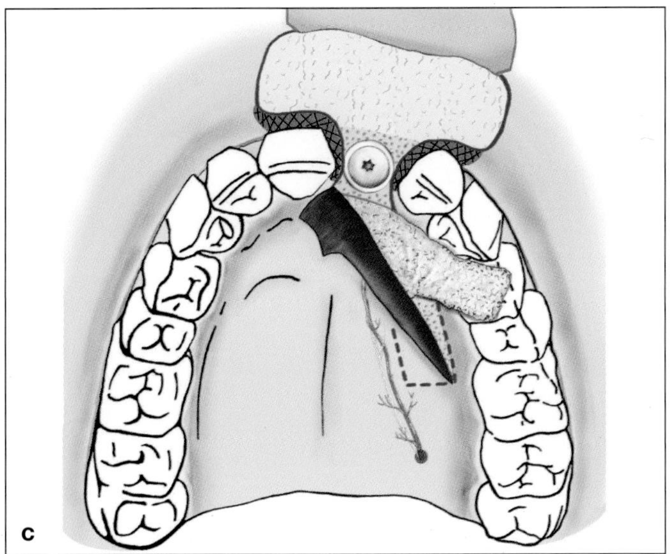

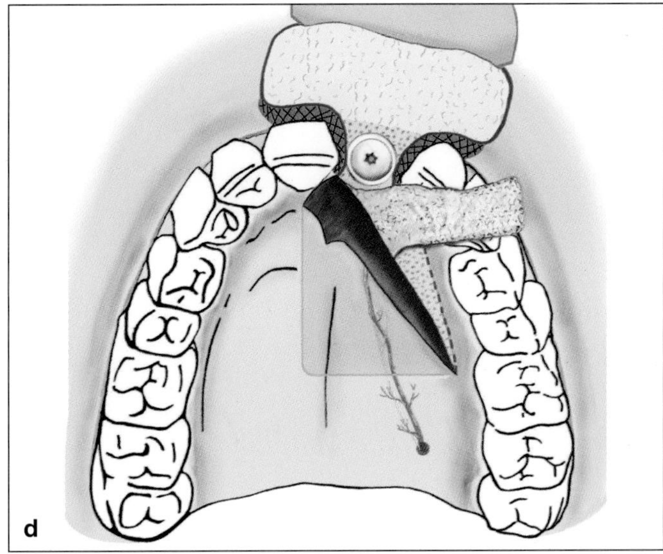

Figs 6-4c and 6-4d Next, the paddle end of a Buser periosteal elevator is used to continue the subperiosteal elevation initiated at the palatal aspect of the recipient site toward the distal extent of the donor-site dissection, defined by the vertical incision made through the connective tissue–periosteal layer. The apical extent of the subperiosteal elevation will again be limited by the height of the palate. The author finds it useful to carefully perform subperiosteal elevation alternately at the mesial and distal extents of the donor site until the dissections converge. This is especially useful if difficulty is encountered in maintaining the integrity of the periosteum when subperiosteal elevation is performed in the palatal rugae area, where inadvertent periosteal tearing is most likely to occur. Adson tissue forceps are then used to apply coronal tension on the resultant connective tissue–periosteal layer while a no. 15C scalpel is used to complete a horizontal incision through the apical extent of the elevated connective tissue–periosteal layer. This incision is initiated at the apical extent of the distal vertical incision and is extended mesially to the distal aspect of the canine. Although the periosteal–connective tissue flap is now defined, passive rotation to an anterior site will usually require subperiosteal undermining at the newly defined base of the flap. Although further extension of the apical horizontal incision will allow further rotation of the flap at this time, this should be reserved for instances when it is determined that subperiosteal undermining does not provide for passive flap rotation. Doing so preserves the maximum amount of circulation to the flap from the subepithelial periosteal–connective tissue vascular plexus derived from the adjacent greater palatine artery.

The paddle end of a Buser periosteal elevator and/or the blunt end of a membrane-placement instrument are used to carefully undermine the base of the flap via extension of the subperiosteal dissection across the midline of the hard palate. In most cases, it is convenient to begin at the distalmost and apicalmost extent of the donor site and move anteriorly toward the incisive foramen *(shaded area).* Adson forceps are periodically used to assess whether passive flap rotation into the recipient site has been achieved or whether additional undermining is necessary. Care must be taken to avoid damage to the neurovascular structures that course through the palate and exit through the incisive foramen. In most instances it is not necessary to extend the apical horizontal incision further or to make a tension-releasing cutback incision to achieve passive rotation of the flap into the recipient site. When it is necessary, the apical horizontal incision should not be extended mesial to the distal aspect of the canine, and any cutback incisions should be limited to approximately 2 to 3 mm in depth.

sion (Fig 6-4d). Nevertheless, when a tension-releasing cutback incision is necessary despite undermining, the surgeon must be careful to limit the length of the incision to avoid embarrassing the circulation. Intraoperative assessment of the area of greatest tension will guide placement of releasing incisions. Next, the flap is rotated into the recipient site and rigidly immobilized with sutures placed apically and/or laterally (Fig 6-4e). Alternatively, the flap can be secured directly to a block bone graft using sutures passed through transosseous perforations in the bone graft as previously discussed. CollaPlug absorbable collagen dressing (Centerpulse Dental, Carlsbad, CA) is used as an aid to hemostasis and to eliminate dead space in the donor harvest area (see Fig 6-4e). Finally, the donor and recipient sites are closed primarily with absorbable sutures, and gentle pressure is applied with moistened saline gauze for 10 minutes (Fig 6-4f).

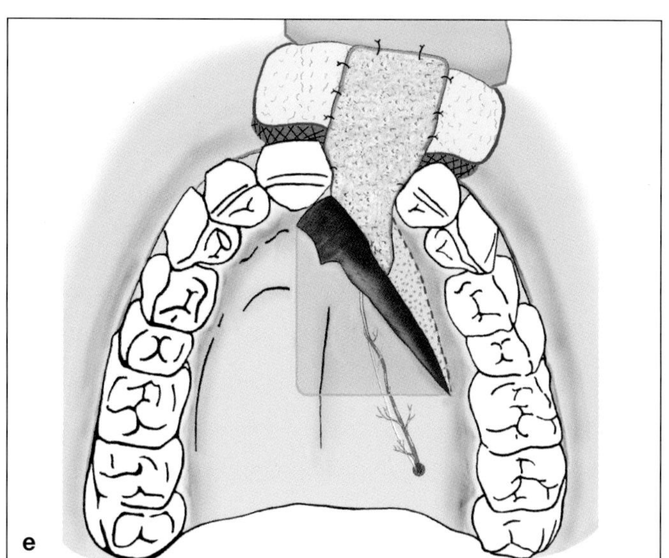

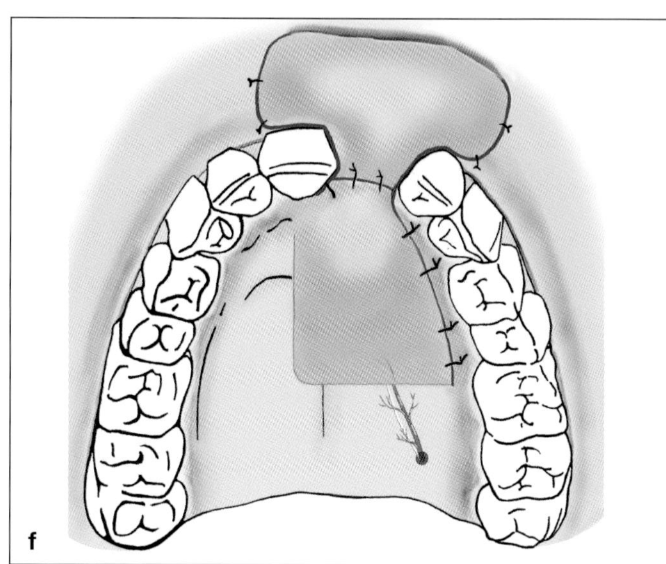

Figs 6-4e and 6-4f Immobilization of the VIP-CT flap. A horizontal mattress suture enters through the attached tissue on each side of the recipient site, passes twice through the flap, and exits through the attached tissue adjacent to the area in which it was initiated, where it is secured with a triple tie. Alternatively, when the adjacent gingival tissues and papillary and col areas have been de-epithelialized, simple interrupted sutures can be used to secure the pedicle through these areas, providing a vascularized recipient site. When a periosteal recipient site is available, additional sutures are secured along the periphery. When hard and soft tissue grafting is performed simultaneously and additional sutures are deemed necessary to achieve rigid immobilization, sutures can also be passed through perforations made through the block bone graft.

Subsequent to immobilization of the VIP-CT flap, the donor and recipient flaps are closed. Because of communication between the donor and recipient sites for interpositional flaps, closure is performed simultaneously. Following placement of CollaPlug absorbable collagen dressing to aid in hemostasis and obliterate dead space at the donor site, closure of the recipient site begins with sutures secured at the mesial and distal extent of the crestal incision. The curvilinear-beveled incisions are then closed with the sutures oriented to maintain the coronal advancement necessary to accommodate the increased buccal and vertical contours resulting from the underlying hard tissue graft, VIP-CT flap, or both. The design of the exaggerated curvilinear-beveled flap will cause some overlapping of the cover flap over the de-epithelialized papilla and col tissues as it is coronally advanced. A suture carefully oriented to pass through the cover flap and to exit through the attached tissue on the palatal aspect of the adjacent tooth will ensure intimate adaptation of the coronally advanced cover flap tissue to the underlying de-epithelialized papillary and col tissue. This results in excellent soft tissue esthetics and in many cases vertical soft tissue augmentation on the adjacent natural tooth. Finally, primary closure of the donor site is achieved by securing sutures in the area of the gingival embrasures of the adjacent canine and premolar teeth. Pressure is then applied over the recipient and donor sites with moistened saline gauze.

Clinical Experience

Use of the VIP-CT flap has consistently yielded excellent results in the correction of large-volume soft tissue esthetic ridge defects at implant sites in the anterior maxillary area. The amount of horizontal soft tissue augmentation obtained is consistently superior to that obtained with free soft tissue grafting techniques (Fig 6-5). In addition, the amount of vertical soft tissue augmentation typically obtained with a single VIP-CT flap exceeds that obtainable even when several free soft tissue grafts are performed (Fig 6-6). This technique has also proven useful in the treatment of compromised sites where existing soft tissues were poor in quality and severely scarred, rendering them inadequate to support required hard tissue site development (Fig 6-7), as well as a predictable means of resubmerging an implant in the anterior area when an unexpected soft tissue dehiscence compromises the final esthetic result (Fig 6-8).

The volume of tissue transfer routinely obtained with the VIP-CT flap has also allowed the camouflaging of small-volume combination hard and soft tissue ridge defects as well as the correction of large-volume soft tissue defects simultaneously with implant placement (Figs 6-9 and 6-10), as previously discussed. Of

Horizontal soft tissue reconstruction with the VIP-CT flap

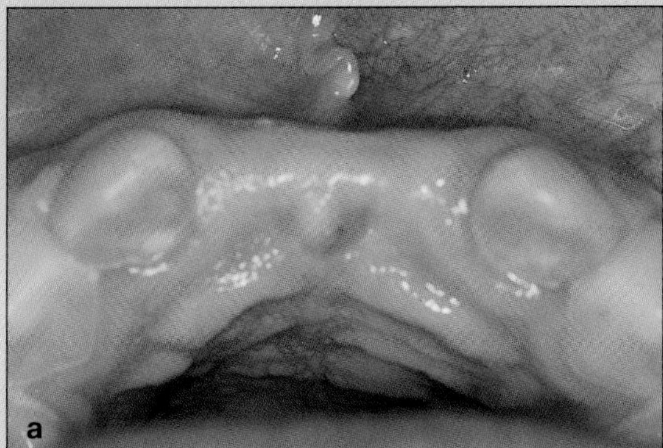

Fig 6-5a Preoperative occlusal view of edentulous maxillary incisor sites with large-volume soft tissue defect. Diagnostic waxup indicated a 3- to 4-mm horizontal deficiency of soft tissue contour needed for esthetic restorative emergence.

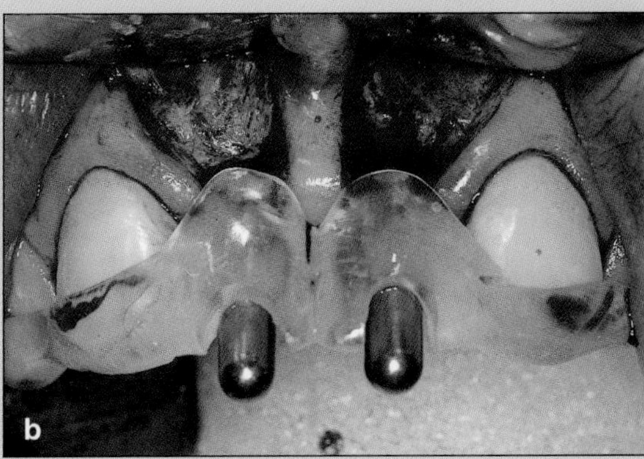

Fig 6-5b Recipient sites were outlined with curvilinear-beveled incisions. Full-thickness subperiosteal elevation was limited to the implant placement area (buccal and palatal ridge crest), while partial-thickness dissection was used to create periosteal recipient sites on the buccal aspect of the alveolar ridge.

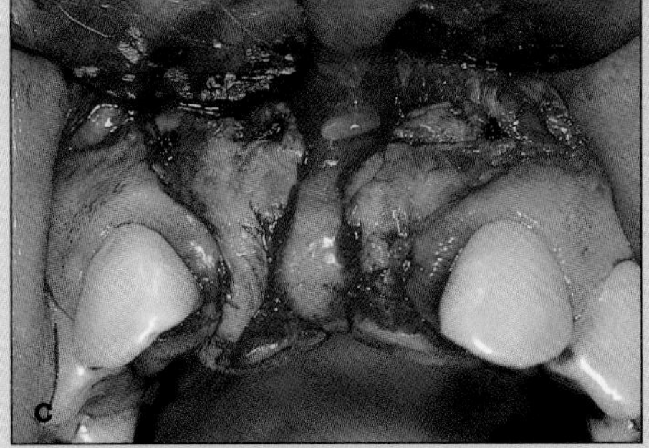

Fig 6-5c Following implant placement, bilateral VIP-CT flaps have been rotated into the recipient sites and secured to periosteum at the apical portion of the recipient sites. A supraperiosteal tunnel was created with sharp dissection under the midline tissues, and the VIP-CT flaps have been secured with a deep horizontal mattress suture.

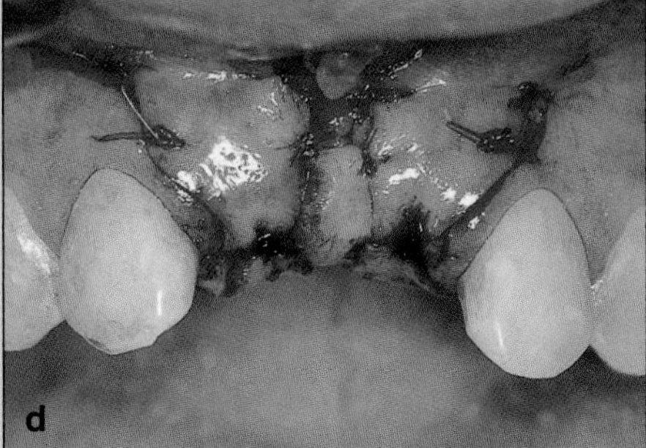

Fig 6-5d Donor and recipient sites were closed beginning with the crestal incision, proceeding with the curvilinear-beveled incisions on the buccal aspect of the ridge, and finishing with the palatal donor site, which had been dressed with CollaPlug absorbable collagen dressing.

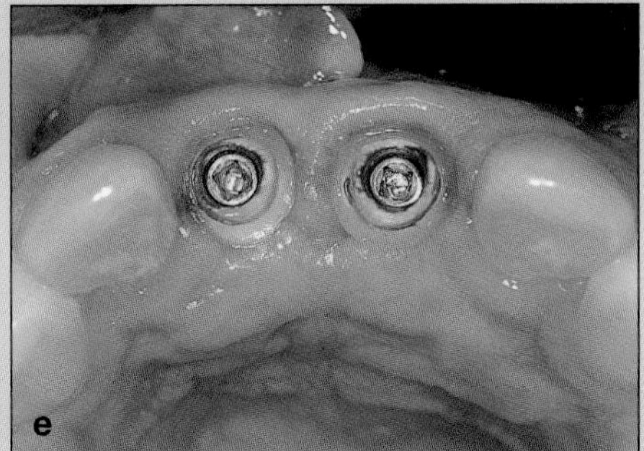

Fig 6-5e Six months after implant placement, tissue-punch exposure was used for delivery of custom abutments and provisional restorations. Six weeks later, the final restorations were delivered. Because no appreciable soft tissue shrinkage occurred, the need for chairside marginal adjustments was eliminated. In this case, 3.5 mm of horizontal soft tissue augmentation was obtained with the VIP-CT flap and midline tunneling technique.

greatest significance, the development and use of this technique provides the implant surgeon with a proven technique for predictable simultaneous hard and soft tissue esthetic implant site development at compromised anterior sites with large-volume combination ridge defects. Finally, the amount of vertical soft tissue augmentation afforded by this technique has allowed the re-creation of positive gingival architecture in situations where previous hard and soft tissue site-development techniques have fallen short.

These improved results are directly related to maintenance of intact circulation to the flap and decreased postsurgical contraction. In fact, resultant vertical soft tissue heights of tissue-punch specimens taken at the time of implant exposure following the use of the VIP-CT flap routinely measured between 6 and 8 mm, compared to presurgical vertical soft tissue dimensions that measured between 3 and 5 mm. While these soft tissue dimensions greatly enhance implant esthetics, they have provided the same prosthetic dilemma presented by excessively deep-placed implants. In the author's experience, these prosthetic challenges have been managed with surgical indexing of submerged implants or introduction of custom healing abutments when nonsubmerged implants were used (Figs 6-11 to 6-15).

Vertical soft tissue reconstruction with the VIP-CT flap

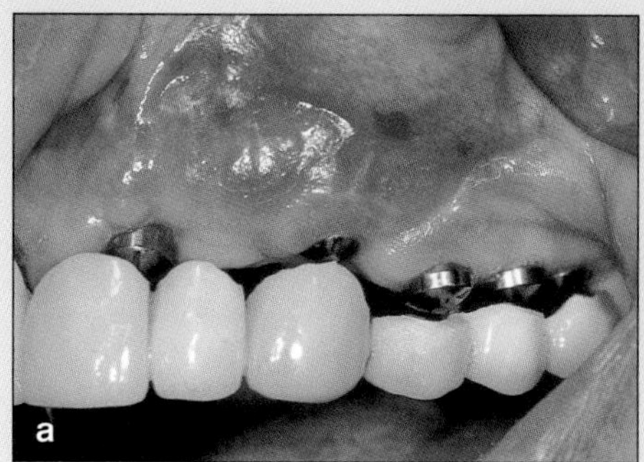

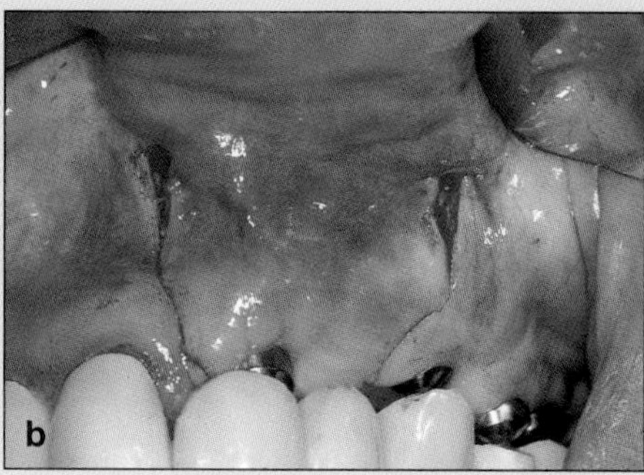

Fig 6-6a Preoperative view demonstrating large-volume soft tissue defect in the area between the central incisor and canine implants 2 months after five two-piece external hex implants (3i, West Palm Beach, FL) were placed via a nonsubmerged approach with temporary healing abutments. There is inadequate crestal bone height distal of the central incisor implant to support an interdental papilla.

Fig 6-6b Curvilinear-beveled incisions outline the recipient site. Sharp dissection is then used to create a periosteal recipient site.

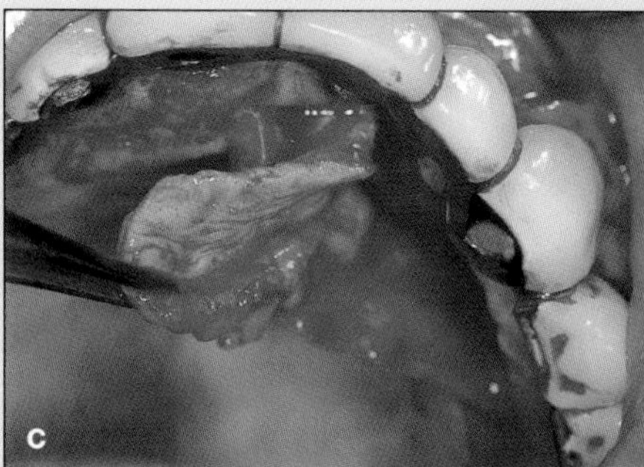

Fig 6-6c Following development of the VIP-CT flap, Adson tissue forceps are used to confirm that subperiosteal undermining is sufficient to achieve passive rotation of the flap into the recipient site.

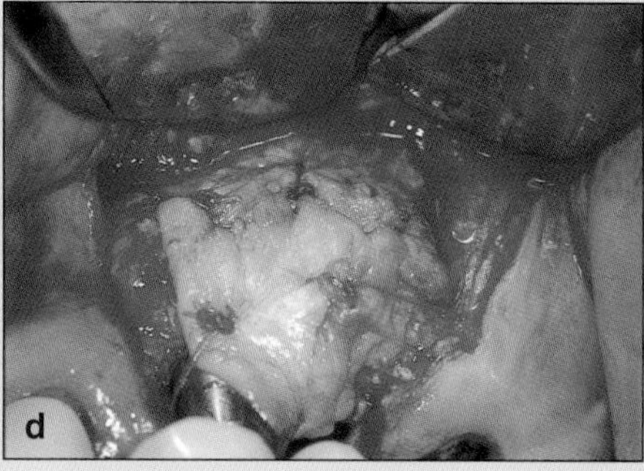

Fig 6-6d The VIP-CT flap has been passively positioned at the site and secured to the periosteum with 4-0 chromic gut sutures. Care is taken to avoid stretching the flap, which would compromise circulation.

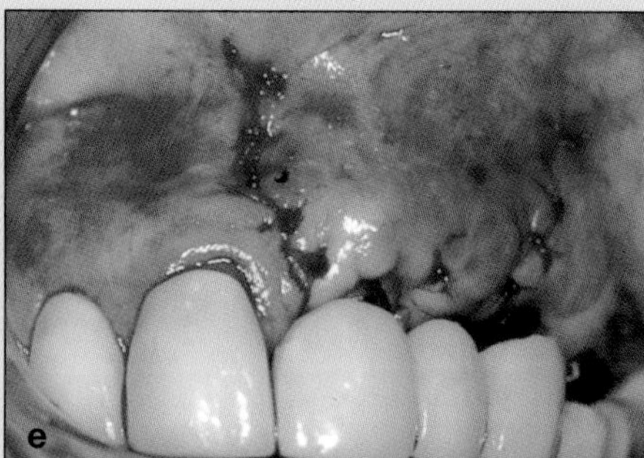

Fig 6-6e After coronal advancement, the cover flap is secured with 4-0 chromic gut sutures.

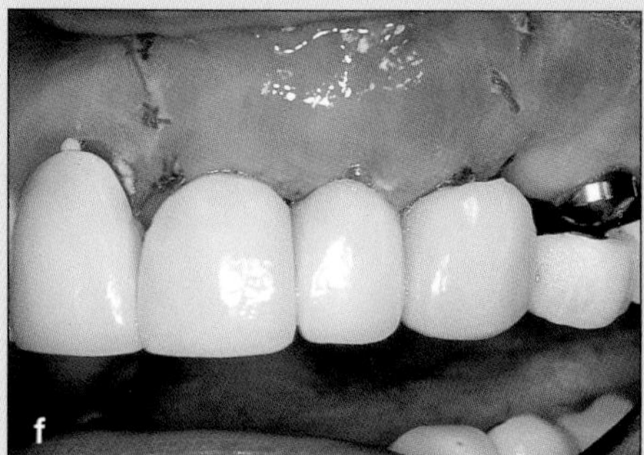

Fig 6-6f Two-week postoperative view demonstrates excellent vertical soft tissue reconstruction in the area between the central incisor and canine implants and no evidence of cover flap retraction.

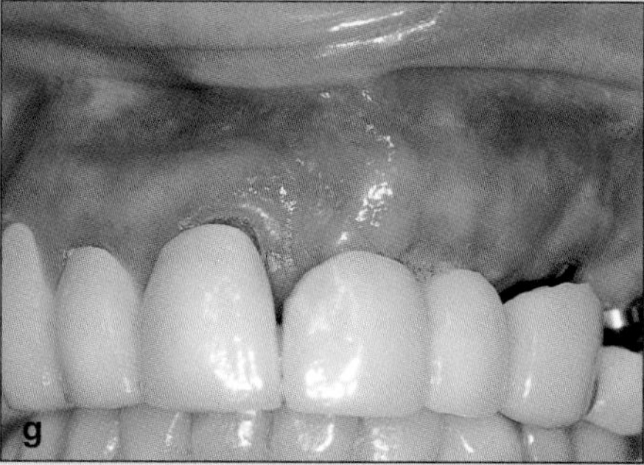

Fig 6-6g Three-month postoperative view demonstrates maintenance of vertical soft tissue levels without evidence of postoperative soft tissue shrinkage.

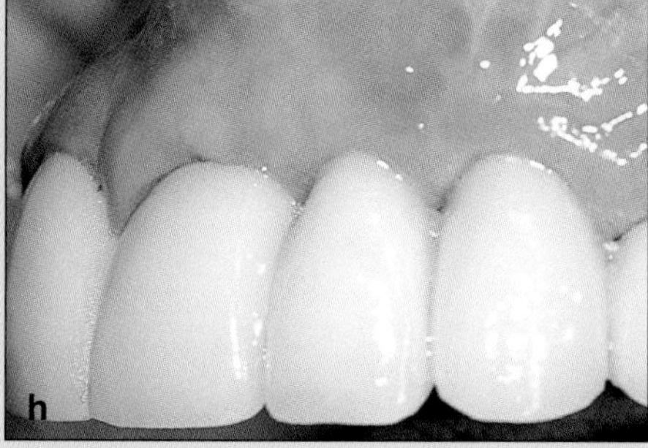

Fig 6-6h One-year postoperative view. Final restoration demonstrates harmonious dental proportions. Esthetic gingival appearance has been restored. (Restoration by Dr Larry Lesperance, South Miami, FL.)

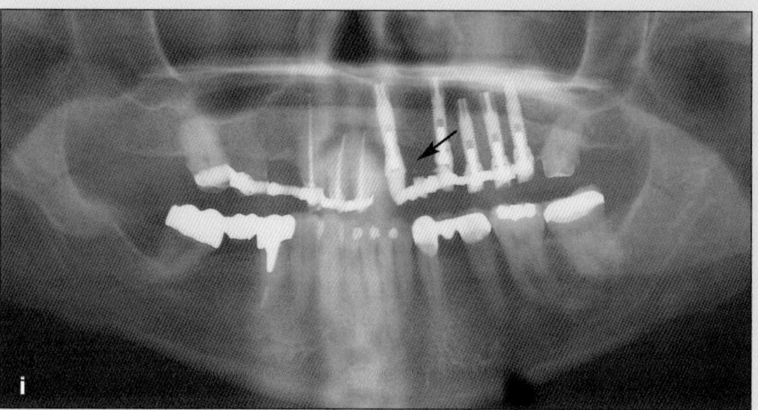

Fig 6-6i Radiograph with final restoration in place demonstrates a compromised vertical level of bone at the distal aspect of the central incisor implant *(arrow)*. Nonetheless, the VIP-CT flap camouflaged the defect and resulted in a final restoration with acceptable gingival esthetics. This amount of vertical augmentation is not achievable even when multiple free soft tissue grafts are performed.

Reconstruction of large-volume soft tissue defect and severely scarred soft tissues with the VIP-CT flap in preparation for subsequent hard tissue site development

Fig 6-7a Preoperative view of interim provisional fixed partial denture with pontic-site defect camouflaged by the addition of a large amount of tissue-colored acrylic resin.

Fig 6-7b Undersurface view of provisional restoration showing the severity of the large-volume combination hard and soft tissue esthetic ridge defect in the area.

Figs 6-7c and 6-7d Preoperative views. Previous failed bone graft attempts led to loss of the lateral incisor. The soft tissue cover at the site is severely scarred and of inadequate quality to support a bone graft. In addition, there is soft tissue recession involving the distal aspect of the adjacent central incisor with loss of papilla and col tissue *(arrow)*. This anatomic defect will usually limit bone grafting outcomes because of failure to achieve and maintain soft tissue cover in this area.

Fig 6-7e Following mechanical and chemical preparation of the adjacent teeth, a closed recipient site was modified to expose the adjacent root surfaces of the central incisor and canine. To avoid sloughing of the thin and extremely scarred tissue site, subperiosteal dissection was performed.

Fig 6-7f A VIP-CT flap was harvested via a dual-incision approach, maintaining an intact epithelial strip. The flap was passively rotated to the site and immobilized in the standard fashion. Note that a large portion of the flap remained exposed. The flap was large enough to allow close adaptation to the adjacent teeth. The interim provisional restoration was adjusted to accommodate the increased soft tissue volume. The epithelium was excised where the flap was submerged.

Figs 6-7g and 6-7h Four-month postoperative views demonstrate tremendous improvement in soft tissue volume and quality at the edentulous site. The missing papillary and col tissues appear partially reconstructed.

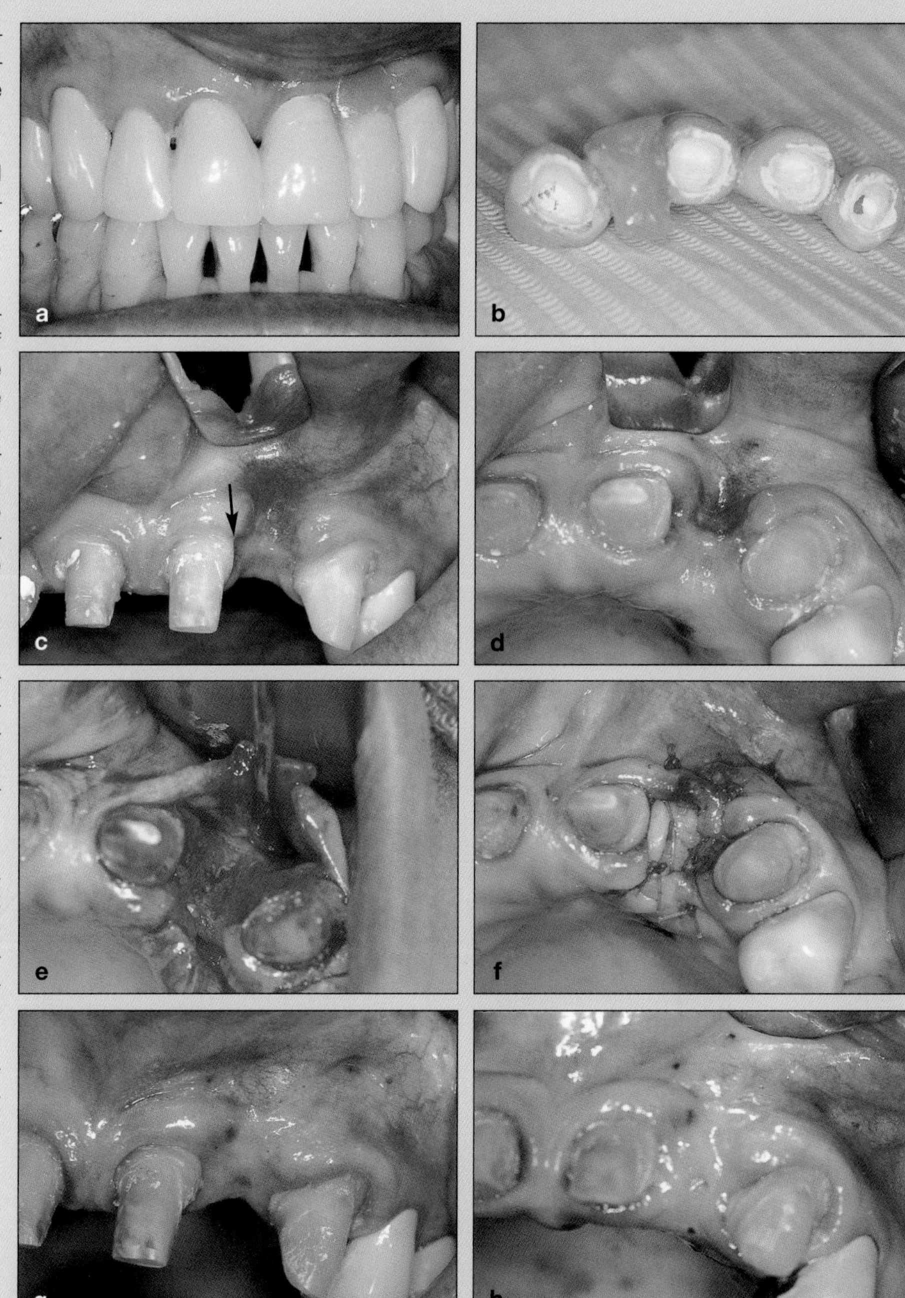

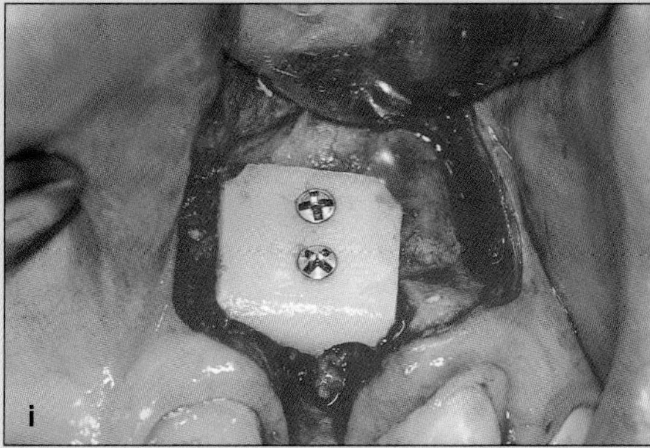

Fig 6-7i A full-thickness curvilinear-beveled flap was elevated for subsequent block and particulate bone grafting procedures. A resorbable collagen membrane was adapted over the bone graft, and tension-free primary closure was obtained.

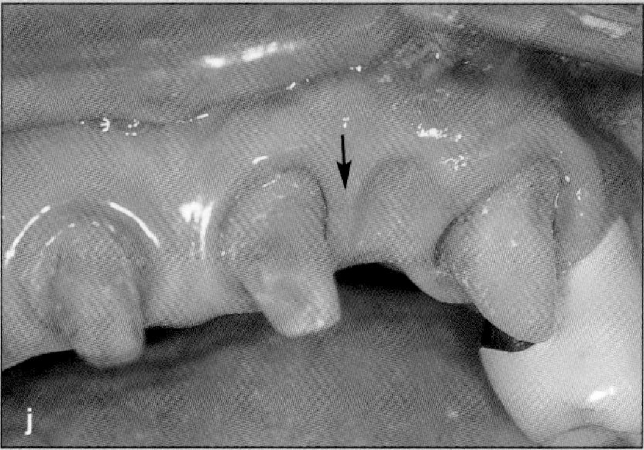

Fig 6-7j Four-month postoperative view shows complete reconstruction of the edentulous site. Ideal restorative contours are present, and soft tissue health is excellent. Notice that the adjacent papillary morphology has been restored in this case *(arrow)*, an outcome that is not always possible even with the VIP-CT flap.

Use of the VIP-CT flap to manage soft tissue dehiscence and exposed metal collar around nonsubmerged maxillary implants

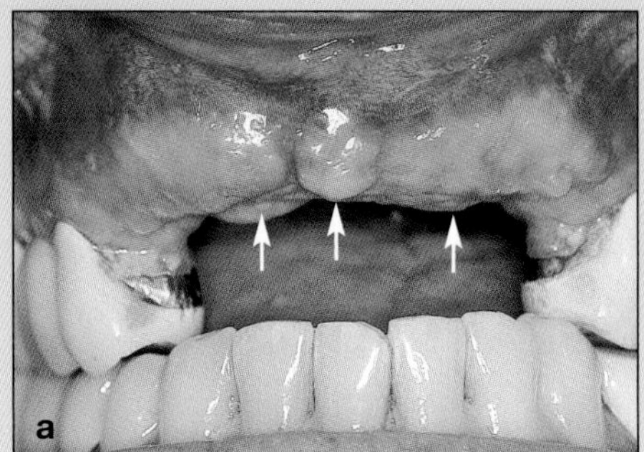

Fig 6-8a Preoperative view of anterior maxillary edentulous area 3 months after bone graft reconstruction was performed to develop the site for placement of canine and central incisor implants eventually to be restored with a six-unit fixed restoration.

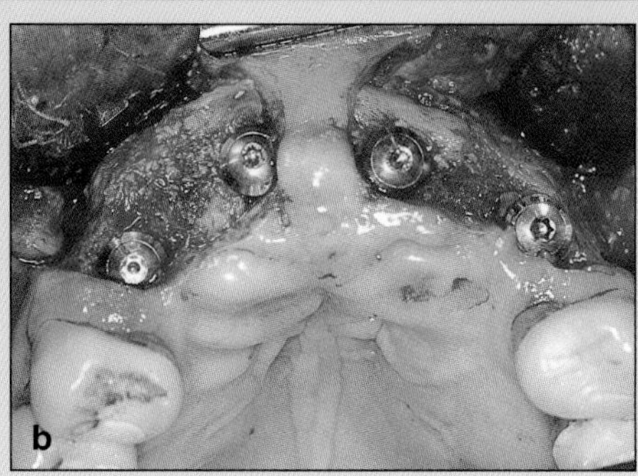

Fig 6-8b Four months later, curvilinear-beveled flaps were elevated to remove Mincro fixation screws (Osteomed) used to immobilize the corticocancellous block grafts. One-piece nonsubmerged implants were placed, and the cover flaps were coronally advanced and reapproximated to submerge the implants.

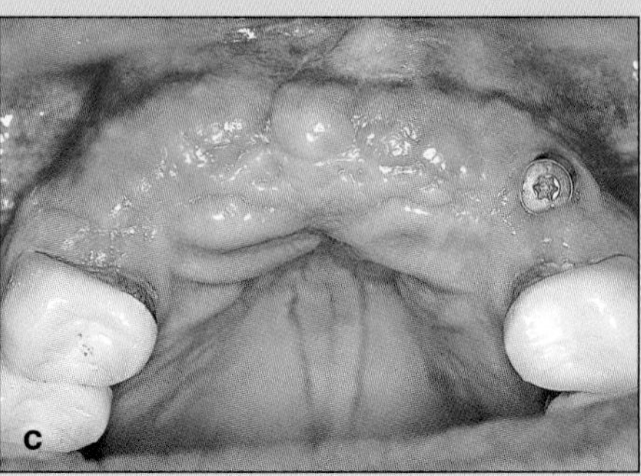

Fig 6-8c Three-month postoperative occlusal view demonstrates complete dehiscence of the soft tissues and exposure of the metal collar around the left maxillary canine implant. This resulted secondary to excessive buccal inclination of the implant.

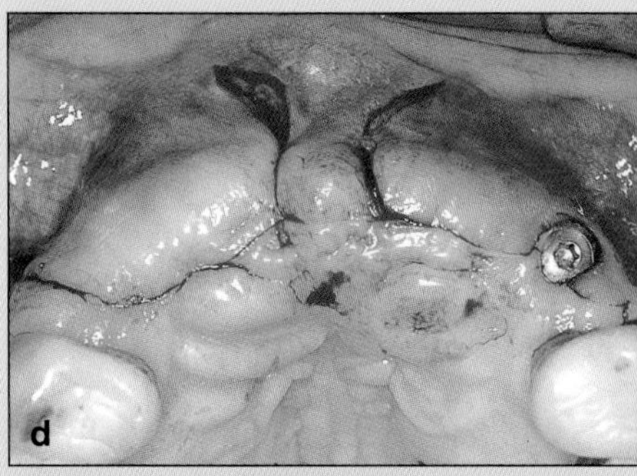

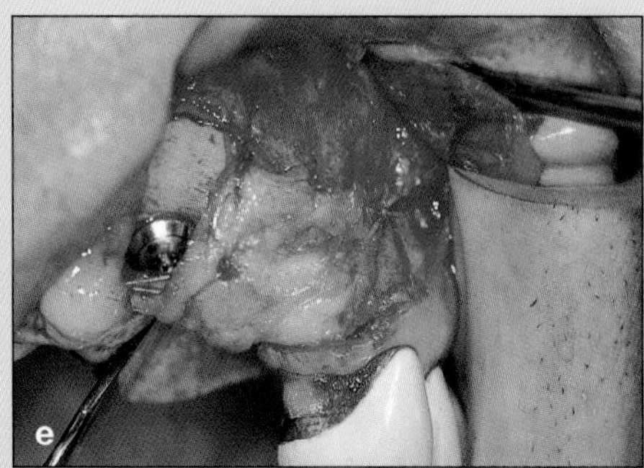

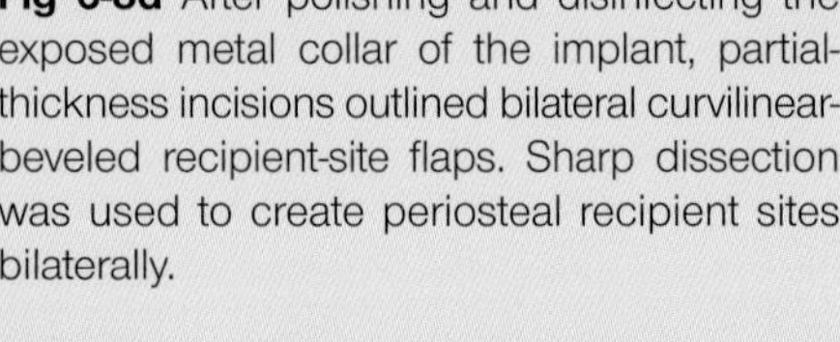

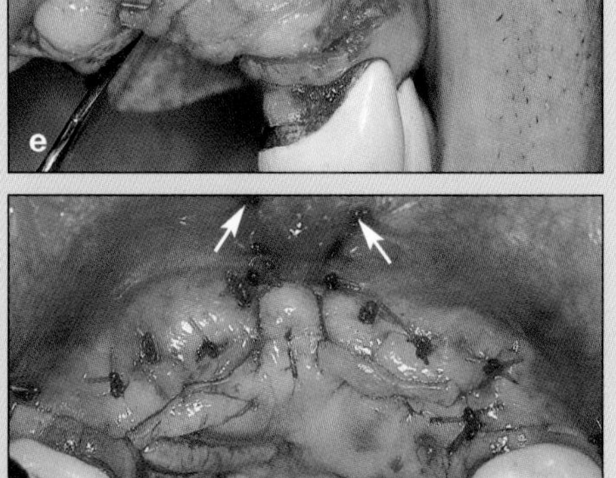

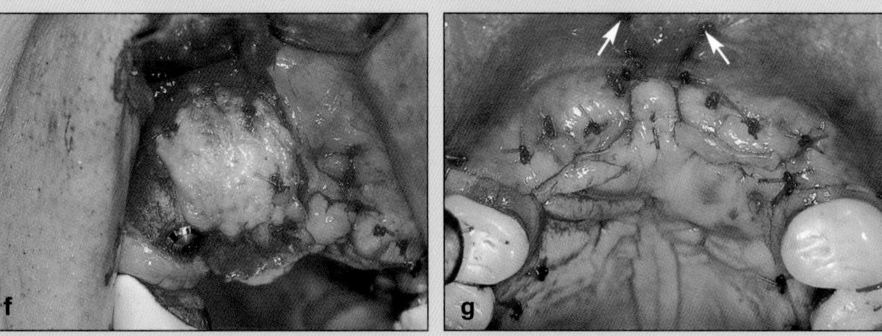

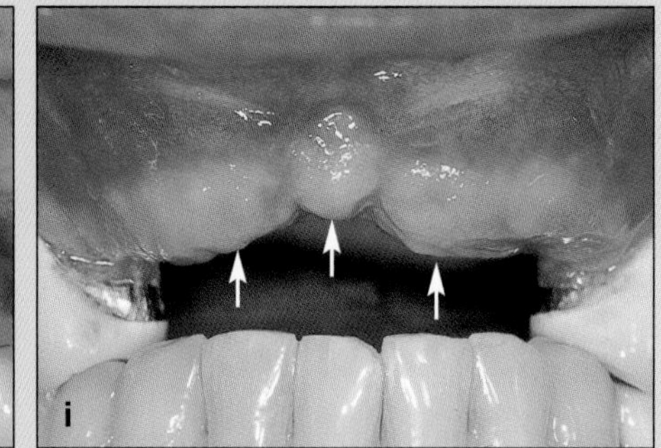

Fig 6-8d After polishing and disinfecting the exposed metal collar of the implant, partial-thickness incisions outlined bilateral curvilinear-beveled recipient-site flaps. Sharp dissection was used to create periosteal recipient sites bilaterally.

Fig 6-8e A VIP-CT flap was developed and passively rotated to the recipient site, adapted over the exposed implant, and secured to the periosteum on the buccal aspect of the ridge. The width of the flap was sufficient to provide vertical soft tissue augmentation over the canine, lateral incisor, and distal aspect of the central incisor.

Fig 6-8f A VIP-CT flap was also developed from the right side of the palate and passively rotated and secured to periosteum at the recipient site. The central and lateral incisor sites were augmented by this flap.

Fig 6-8g The recipient and donor sites were closed bilaterally. Tension-releasing cutback incisions *(arrows)* facilitated the necessary coronal advancement of the recipient-site flaps to allow tension-free closure and accommodation of the increased ridge contours that resulted from the VIP-CT flaps.

Fig 6-8h Three-month postoperative occlusal view demonstrates complete coverage of previously exposed left maxillary canine implant. Note the increased thickness of the attached tissues enveloping the ridge crest.

Fig 6-8i Three-month postoperative frontal view demonstrates vertical soft tissue augmentation in the areas where the VIP-CT flaps were performed. Using the central papilla as a reference (see Fig 6-8a), approximately 4.0 mm of vertical soft tissue augmentation was obtained *(arrows)*, exceeding the amount obtainable even with sequential free soft tissue grafts. Correction of this discrepancy was necessary prior to implant emergence.

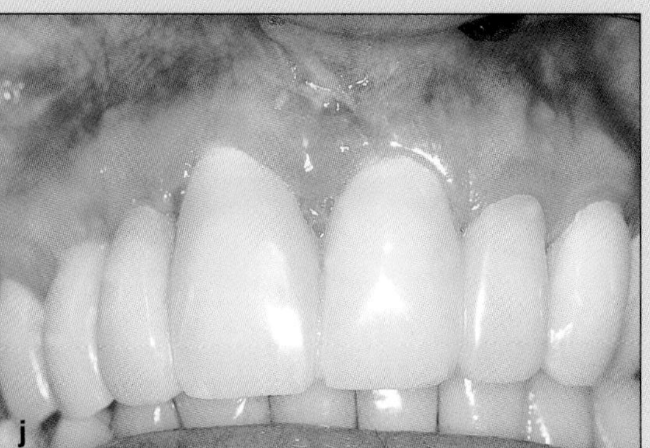

Fig 6-8j One-year postoperative view demonstrates esthetic emergence and acceptable gingival contouring. Soft tissue coverage of the implant collar was maintained. (Restoration by Dr Carlos Interian, Miami, FL.)

VIP-CT flap for simultaneous correction of a small-volume combination esthetic ridge defect simultaneous with esthetic implant placement

Figs 6-9a and 6-9b Preoperative views of edentulous maxillary canine site with removable interim provisional restoration. The restoration has a ridge lap pontic to camouflage a small-volume combination esthetic ridge defect. Note that the papilla mesial of the canine site is blunted and that there is vertical and horizontal ridge deficiency.

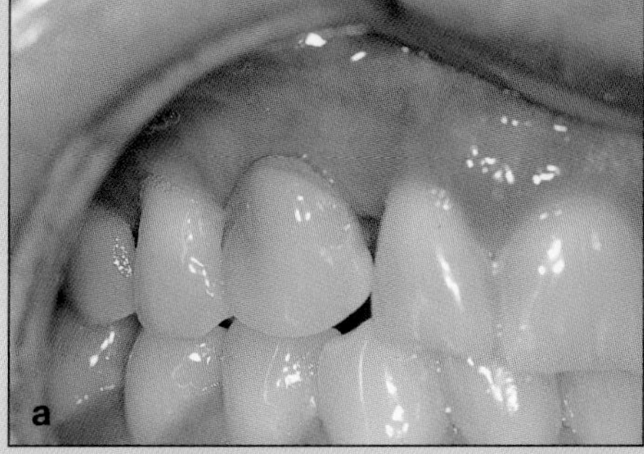

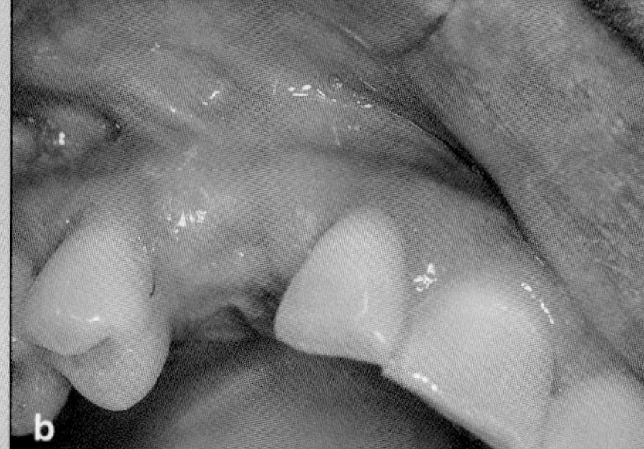

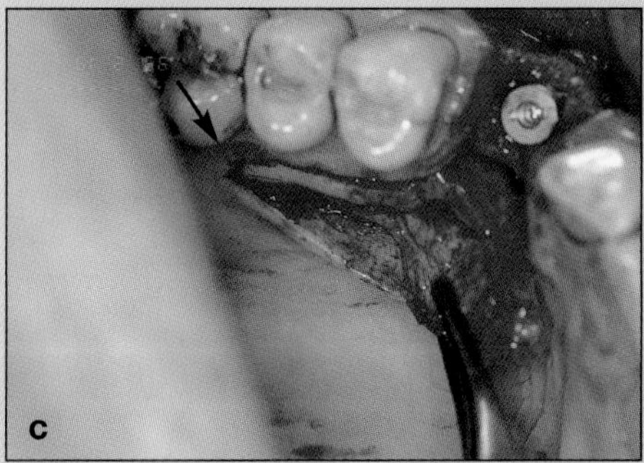

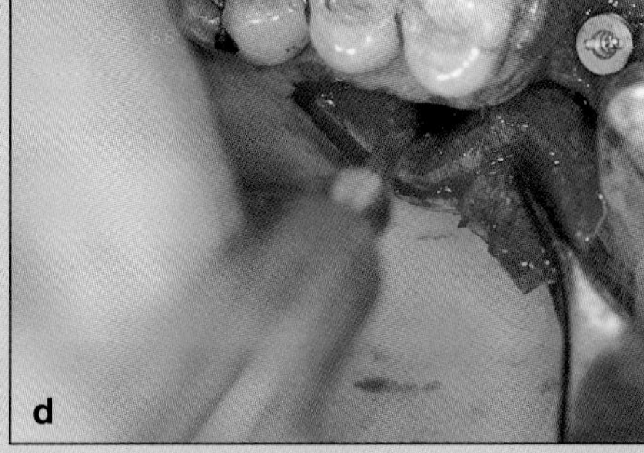

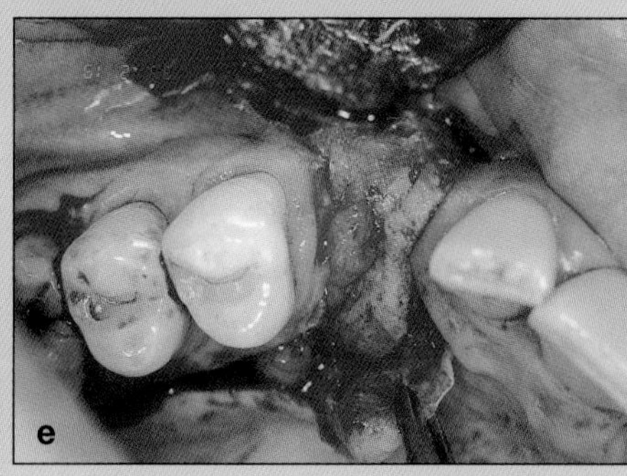

Fig 6-9c After placement of a submerged implant (Frialit-2; Dentsply, York, PA), sharp dissection was used to define the subepithelial plane of dissection. The margin of the VIP-CT flap was defined by a vertical incision made through the connective tissue and periosteum at the distal aspect of the dissection *(arrow)*.

Figs 6-9d and 6-9e A Buser periosteal elevator was used to define the subperiosteal plane of dissection, and an apical horizontal incision completed the outline of the pedicle flap. Subsequent subperiosteal undermining of the newly defined base of the flap allows passive rotation to the recipient site without the need for a tension-releasing cutback incision.

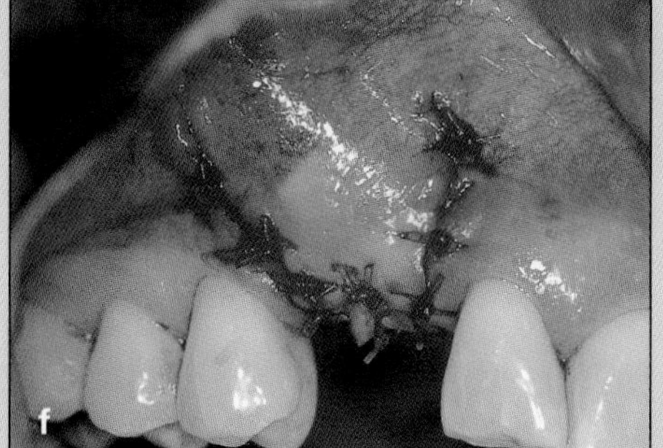

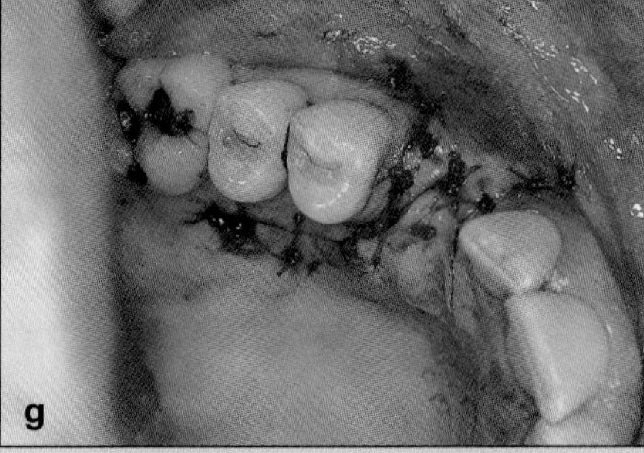

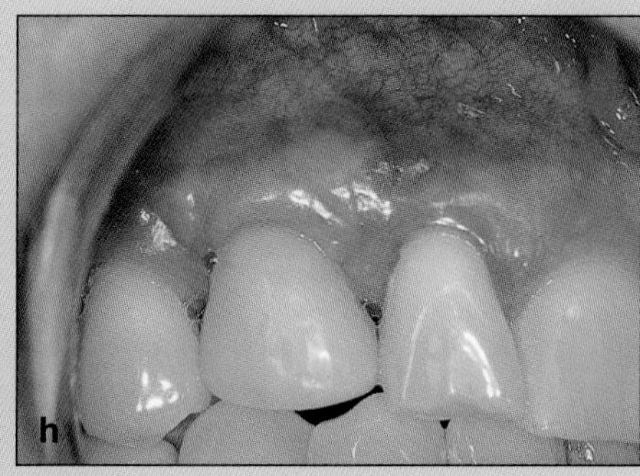

Figs 6-9f and 6-9g The recipient-site flap was coronally advanced to accommodate the increased soft tissue bulk created by the flap and then secured with 4-0 chromic gut sutures. Primary closure was obtained at the donor site after obliteration of dead space with CollaPlug absorbable collagen dressing.

Fig 6-9h Provisional restoration delivered via a tissue punch 4 months after implant placement simultaneous with a VIP-CT flap. Note improvement in ridge contours and morphology of mesial papilla compared to Fig 6-9a.

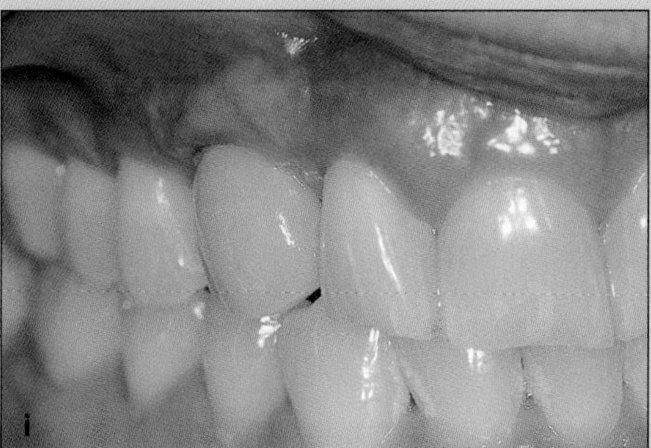

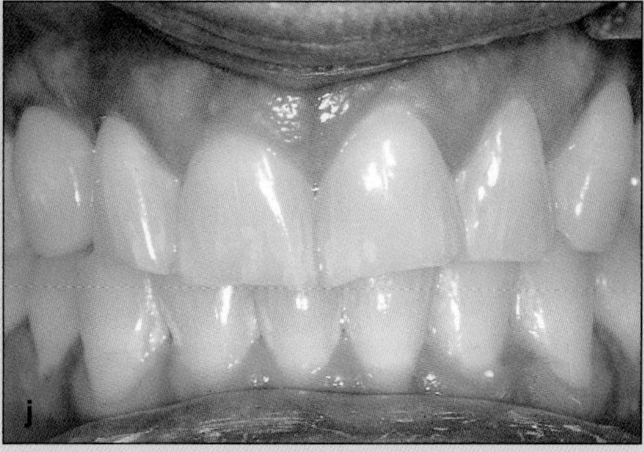

Figs 6-9i and 6-9j One year after delivery of the final restoration, esthetic restorative emergence and improved papillary morphology have been achieved. Recommended laser soft tissue contouring and resurfacing was declined by this patient. (Restoration by Dr Cecil Abraham, Miami, FL.)

Simultaneous correction of large-volume soft tissue defect with esthetic implant placement

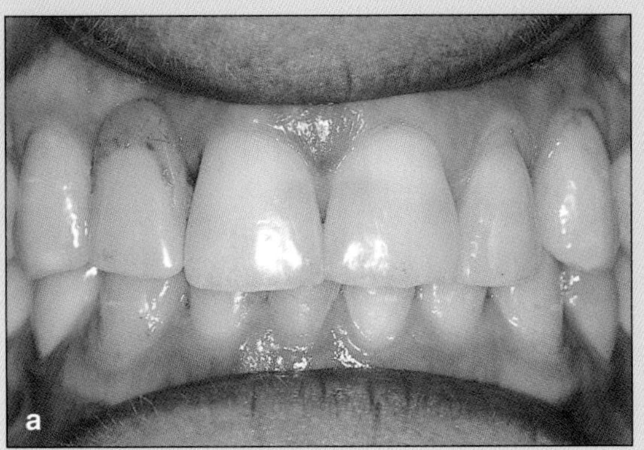

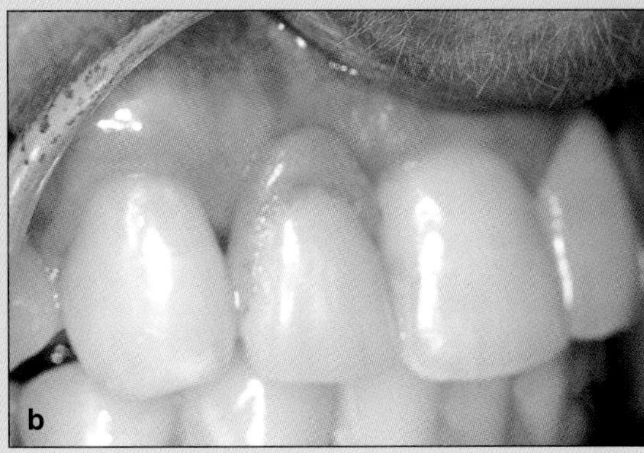

Figs 6-10a and 6-10b Preoperative views of lateral incisor implant site with large-volume soft tissue esthetic ridge defect. A large amount of tissue-colored resin material was needed to camouflage the defect with the interim removable restoration. Vertical and horizontal soft tissue augmentation are required for esthetic emergence of the planned implant restoration.

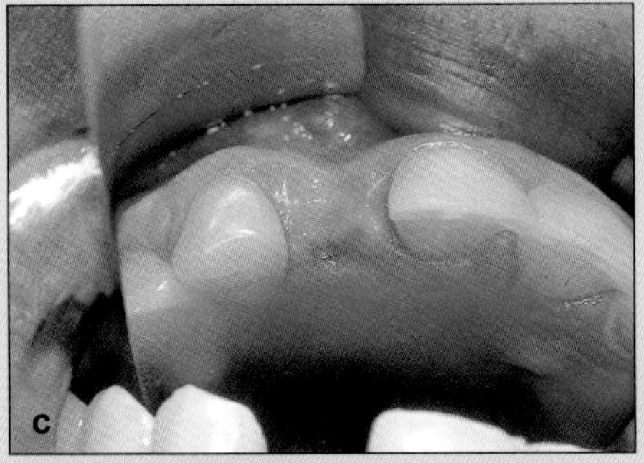

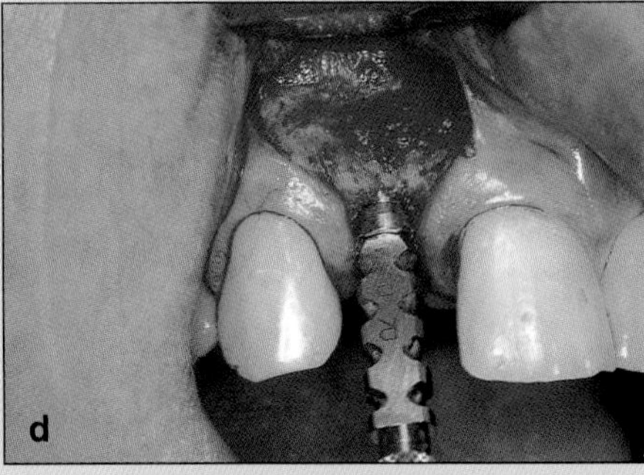

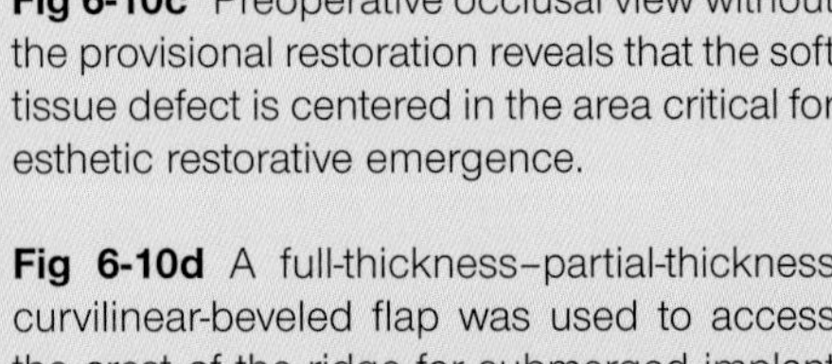

Fig 6-10c Preoperative occlusal view without the provisional restoration reveals that the soft tissue defect is centered in the area critical for esthetic restorative emergence.

Fig 6-10d A full-thickness–partial-thickness curvilinear-beveled flap was used to access the crest of the ridge for submerged implant placement (Nobel Biocare, Yorba Linda, CA) and subsequent fixture-level impression. The full-thickness dissection was limited to the ridge crest and the partial-thickness dissection was performed apically to create a periosteal recipient site on the buccal aspect of the alveolar ridge.

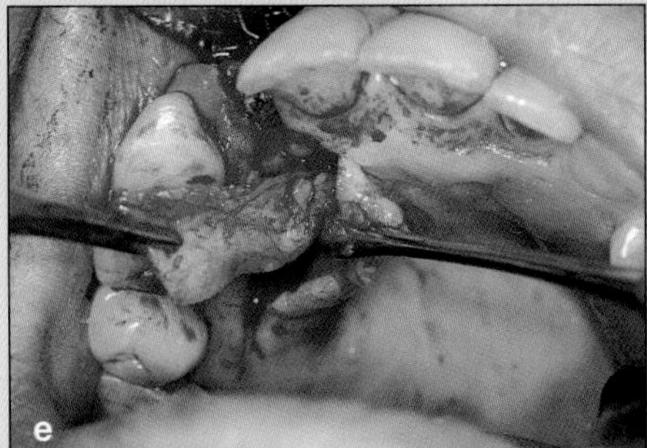

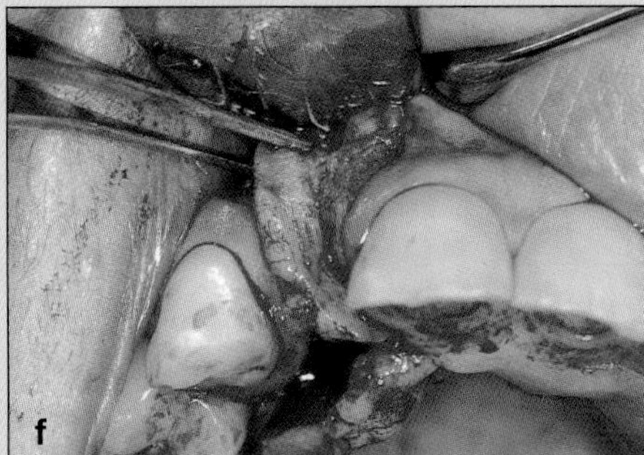

Figs 6-10e and 6-10f After placement of the cover screw, the VIP-CT flap was surgically developed via a single-incision approach at the palatal donor site, rotated over the ridge crest, and passively adapted over the periosteal recipient site on the buccal aspect of the alveolar ridge.

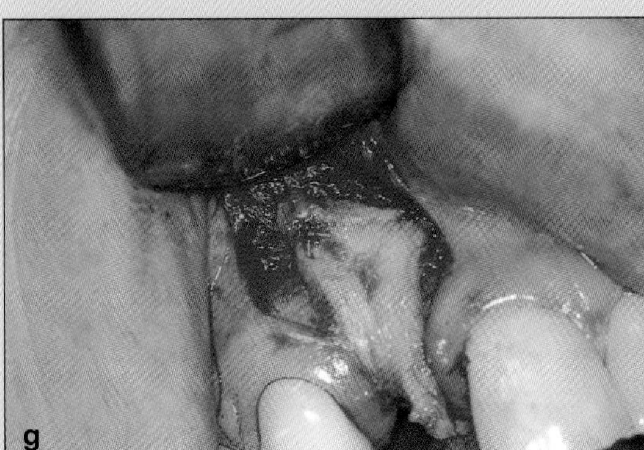

Fig 6-10g The VIP-CT flap was secured to the periosteum at the recipient site with 4-0 chromic gut sutures. Tension-free closure of the recipient- and donor-site flaps was obtained.

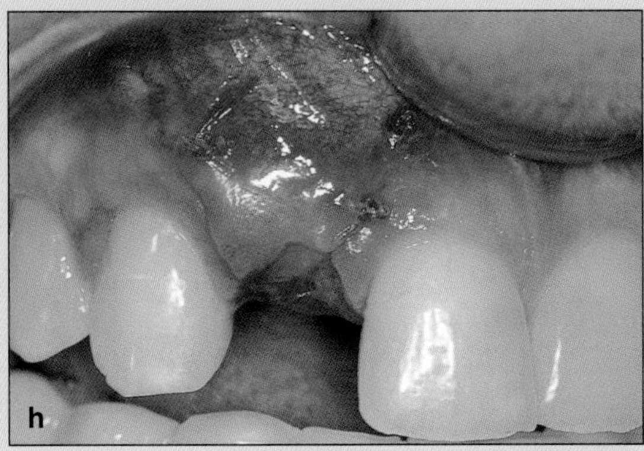

Fig 6-10h Two-week postoperative view of the lateral incisor site. Note the tremendous increase in soft tissue volume at the site. Sufficient vertical and horizontal soft tissue reconstruction was achieved to ensure esthetic emergence of the final restoration. An Essex-type tooth-borne interim provisional restoration that provided coverage of the palatal donor site and housed an abbreviated ovate pontic for support of the adjacent papilla was used during the initial 2-week postoperative period.

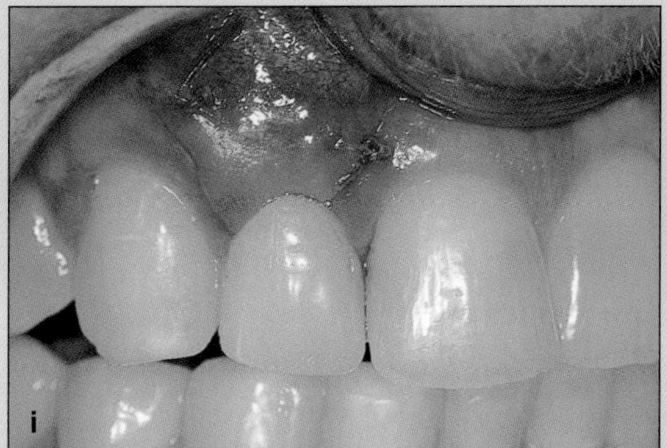

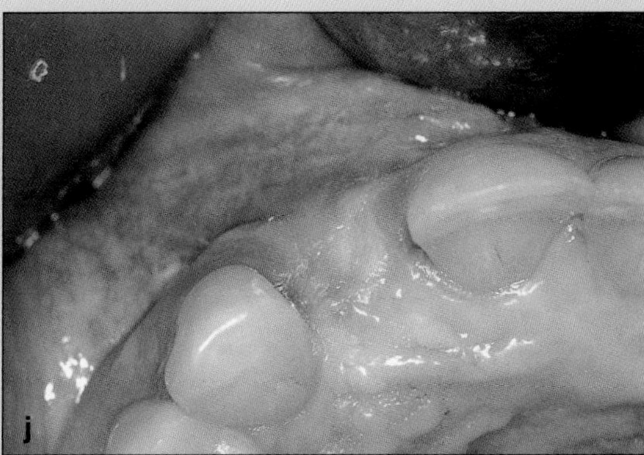

Fig 6-10i Two-week postoperative view of the original removable provisional restoration in place after significant modification to accommodate the soft tissue augmentation at the site and the excess tissue bulk in the palate. In addition to removing all of the tissue-colored resin material from the prosthesis, the cervical portion of the lateral incisor pontic also was reduced (see Fig 6-10b).

Fig 6-10j Four-month postoperative view. Minimal soft tissue shrinkage has occurred. In some cases, the excess palatal soft tissue bulk created by the interpositional flap as it courses into the recipient site may need to be debulked if patient comfort or phonetics is adversely affected.

Fig 6-10k An open flap was used to debulk the palatal tissues and gain access for delivery of a custom abutment and provisional restoration.

Figs 6-10l and 6-10m Six weeks after abutment connection, excess soft tissue bulk is evident on the facial aspect of the restoration. Laser soft tissue contouring and resurfacing will be performed to optimize gingival esthetics.

Fig 6-10n Provisional restoration 3 months after abutment connection and 6 weeks after esthetic laser sculpting and resurfacing of buccal tissues at the recipient site.

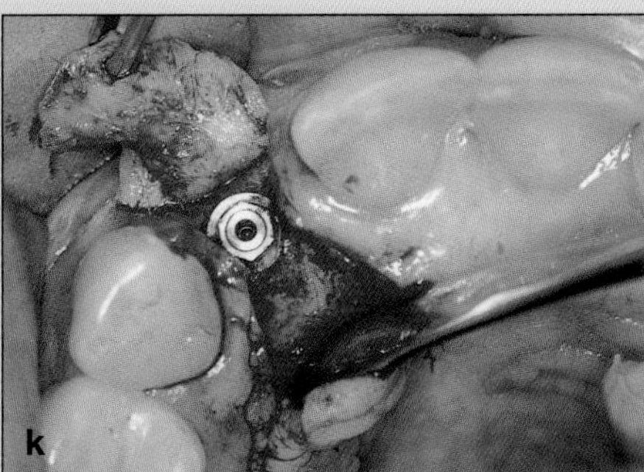

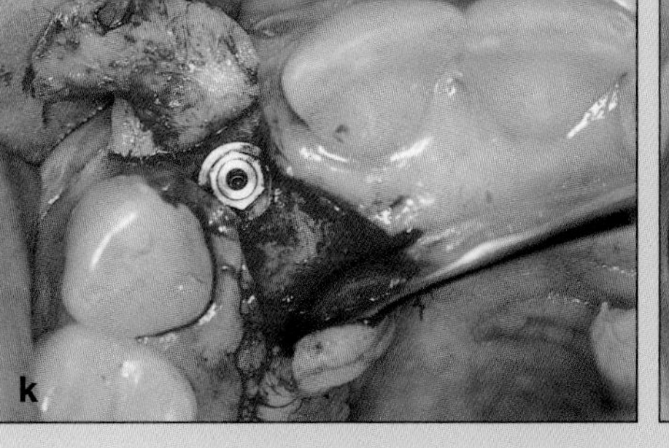

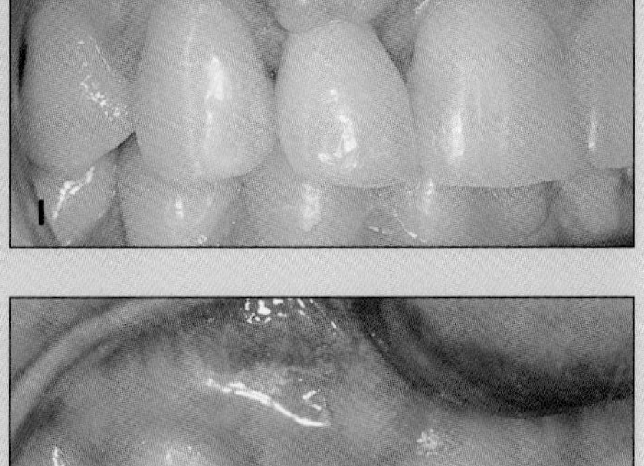

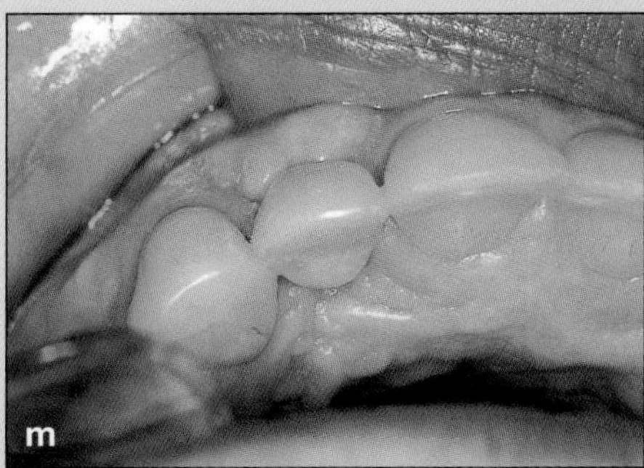

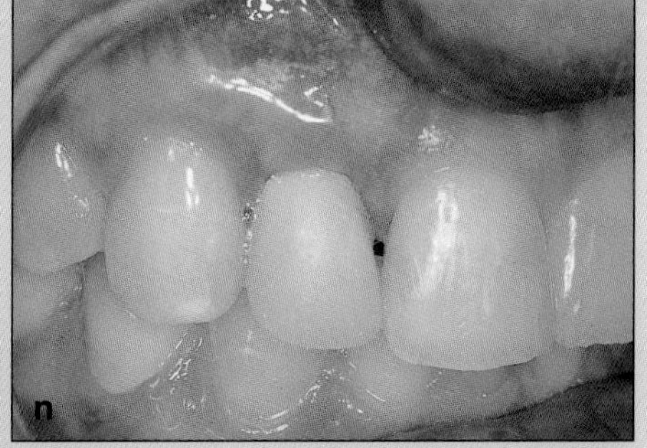

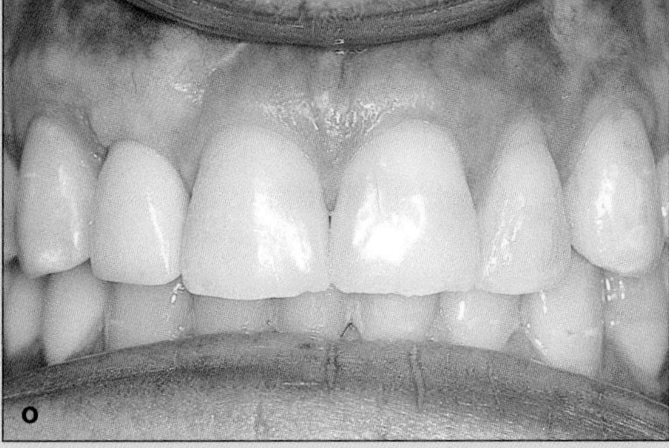

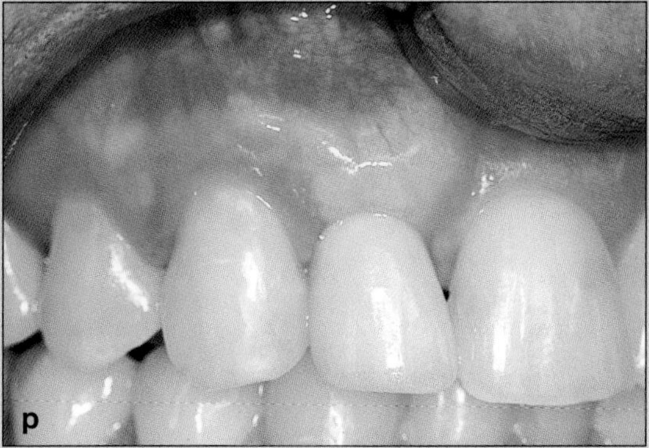

Figs 6-10o and 6-10p One year after delivery of final restoration.The lateral incisor implant restoration is harmonious with the adjacent dentition, and peri-implant soft tissue health is excellent. (Restoration by Dr Doug Deam, Coral Gables, FL.)

Simultaneous hard and soft tissue site development with the VIP-CT flap

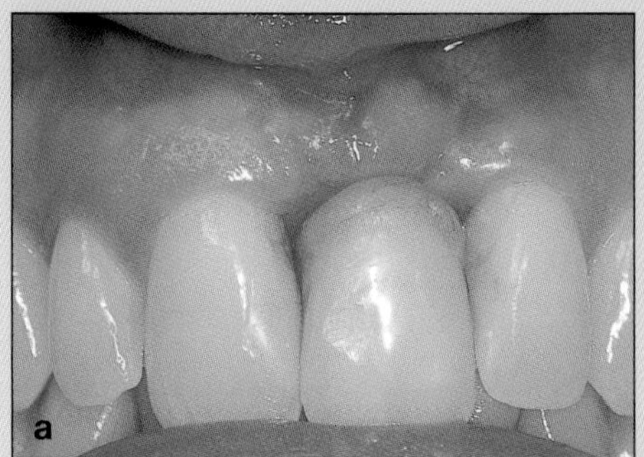
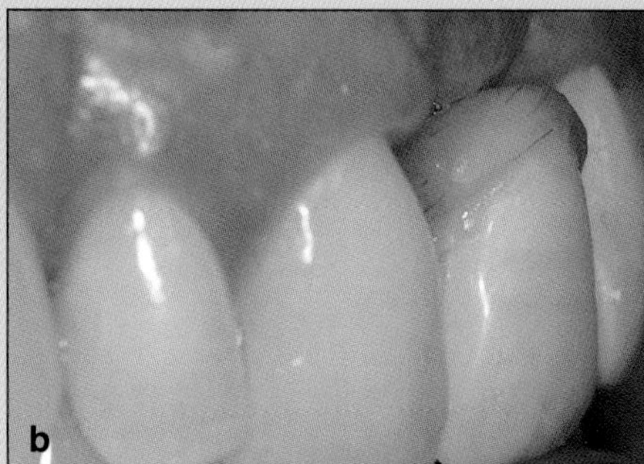

Figs 6-11a and 6-11b Preoperative views of edentulous maxillary central incisor implant site with large-volume combination hard and soft tissue esthetic ridge defect with significant vertical and horizontal components. In addition, the crestal bone levels on the adjacent central and lateral incisors, which are not adequate to support a papilla, present an anatomic limitation that will prevent ideal esthetics. Esthetic crown lengthening and cosmetic restorations of adjacent teeth will be required to camouflage these residual esthetic defects.

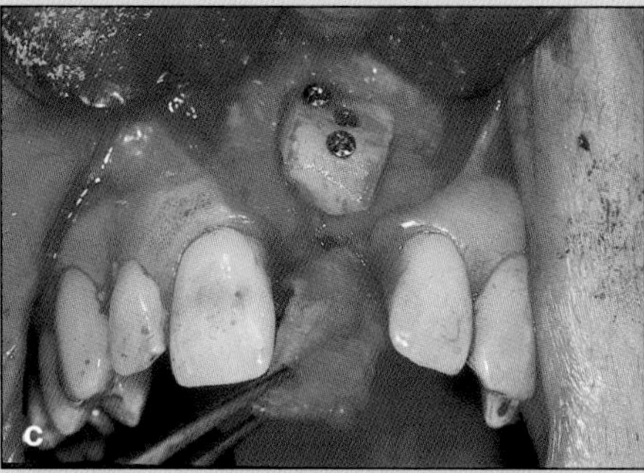
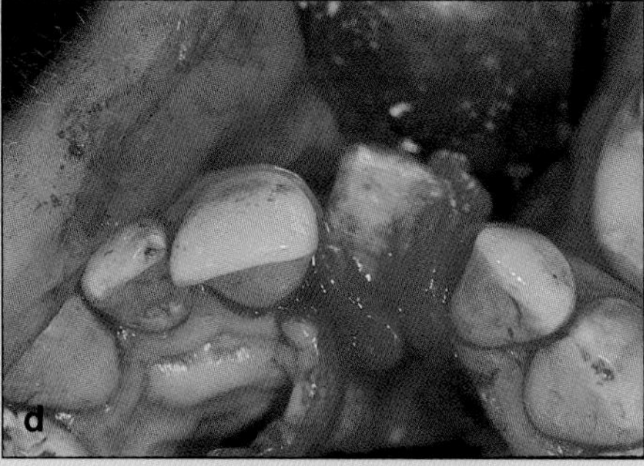
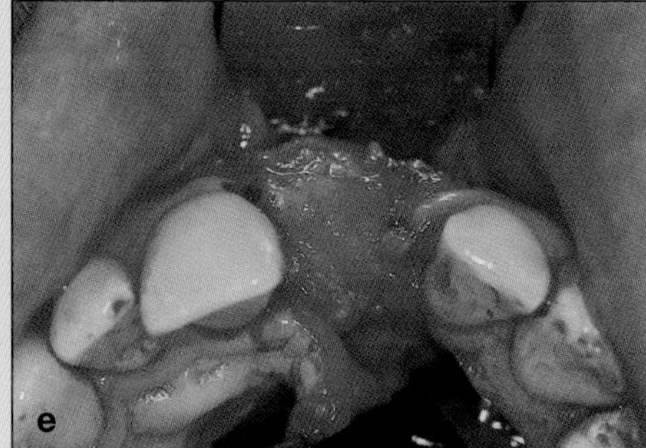

Figs 6-11c to 6-11e Access to the site was obtained with an exaggerated curvilinear-beveled flap with tension-releasing cutback incisions elevated subperiosteally. The adjacent attached tissues and papillary areas are de-epithelialized. After the block bone graft has been secured, the VIP-CT flap is developed, passive rotation over the block bone graft is verified, and any portion of the bone graft that will not be covered by the flap is noted. In this case, the flap is large enough to cover the bone graft but not wide enough to expect any significant enhancement of tissue levels on the adjacent teeth. Passive coaptation of the recipient-site flap over the block bone graft and VIP-CT flap is also verified at this time. Tension-releasing cutback incisions are extended if necessary. Next, the particulate bone graft is condensed around the periphery of the block bone graft, and a resorbable membrane is adapted over any portion of the bone graft that will not be covered by the periosteal–connective tissue flap. The flap is positioned over the bone graft and secured with horizontal mattress sutures passed through the flap and the adjacent attached tissues or to the adjacent de-epithelialized areas with interrupted sutures, as shown here.

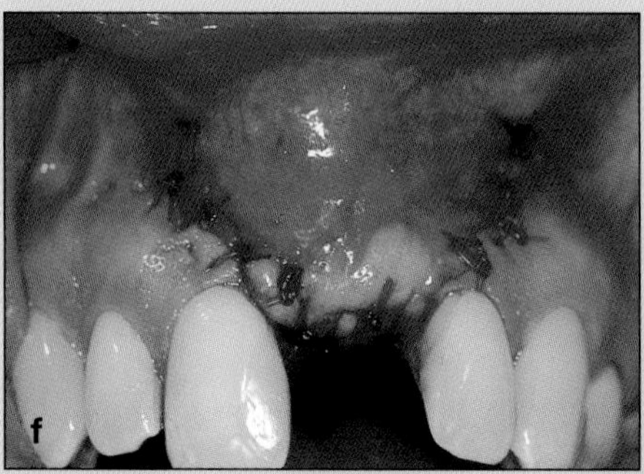
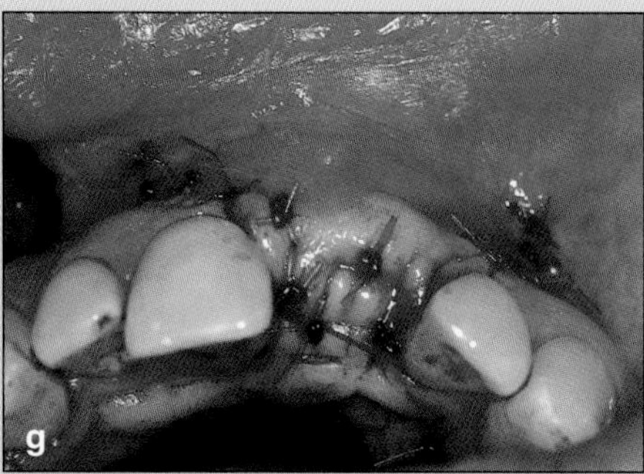

Figs 6-11f and 6-11g The exaggerated curvilinear-beveled flap design with tension-releasing cutback incisions passively accommodated the large-volume hard and soft tissue augmentation and allowed for tension-free closure.

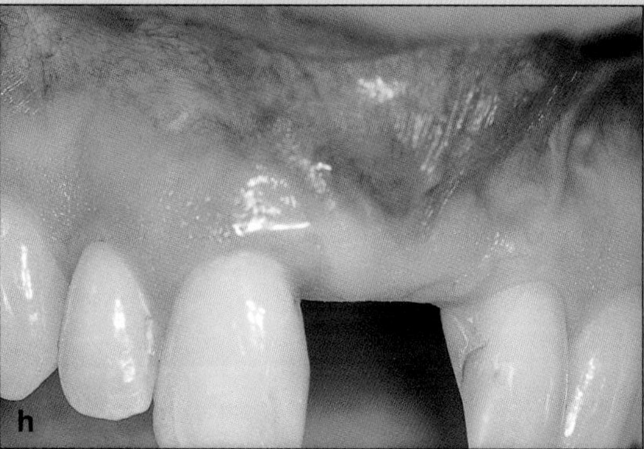
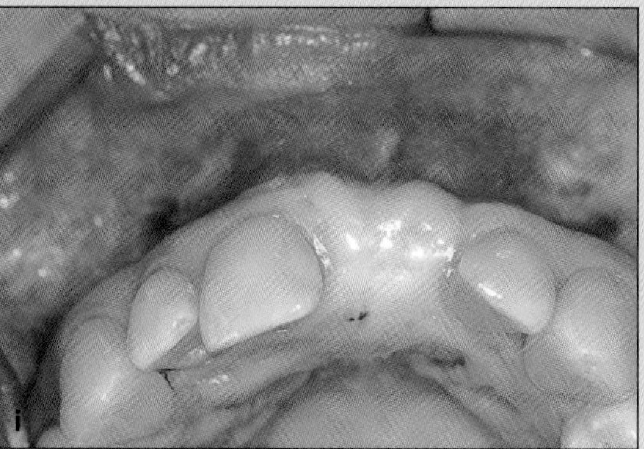

Figs 6-11h and 6-11i Four-month postoperative view demonstrates significant vertical ridge augmentation limited only by the compromised crestal bone levels on adjacent teeth. An impressive degree of horizontal ridge augmentation has also been achieved. Site development has been successfully completed with a single surgery and in less time than would be required for conventional staged implant site development. The site is ready for nonsubmerged implant placement after merely 4 months.

Simultaneous hard and soft tissue site development for correction of large-volume combination esthetic ridge defect at central incisor site

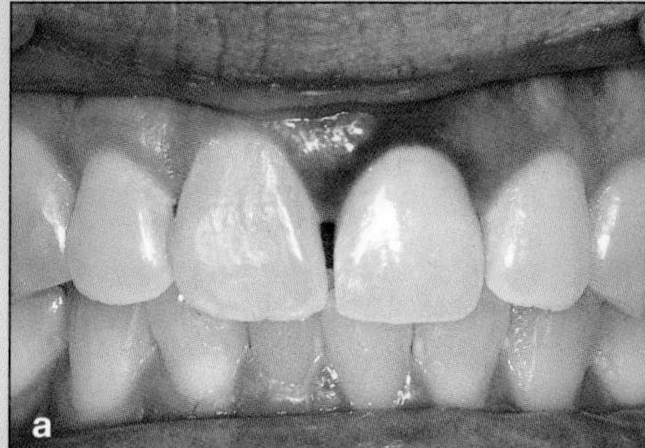

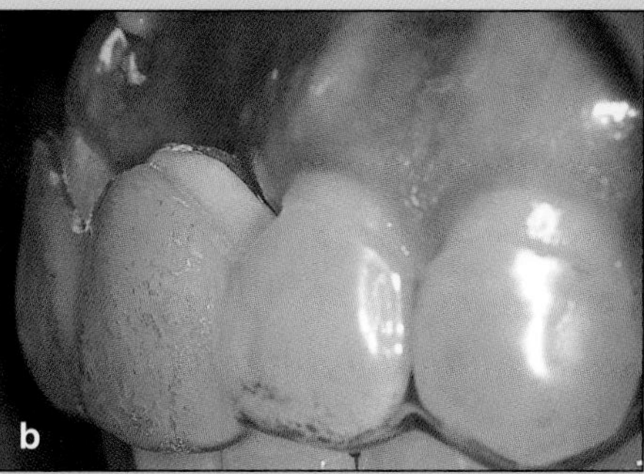

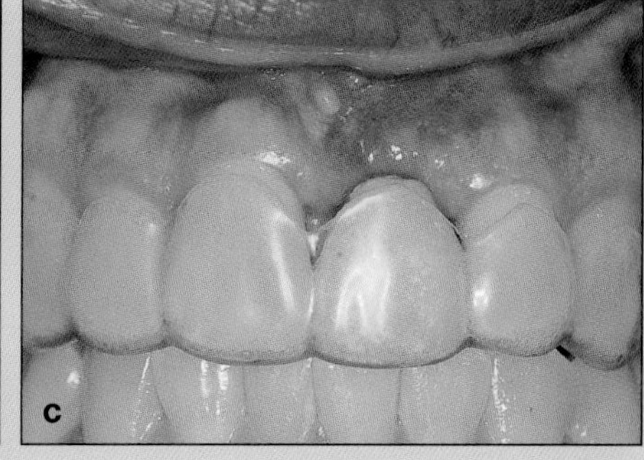

Fig 6-12a Preoperative view of failing left central incisor exhibiting tremendous soft tissue edema and inflammation involving the marginal gingival tissues. Loss of hard and soft tissue volume is predictable despite efforts to preserve the alveolar ridge when tooth mobility is accompanied by such an inflammatory soft tissue response.

Figs 6-12b and 6-12c Two months after tooth removal with the Bio-Col technique, a large-volume combination hard and soft tissue esthetic ridge defect is evident. A large dehiscence (wider than one third the mesiodistal width of the site) was noted, involving the buccal plate at the time of tooth removal. The Bio-Col technique was performed to prevent soft tissue collapse and scarring into the defect, thereby maintaining the volume of the reconstructive soft tissue envelope.

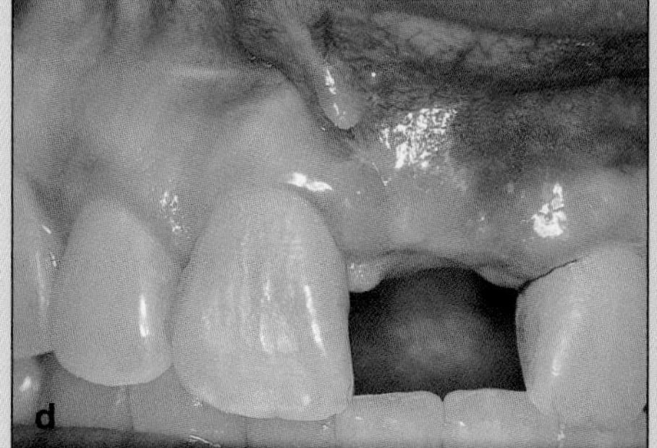

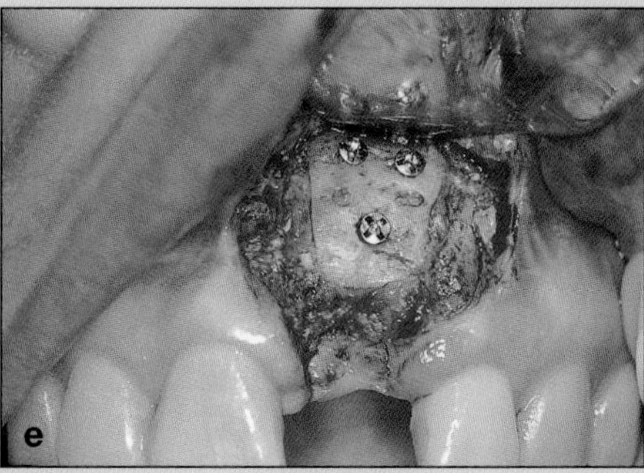

Fig 6-12d Four months after simultaneous hard and soft tissue site development with autogenous corticocancellous block and particulate bone grafts combined with the VIP-CT flap, natural alveolar ridge contours have been completely restored.

Figs 6-12e and 6-12f Four months after site development, the site was re-entered for removal of bone graft fixation screws and for implant placement. Multiple bleeding points were noted on the surface of the block graft and no loss of volume or contour was found around the fixation screws. The particulate bone graft showed evidence of advanced integration *(arrows)*.

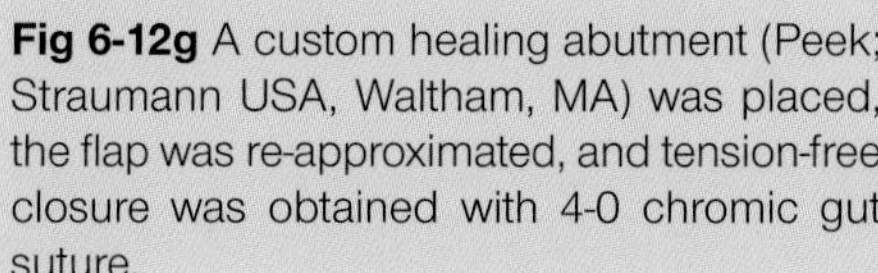

Fig 6-12g A custom healing abutment (Peek; Straumann USA, Waltham, MA) was placed, the flap was re-approximated, and tension-free closure was obtained with 4-0 chromic gut suture.

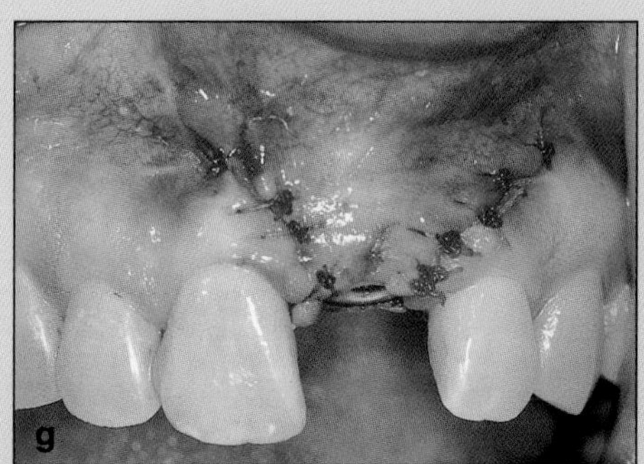

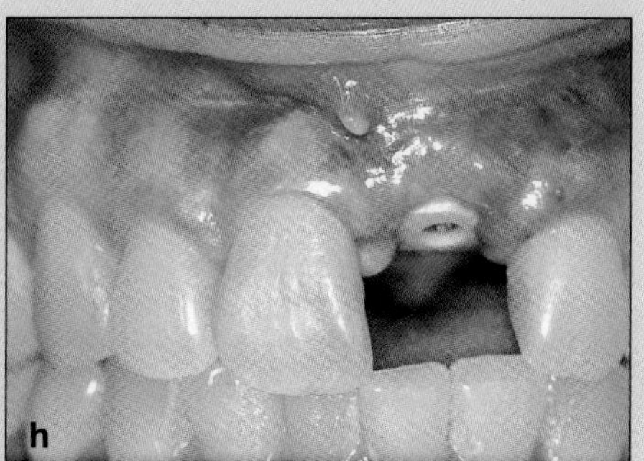

Fig 6-12h Three months after implant placement, it is apparent that esthetic ridge contours have been restored. The adjacent papillae are supported and the marginal gingival tissues are symmetrical with the adjacent central incisor.

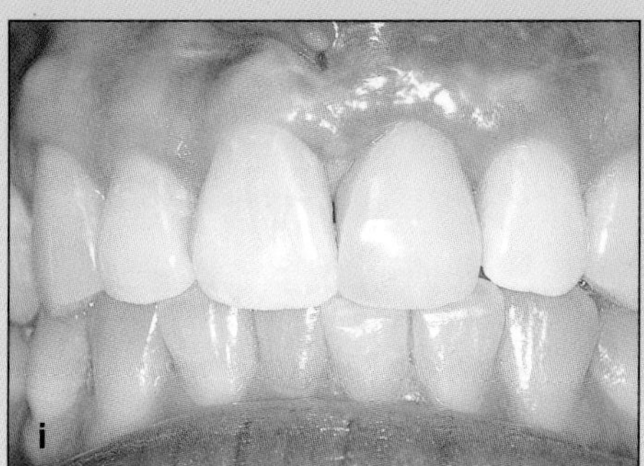

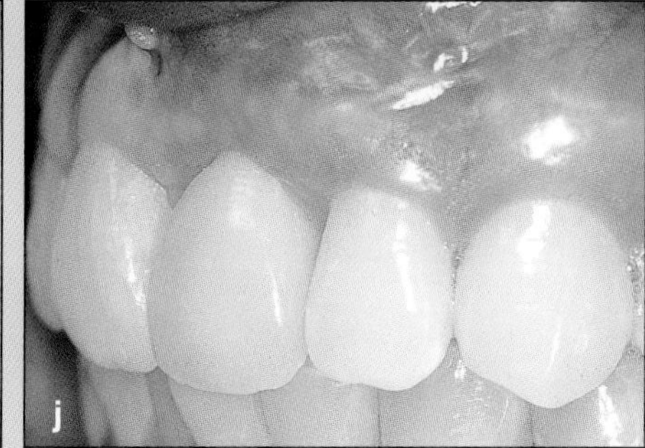

Figs 6-12i and 6-12j One-year postoperative frontal and side views demonstrate central incisor implant restoration of harmonious proportions and the restoration of an esthetic gingival appearance despite the pre-existence of a large-volume combination defect at this compromised site. (Restoration by Dr Paul Moo Young, Miami, FL.)

Simultaneous hard and soft tissue site development for correction of large-volume combination esthetic ridge defect at central incisor site

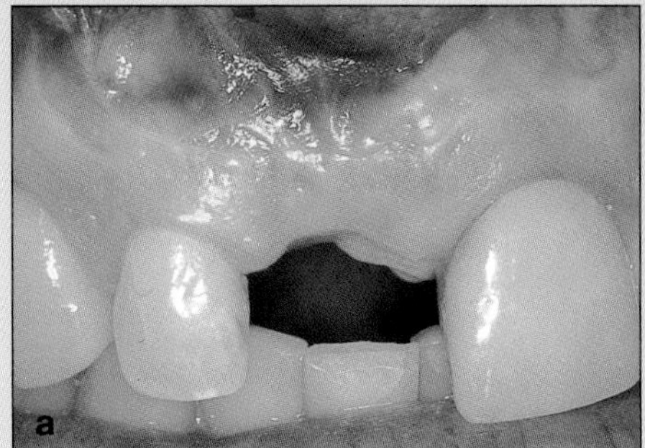

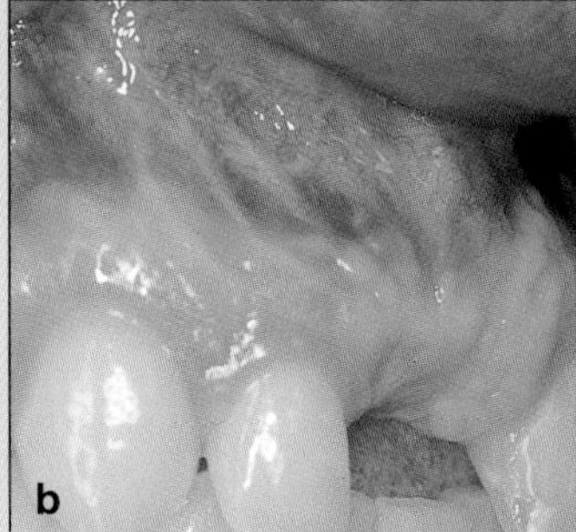

Figs 6-13a and 6-13b Preoperative view of maxillary central incisor implant site with large-volume combination hard and soft tissue esthetic ridge defect. The regenerative potential of the site is compromised by previous trauma and multiple surgical endodontic interventions leading to eventual loss of the tooth. Note unesthetic soft tissue tattoo at the site.

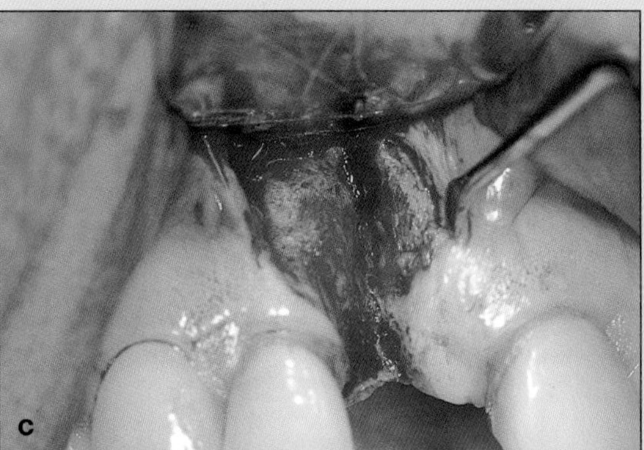

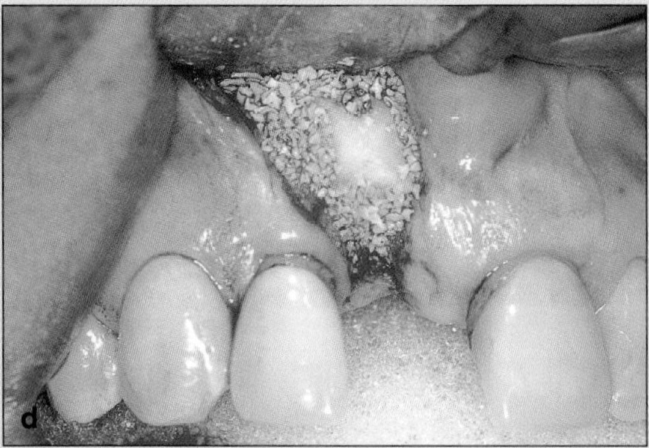

Figs 6-13c and 6-13d Curvilinear-beveled full-thickness flap provided access to the site for simultaneous hard and soft tissue site development. Though complete loss of the buccal plate was noted, the defect has a favorable morphology. A corticocancellous block graft has been secured at the site, and particulate bone graft has been condensed around the periphery. The site demonstrates compromised circulation with little evidence of bleeding.

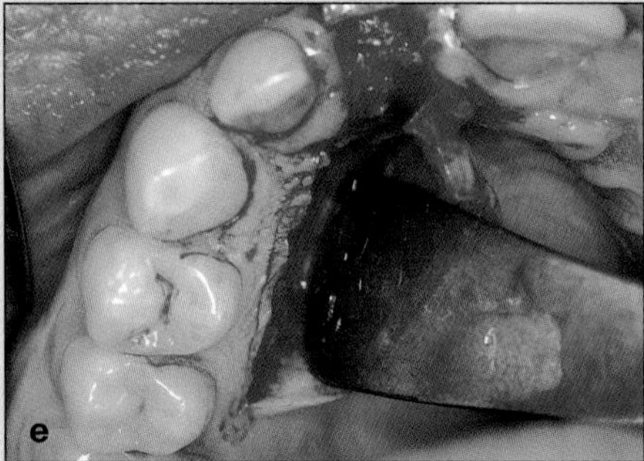

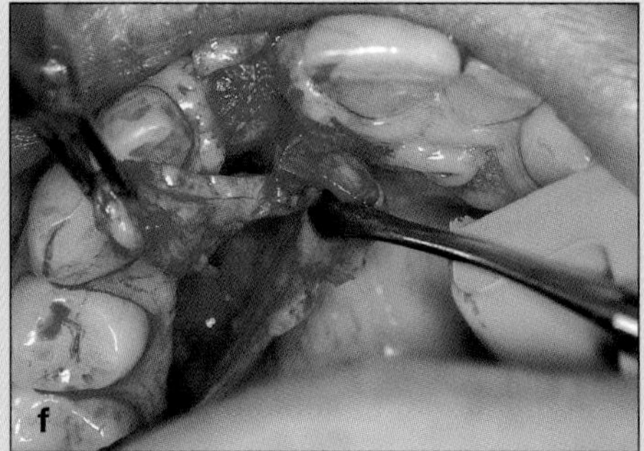

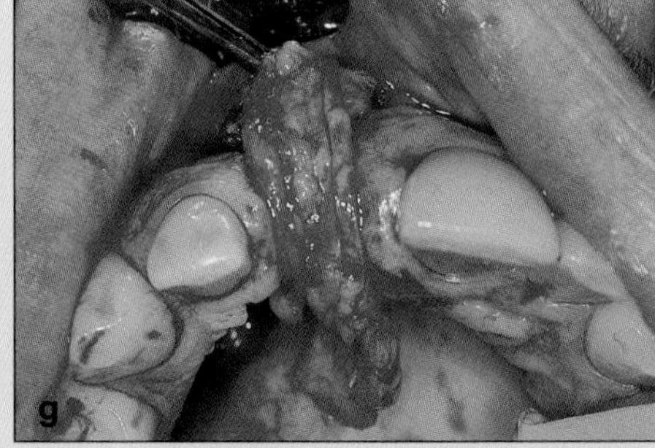

Figs 6-13e to 6-13g The VIP-CT flap was developed at the donor site and, after subperiosteal undermining, was passively rotated over the bone graft. In this case, the apical horizontal incision was extended to achieve complete periosteal coverage of the bone graft at the recipient site. Bleeding from the flap margin after rotation indicated maintenance of sufficient perfusion circulation.

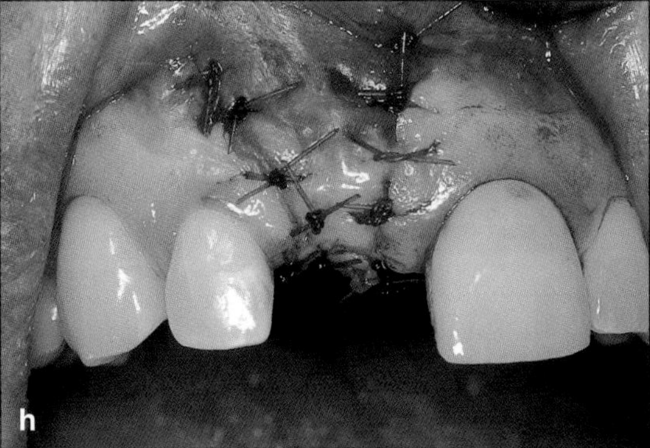

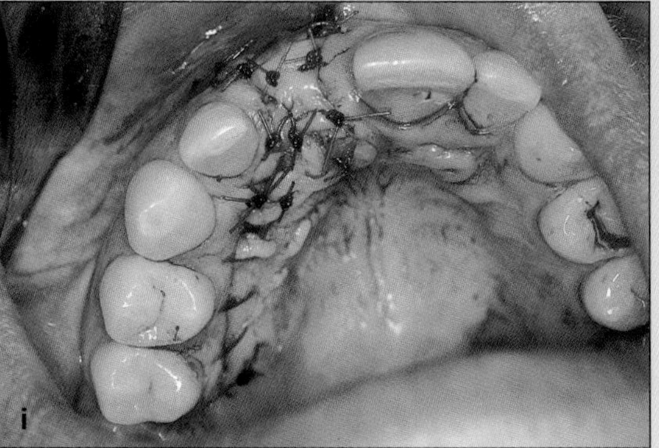

Figs 6-13h and 6-13i Tension-free primary closure was obtained at the contiguous donor and recipient sites.

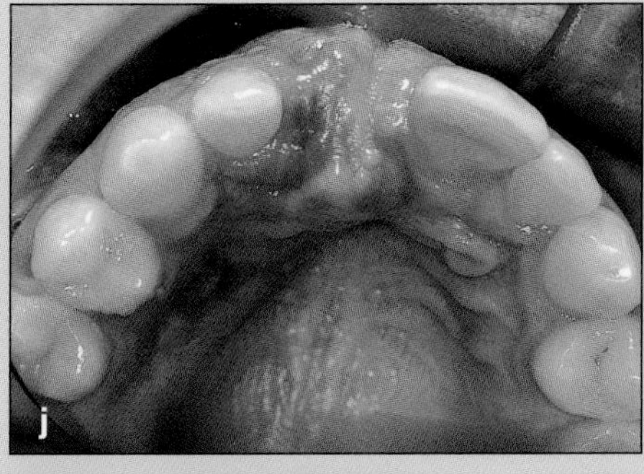

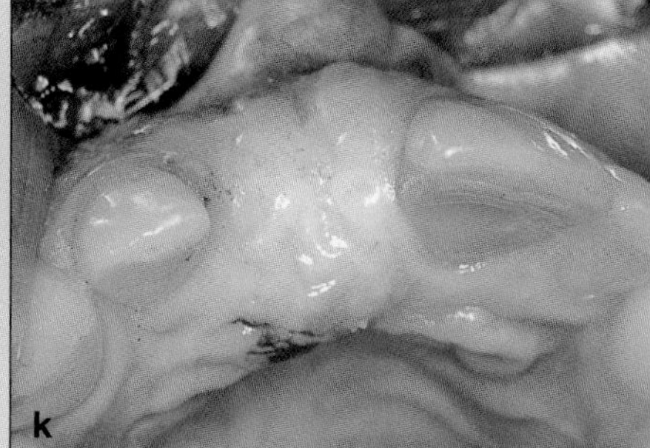

Fig 6-13j Two-week postoperative view demonstrating complete restoration of deficient alveolar ridge contours. All wounds except a small area of the donor-site cover flap healed by primary intention.

Fig 6-13k Four-month postoperative view shows negligible soft tissue shrinkage. This is the norm when the VIP-CT flap is used and presents a tremendous advantage over free soft tissue grafting techniques.

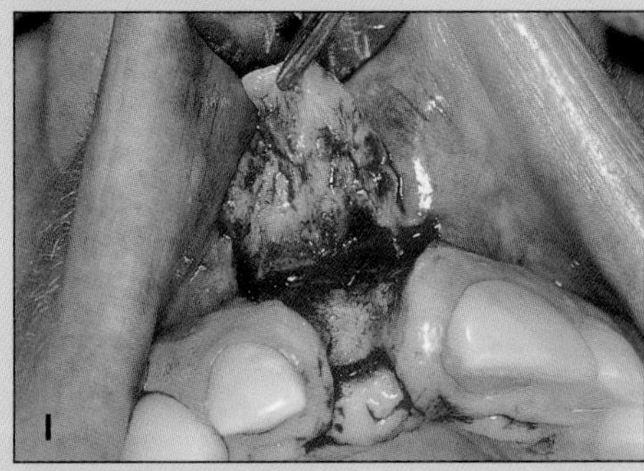

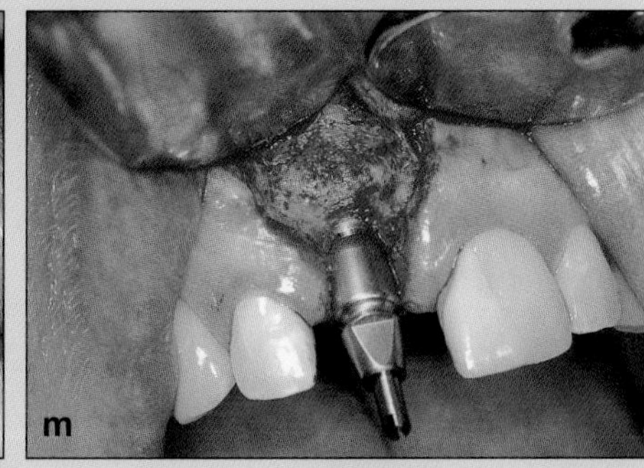

Figs 6-13l and 6-13m The site was re-entered after 4 months of healing. Fixation screws were removed, a submerged implant (Frialit-2, Dentsply) was placed, and a fixture-level impression was taken.

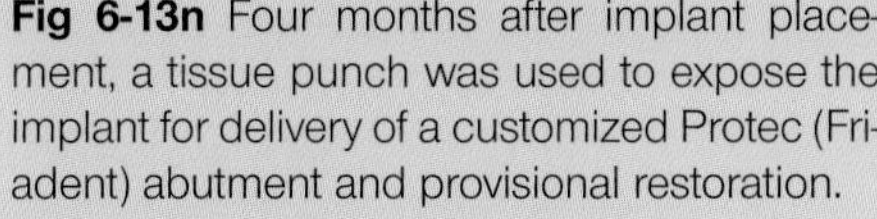

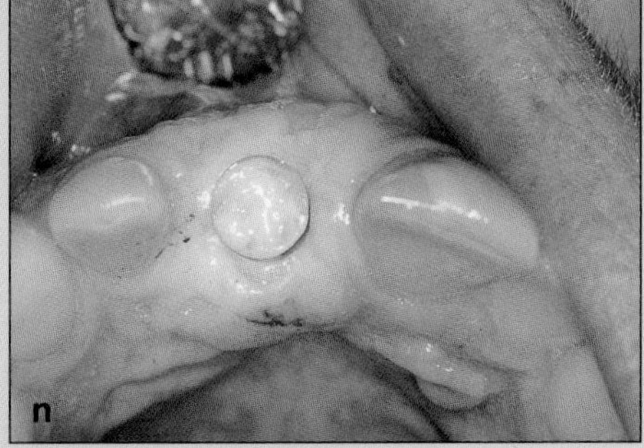

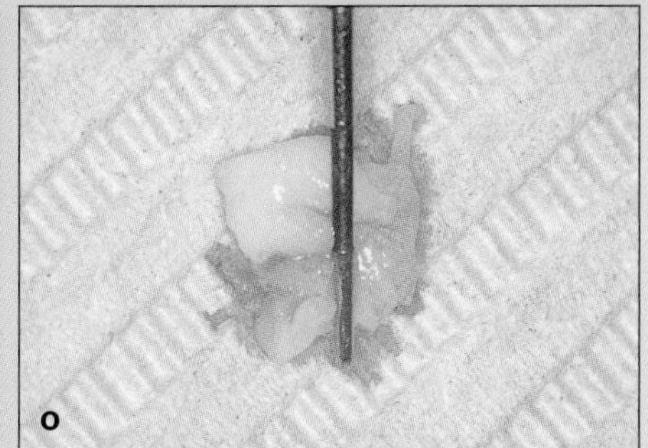

Fig 6-13n Four months after implant placement, a tissue punch was used to expose the implant for delivery of a customized Protec (Friadent) abutment and provisional restoration.

Fig 6-13o The vertical soft tissue augmentation that resulted from the use of the VIP-CT flap far surpasses that obtainable even with sequential free soft tissue grafts. This tissue-punch specimen measured approximately 8.0 mm in height. Tissue heights of 6 to 8 mm are routinely obtained in the anterior maxillary area following use of the VIP-CT flap.

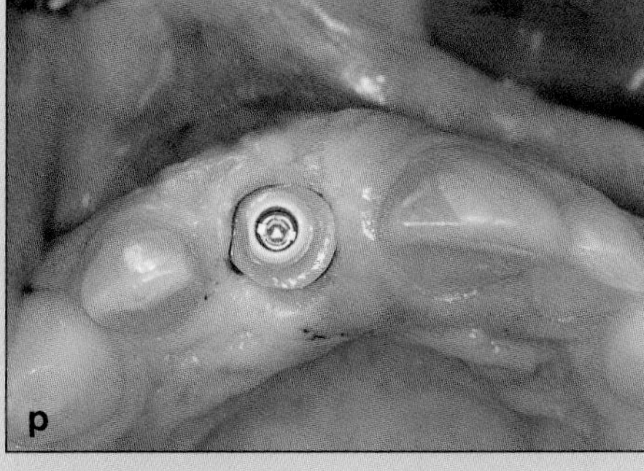

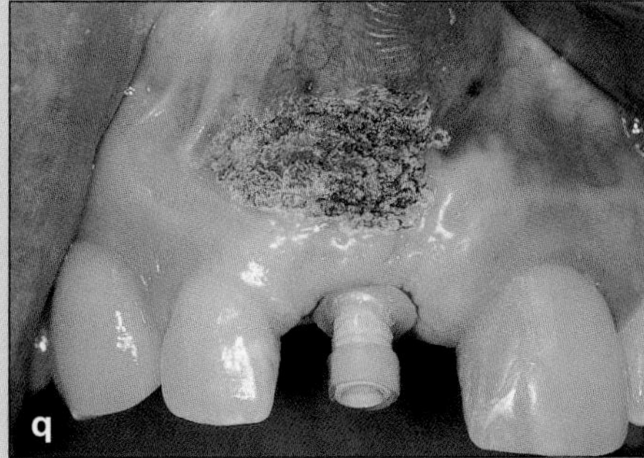

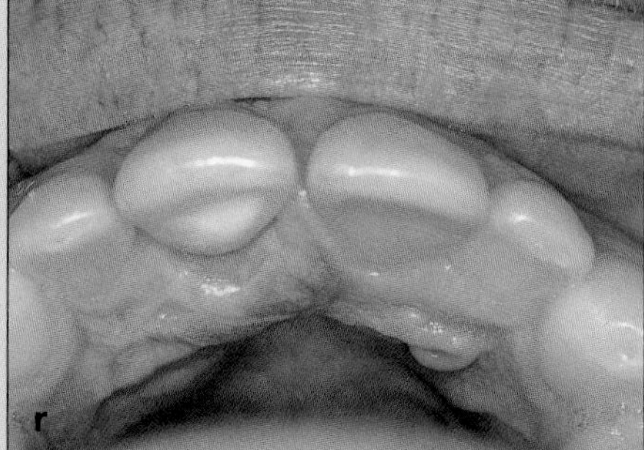

Figs 6-13p to 6-13r The custom abutment was delivered and laser resurfacing was performed to diminish the superficial tissue discoloration in the area.

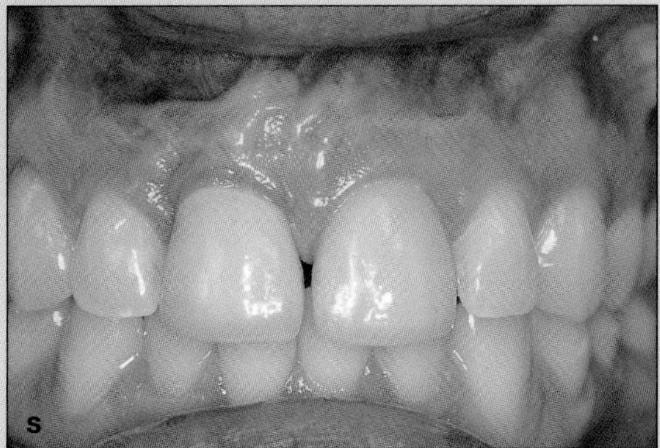

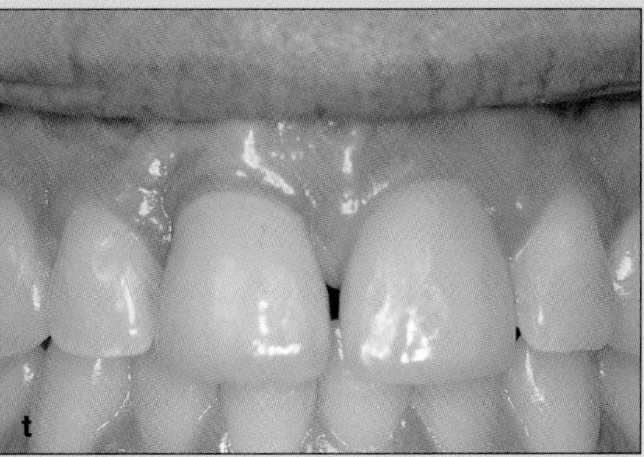

Figs 6-13s and 6-13t Six months after delivery of the final implant restoration, harmonious dental proportions and an esthetic gingival appearance have been restored. Total treatment time for this case was reduced to 10 months: 4 months for site development, 4 months for osseointegration, and 2 months for provisionalization and delivery of the all-ceramic restoration. (Restoration by Dr Stephen Parr, Coconut Grove, FL.)

Simultaneous hard and soft tissue site development of large-volume combination esthetic ridge defects at severely compromised sites

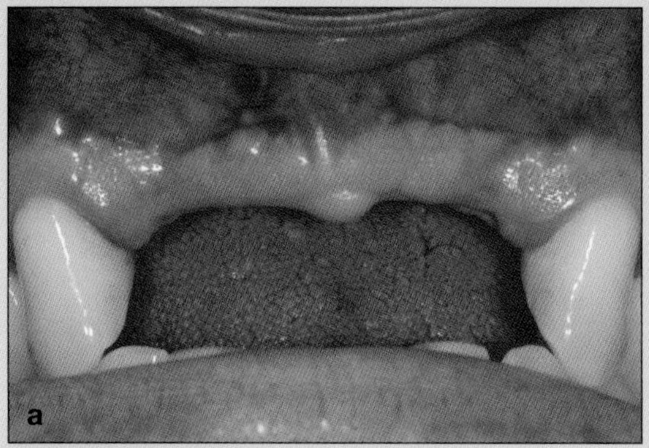

Fig 6-14a Preoperative view of maxillary incisor implant sites with large-volume combination hard and soft tissue defects. The sites are compromised secondary to multiple endodontic procedures and development of osseous periodontal defects. Note significant tissue discoloration secondary to previous surgical endodontic procedures.

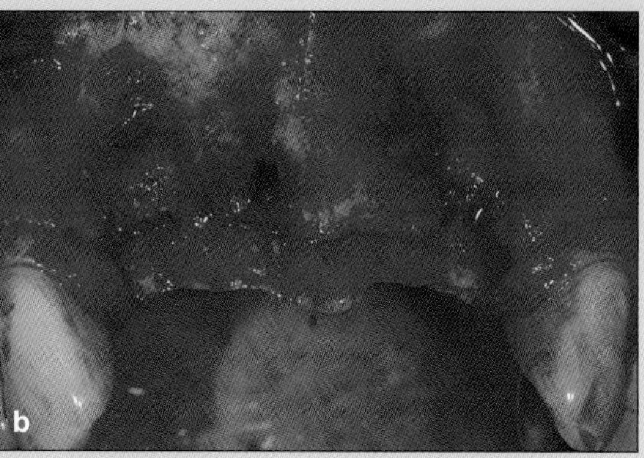

Fig 6-14b A full-thickness exaggerated curvilinear-beveled flap with tension-releasing cutback incisions was used to expose the deficient edentulous alveolar ridge. Note unfavorable through-and-through osseous defects. The adjacent buccal attached tissues and the papillary and col areas have been de-epithelialized.

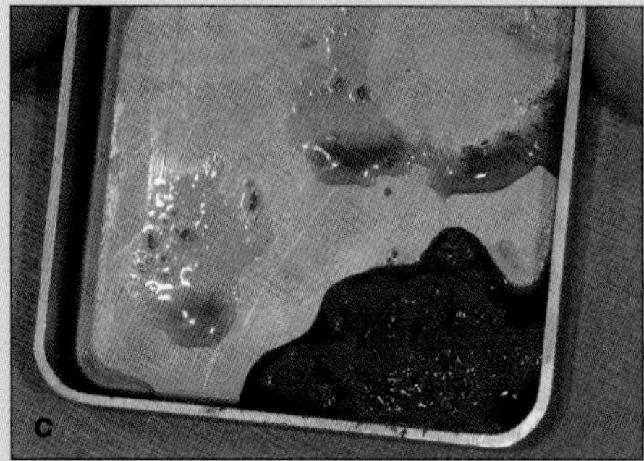

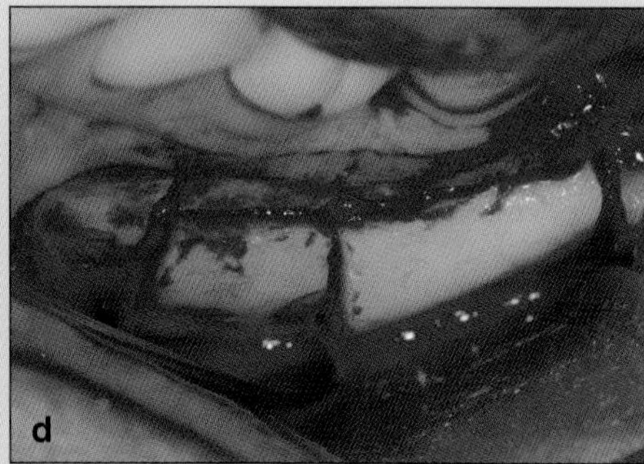

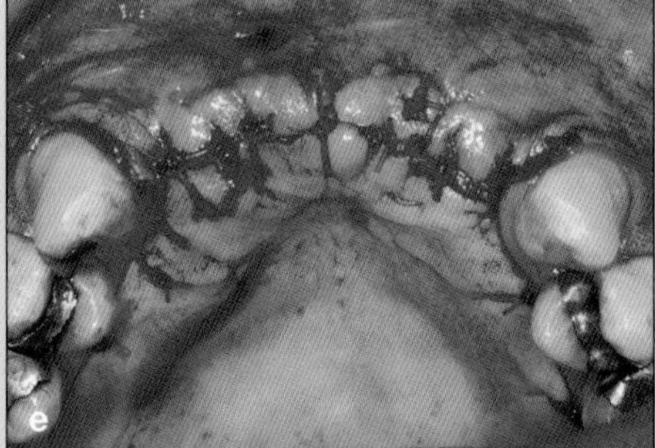

Figs 6-14c to 6-14e Autogenous corticocancellous block and particulate cancellous bone grafts were harvested from intraoral sites and secured at the prepared recipient sites, after which bilateral VIP-CT flaps were developed within the palate and passively rotated and secured over the bone grafts. Exaggerated curvilinear-beveled flap with tension-releasing cutback incisions facilitated tension-free closure at recipient sites. Donor sites were closed after CollaPlug (Centerpulse) absorbable collagen dressing was applied to each site.

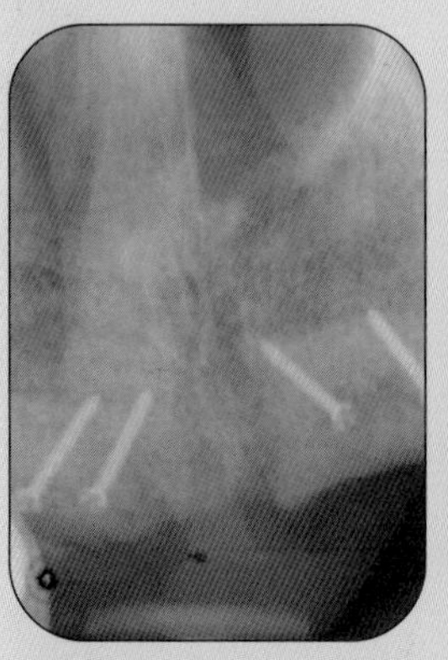

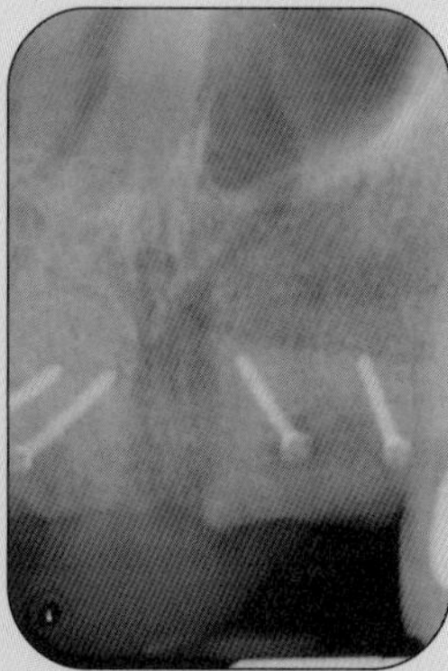

Fig 6-14f Radiographs demonstrating secured corticocancellous bone grafts. A mixture of autogenous cancellous bone and Bio-Oss was used to fill in the areas between the block grafts. Vascularized periosteal connective tissue flaps were then passively rotated and rigidly immobilized over the bone grafts.

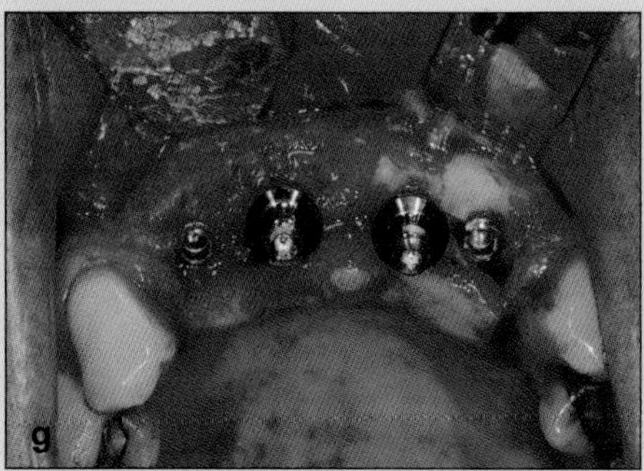

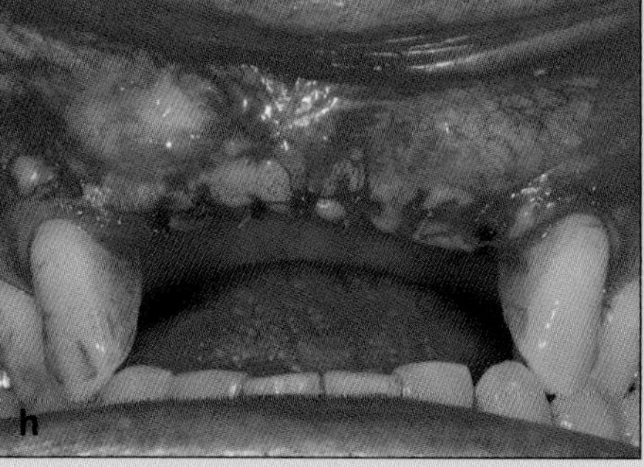

Fig 6-14g The flap used for hard and soft tissue site development was deliberately retraced to provide access for removal of bone graft fixation screws and placement of four submerged external hex implants (3i). To ensure appropriate inter-implant bone width, small-diameter implants were placed at the lateral incisor sites.

Fig 6-14h Tension-free closure over submerged implants and esthetic soft tissue reapproximation is evident.

Fig 6-14i Radiographs taken 4 months after submerged implant placement demonstrate evidence of osseointegration and further incorporation of the bone grafts.

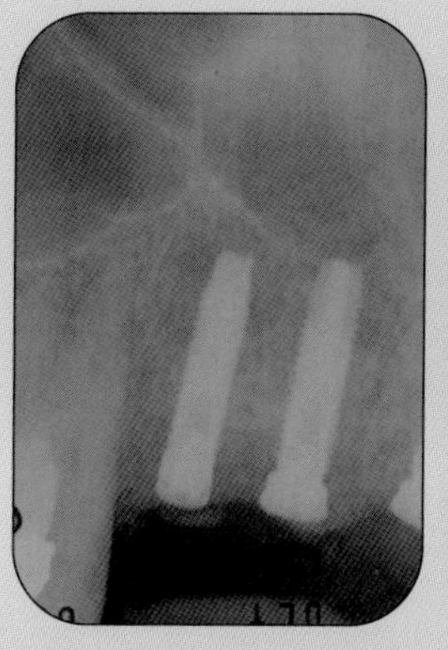

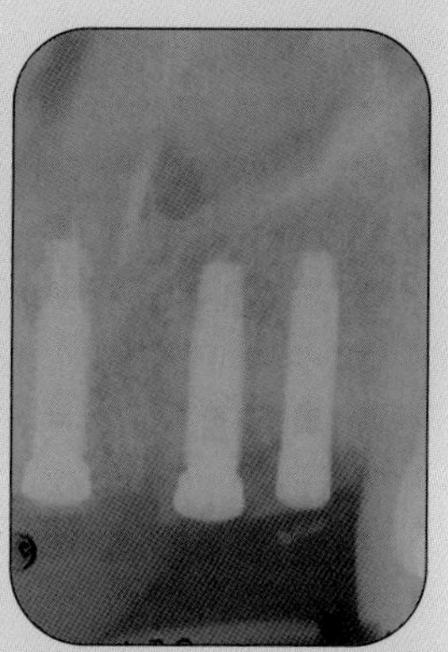

Fig 6-14j Frontal view of implant sites 4 months following implant placement demonstrating successful reconstruction of large-volume combination defects at these severely compromised esthetic sites. Note the successful augmentation of horizontal and vertical ridge contours.

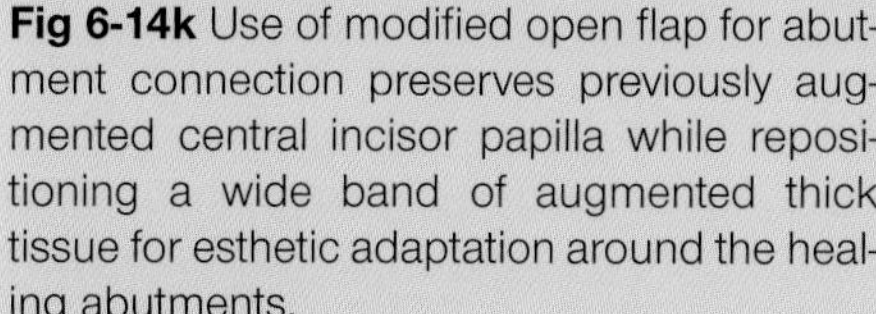

Fig 6-14k Use of modified open flap for abutment connection preserves previously augmented central incisor papilla while repositioning a wide band of augmented thick tissue for esthetic adaptation around the healing abutments.

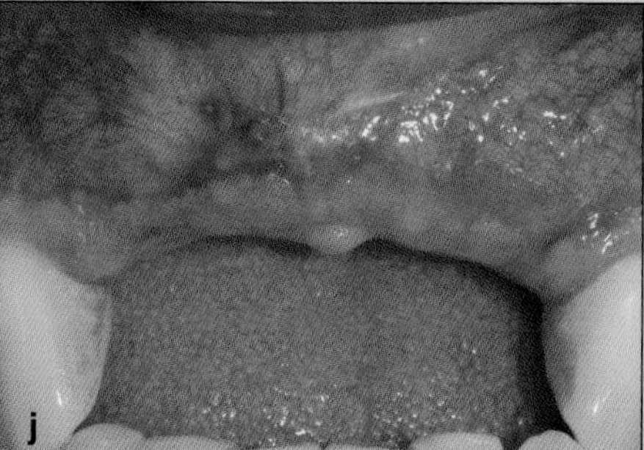

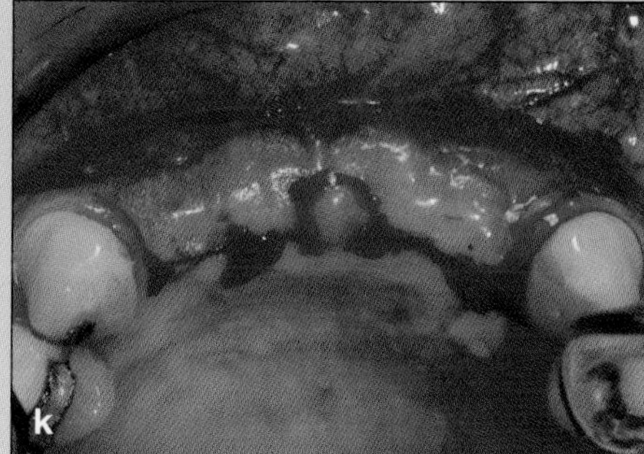

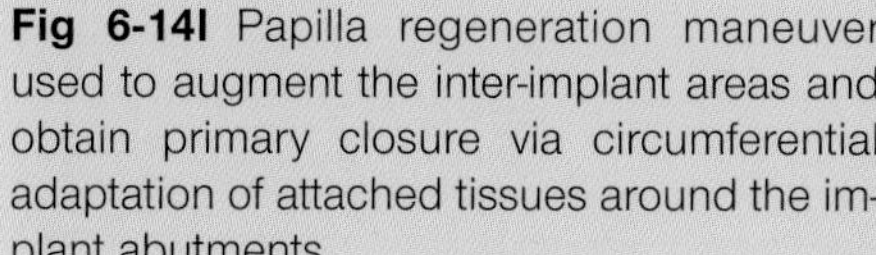

Fig 6-14l Papilla regeneration maneuver used to augment the inter-implant areas and obtain primary closure via circumferential adaptation of attached tissues around the implant abutments.

Fig 6-14m Occlusal view 2 months following implant exposure and abutment connection demonstrating abundant attached tissues surrounding the emerging healing abutments and restoration of ridge contours.

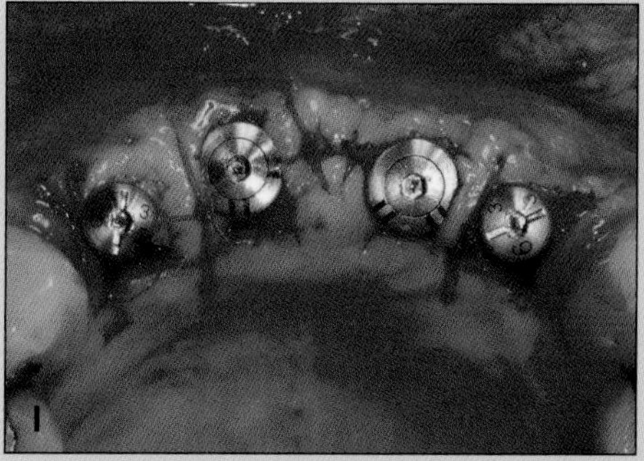

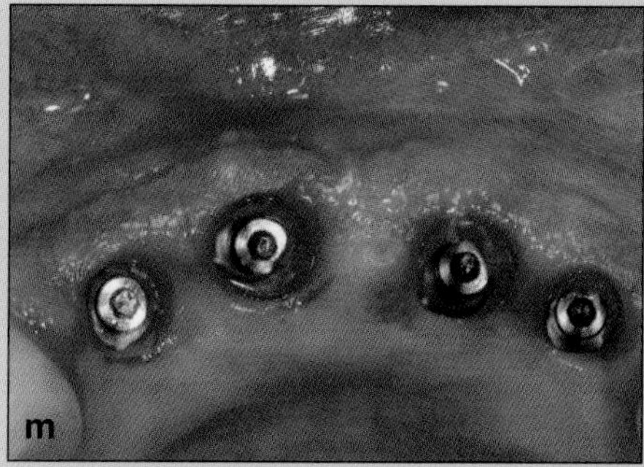

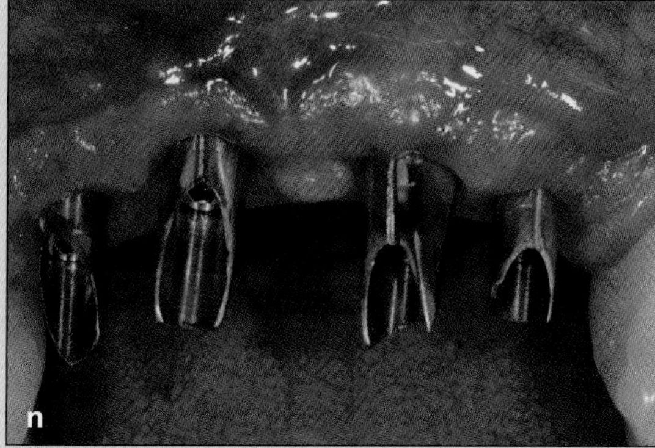

Fig 6-14n Two months after exposure of implants, the temporary abutments have been replaced by permanent abutments. Positive soft tissue architecture has been restored and adequate soft tissue thickness buccal to the implants will allow esthetic restorative emergence. A healthy peri-implant soft tissue environment is evident.

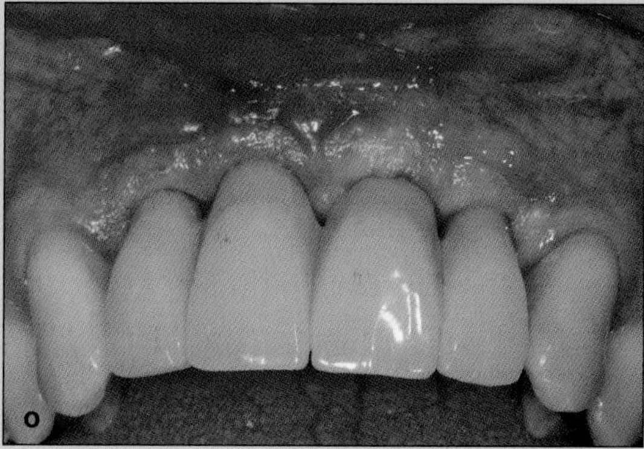

Fig 6-14o Provisional restoration in place. Note that the successful vertical soft tissue augmentation realized by performing the VIP-CT flap in conjunction with hard tissue grafting allows for esthetic restorative emergence and a straight gingival pattern bilaterally. Tissue bulk in the inter-implant areas allows for further development of the positive gingival architecture via guided soft tissue healing. (Restoration by Dr Michael Robinson, South Miami, FL.)

Use of VIP-CT flaps for simultaneous hard and soft tissue site development at anterior esthetic implant sites compromised by significant vertical maxillary deficiency

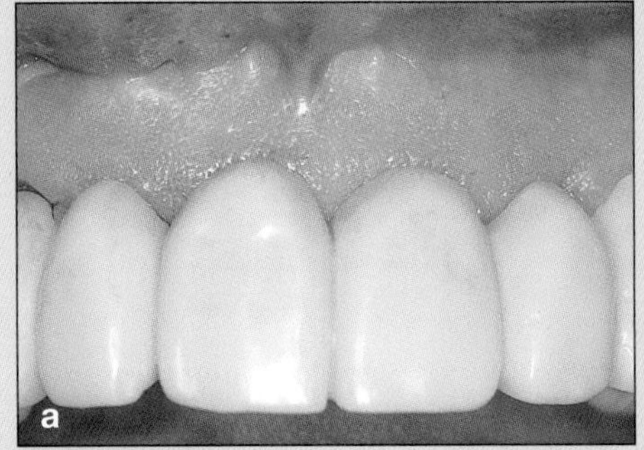

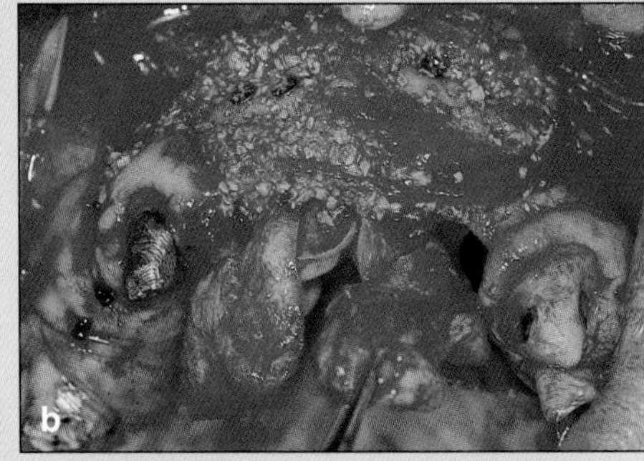

Fig 6-15a Preoperative view of central and lateral incisor implant sites with large-volume combination hard and soft tissue esthetic ridge defect. The esthetic outcome from site development and implant therapy is highly uncertain because of the significant vertical maxillary deficiency and the possibility for limited coronal movements of soft tissue at these sites.

Fig 6-15b An exaggerated full-thickness curvilinear-beveled flap was initiated at the depth of the vestibule in the premolar area to incorporate as much elastic mucosal tissue as possible into the recipient-site flap. Large tension-releasing apical cutback incisions (3 to 4 mm in depth) were performed bilaterally. Corticocancellous block grafts were secured, the VIP-CT flaps were developed as previously described, and particulate bone was condensed around the periphery of the block grafts.

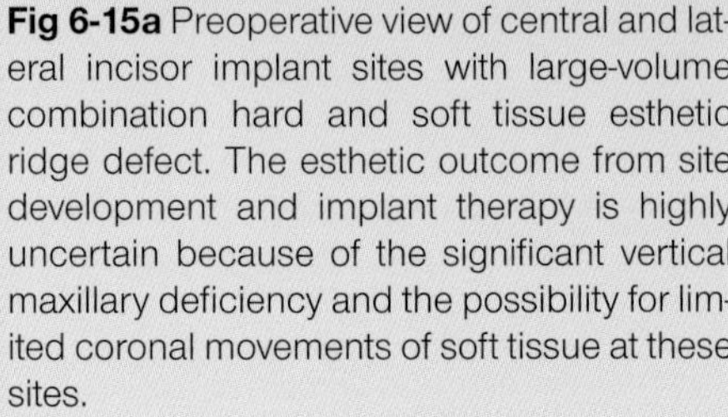

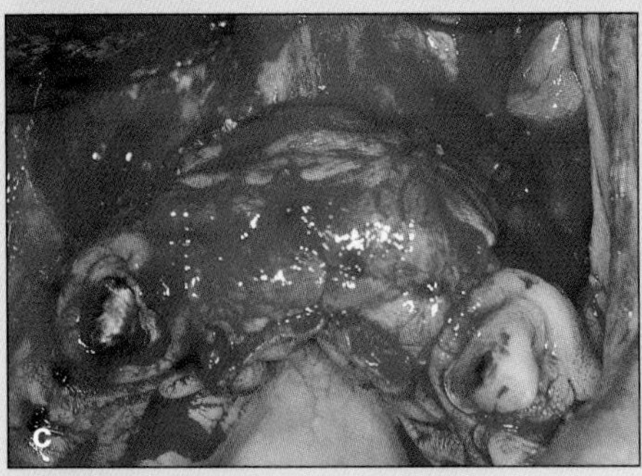

Fig 6-15c A Bio-Gide membrane (Osteohealth) was adapted over the buccal portion of the bone graft, which was not covered by the VIP-CT flaps since vertical soft tissue augmentation was the primary treatment goal. The VIP-CT flaps were sutured together at the midline to create a midline prominence of soft tissue. Additional sutures were passed through transosseous holes previously made in the block grafts with a small wire-passing bur (Osteomed).

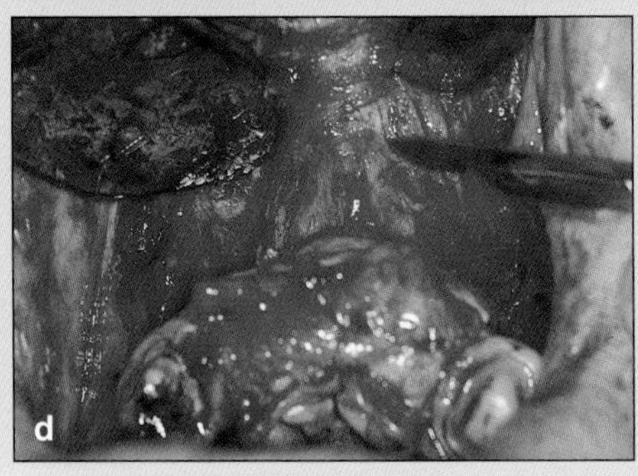

Fig 6-15d Flap design and tension-releasing cutback incisions were insufficient to achieve passive recipient flap accommodation over VIP-CT flaps secured over the crest of the ridge. Due to the severity of the vertical maxillary deficiency, osseous reduction of the anterior nasal spine and periosteal releasing incisions at the confluence of the alveolar ridge and nasal floor periosteum were also necessary.

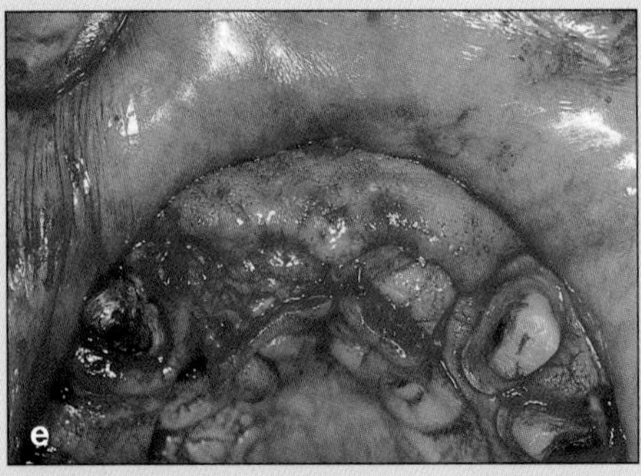

Fig 6-15e Vertical movement of the soft tissues at the midline is evident. Tension-free closure is now possible.

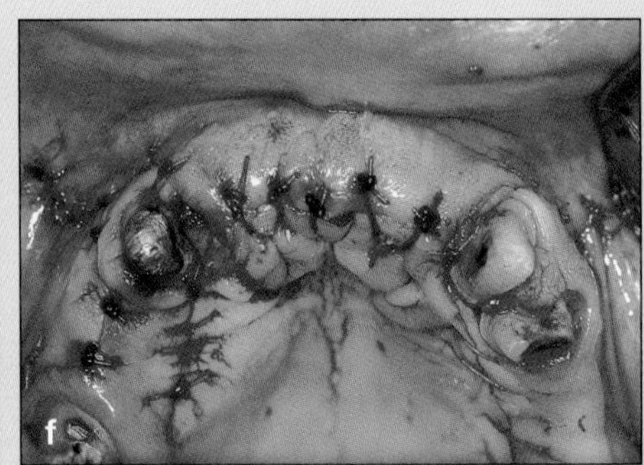

Fig 6-15f Tension-free closure of the recipient site and the bilateral palatal donor sites was achieved using 4-0 chromic gut suture on a P3 needle. Donor sites were also closed after dressing with CollaPlug absorbable dressing.

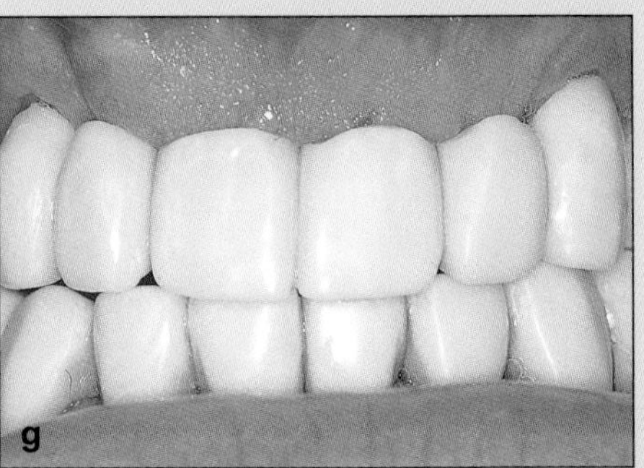

Fig 6-15g Four-month postsurgical view. Note the unprecedented amount of vertical soft tissue augmentation that resulted from use of the VIP-CT flaps when compared to the preoperative condition. This is the key to establishing an esthetic gingival appearance when multiple successive implants are used for restoration of maxillary anterior dentition.

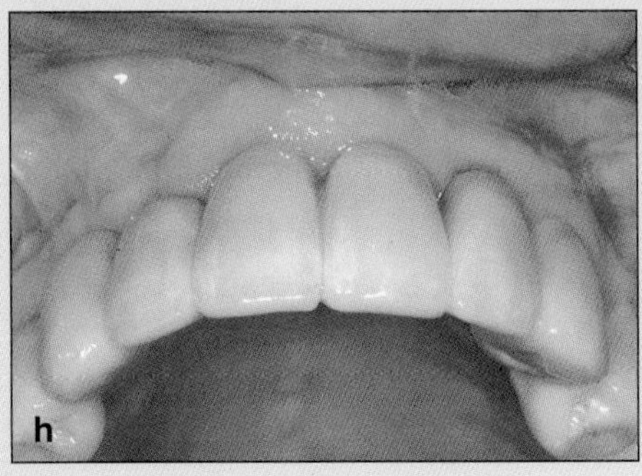

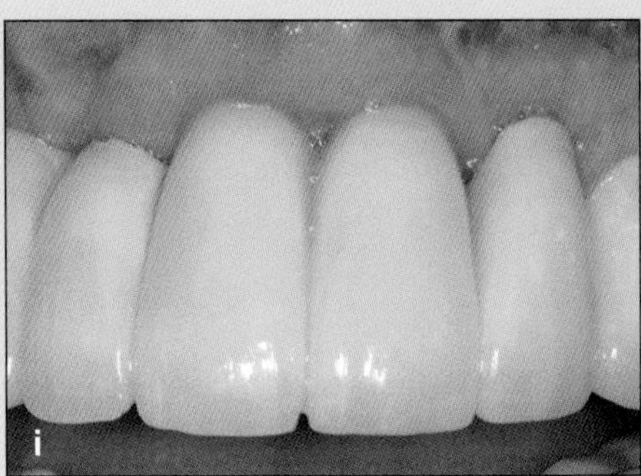

Fig 6-15h Occlusal view 1 year postdelivery demonstrating the severity of the vertical maxillary deficiency and the large amount of horizontal augmentation that resulted from the use of the VIP-CT flap.

Fig 6-15i Frontal view 1 year postdelivery demonstrating esthetic emergence of the four incisor implants with a stable and healthy soft tissue environment despite the compromise imposed by the anatomic limitation.

Summary

The VIP-CT flap is an innovative technique that is extremely useful for large-volume soft tissue augmentation and simultaneous hard and soft tissue site development of deficient alveolar ridges in conjunction with implant therapy. The pedicled blood supply derived from the connective tissue–periosteal plexus within the flap provides the biologic basis for predictable simultaneous hard and soft tissue grafting procedures during esthetic implant site development, even at compromised sites. This significantly reduces treatment time and patient inconvenience. Additional advantages of the technique include the ability to reconstruct large-volume soft tissue defects with a single procedure, negligible postoperative soft tissue shrinkage, and enhanced results realized from hard tissue grafting procedures due to the supplemental source of circulation and the contribution to phase-two bone graft healing provided by the mesenchymal cells transferred with the flap. In addition, when hard and soft tissue site-development procedures are necessary, treatment time and patient inconvenience are minimized.

The VIP-CT flap was used at 126 esthetic implant sites for simultaneous hard and soft tissue site development between March 1995 and December 2001. Additional bone grafting was not necessary in any of these cases, and an osseointegration rate of 99.2% was achieved with a follow-up period ranging from 12 to 54 months. The volume of soft tissue transfer obtained from this technique is consistently superior to that of previously described free soft tissue grafting techniques. The VIP-CT flap was used at 229 esthetic implant sites for large-volume soft tissue reconstruction prior to and simultaneous with implant placement. Tissue-punch specimens obtained at anterior maxillary sites consistently demonstrated vertical tissue heights between 6 and 8 mm following the VIP-CT flap procedure.

One limitation of the technique is the necessity to use a toothborne provisional restoration during the healing period. During initial healing, a customized toothborne interim provisional restoration designed to house pontics at the edentulous site(s) and also protect the palatal donor site (eg, Essex retainer) is recommended. Subsequently, the restorative dentist may provide a more definitive interim restoration that allows the patient to resume function. As with the harvesting of free connective tissue grafts, the VIP-CT flap is also limited by the size and shape of the donor palate and the thickness of the tissue present in the premolar region. The excess soft tissue that results on the palatal aspects of the alveolar ridge adjacent to the recipient site may require secondary debulking. Finally, soft tissue plasty is often needed to re-establish vestibular depth at sites where large-volume alveolar ridge defects were reconstructed. The routine use of this technique as part of esthetic implant site development has provided a level of esthetic predictability in the restoration of deficient implant sites in the maxillary anterior region not routinely obtainable with previously described techniques.

CHAPTER 7

Esthetic Implant Therapy: A Comprehensive Approach

This chapter presents a comprehensive approach to the surgical management of a wide range of clinical case types encountered in esthetic implant therapy. A specific philosophy of care is presented to give the implant surgeon a perspective on how to approach and manage patients who desire esthetic implant replacements. The rationale for the use of "site-preservation" techniques is emphasized. The techniques for providing inconspicuous restoration of large- and small-volume hard tissue defects at esthetic implant sites are presented in detail. The indications for specific hard and soft tissue site-development techniques are correlated with the six individual types of esthetic ridge defects previously outlined in chapter 2. The importance of taking advantage of recent advances in surgical biotechnology, close coordination of surgery and prosthetics, use of guided soft tissue–healing techniques, use of cosmetic laser soft tissue sculpting and resurfacing, and use of cosmetic periodontal surgery to enhance outcomes in esthetic implant therapy is discussed. In addition, the rationale and protocols for the use of platelet-rich plasma (PRP) to enhance wound healing, to maximize volume yields from site-development procedures, and to minimize soft tissue shrinkage at esthetic implant sites are presented. Finally, a conceptual framework for implant site development is presented to aid the surgeon in selecting and sequencing indicated procedures and in estimating the average time necessary to treat common clinical case types. The reader should realize that the information and concepts presented in this chapter rely on an understanding of the information already presented in chapters 1 through 6.

Philosophy of Care

The placement of an osseointegrated implant is a reconstructive procedure that forms the foundation for subsequent functional and esthetic dental rehabilitation. When the esthetic concerns of implant therapy demand inconspicuous dental and periodontal esthetics, the surgical site-development procedures are by definition plastic and reconstructive in nature. Therefore, adoption of the plastic and reconstructive surgery "mindset," which embraces the need for a sequence of surgical procedures performed to achieve the desired result, is appropriate in esthetic implant therapy and forms the basis for a philosophy of care.

Recent biotechnologic advances have both expanded the options for and simplified hard and soft tissue site development. Combined with sound surgical principles and the plastic and reconstructive surgery mindset, we are now able to provide functional and esthetic implant restorations with impressive predictability. Even more important is our understanding of the factors that limit the volume yields from various reconstructive procedures. This insight guides our selection of treatment-planning options and surgical approaches that have an anatomic and biologic basis for success. Perhaps of greatest significance is the recognition of individual anatomic limitations and their effect on the final esthetic results.

Consequently, before treatment is initiated, comprehensive treatment planning is essential. This process begins with a thorough functional and esthetic periodontal examination, as described in chapter 2, and should include a determination of periodontal phenotype; identification and classification of soft tissue recession defects; classification of existing alveolar ridge defects; evaluation of tooth positions and proportions; evaluation of occlusal considerations; evaluation of gingival and incisal plane morphologies; and careful study of lip position at rest, relaxed-smile, and full-animation positions. In addition, the implant surgeon should take time to obtain a detailed history of the events leading to loss of teeth in the areas involved. This will aid in assessing the regenerative potential of the site. Implant sites with a history of trauma such as intrusion, subluxation, avulsion with reimplantation, infection, or multiple surgical or endodontic procedures often have diminished circulation available to support osseointegration or to sustain hard or soft tissue grafts, resulting in implant failure or in reduced volume yields or complications from grafting procedures.

Based on the findings of the pretreatment evaluation and history of the site, the implant team is able to quantify existing dental and periodontal esthetic deficiencies and select and sequence the therapeutic modalities that will be required to achieve an implant restoration in harmony with the adjacent dentition. Realistic expectations for the final result are established, and the number of procedures and total treatment time are estimated. This information is then reviewed with the patient, the restorative dentist, and, when appropriate, the laboratory technician. Achieving ideal implant esthetics can be as simple as removing a failed tooth with immediate implant replacement in a manner that preserves the soft tissue architecture at the site, or as complex as a multiple therapeutic sequence that includes orthodontic therapy, staged hard and soft tissue reconstruction of the implant site, and the use of cosmetic periodontal surgery to ensure harmony with the adjacent dentition. Correspondingly, the treatment time required to obtain an esthetically pleasing result for the implant patient may be as short as 3 months for uncomplicated immediate implant replacements, or as long as 2 years or more for complex cases requiring a comprehensive multidisciplinary approach.

Rationale for Site Preservation

As discussed in chapter 4, preservation or re-creation of natural alveolar ridge anatomy is a prerequisite for success in esthetic implant therapy. Natural hard and soft tissue contours allow both ideal implant placement and the emergence of a restoration that is harmonious with the adjacent dentition and free of prosthetic compensations. The successful application of surgical techniques designed either to preserve existing alveolar ridge contours or to reconstruct missing hard and soft tissues at an implant site is based on a clear understanding of both periodontal and peri-implant soft tissue anatomy (see chapter 2) and their individual responses to the multitude of surgical and prosthetic interventions often required in esthetic implant therapy. Armed with this knowledge, the implant surgeon can successfully apply plastic and reconstructive tech-

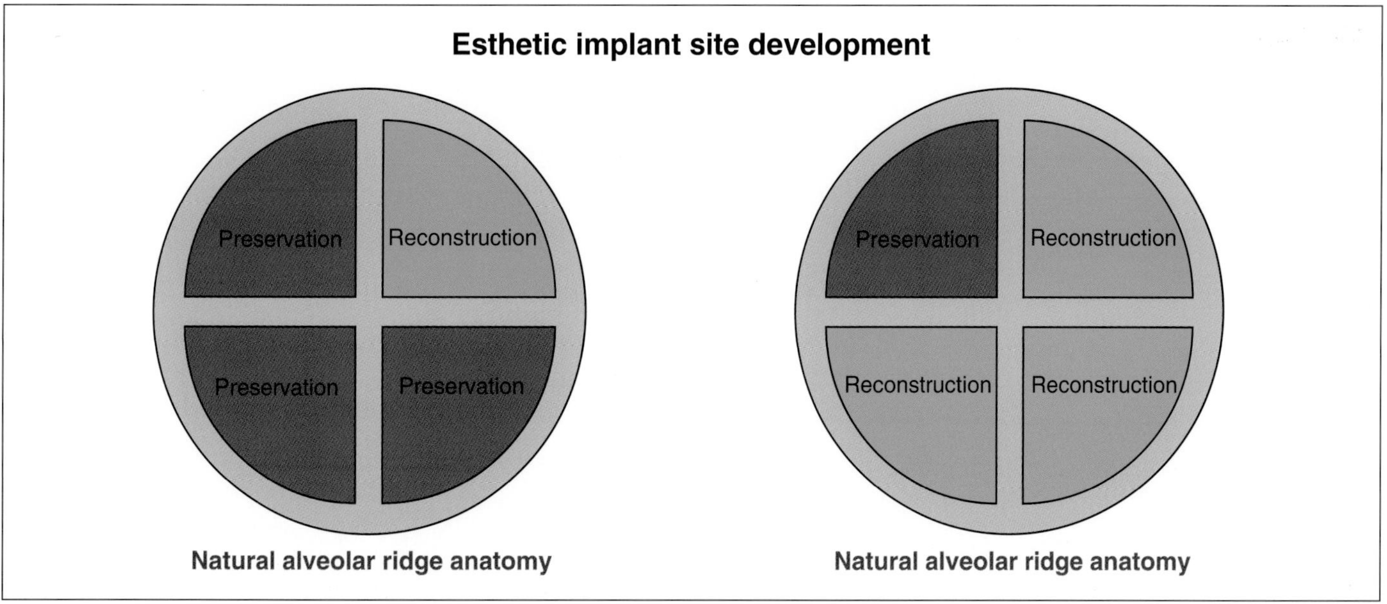

Fig 7-1 The concept of site preservation is an integral part of esthetic implant therapy. Site-preservation techniques minimize the number and/or complexity of subsequent reconstructive procedures required to obtain the desired esthetic results.

niques to restore missing hard and soft tissues in an inconspicuous fashion, providing the restorative dentist with the foundation necessary for the creation of a beautiful implant restoration.

Site preservation is an extremely important concept for the surgeon, the restorative dentist, and the patient to embrace when implant therapy is contemplated in an area of esthetic concern. The use of site-preservation techniques often reduces or even eliminates the need for subsequent reconstructive procedures. Of greater significance, failure to use surgical and prosthetic site-preservation techniques when applicable inevitably increases the number of reconstructive procedures ultimately required to achieve acceptable esthetic results (Fig 7-1). It is important to emphasize that in esthetic implant therapy, the primary objective of site preservation is maintenance of the reconstructive soft tissue envelope and scalloped soft tissue architecture at the site. Allowing the soft tissue envelope to contract severely limits the outcome of subsequent site-development procedures. Just as the volume of the soft tissue envelope and the ability to expand this envelope often represents the limiting factor in plastic and reconstructive surgery, the reconstructive soft tissue envelope is a prime determinant of our ability to surgically reconstruct hard and soft tissue alveolar defects in implant therapy.

Site preservation often begins at the time of tooth removal. As described in chapter 4, the Bio-Col alveolar ridge preservation technique is used to preserve hard and soft tissue alveolar ridge anatomy in preparation for immediate or delayed implant placement in esthetic areas. This proven technique combines both surgical and prosthetic protocols to consistently improve functional and esthetic results. Alveolar ridge resorption is reduced or avoided by minimizing trauma during tooth removal, preparation, and grafting of the extraction sockets. Isolation of the grafted socket prevents the need for flap elevation and primary closure, thereby preserving surrounding soft tissue volume. Most importantly, the scalloped soft tissue architecture is preserved by the prosthetic protocol, which provides support to the marginal tissues and interdental papillae and thereby preserves natural soft tissue anatomy at the site.

The cosmetic incisions, innovative flap designs, and conservative exposure techniques described in chapter 3 represent additional site-preservation techniques. These surgical approaches preserve soft tissue circulation and minimize soft tissue shrinkage in areas critical for esthetic restorative emergence. The exaggerated curvilinear flap design with tension-releasing cutback incisions effectively increases the elastic limit of the cover flap used for site-development procedures while preserving circulation to flap margins. As a result, coronal flap repositioning is facilitated and soft tissue accommodation over large-volume grafts is accomplished with tension-free closure, which is not routinely obtainable with traditional flap designs without some compromise in circulation to flap margins. The expanded soft tissue envelope that results from this flap design maximizes volume yields obtained from hard and soft tissue grafting procedures. Similarly, routine beveling of incisions and de-epithelialization of papillary areas adjacent to deficient implant sites extends the area of flap coaptation upon closure. This improves the stability of the postoperative wound complex following site-development procedures and decreases the incidence of wound dehiscence and unwanted retraction of the soft tissues at the site. In addition, the transverse orientation of the beveled incisions enhances incision line esthetics by improving light transmission through the resultant scar and by minimizing surface irregularities at the incision area. The conservative U-shaped peninsula flap provides access to and visibility of the alveolar crest during implant placement without consequence to the soft tissues in the area critical for esthetic restorative emergence. Circulation to the soft tissues at the site is preserved and soft tissue volume and architecture are maintained by this approach. Finally, the use of a tissue punch is a conservative approach to implant exposure. This approach has its greatest value at sites where hard and soft tissue grafting have previously been used to restore appropriate volume for esthetic implant restoration. The tissue punch avoids an additional incision and allows for the implementation of prosthetic-guided soft tissue healing via the delivery of customized provisional restorations or "tooth-form" healing abutments.

Implant Site Development Techniques

In cases where site-preservation techniques were not used or were unsuccessful in maintaining natural alveolar ridge anatomy at esthetic sites, the implant surgeon is faced with the need to restore missing hard and soft tissues in an inconspicuous fashion in preparation for implant replacements. As discussed in chapter 2, esthetic ridge defects are classified according to the volume and nature of the defect. Correlation of treatment options with specific defect types simplifies the selection of site-development procedures for the surgeon and enhances the predictability of esthetic results. In addition to presenting the specific bone-grafting techniques used by the author to restore hard tissue volume defects at esthetic sites, the indications for specific hard and soft tissue grafting procedures are correlated with the various types of esthetic ridge defects. Furthermore, the role of forced orthodontic eruption as a means of nonsurgical hard and soft tissue site development is discussed in the section below.

Surgical restoration of hard tissue volume at esthetic sites

When reconstructing hard tissue alveolar ridge defects at esthetic sites, the implant surgeon should take advantage of the advances in biotechnology that have greatly improved our ability to predictably reconstruct osseous defects in a minimally invasive fashion. Advances in instrumentation and grafting biomaterials allow the implant surgeon to harvest sufficient quantities of viable autogenous bone (particulate marrow and corticocancellous block grafts) via minimally invasive intraoral approaches, which, when expanded by xenografts, allow the surgeon to treat up to six sites with large-volume hard tissue alveolar ridge defects without the inconvenience of iliac and tibial bone graft harvests. Instrumentation for rigid internal fixation of small block bone grafts at implant sites has been refined to further simplify the surgical procedures. Long-lasting absorbable collagen membranes have improved outcomes of guided bone regeneration techniques while minimizing inconvenience to both patient and surgeon from complications or secondary procedures associated with first-generation nonresorbable membranes.

Recently, the ability to harvest autogenous particulate bone as well as corticocancellous block bone from the oral cavity has been greatly simplified both for the surgeon and for the patient by the development of new instrumentation. The author routinely harvests autogenous particulate bone grafts from the retromolar, buccal shelf, and symphyseal regions of the mandible using the OsteoHarvester (Osteomed, Addison, TX), which harvests, morselizes, and collects viable bone (Fig 7-2). Since the initial degree of bone regeneration at the recipient site is directly proportional to the amount of viable autogenous bone cells transferred with the graft, the surgeon should be aware that maintaining cellular viability during the harvest, collection, and storage of the bone graft requires a sensitive handling technique. To collect viable particulate bone, the author routinely uses the OsteoHarvester at slow speeds (500 to 700 rpm) under gentle pressure with copious amounts of sterile saline irrigation. This device is connected to a dedicated source of suction, which draws the harvested cortical and cancellous bone particles into the collecting reservoir. Once the cortical bone is perforated, the author recommends using a rotary motion to expand the volume of cancellous bone collected. Dessication of the graft must be avoided during collection to maintain graft viability. This is best accomplished by immediate clamping of the dedicated suction line by the circulating assistant or nurse when the bone harvest is complete or when the tip of the collecting reservoir is not immersed either in blood from the site or in saline (see Fig 7-2c). The subsequent transfer and storage of the autogenous particulate bone is also technique sen-

Bone-grafting biotechnology: Intraoral harvesting of viable autogenous particulate bone

Fig 7-2a The OsteoHarvester safely harvests viable autogenous particulate bone from intraoral sites. The device uses specially designed burs (7 or 11 mm in length) to morselize the bone as it is collected and stored.

Fig 7-2b Three 7-mm-deep donor sites usually yield sufficient particulate bone for use around two block bone grafts or a small sinus lift bone graft when used in a 1:1 ratio with deproteinized bovine bone (Bio-Oss; Osteohealth, Shirley, NY).

Fig 7-2c Typical volume yield of autogenous particulate bone obtained from three 7-mm-deep donor sites in the mandible. By avoiding desiccation of the morselized bone, cellular viability was maintained.

Fig 7-2d The ease of setting up and using the OsteoHarvester facilitates the harvest of bone from adjacent sites when an unanticipated peri-implant osseous defect occurs during implant placement.

Fig 7-2e Autogenous particulate bone grafts should be stored in a plastic container, where they can be kept moist in anticoagulated PRP solution or sterile saline. Storage in activated PRP (blood clot) or immersion in saline solution is detrimental to graft survival.

Fig 7-2f A 1:1 ratio of autogenous particulate cancellous bone and Bio-Oss is used for guided bone regeneration procedures, around block bone grafts, and for sinus lift bone grafts. The addition of Bio-Oss may provide an inclusive barrier function and greatly improves the handling characteristics and condensability of the graft.

Fig 7-2g Immediately before use, the particulate bone graft mixture is moistened in activated PRP solution to facilitate transfer and condensation at the recipient site.

Fig 7-2h A moldable bone graft that is easily transferred to the site results when the particulate graft mixture is moistened with activated PRP solution. Condensation at the recipient site will disrupt the osteoconductive network of fibrin formed within the graft, necessitating reapplication of activated PRP solution.

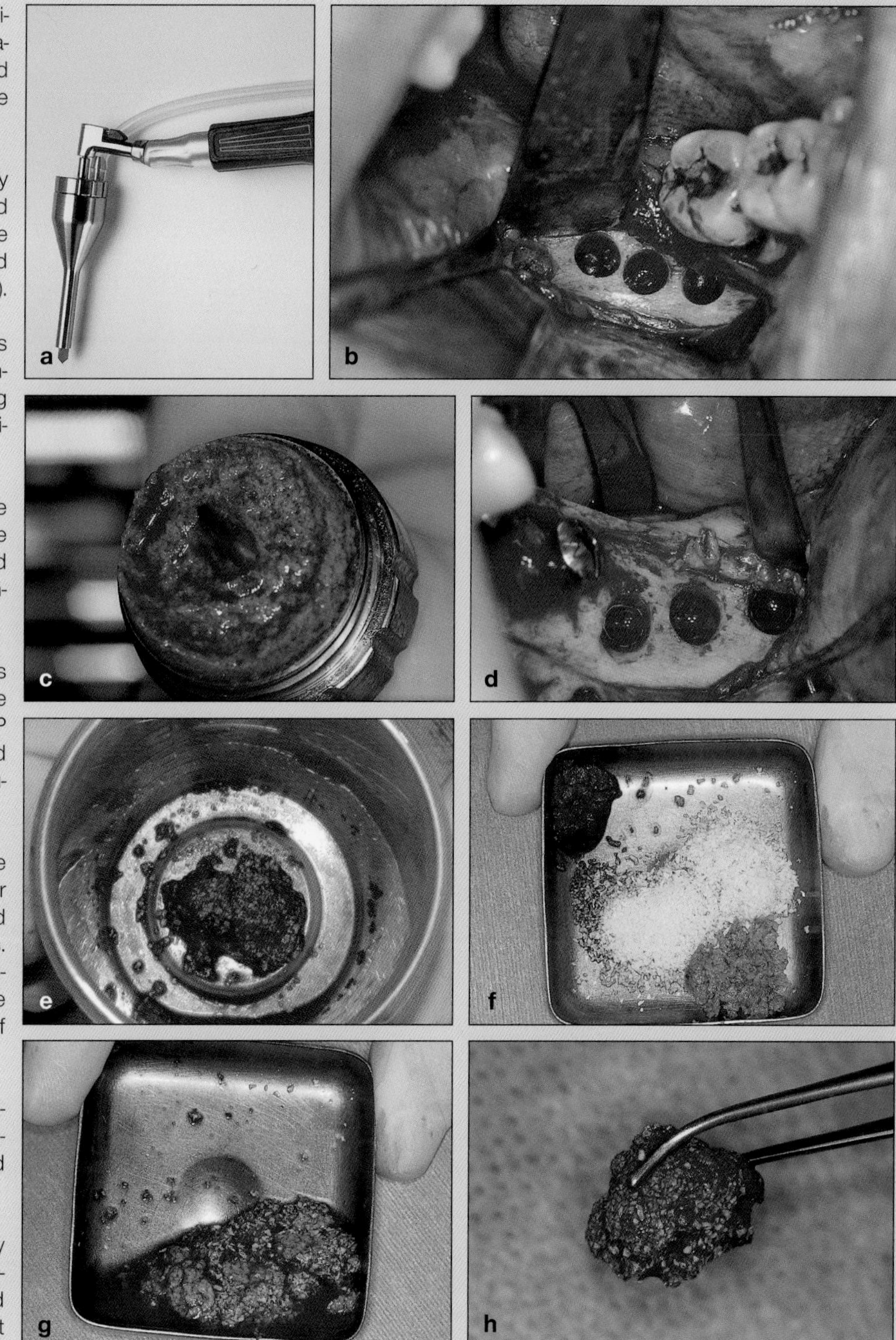

sitive; the author prefers to use a sterile plastic container to which a small amount of anticoagulated PRP solution has been added (see Fig 7-2e). This provides a physiologic medium for storage of the graft and takes advantage of the theoretical uptake of growth factors contained in PRP by the viable bone graft cells. After several minutes, some activation of the solution can be observed within the harvested graft in the form of a thin film of coagulum within the substance of the graft. Activation and degranulation of platelets immediately surrounding the graft particles has the potential to release growth factors to which the cancellous marrow graft particles can respond via their cell membrane receptors. Theoretically, the response of these graft cells can enhance phase-one bone graft maturation and ultimately the volume yield and density of bone achieved by the graft. Because clotted blood is not an ideal storage medium for these grafts, activated PRP solution is not applied to the graft until immediately before delivery to the site or directly at the site after graft conden-

Intraoral donor sites for harvesting of autogenous block and particulate bone from the mandible

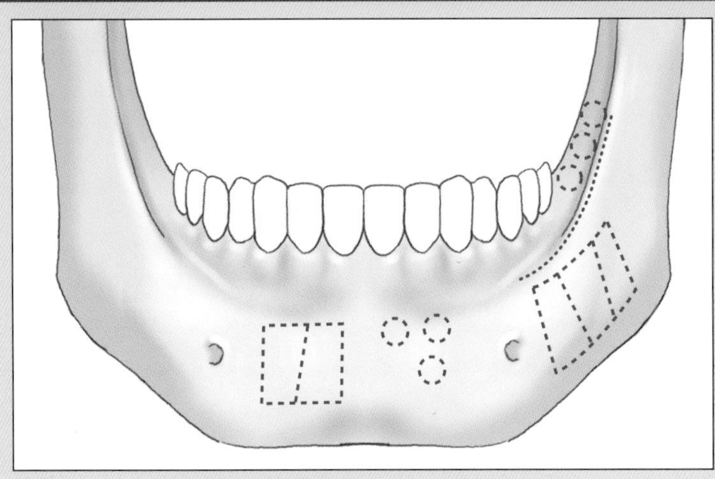

Fig 7-3 Commonly used intraoral donor sites for harvesting corticocancellous block grafts and particulate cancellous grafts from the mandible. Note that three block grafts can usually be harvested from each side of the body of an average-sized mandible. Three or more particulate bone graft donor sites are available from the buccal shelf and retromolar areas bilaterally. A conservative incision *(blue dotted line)* provides access for the harvest. In addition, the mandibular symphysis provides an additional donor site for harvesting block and particulate bone.

sation. Alternatively, the graft can be transferred to and stored in a sterile container. Sterile saline can be used to moisten the graft if needed, but immersion of the particulate graft in saline should be avoided because growth factors can be washed out of the graft.

Deproteinized bovine bone mineral (Bio-Oss) is another product of bone-grafting technology that can be used to expand the volume of autogenous particulate grafts and limit bone graft harvesting at intraoral sites in many cases. This bone graft volume expander is porous, hydrophilic, and osteoconductive; when mixed with autogenous bone, it not only expands graft volume but also improves the working properties of the particulate graft. In addition, as discussed in chapter 4, when Bio-Oss is combined with autogenous particulate cancellous bone, an inclusive barrier effect is obtained. To create a graft, the author prefers to mix a 1:1 ratio of deproteinized bovine bone mineral and harvested autogenous particulate bone. This can be performed in a separate container (see Fig 7-2f). The volume expander is moistened with sterile saline or anticoagulated PRP solution before it is combined with the autogenous bone to create the graft mixture (see Fig 7-2g). The mixture is then carried to and mechanically condensed at the recipient site. When PRP is used, it is added to the mixture to create a moldable bone graft that is immediately transferred to the site (see Fig 7-2h).

Corticocancellous block grafts harvested from intraoral sites offer tremendous advantages over conventional monocortical grafts. While monocortical grafts are valuable for reconstructing deficient osseous contours at implant sites, there is no biologic basis to expect any significant contribution to subsequent osseointegration of an implant placed at that site. Corticocancellous block grafts, on the other hand, are biologically superior since the viable cancellous marrow cells transferred with the graft contribute to phase-one bone regeneration at the recipient site. In addition, the cancellous bone improves the intimacy with which the graft can be adapted at the prepared recipient site, the rate of incorporation of the graft, and its theoretical response to growth factors contained in PRP, as discussed above. To reduce the trauma of bone handling, the author recommends harvesting corticocancellous grafts to match the exact dimensions of the prepared recipient site. This will eliminate the need to modify the graft with rotary instrumentation under saline irrigation and potentially devitalize graft cells from heat, desiccation, or repeated washing with saline irrigation.

The body of the mandible in the areas adjacent to the second premolar and first and second molars are the author's preferred intraoral sites for harvesting these grafts. It is generally possible to procure sufficient block graft(s) to restore three individual or contiguous implant sites from each side of the average-sized mandible. The recipient site is exposed and prepared prior to donor-site surgery. A minimally invasive surgical approach is used to harvest the grafts. A 4- to 5-cm horizontal incision is made through the buccal mucosa approximately 1 cm lateral to the free gingival margins of the premolar and molar teeth in the area. The incision is extended posteriorly parallel to and directly over the external oblique ridge of the mandible if harvesting of particulate bone from the adjacent retromolar area is planned (Fig 7-3). Otherwise, the incision is confined to the area of block bone graft harvesting. Subperiosteal dissection is carried anteriorly to identify the mental nerve and to the inferior border of the mandible. In some cases it is necessary to strip the attachments from the inferior border with a modified Freer elevator.

A periodontal probe is used to transfer the dimensions of the prepared recipient site(s) to the donor area. Using a microsaw (Friadent; Dentsply, York, PA) (Figs 7-4a and 7-4b) or a no. 701 fissure bur (Osteomed), a horizontal osteotomy is made superiorly to define the coronal width of the graft(s). The osteotomy cut should be sufficiently deep and oriented to include several millimeters of cancellous bone. Using the same

Bone-grafting biotechnology: Intraoral harvesting of autogenous corticocancellous block bone grafts

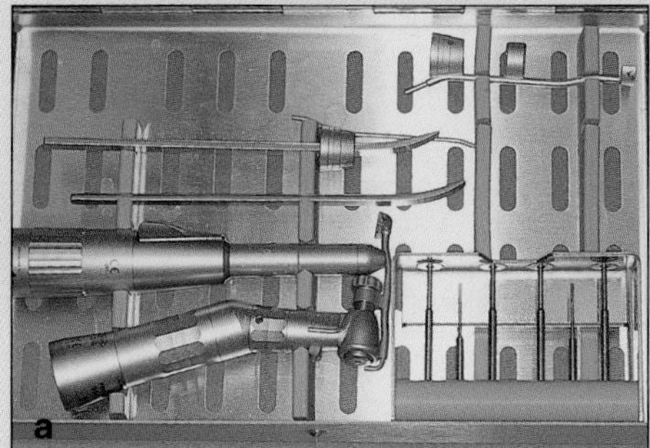

Fig 7-4a Microsaw bone graft harvest set (Friadent) includes straight and contra-angle instrumentation, several diamond saw discs, and bone chisels for harvesting block bone grafts.

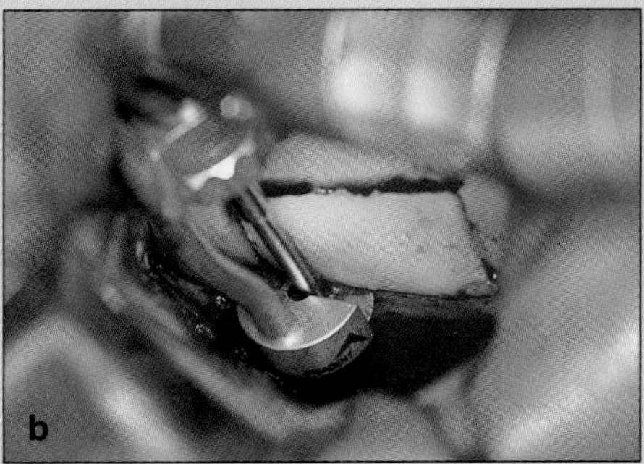

Fig 7-4b The contra-angle handpiece facilitates the harvesting of corticocancellous block grafts from the body of the mandible via a conservative incision and minimal tissue stripping.

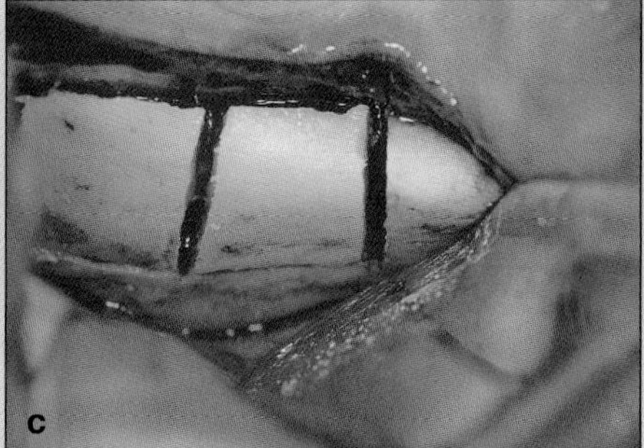

Fig 7-4c A no. 701 bur (Osteomed) is used to ensure the harvesting of customized individual block grafts sized and shaped according to the intended recipient site.

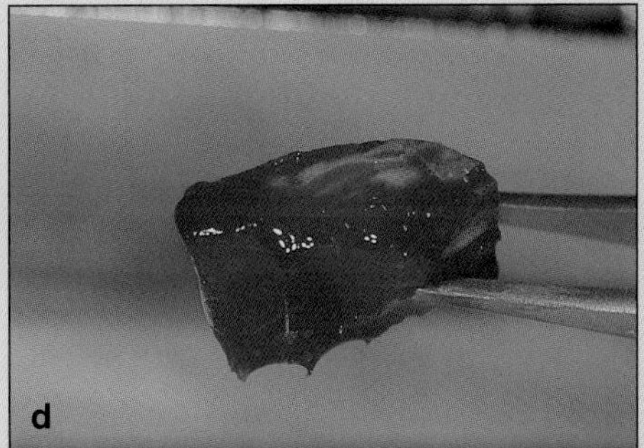

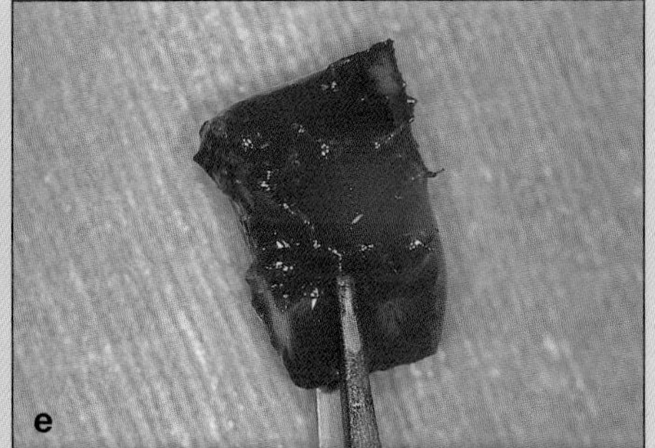

Figs 7-4d and 7-4e Typical corticocancellous block bone graft harvested from the body region of the mandible. Note the thickness of the cancellous bone portion of the graft. The cancellous bone facilitates intimate adaptation to the prepared recipient site and contributes to phase-one bone regeneration and subsequent osseointegration of an implant placed at the graft site.

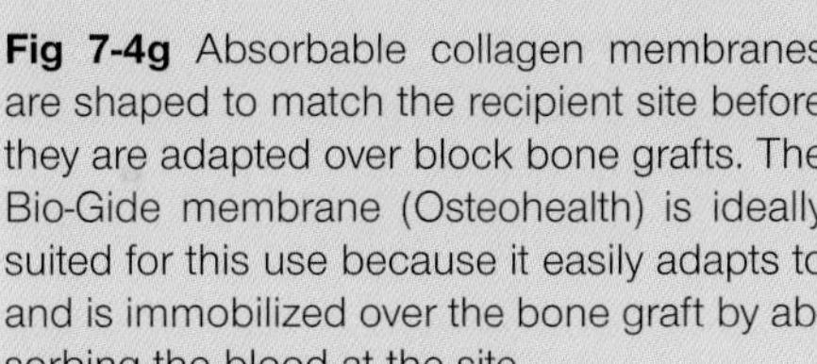

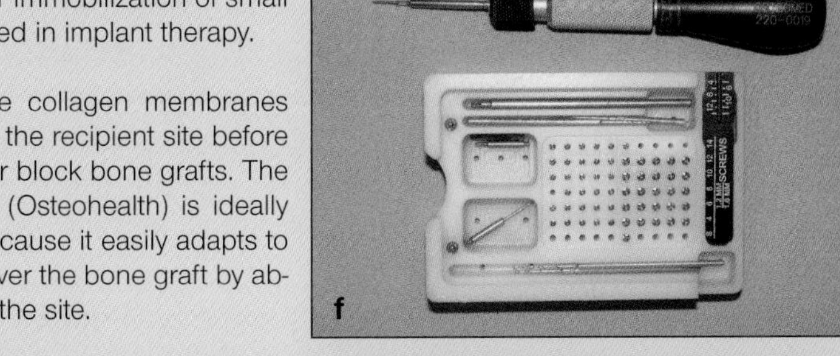

Fig 7-4f Mincro rigid fixation screw set (Osteomed) designed for immobilization of small block bone grafts used in implant therapy.

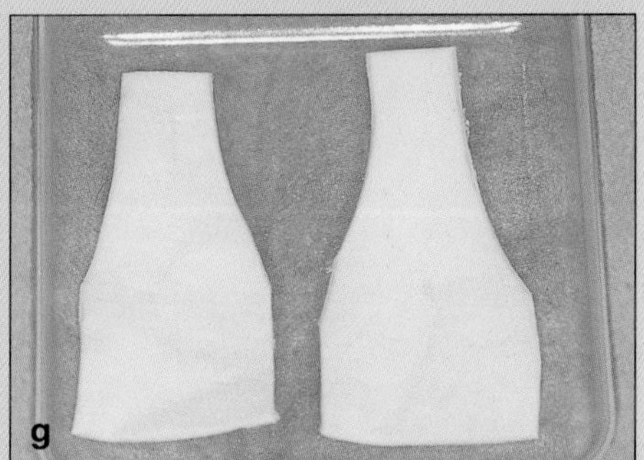

Fig 7-4g Absorbable collagen membranes are shaped to match the recipient site before they are adapted over block bone grafts. The Bio-Gide membrane (Osteohealth) is ideally suited for this use because it easily adapts to and is immobilized over the bone graft by absorbing the blood at the site.

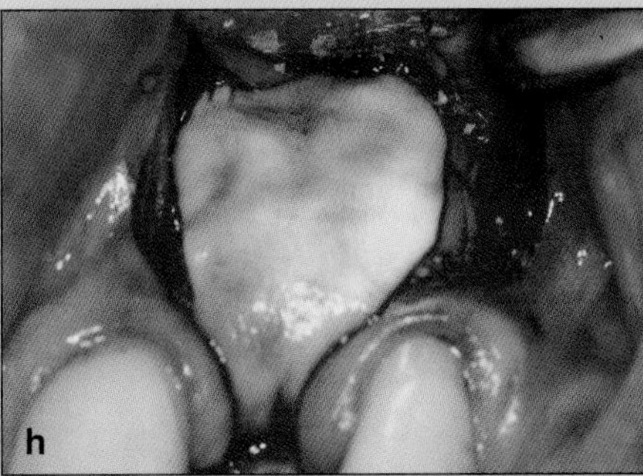

Fig 7-4h Passive adaptation of a Bio-Gide membrane over the crest of the alveolar ridge is achieved at this esthetic site, where block and particulate bone grafting were performed. When the cover flap is adequately developed, the soft tissues are easily closed without displacing the underlying membrane. Fixation of the Bio-Gide membrane is rarely necessary because it lacks memory once moistened in saline or (preferably) blood.

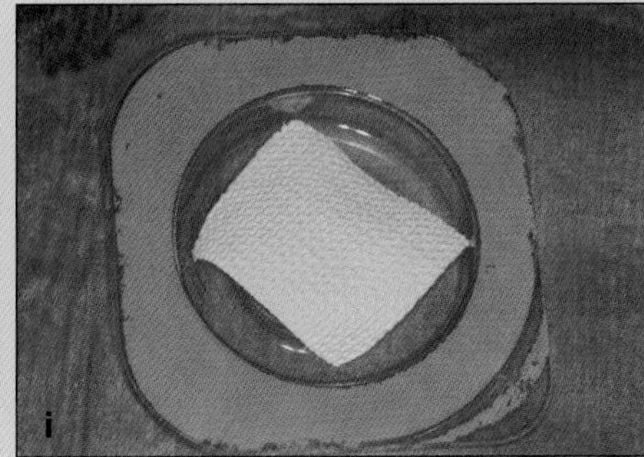

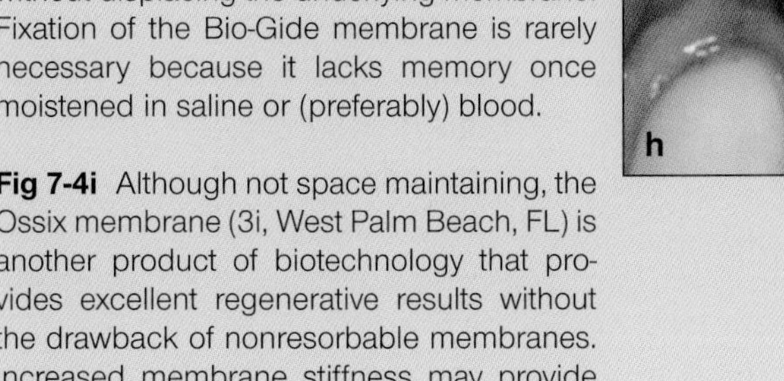

Fig 7-4i Although not space maintaining, the Ossix membrane (3i, West Palm Beach, FL) is another product of biotechnology that provides excellent regenerative results without the drawback of nonresorbable membranes. Increased membrane stiffness may provide an advantage when used for correction of fenestration defects via either an open flap or a subperiosteal pouch approach.

instrumentation, vertical osteotomies are extended inferiorly at the anterior and posterior ends of the superior horizontal osteotomy. The author prefers to diverge these vertical osteotomies to approximate the dimensions of trapezoidal recipient-site preparation. The microsaw is then used to make a second inferior horizontal osteotomy, which completes the outline of the graft.

An innovative product of biotechnology, the microsaw greatly improves the predictability and accuracy of intraoral harvesting of block bone grafts from the mandible by facilitating perpendicular orientation of the inferior horizontal osteotomy through a minimally invasive approach. Use of the microsaw also significantly decreases surgical time and improves postoperative recuperation and patient comfort. The microsaw has a soft tissue guard that effectively avoids injury to the soft tissues. The depth of cutting is defined or limited for safety. In most cases, the saw cut includes several millimeters of cancellous bone as long as the harvest does not extend close to the inferior border, where the cortical bone is much thicker.

The osteotomies are then inspected to ensure that they extend to sufficient depth to include bone marrow. If multiple block grafts are needed, a small fissure bur (no. 701) or the microsaw can be used to define the exact width of each block both coronally and apically to match the prepared recipient sites (Fig 7-4c). Although the microsaw can be used to perform all osteotomies, the author generally prefers to improve visibility of the depth of the cuts by using a small fissure bur for all of the osteotomies except the inferior horizontal osteotomy. The one exception is when multiple blocks are needed from a small donor mandible, because each vertical osteotomy made with a bur occupies close to 2 mm. In some cases this may limit the harvest to two blocks instead of the three corticocancellous block grafts that usually can be harvested from each side of the mandible. Once the block graft(s) has been outlined and inspected, a small bone chisel or osteotome is used to carefully lift the graft, elevating marrow with the cortex. The corticocancellous grafts are inspected for uniformity of the cancellous bone included with the graft (Figs 7-4d and 7-4e) and briefly stored in nonactivated PRP solution before they are transferred to and secured at the recipient site with rigid fixation screws. Alternatively, when PRP is not used, the graft is immediately delivered and secured at the previously prepared recipient site after its harvest.

As noted earlier, when possible the recipient site is prepared in the shape of a trapezoid, with the wider side positioned apically to take advantage of peripheral circulation provided by the extended recipient site (similar to that previously described for soft tissue grafting). In addition, this modification often allows for the placement of two apical fixation screws, which are helpful when the crestal portion of the residual ridge is extremely thin and fixation is questionable. The graft must be intimately adapted to the recipient site before fixation. Should there be a mismatch between the surfaces of the graft and recipient site, the graft should either be returned to the donor site or placed in nonactivated PRP solution while the recipient site is modified to ensure intimate adaptation. Fixation of the graft is then accomplished in the following fashion. The surgical assistant loads a 1.2-mm screw (Osteomed) (Fig 7-4f) of the appropriate length based on observed or measured thickness of the recipient site and graft. While the assistant gently retracts the cover flap, the surgeon stabilizes the graft with the spear end of a no. 9 periosteal elevator and drills the screw hole through the graft and recipient site. The author routinely enlarges the size of the hole in the graft. Subsequently, a lag effect is obtained upon placement of the fixation screw(s). The surgical assistant confines the saline irrigation to the drilling area and avoids excessive washing of the graft during this process. Following fixation of the block graft and prior to delivery of the particulate bone graft and adaptation of the resorbable barrier membrane, the author recommends confirming that passive flap reapproximation is possible. In most instances the exaggerated curvilinear flap design with tension-releasing cutback incisions ensures this even when large-volume defects are being corrected. Nevertheless, at severely scarred sites, extension of the depth of the cutback incisions may be necessary. Next, the prepared particulate graft mixture is carefully condensed around the periphery of the graft and recipient site to fill any voids, similar to the way in which mortar is used to set a brick in a wall.

Long-lasting resorbable collagen membranes represent another important advancement in grafting biotechnology. These membranes provide all of the well-documented benefits of nonresorbable membranes without their attendant problems, namely a high rate of exposure, secondary infections, and undesirable changes in the color and character of the overlying soft tissues. The author trims or fashions these membranes for a precise fit before delivering them to the site(s), where they are stabilized by blood absorption as they are adapted over the particulate or block and particulate composite grafts (Figs 7-4g to 7-4i). Alternatively, the application of activated PRP at the site will physically stabilize the membrane over a particulate bone graft or composite corticocancellous-particulate graft. Following membrane adaptation and stabilization, tension-free closure of the soft tissues and protection of the site are prerequisites for a successful outcome.

Surgical technique for restoring a small-volume hard tissue defect at an esthetic implant site

While small-volume hard tissue defects located away from the crest of the ridge may be reconstructed simultaneously with implant placement in esthetic areas, the author recommends staged reconstruction of these defects when they involve the area critical for prosthetic emergence. When the defect involves or jeopardizes the buccal ridge crest, simultaneous correction at the time of implant placement with a guided bone regeneration procedure carries a significant risk of compromising esthetics. Often this is not appreciated until after a provisional or final restoration has been delivered. In these instances, soft tissue recession often follows delivery of the restoration and in certain instances will continue to progress. Correction of the resultant recession defect can be challenging since a loss of underlying bone can lead to a compromised recipient site for a corrective soft tissue graft. Furthermore, soft tissue recipient-site preparation may further compromise the circulation to the immature regenerated bone occupying the previous buccal crestal defect, resulting in additional bone loss. When this occurs, metal showthrough will compromise final esthetics despite the corrective soft tissue graft. In the worst-case scenario, recession will be progressive, resulting in both an esthetic and a functional compromise that will usually require removal of the implant and a complicated series of procedures to develop the site in preparation for placement of a second implant. In many cases, patients will refuse such a sequence of events and will choose a conventional dental restoration. In the author's experience, staged reconstruction of small-volume hard tissue defects involving or jeopardizing the crest of the ridge at esthetic sites virtually eliminates the above risks, yields a high degree of predictability, and is always indicated when esthetics is a high priority.

When small-volume hard tissue defects do not jeopardize the integrity of the ridge crest, simultaneous correction of the defect at the time of implant placement yields excellent results with a high degree of predictability. The surgical protocol for reconstructing these defects begins with an exaggerated curvilinear beveled flap with apical tension-releasing cutback incisions, as described in chapter 3. Next, the implant is ideally placed with the help of a surgical guide. Once the size of the fenestration defect has been determined, an appropriate amount of autogenous particulate cancellous marrow bone is harvested from the retromolar, buccal shelf, or symphyseal region of the mandible, as previously described using the OsteoHarvester. The harvested bone is transferred to and stored in a sterile plastic container. The graft is saturated in a small amount of nonactivated PRP solution, if available. Next, an equal quantity of deproteinized bovine bone mineral is delivered to a separate container on the sterile field. An absorbable collagen membrane is fashioned with curved Iris tissue scissors to match the size and shape of the recipient site. Prior to grafting, the surgeon repositions the flap and verifies passive flap coaptation. For a nonsubmerged implant, an anatomic healing abutment is placed, and the surgeon verifies that the flap passively adapts around the emerging abutment. If indicated, resective contouring is performed prior to grafting the defect. Next, the stored autogenous bone is mixed with an equal amount of deproteinized bovine bone mineral, and, if available, activated PRP is added to form a moldable bone graft, which is transferred to the site and condensed until the defect is restored. Additional activated PRP is applied to the site, and the absorbable collagen membrane is then adapted over and secured at the graft site by absorbing the PRP solution. Alternatively, when PRP is not used, the dry membrane is adapted over the graft and stabilized by absorbing blood at the site. Proper development of the flap with apical cutback incisions ensures passive coaptation over the grafted defect and eliminates the need to secure the membrane. The cover flap is then passively readapted and secured in a standard fashion (Fig 7-5).

Surgical technique for restoring a large-volume hard tissue defect at an esthetic implant site

Large-volume hard tissue defects should always be reconstructed in a staged fashion prior to implant placement. In most cases this involves a corticocancellous block graft procedure followed by a soft tissue graft performed 4 to 6 months later to compensate for the loss of soft tissue volume resulting from the bone graft procedure. The defect site is accessed with an exaggerated curvilinear flap design with beveled incisions, and adjacent papillary areas are denuded using a fresh no. 15C scalpel. As described in chapter 3, this improves the early integrity of the wound margins and improves incision line esthetics. A no. 8 round bur (Osteomed) operating at slow speeds (500 to 700 rpm) is then used under copious sterile saline irrigation to prepare the recipient site in the shape of a trapezoid. An inline suction bone trap can be used during this process to collect additional autogenous bone, provided the bone is not desiccated and saliva is not suctioned through the filter because this will devitalize the harvested bone. The cortical bone is thinned to obtain a flat, uniform surface and may even be perforated in some areas. Definitive butt-joint margins are created in the periphery of the recipient site. This not only aids in the integration of the graft

Restoration of a small-volume hard tissue esthetic ridge defect simultaneous with implant placement

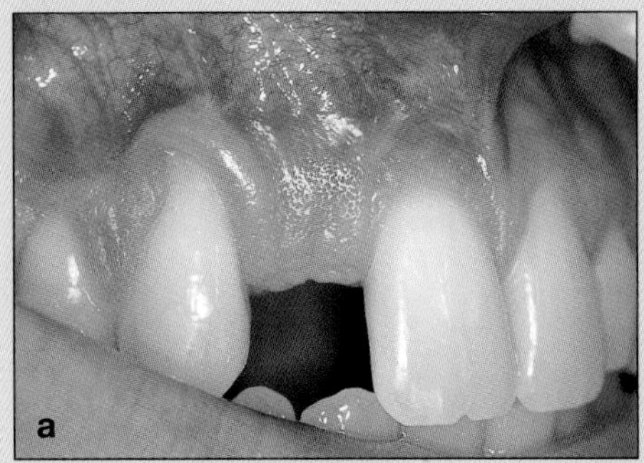
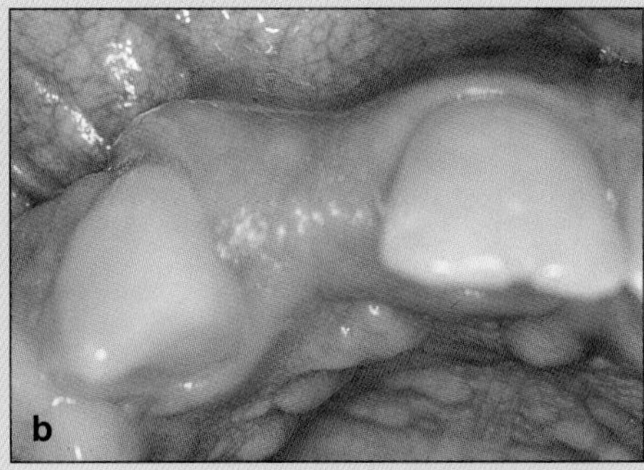
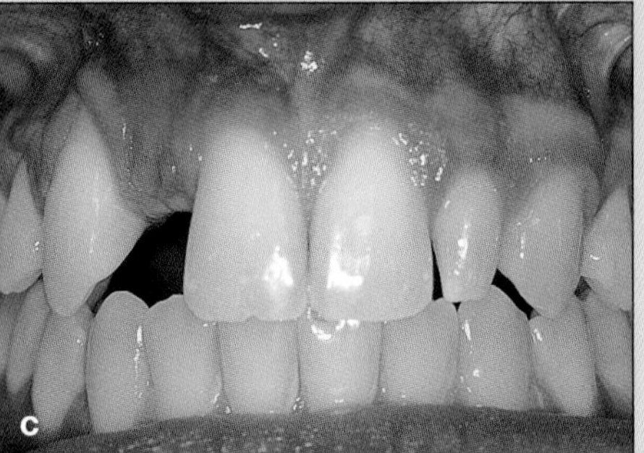

Figs 7-5a to 7-5c Preoperative views of lateral incisor implant site with a small-volume hard tissue esthetic ridge defect that will not interfere with ideal implant placement. The ridge contour at the crest is adequate, and there is a Miller class I recession defect on the adjacent canine.

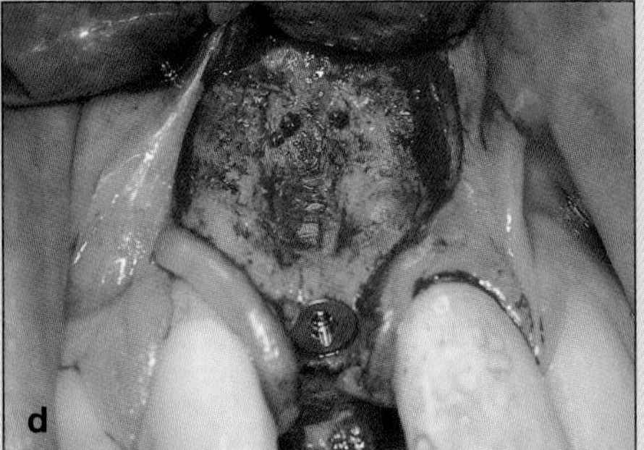

Fig 7-5d Submerged implant (Friadent) placed via the curvilinear-beveled flap technique. The dehiscence defect did not jeopardize the integrity of the buccal ridge crest.

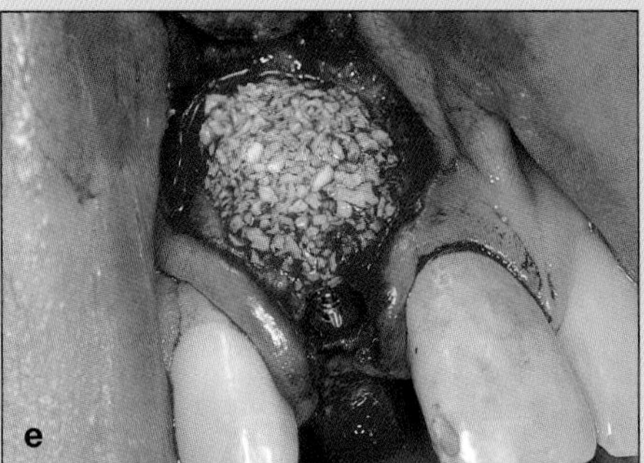

Fig 7-5e A particulate bone graft is condensed at the site over the defect but stops short of the periphery of the recipient site.

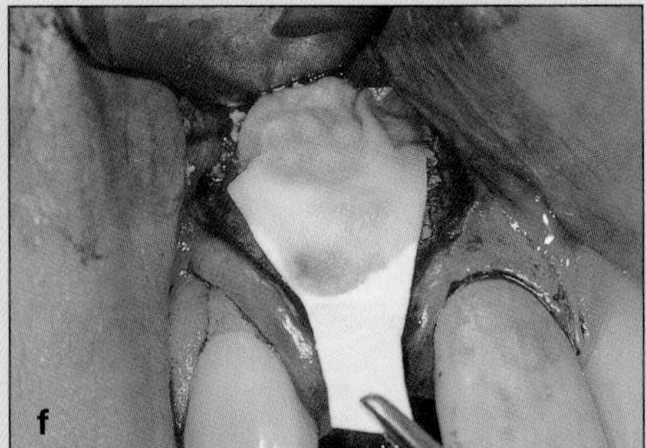

Fig 7-5f An absorbable collagen membrane easily adapts over the graft.

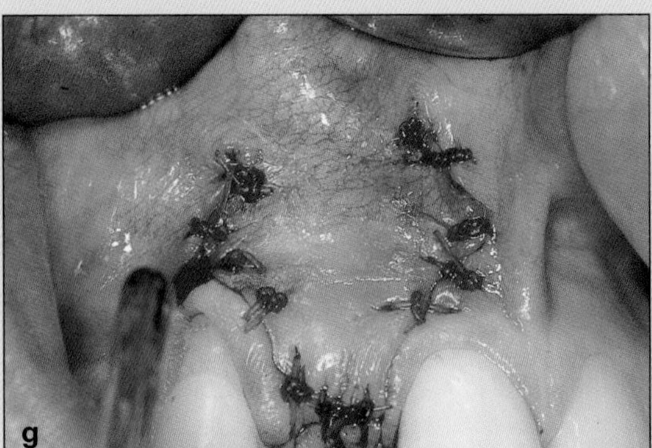

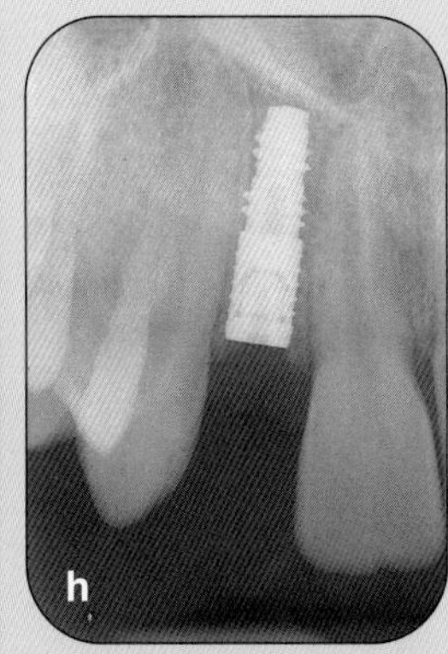

Fig 7-5g Passive flap adaptation and tension-free closure are obtained.

Fig 7-5h Postoperative radiograph demonstrates the advantage of using a tapered implant at this site.

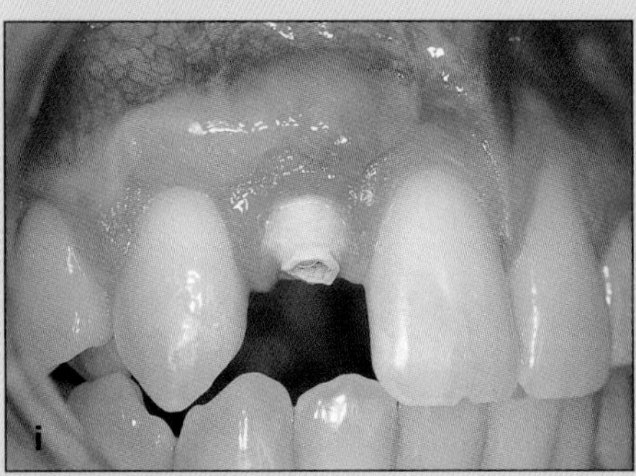
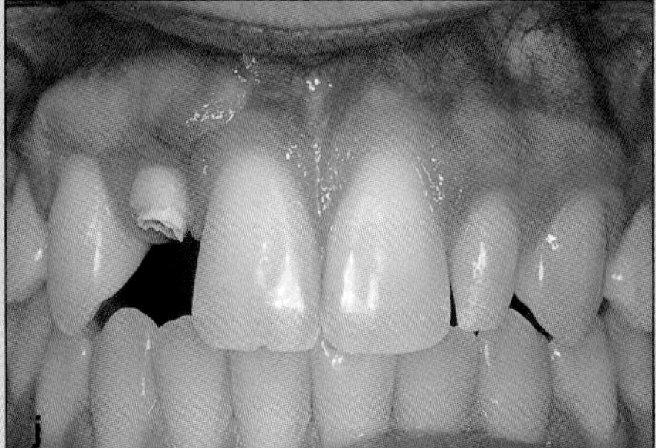

Figs 7-5i and 7-5j At second-stage surgery, a customized Protec healing abutment (Friadent) was delivered to support the adjacent papilla. Root coverage of the denuded canine root was accomplished with a subepithelial connective tissue graft. Note the maintenance of esthetic scalloped soft tissue architecture and papillary morphology at the 8-month postoperative visit.

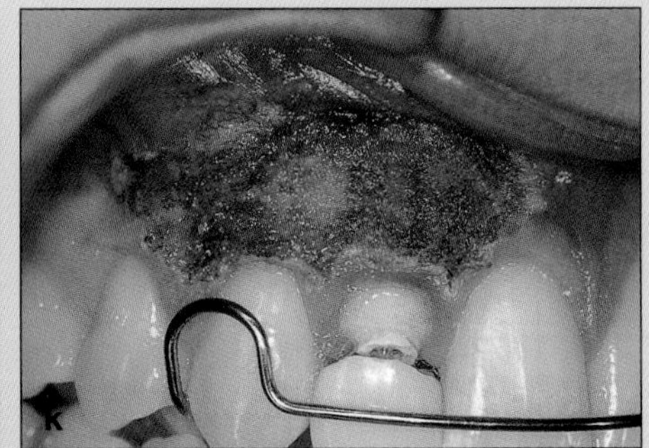

Fig 7-5k Laser soft tissue resurfacing was performed to blend the grafted site with the adjacent areas.

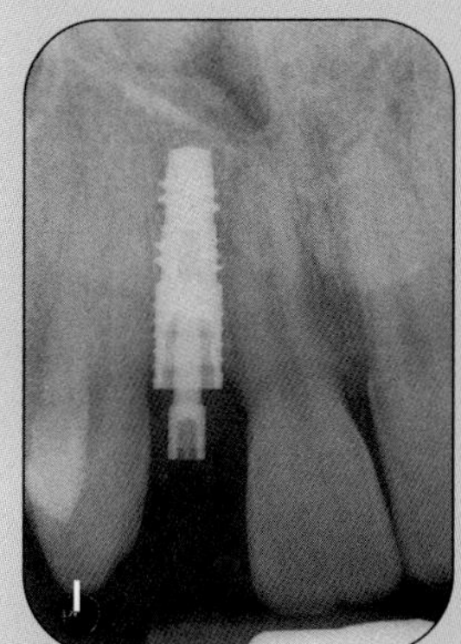

Fig 7-5l Abutment connection radiograph.

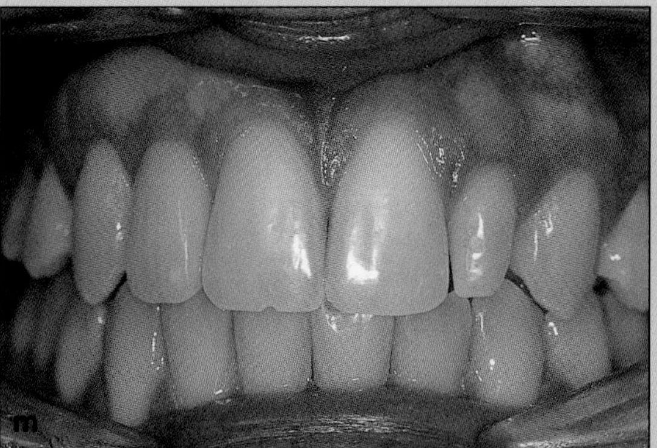

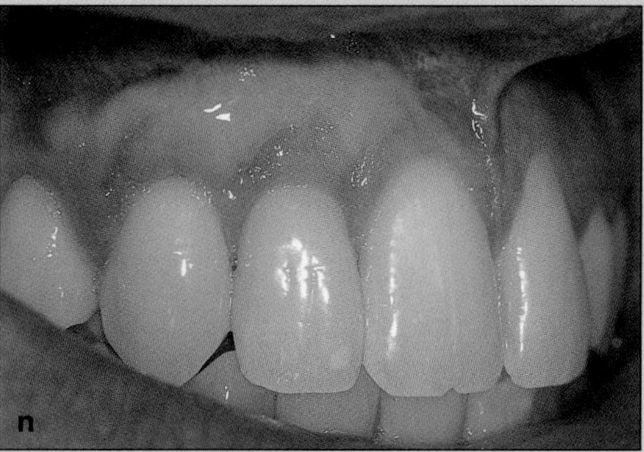

Figs 7-5m and 7-5n Frontal and close-up views of final restoration demonstrating harmonious proportions and an esthetic gingival appearance. Long-term esthetic success is predictable since the repaired osseous defect did not jeopardize the buccal crest of the ridge. Esthetic crown lengthening of the left lateral incisor, canine, and first premolar would complete the smile makeover. (Restoration by Dr Cesar Sabates Jr, Miami, FL.)

at the site but greatly facilitates the fixation of the graft at the time of surgery. The dimensions of the recipient site are then measured using a periodontal probe. The thickness of the recipient-site bone available for screw fixation is also estimated at this time. Next, the corticocancellous block graft and the particulate marrow graft are harvested from the lateral aspect of the body of the mandible and from the retromolar, buccal shelf, or symphyseal area of the mandible, respectively, as previously described. The grafts may be briefly stored in nonactivated PRP solution or moistened with sterile saline prior to transfer to the recipient site. The block graft is first secured obtaining a lag-screw effect using a minimum of two fixation screws. A 1:1 ratio of Bio-Oss and autogenous cancellous bone is then condensed at the periphery of the graft-recipient site after confirming passive reapproximation of the cover flap.

Next, the pre-shaped resorbable collagen membrane is adapted over the graft and secured by absorbing blood or activated PRP solution at the site. Finally, the cover flap is reapproximated and secured in a standard fashion (Fig 7-6). When a VIP-CT flap is performed simultaneously with the correction of a large-volume hard tissue defect in the anterior maxilla, the palatal periosteal-connective tissue flap is developed prior to the delivery of the particulate graft and then returned to the donor site until after the particulate graft has been adapted around the block graft. Subsequently, the flap is rotated and immobilized over the graft, as discussed in chapter 6. In instances where a portion of the block or particulate bone graft is not covered by the periosteal-connective tissue flap, a resorbable collagen membrane is used as described above.

Surgical restoration of soft tissue volume at an esthetic implant site

When restoration of deficient soft tissues is indicated at esthetic sites, the surgeon must select the appropriate soft tissue augmentation procedure based on the volume of the defect encountered and the esthetic outcome expected from the procedure. In addition to the volume of the soft tissue defect, the coexistence of hard tissue ridge defects, periodontal phenotype, and previous history leading to tooth loss will have an impact on the selection and sequencing of the soft tissue augmentation technique most appropriate for the situation. Generally, soft tissue augmentation at esthetic sites is managed with either one or more subepithelial connective tissue grafts or a single VIP-CT flap. As discussed in chapters 5 and 6, these procedures are highly predictable and yield excellent color matching at the recipient sites. Subsequently, soft tissue refinement techniques described later in this chapter are used as needed to further maximize soft tissue esthetics. Nevertheless, thick split-thickness or even full-thickness palatal mucosal grafts may be indicated for correction of large-volume soft tissue defects in esthetic areas. When avulsive trauma or resective tumor surgery results in poor-quality mucosal soft tissues at a site where bone grafting is necessary, the use of palatal mucosal grafts has the advantage of providing good-quality keratinized tissue in a short period of time. As described in chapter 5, these grafts are staged to restore tissue width followed by vertical tissue height. Along with the proper selection of the indicated soft tissue grafting technique, careful attention to the principles of soft tissue grafting outlined in

Restoration of a large-volume hard tissue esthetic ridge defect in preparation for implant placement

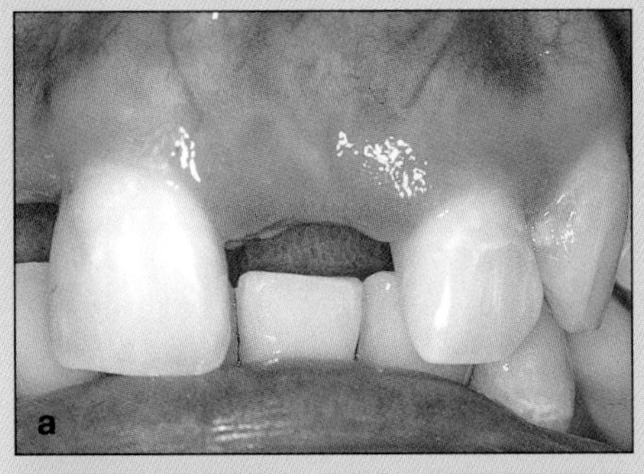

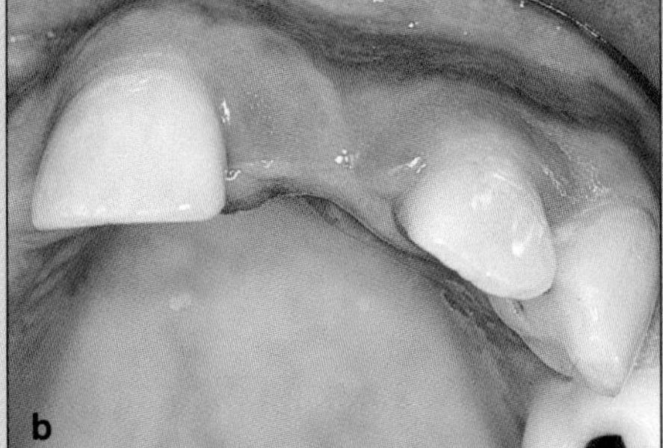

Figs 7-6a and 7-6b Preoperative view of maxillary central incisor implant site requiring staged reconstruction of a large-volume hard tissue esthetic ridge defect. Block and particulate bone grafts are planned followed by implant placement with synchronous soft tissue grafting to counteract anticipated soft tissue shrinkage that usually follows block bone graft procedures.

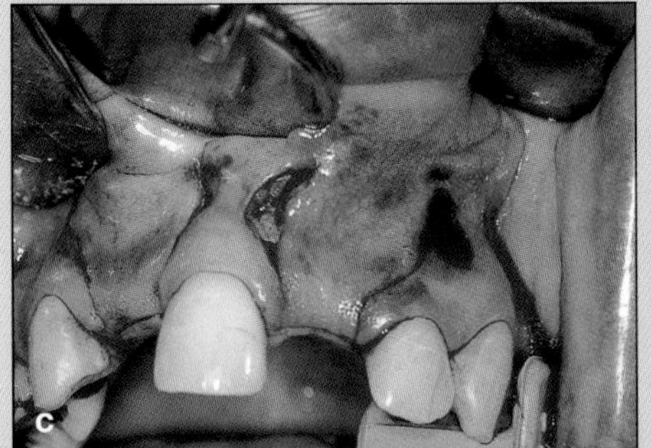

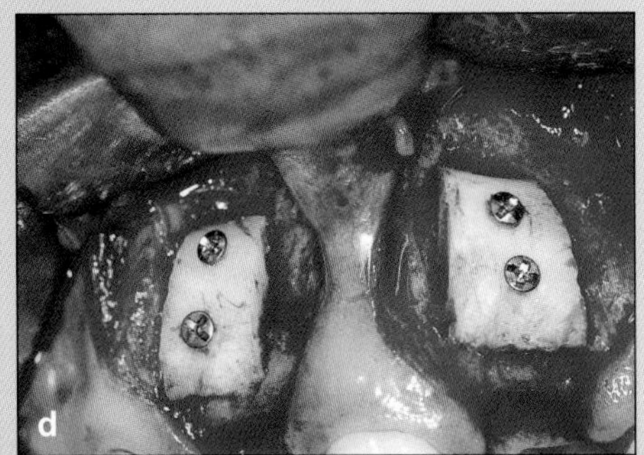

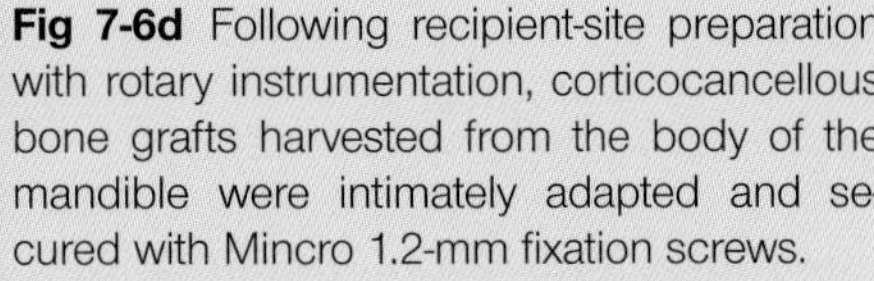

Fig 7-6c A curvilinear-beveled flap used for access to recipient site.

Fig 7-6d Following recipient-site preparation with rotary instrumentation, corticocancellous bone grafts harvested from the body of the mandible were intimately adapted and secured with Mincro 1.2-mm fixation screws.

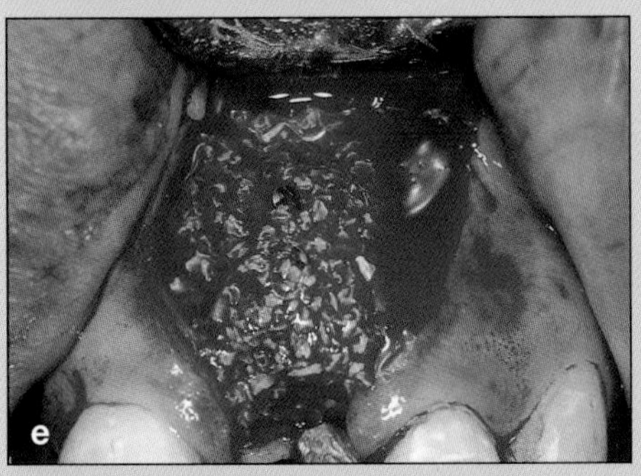

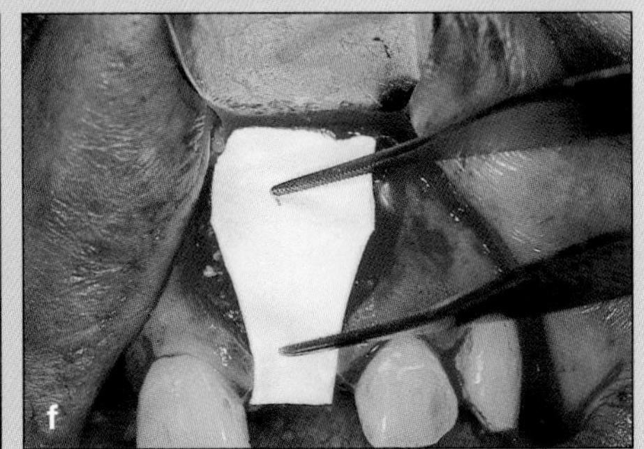

Fig 7-6e Particulate bone graft, consisting of a 1:1 ratio of autogenous cancellous bone harvested from the retromolar area of the mandible and Bio-Oss, was condensed around the periphery of the site.

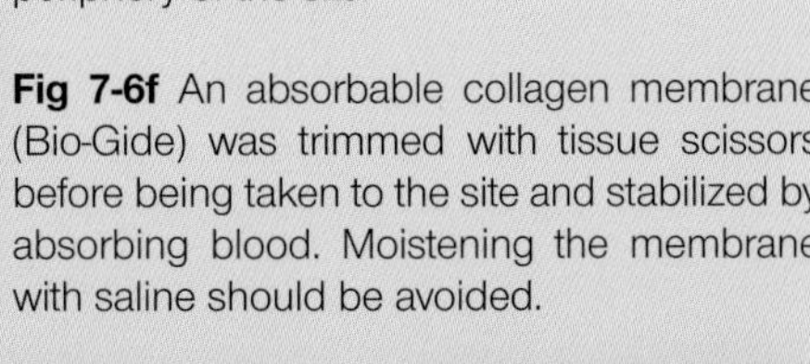

Fig 7-6f An absorbable collagen membrane (Bio-Gide) was trimmed with tissue scissors before being taken to the site and stabilized by absorbing blood. Moistening the membrane with saline should be avoided.

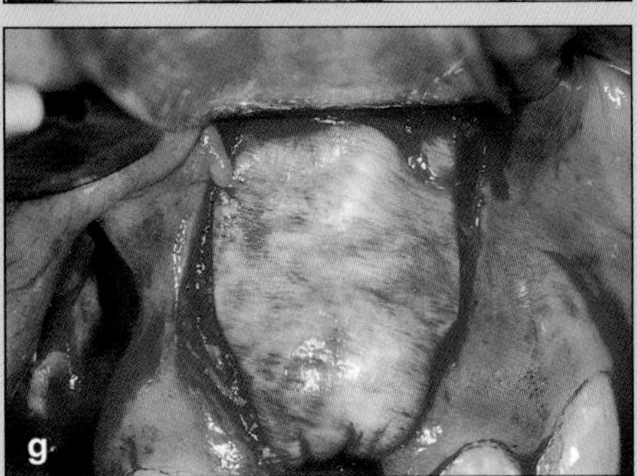

Fig 7-6g The membrane is adapted over the bone graft and the crest of the ridge and tucked under the palatal flap.

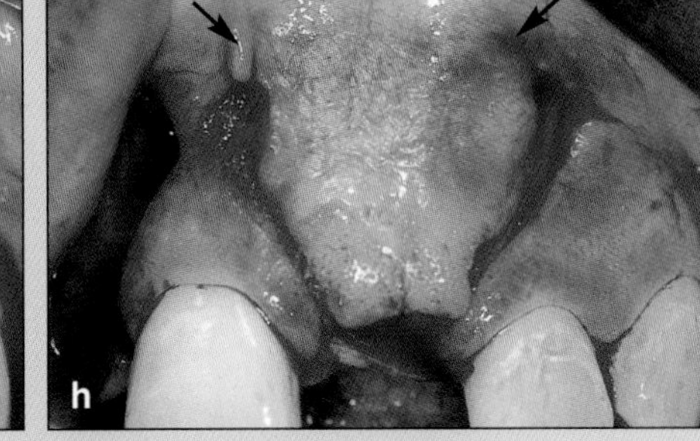

Fig 7-6h Passive flap accommodation is facilitated by the inclusion of tension-releasing cutback incisions *(arrows)*. Fixation of the membrane is unnecessary when the flap is properly developed and when the membrane lacks memory after absorbing blood at the site.

Fig 7-6i Tension-free closure with 4-0 chromic gut suture on a P3 needle.

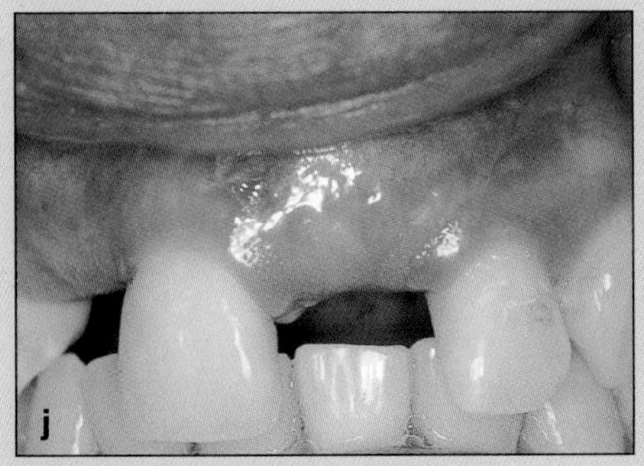

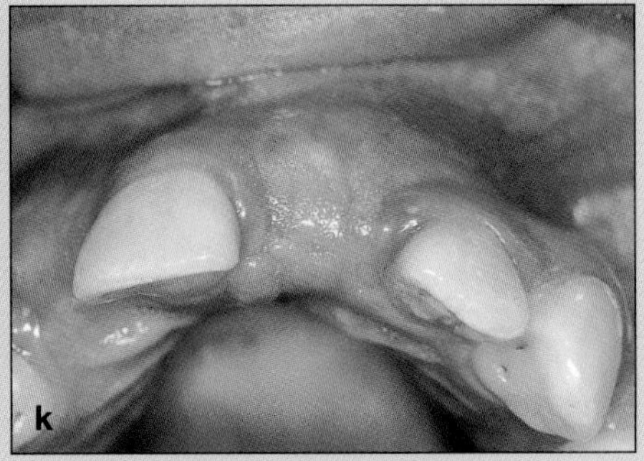

Figs 7-6j and 7-6k Four-month postoperative views demonstrate complete restoration of the large-volume hard tissue defect. Note that the use of beveled incisions resulted in excellent incision line cosmesis.

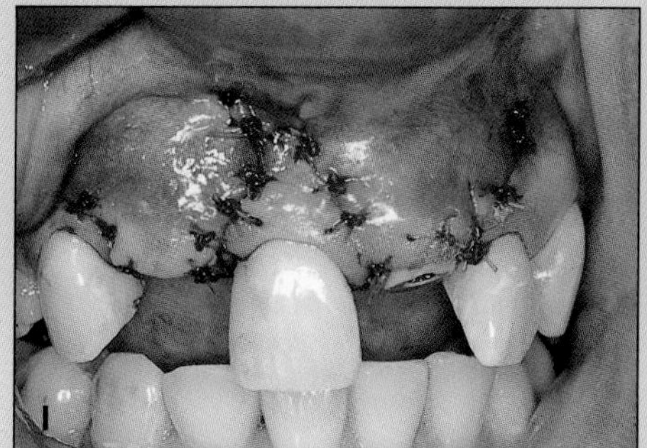

Fig 7-6l Nonsubmerged implant (Straumann USA, Waltham, MA) placed with customized healing abutment. Subepithelial connective tissue graft was performed simultaneously to offset predictable soft tissue recession that will occur when access flap for screw removal and implant placement is readapted at the site. The dissection is modified to be partial thickness over the buccal aspect of the site.

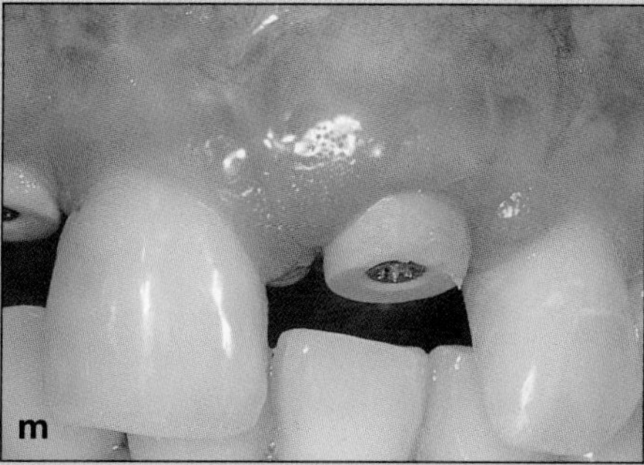

Figs 7-6m and 7-6n Three-month postoperative views of central incisor site. Inconspicuous reconstruction of the deficient alveolar ridge contour was accomplished. The customized healing abutment was shaped to support the adjacent papilla, and a labial bevel established gingival symmetry with the adjacent central incisor.

Figs 7-6o and 7-6p Three-month postoperative views following removal of the customized healing abutment. The implant was not deeply placed; instead, the site-development procedures allowed an optimal balance between fixture depth and esthetic emergence, thereby facilitating prosthetic access and preserving the protective peri-implant soft tissue seal.

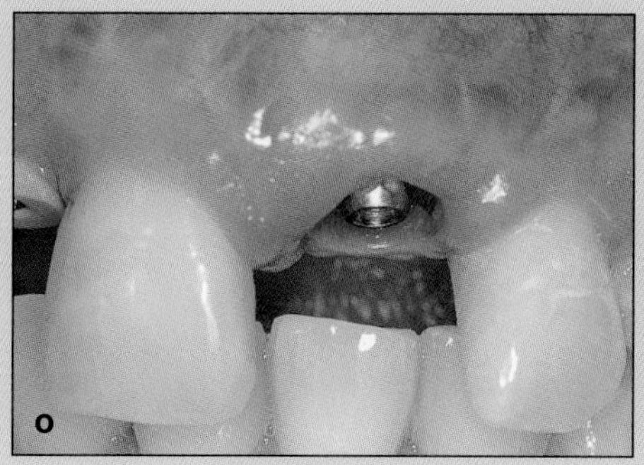

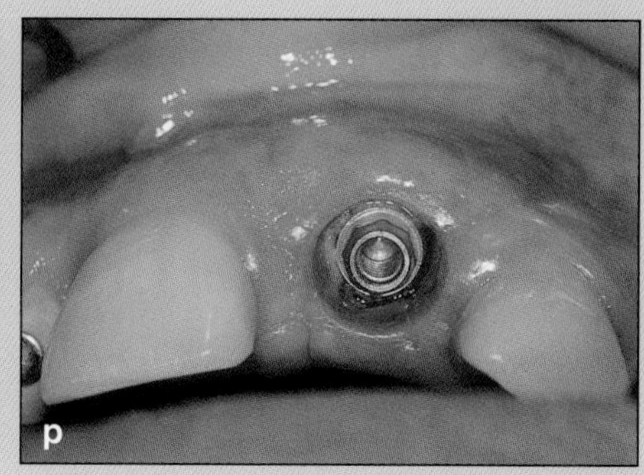

chapter 5 will increase the predictability and success of the procedure. In addition, as with any grafting procedure, measures must always be taken to avoid transmission of micromotion from interim provisional restorations during initial healing following soft tissue augmentation procedures. Failure to do so will result in shrinkage or even sloughing of the graft. Whenever possible, the surgeon should also consider the synergistic benefits of combining prosthetic-guided soft tissue healing with soft tissue augmentation procedures. Finally, the surgeon should take advantage of available biotechnology to improve surgical predictability and patient comfort. Although technique sensitive, the use of PRP appears, based on initial clinical observations, to have a role in maximizing volume yields and minimizing secondary shrinkage or cover flap retraction when properly used in conjunction with soft tissue grafting procedures. The author also recommends that surgeons educate patients undergoing soft tissue grafting procedures about the occasional need for touch-up procedures or additional grafting.

Surgical technique for restoring a small-volume soft tissue defect at an esthetic implant site

Small-volume soft tissue defects at esthetic implant sites are usually managed with a subepithelial connective tissue graft performed either prior to implant placement, simultaneous with implant placement, or after implant emergence. As discussed in chapter 5, grafting prior to emergence of the implant provides the advantage of allowing the surgeon to prepare a larger recipient site that extends over the crest and onto the palatal aspect of the alveolar ridge, providing additional circulation to support a free graft in the area critical for prosthetic emergence. Nevertheless, a subepithelial connective tissue graft can be performed at abutment connection or simultaneous with nonsubmerged implant placement to successfully reconstruct small-volume soft tissue defects in the area critical for prosthetic emergence (Fig 7-7). The predictability of such procedures is improved when abundant vestibular depth exists, allowing coronal advancement of recipient-site flaps over the free connec-

Restoration of a small-volume soft tissue esthetic ridge defect simultaneous with nonsubmerged implant placement

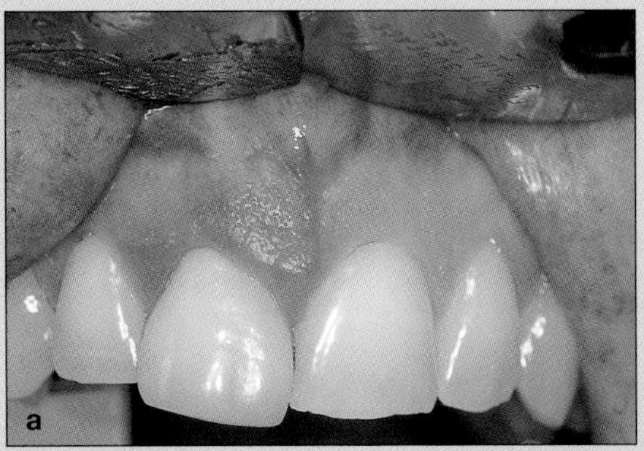

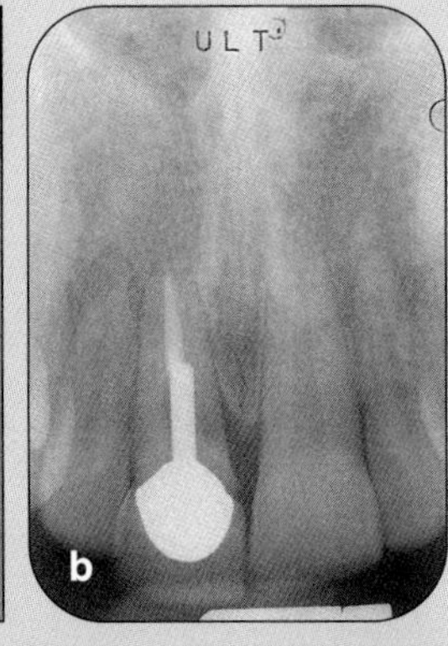

Fig 7-7a Preoperative view of failing right central incisor. Significant soft tissue edema correlated with chronic irritation of failing restoration and tooth mobility precludes immediate implant placement since the loss of soft tissue volume following tooth removal presents a significant esthetic risk.

Fig 7-7b Preoperative radiograph of failing central incisor.

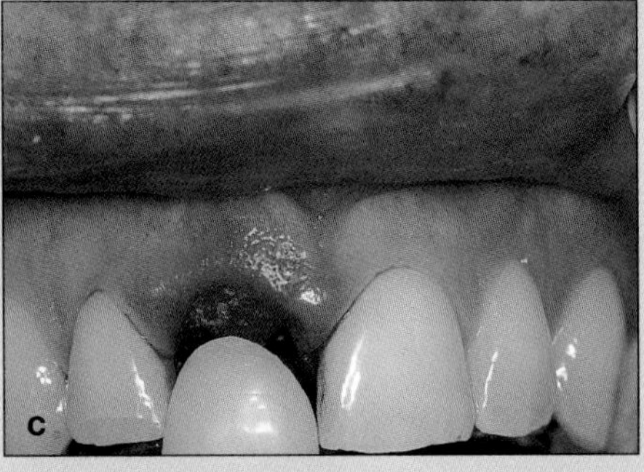

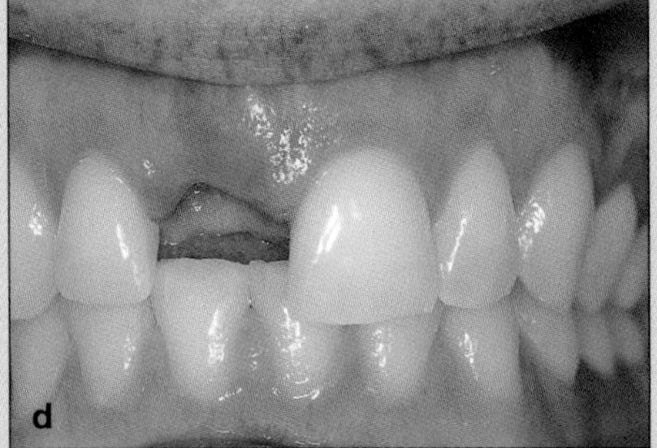

Fig 7-7c Tooth removal with the Bio-Col technique was performed in preparation for delayed implant placement.

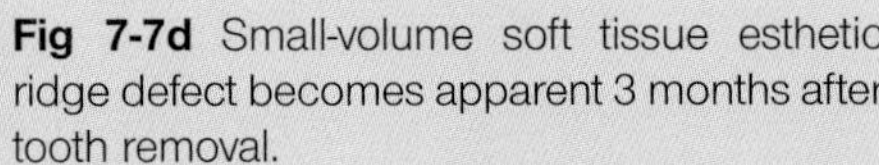

Fig 7-7d Small-volume soft tissue esthetic ridge defect becomes apparent 3 months after tooth removal.

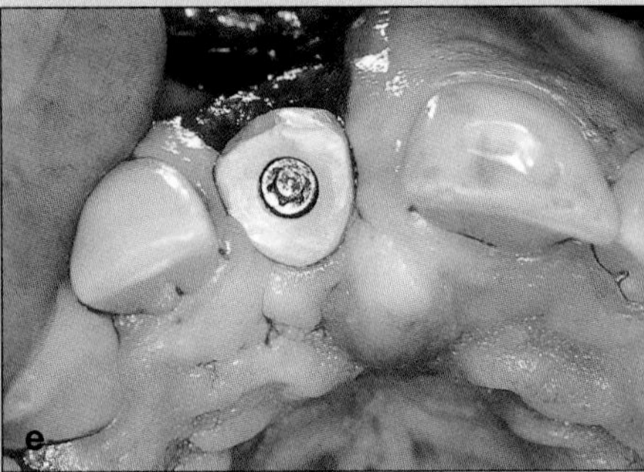

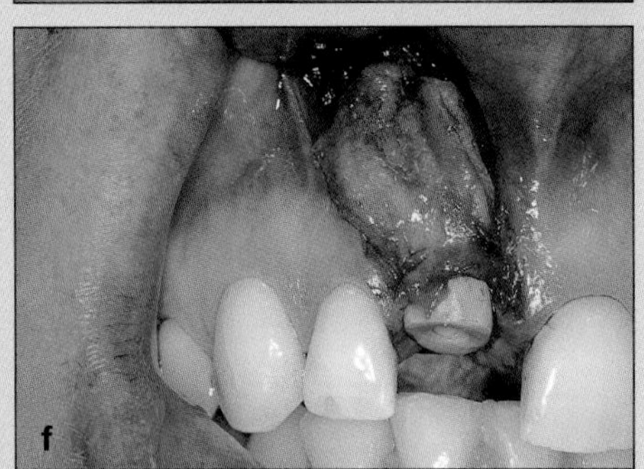

Fig 7-7e Nonsubmerged implant placed with customizable healing abutment (Straumann USA) via a full-thickness (ridge crest)–partial-thickness (buccal ridge) flap.

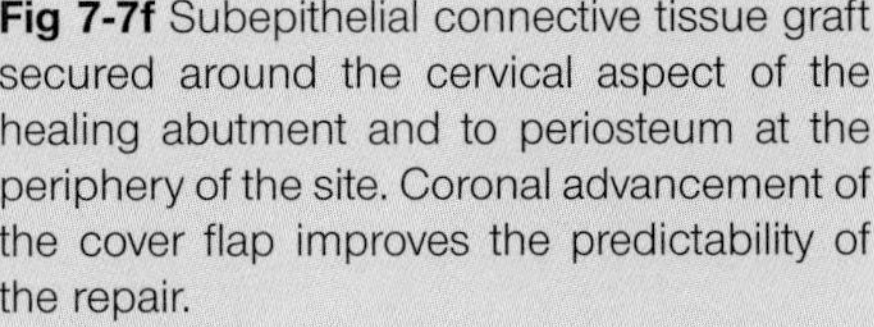

Fig 7-7f Subepithelial connective tissue graft secured around the cervical aspect of the healing abutment and to periosteum at the periphery of the site. Coronal advancement of the cover flap improves the predictability of the repair.

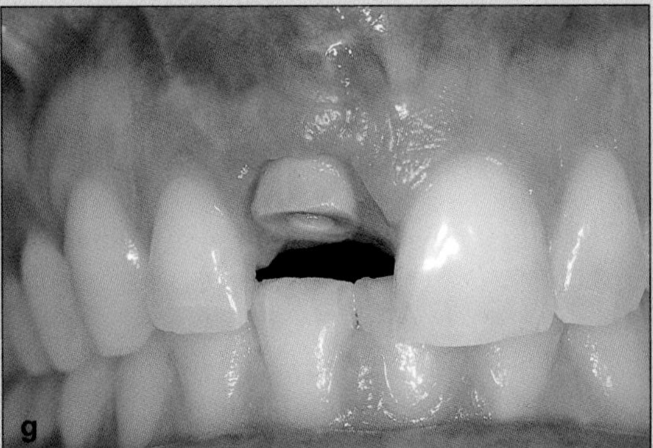

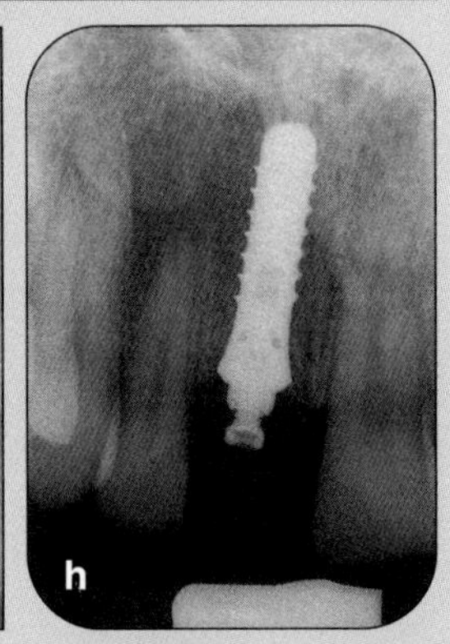

Fig 7-7g Three-month postoperative view demonstrates correction of the small-volume soft tissue esthetic ridge defect and maintenance of scalloped gingival architecture.

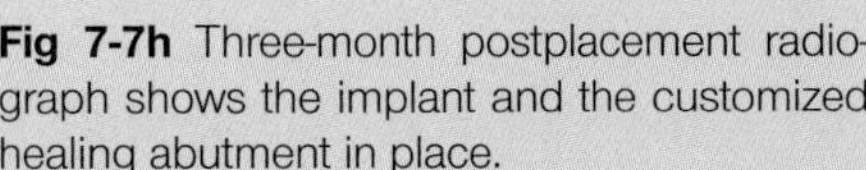

Fig 7-7h Three-month postplacement radiograph shows the implant and the customized healing abutment in place.

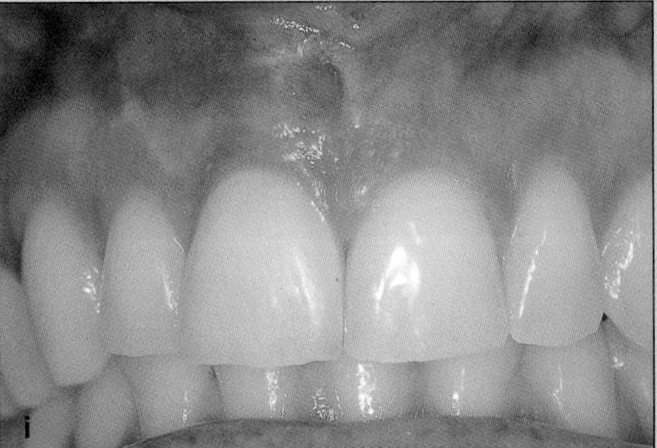

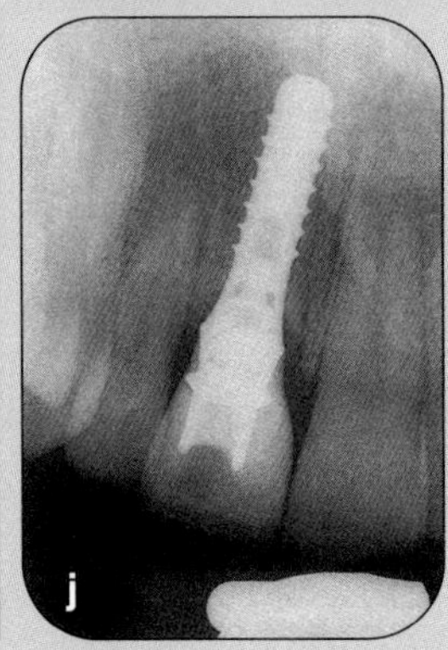

Fig 7-7i One-year postoperative view of inconspicuous final implant restoration with harmonious dental proportions and natural gingival esthetics. (Restoration by Dr Mark Fisher, Miami, FL.)

Fig 7-7j One-year postoperative radiograph demonstrates stable crestal bone levels and maintenance of adjacent interdental bone volume.

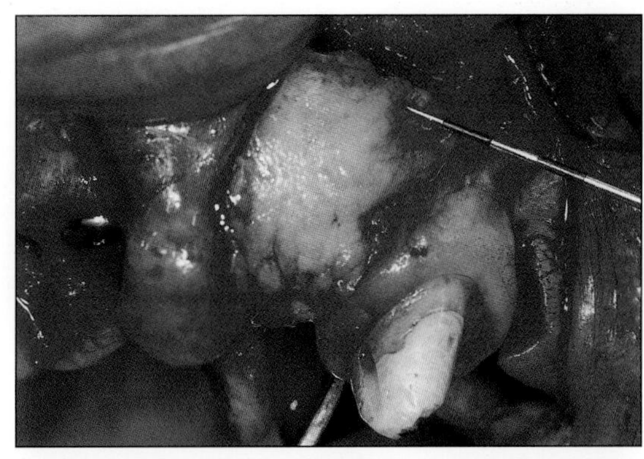

Fig 7-8 Intraoperative view of partially edentulous maxilla during placement of multiple implants at sites requiring soft tissue grafting. Bilateral VIP-CT flaps will be performed to augment central and lateral incisor sites. The right first premolar to canine can be augmented simultaneously with AlloDerm or delayed and subsequently grafted with autogenous tissue after 3 months have been allowed for the palatal donor sites to heal.

Subepithelial connective tissue grafting: Second-harvest effect

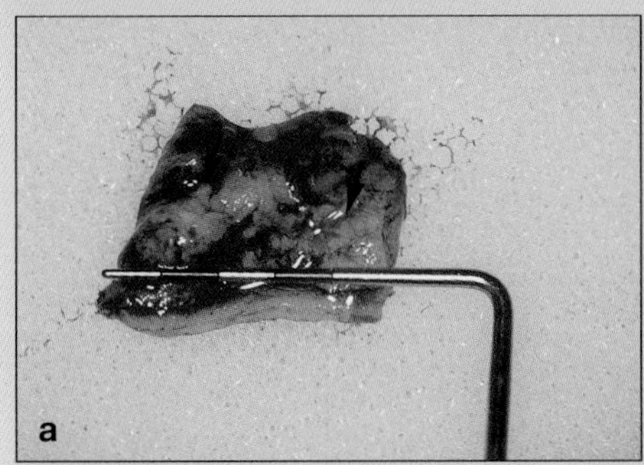

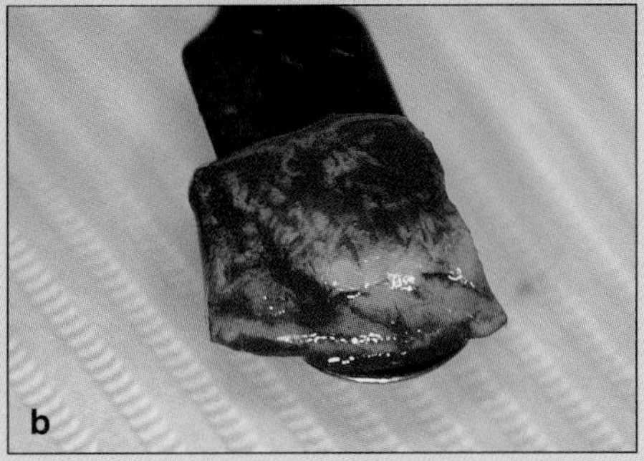

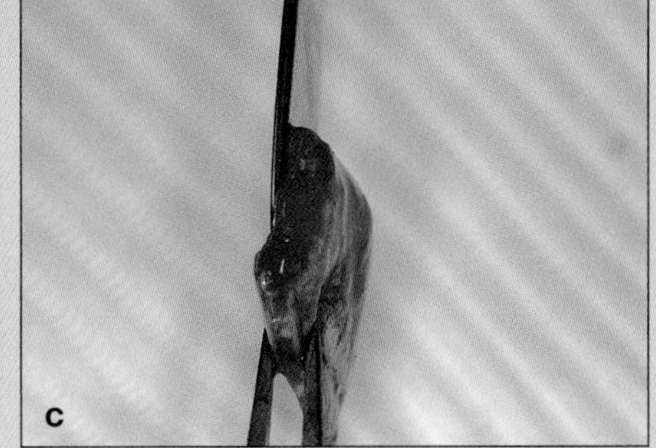

Fig 7-9a Subepithelial connective tissue graft harvested for the first time from a premolar palatal donor site. Note the significant amount of fatty tissue *(arrows)* that makes up the apical portion of the graft.

Figs 7-9b and 7-9c A second subepithelial graft harvested from the same site 3 months after the first harvest demonstrates a significant improvement in the thickness and volume of good-quality connective tissue obtained. There is no fatty tissue in the second graft. The absorbable collagen dressing (CollaPlug; Centerpulse Dental, Carlsbad, CA) used at the donor site may contribute to this clinical observation.

tive tissue grafts. The surgical technique for performing a subepithelial connective tissue graft and the choice of an open versus closed recipient site are described in chapter 5.

Surgical technique for restoring a large-volume soft tissue defect at an esthetic implant site

Large-volume soft tissue defects at esthetic sites can be reconstructed with multiple interpositional subepithelial connective tissue grafts, with multiple onlay palatal mucosal grafts, or with a single VIP-CT flap. The selection of the appropriate soft tissue augmentation procedure depends on the specific findings of the pretreatment evaluation as well as the history that led to loss of dentition in that area. For instance, when the patient has a small and shallow palate, the subepithelial connective tissue graft and VIP-CT flap may not be appropriate. Instead, sequential gingival grafts can be performed to accomplish horizontal augmentation followed by vertical augmentation. Although color matching may be poor, this may be the best approach in this situation. Although the VIP-CT flap yields superior volume, free soft tissue grafting techniques are sometimes indicated because of other limitations. For example, even in high vaulted palates, the width of the VIP-CT flap usually limits its use to two contiguous sites. Therefore, when multiple sites (3 or more) in the anterior maxillary area require soft tissue augmentation, selecting an alternate technique or staging multiple VIP-CT flaps becomes necessary. If a patient with a thin, scalloped periodontium and pre-existing gingival recession needs implant replacement of a missing maxillary right first premolar, canine, lateral incisor, and central incisor, for example, the author would use the VIP-CT flap to reconstruct missing soft tissues at the central incisor and possibly at the lateral incisor sites (provided adequate palatal height yielded a wide enough periosteal–connective tissue pedicle). For the remaining areas, the author would use a subepithelial connective tissue graft harvested from the contralateral side of the palate or an AlloDerm graft (LifeCell, Branchburg, NJ) (Fig 7-8). Due to the so-called second-harvest effect, repeat harvesting of subepithelial connective tissue grafts from the same donor site improves both the quality and quantity of connective tissue obtained at the second harvest (Fig 7-9). Therefore, when a single connective tissue graft fails to significantly improve a large-volume defect, repeat grafting can often resolve the situation, provided the procedures are

Restoration of a large-volume esthetic ridge defect simultaneous with submerged implant placement

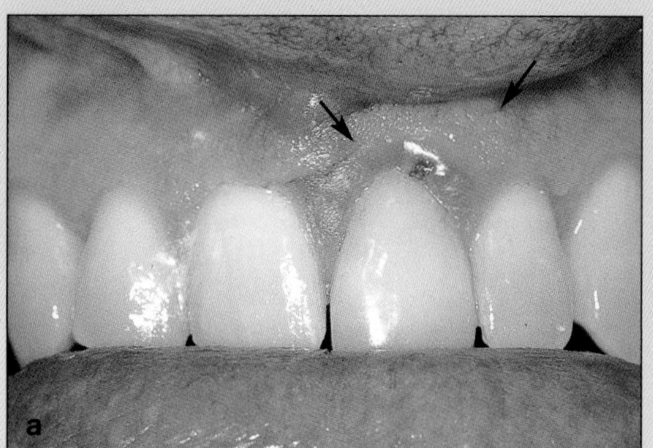

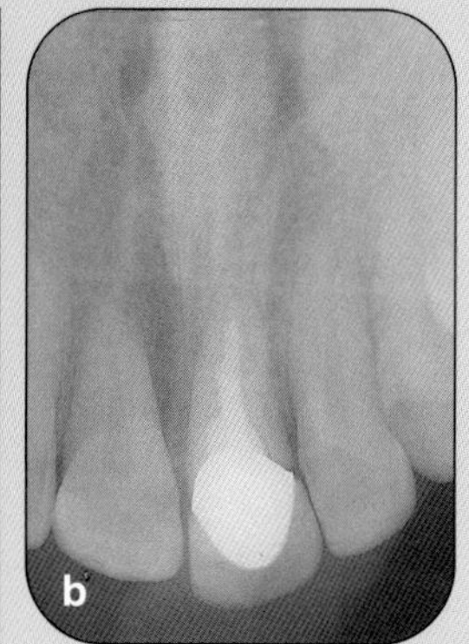

Fig 7-10a Preoperative view of failing maxillary central incisor. Tissue edema associated with chronic irritation from failing restoration and tooth mobility precludes immediate implant placement. Demarcation of pathologic tissue *(arrows)* indicates that a large-volume soft tissue defect is likely following tooth removal.

Fig 7-10b Preoperative radiograph of failing central incisor.

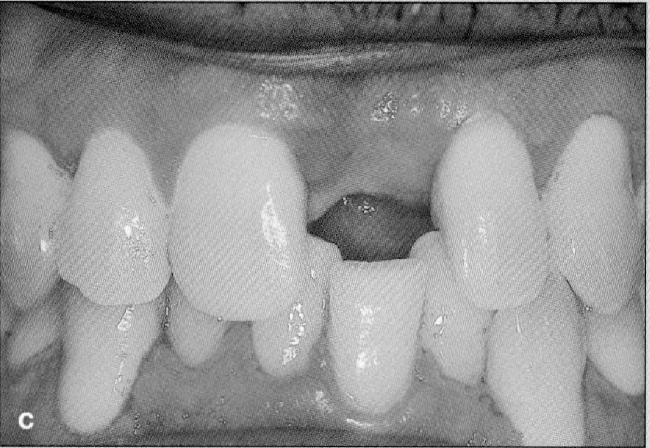

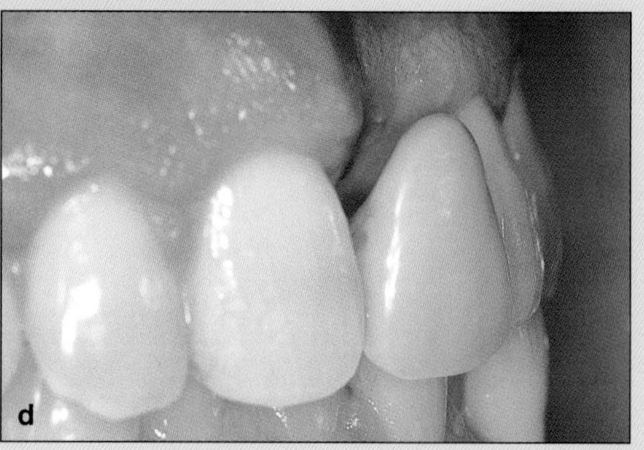

Figs 7-10c and 7-10d Three months following the removal of the tooth with the Bio-Col technique, a large-volume soft tissue esthetic ridge defect became apparent. No defect in the buccal socket wall was noted at the time of tooth removal. This ridge defect is entirely soft tissue in nature.

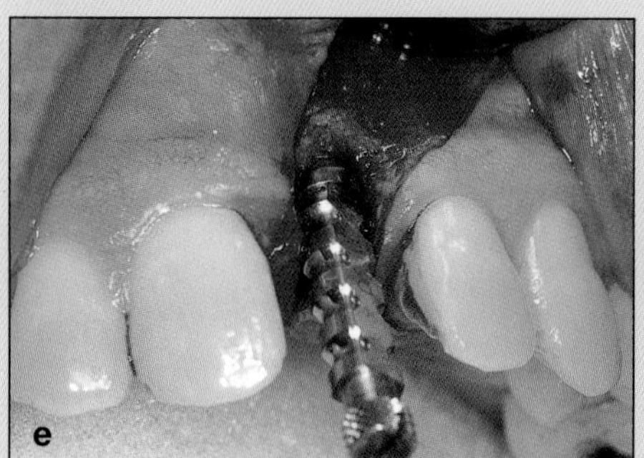

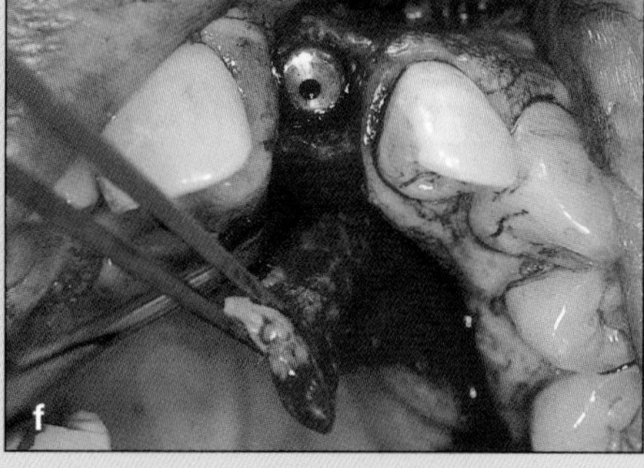

Fig 7-10e Three months after tooth removal, a submerged implant (Nobel Biocare, Yorba Linda, CA) was placed, and surgical indexing was performed via a full-thickness (ridge crest)–partial-thickness (buccally ridge) access flap.

Fig 7-10f After placement of the cover screw, a palatal incision was extended and a VIP-CT flap was developed and rotated over the crest of the ridge onto the buccal aspect of the ridge.

scheduled at least 3 months apart. Nevertheless, use of the VIP-CT flap technique as described in chapter 6 is the author's preferred method for reconstructing large-volume soft tissue defects at single-tooth and multiple-tooth sites in the anterior maxilla (Fig 7-10). The amount of vertical soft tissue augmentation realized with this technique is superior to that obtained even when multiple free soft tissue grafts are performed.

Combination hard and soft tissue defect at an esthetic implant site

Combination hard and soft tissue defects are the most common types of defects encountered at esthetic sites. As discussed in chapter 2, these defects can prevent ideal implant positioning, the development of a stable peri-implant soft tissue environment, or esthetic restorative emergence. These defects also are distinguished as small or large in volume. While large-volume combination defects are common, small-volume combination defects are more difficult to detect on clinical examination. Treatment of small-volume combination defects in esthetic areas depends on the location of the hard tissue component. If the hard tissue component of a small-volume combination defect will not jeopardize the integrity of the buccal ridge crest after ideal implant placement, then a camouflage procedure (hard or soft tissue graft) can be performed prior to

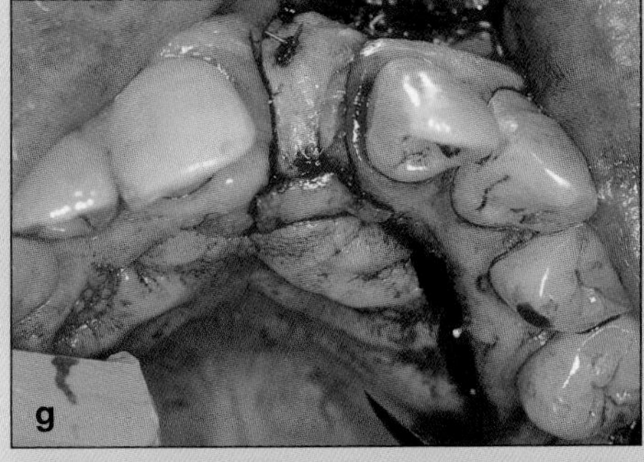

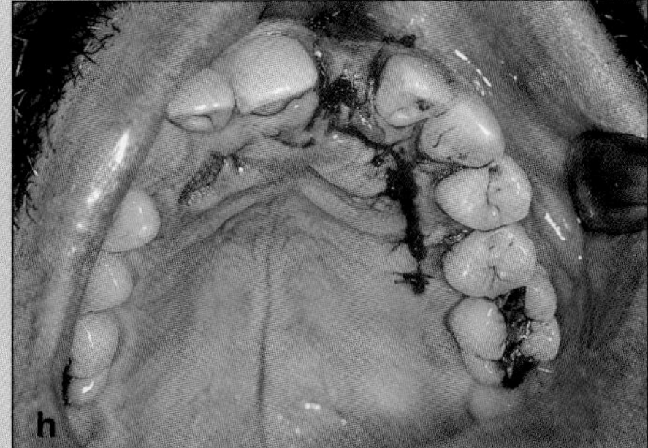

Fig 7-10g The VIP-CT flap was secured to the periosteum at the recipient site and by horizontal mattress sutures laterally.

Fig 7-10h Tension-free closure of contiguous donor- and recipient-site flaps was obtained.

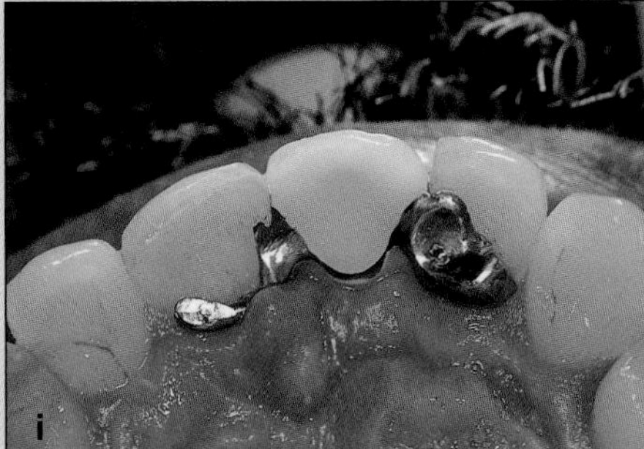

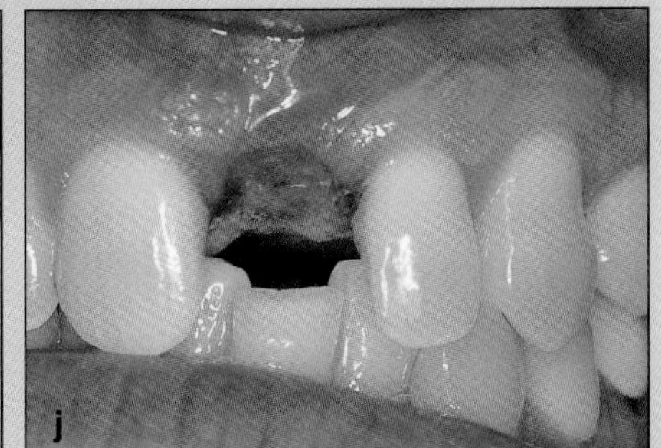

Fig 7-10i A resin-bonded toothborne interim provisional restoration was used to support the adjacent papilla and prevent transmission of micromotion to the underlying flap during initial healing.

Fig 7-10j Six months following implant placement and simultaneous correction of large-volume soft tissue esthetic ridge defect, the interim provisional was removed and a custom abutment and provisional restoration were delivered via a palatal peninsula flap.

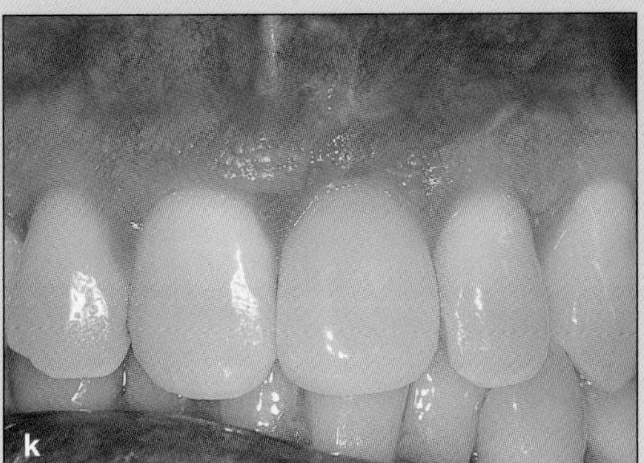

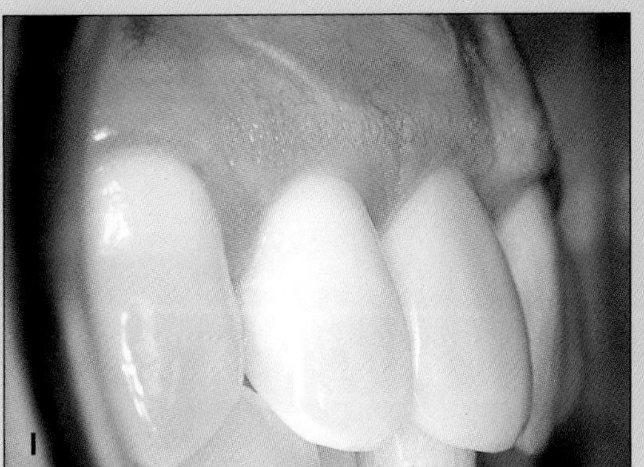

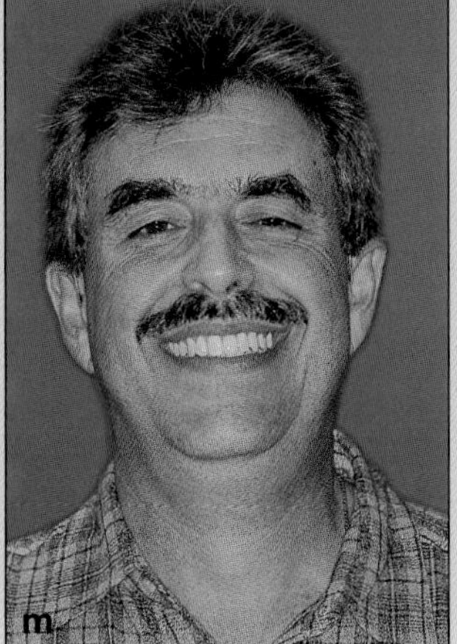

Figs 7-10k to 7-10m Final restoration 1 year after delivery. Complete restoration of large-volume soft tissue esthetic ridge defect was obtained with the VIP-CT flap. Vertical and buccal soft tissue augmentation of this volume is not routinely obtainable even when multiple free soft tissue grafts are performed. The implant restoration is inconspicuous and harmonious in proportion. The patient's high smile line is unencumbered. (Restoration by Dr Cecil Abraham, Miami, FL.)

or simultaneous with implant placement. Conversely, when the hard tissue component of the defect will jeopardize the buccal crest of the ridge, staged reconstruction is indicated (as previously discussed for isolated small-volume hard tissue defects). Because it is extremely difficult to determine whether the buccal crest will be jeopardized based on the clinical examination and bone sounding alone, these defects are usually reconstructed in stages to improve esthetic predictability. Nevertheless, techniques to camouflage small-volume combination defects are discussed below. In contrast, large-volume combination defects in esthetic areas are always reconstructed in stages, as discussed below.

Surgical technique for camouflaging a small-volume combination defect at an esthetic implant site

Small-volume combination defects at esthetic sites can be camouflaged either with a soft tissue graft or with synthetic bone graft material placed subperiosteally at the site, provided that the hard tissue component of the defect will not jeopardize the ridge crest after ideal implant placement. The decision of whether to use a soft tissue graft or a synthetic bone graft material is based on the health and thickness of the soft tissue cover at the site and the periodontal phenotype of the patient. When the soft tissues at the site are of adequate thickness, subperiosteal hydroxyapatite grafts have been used successfully to camouflage small-volume defects. Nevertheless, the author's preference is to camouflage these small-volume combination esthetic ridge defects with one or more subepithelial connective tissue grafts or with a VIP-CT flap (Fig 7-11). Finally, when unexpected dehiscence of bone occurs during osteotomy preparation at the buccal crest of the ridge at an esthetic site, these small-volume defects are initially managed with a guided bone regeneration procedure as previously described. Afterward, a soft tissue graft is performed to restore acceptable soft tissue contour and color at the site.

Surgical technique for restoring a large-volume combination defect at an esthetic implant site

For large-volume combination defects in the anterior maxillary area, the author prefers simultaneous hard and soft tissue site development with autogenous block and particulate bone grafts as described above and the VIP-CT flap as described in chapter 6. The use of the VIP-CT flap provides sufficient vertical soft tissue augmentation to reconstruct or re-create inter-implant papillae even at multiple implant sites that present with large-volume combination defects (Fig 7-12). In addition, the transfer of a vascularized periosteal–connective tissue flap into the bone graft area improves the vascularity and cellularity of the recipient site, thereby improving phase-two bone formation and long-term maintenance of transplanted bone volume at the site. Implants are then placed 4 months after site development in either a submerged or nonsubmerged fashion and allowed to integrate for an additional 4 months before provisional restorations are delivered. Soft tissue refinement procedures such as laser sculpting or resurfacing, if indicated, may be performed as early as 3 months after site-development procedures. On average, definitive esthetic restorations are delivered 2 to 3 months following delivery of the provisional restorations. When nonsubmerged implants are placed, healing abutments that can support the adjacent papillae or inter-implant tissues are recommended to re-create positive scalloped soft tissue architecture. This early employment of prosthetic guided soft tissue healing allows time for the development of a stable sulcus and, in the author's experience, consistently improves the final esthetic outcome. Simultaneous hard and soft tissue site development as described above greatly simplifies the treatment of large-volume combination defects in esthetic areas for both surgeon and patient.

Alternatively, these large-volume combination defects can be reconstructed in a staged fashion. As the initial site-development procedure, bone grafting can be performed provided the soft tissues at the site are of adequate quality. After 4 to 6 months of maturation, one or more free soft tissue grafts can be performed prior to or at the time of implant placement. If indicated, additional soft tissue grafting can be performed during the osseointegration period prior to implant emergence. Finally, soft tissue refinement procedures are performed 3 months after emergence of the implants in preparation for provisional and eventual definitive restorations. Although successful, this staged approach to restoration of combination hard and soft tissue defects requires additional surgical procedures and treatment time when compared to the predictable simultaneous technique afforded by the use of the VIP-CT flap.

Hard and soft tissue site development via forced orthodontic eruption

As discussed in chapter 2, orthodontic therapy is often indicated in preparation for esthetic implant rehabilitation. Obtaining proper tooth position and rotation, progressive medial tipping, and appropriate spacing prior to implant therapy greatly improves the likelihood that the implant restorations will be harmonious with the adjacent dentition and that pleasing tooth proportions and relationships will be possible. In addition, such detailing allows the implant team to identify the need for cosmetic periodontal surgery or cosmetic enhancements of adjacent natural dentition as part of an ideal esthetic treatment plan.

The implant surgeon should be aware that forced orthodontic eruption of selected teeth is a nonsurgical hard and soft tissue site-development technique that has two distinct indications in esthetic implant therapy. The first indication is to increase the hard and soft tissue volume around a hopeless tooth prior to its removal when implant placement or subsequent site development is planned. The second indication is to improve the vertical bone levels and soft tissue height when a pre-existing periodontal defect is identified on a natural tooth adjacent to an implant site that will require hard and soft tissue site development in preparation for eventual implant replacement. The most important issue to recognize is that these pre-existing periodontal defects impose anatomic limitations on the potential results obtainable from currently available site-development techniques (see chapter 2). As previously discussed, regeneration of periodontal tissues (cementum, periodontal ligament, and bone) beyond the level of the adjacent osseous tissues is not predictable. Therefore, whenever such a defect is identified around a tooth adjacent to a deficient esthetic implant

Camouflage of a small-volume combination hard and soft tissue esthetic ridge defect with the VIP-CT flap

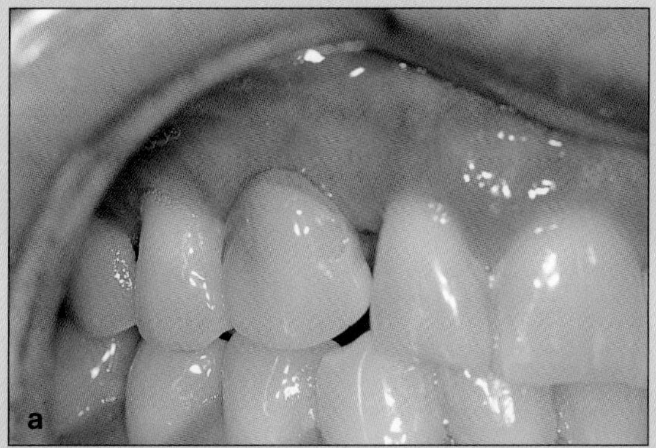

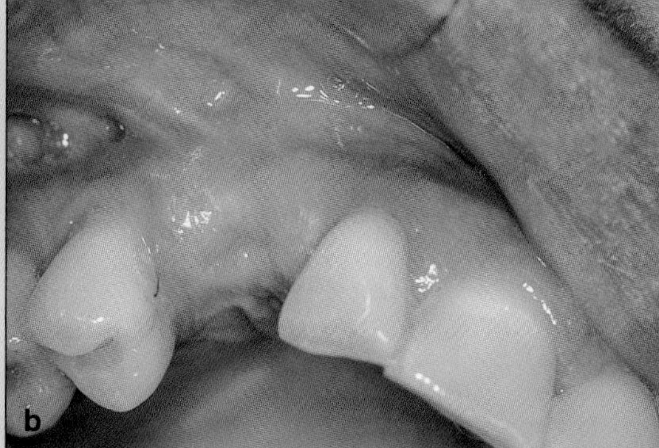

Figs 7-11a and 7-11b Preoperative views of maxillary canine implant site with small-volume combination esthetic ridge defect that will be camouflaged with a VIP-CT flap simultaneous with implant placement.

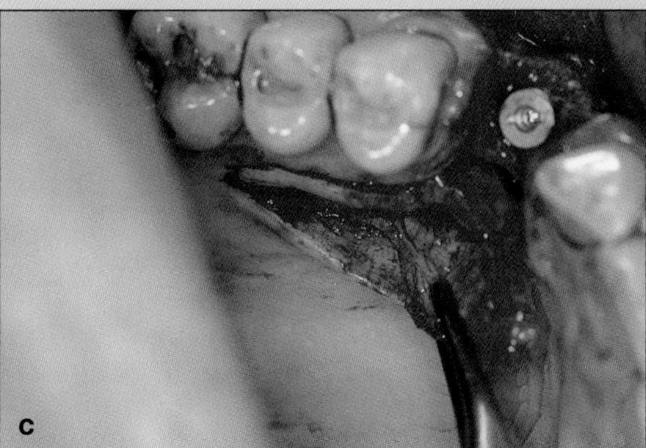

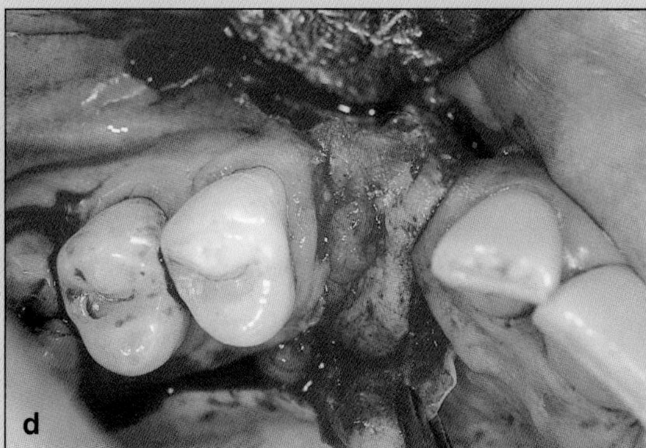

Figs 7-11c and 7-11d After ideal implant placement, the VIP-CT flap is developed within the adjacent palatal donor site, rotated and adapted over the crest of the ridge, and secured to the periosteum on the buccal aspect of the recipient site. Note the distinct subepithelial and subperiosteal planes of dissection that define the VIP-CT flap.

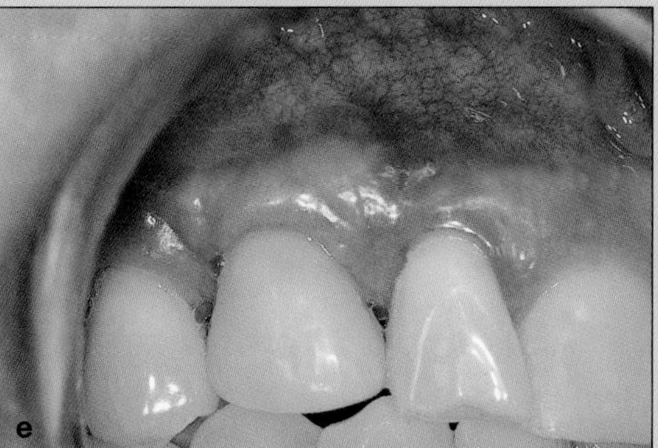

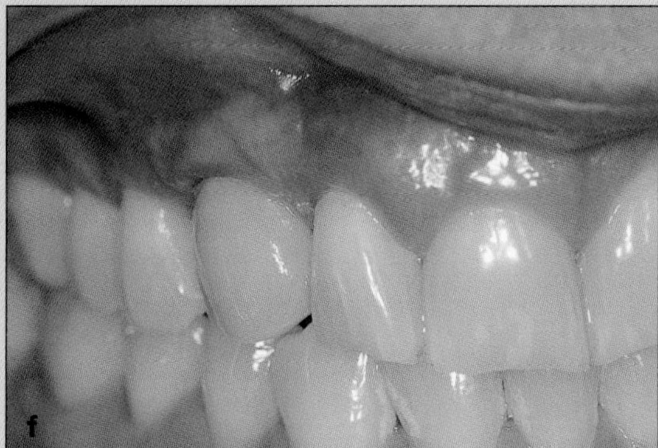

Figs 7-11e and 7-11f One-year postoperative view demonstrates camouflaging of the small-volume combination defect with natural emergence of the implant restoration, natural gingival esthetics, and excellent peri-implant health.

site, the long-term prognosis of that tooth should be determined and the options of forced orthodontic eruption to improve the recipient-site anatomy at the implant site, or tooth removal with orthodontics and replacement with an additional implant should be discussed with the patient. Failure to identify such preexisting periodontal defects may create false expectations for the results obtainable from subsequent site-development procedures (Fig 7-13). Furthermore, these defects may be exacerbated by the adjacent site-development surgery, leading to further blunting or complete loss of adjacent papillae and severely compromising esthetic results for patients with high smile lines.

Reconstruction of a large-volume combination esthetic ridge defect via simultaneous hard and soft tissue grafting

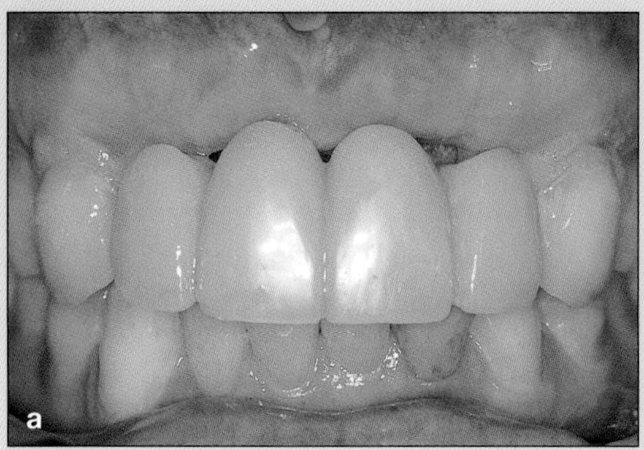

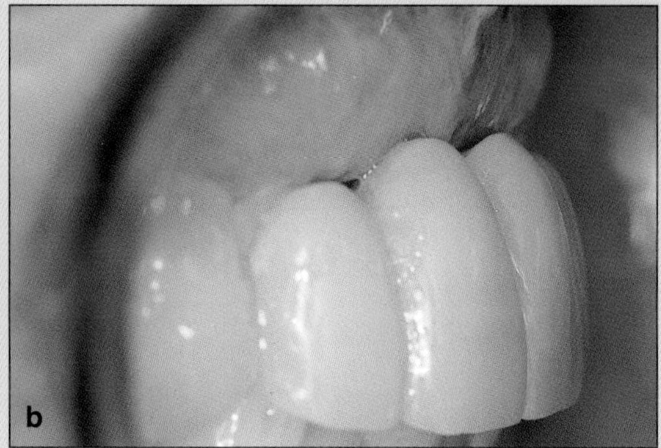

Figs 7-12a and 7-12b Preoperative views of maxillary incisor sites with large-volume combination defect. Note the significant deficiency in the vertical and horizontal ridge contours. The sites are compromised as a result of a previous history leading to tooth loss and an attempt at bone grafting, which failed.

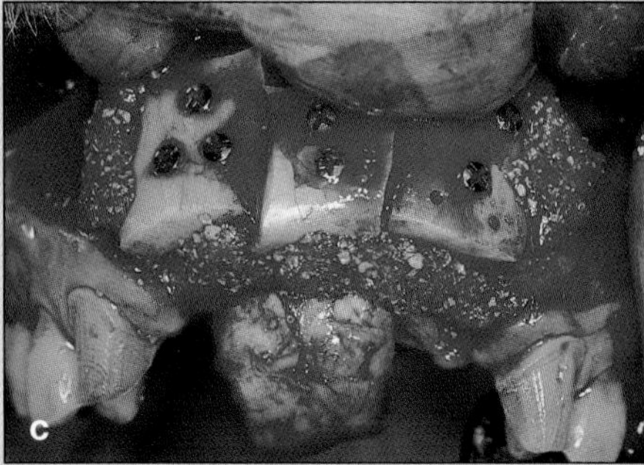

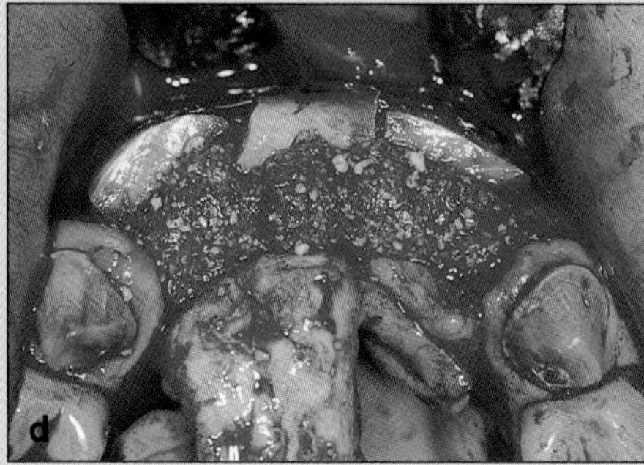

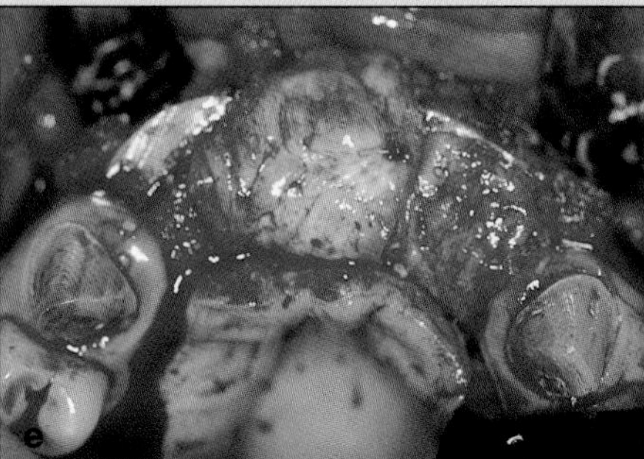

Figs 7-12c to 7-12e Three thick corticocancellous block grafts harvested from the body of the mandible were intimately adapted to the prepared recipient site and secured with fixation screws. Bilateral VIP-CT flaps were then developed from the palatal donor sites. Passive coaptation of the access flap was confirmed. The particulate graft was then condensed around the periphery of the block grafts, and the VIP-CT flaps were secured over the crest of the ridge to achieve vertical soft tissue height for emergence of harmonious implant restorations. A large resorbable collagen membrane (Bio-Gide) was adapted over the portions of the bone graft not covered by the periosteum of the VIP-CT flaps. Note the emphasis on midline vertical soft tissue augmentation.

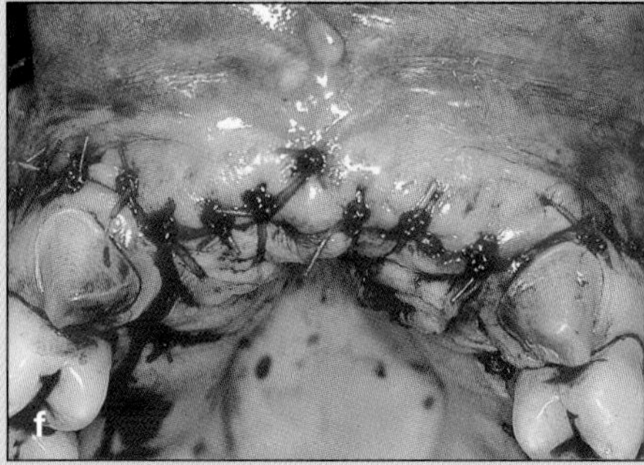

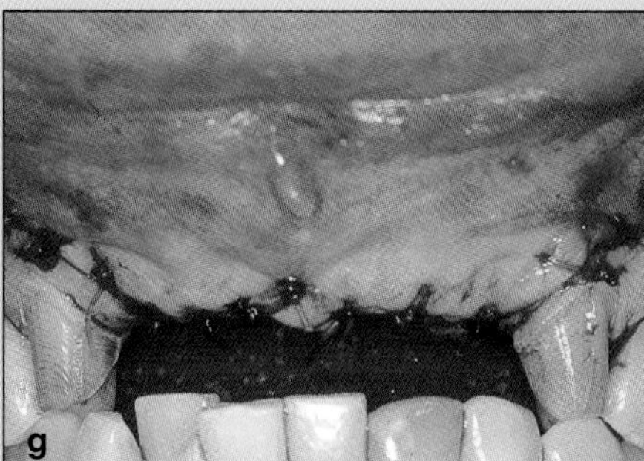

Figs 7-12f and 7-12g Exaggerated curvilinear-beveled flaps with tension-releasing cutback incisions facilitated tension-free closure of the buccal flap without the need for periosteal releasing incisions, which compromise circulation. The donor site was also closed primarily.

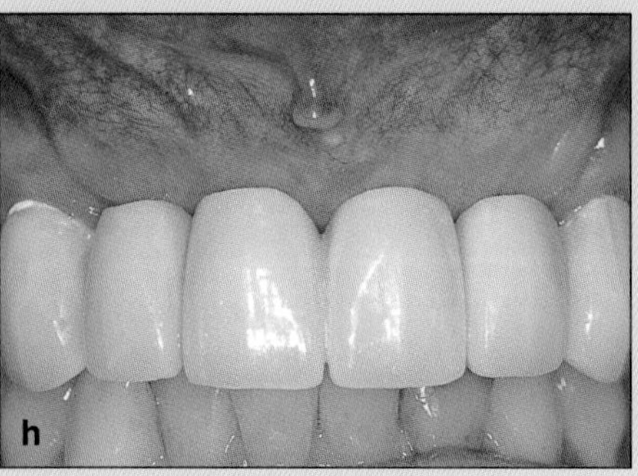

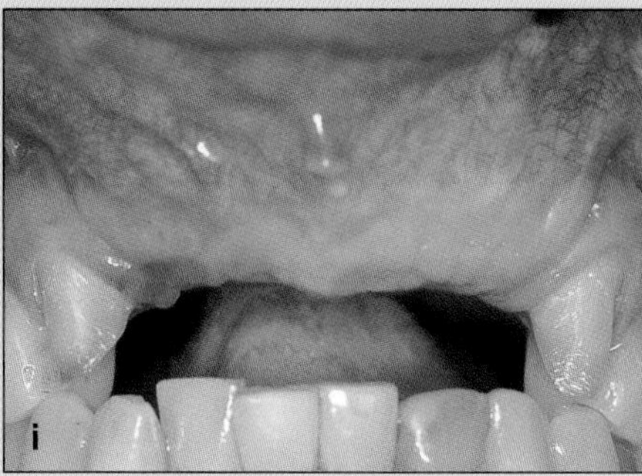

Figs 7-12h and 7-12i Three-month postoperative views, with and without modified interim provisional restoration in place, demonstrate successful reconstruction of large-volume combination defect. The natural alveolar ridge contours have been restored.

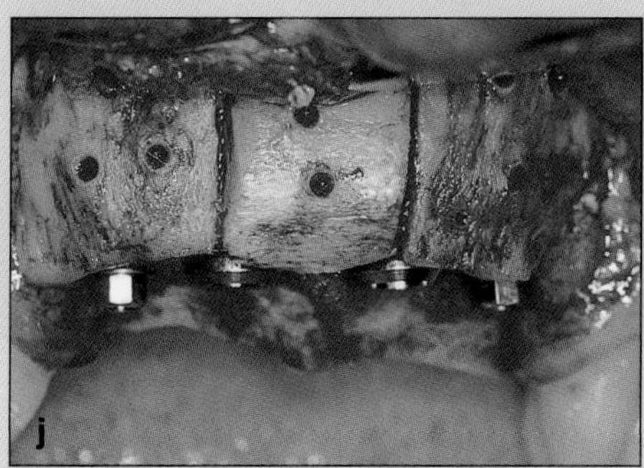
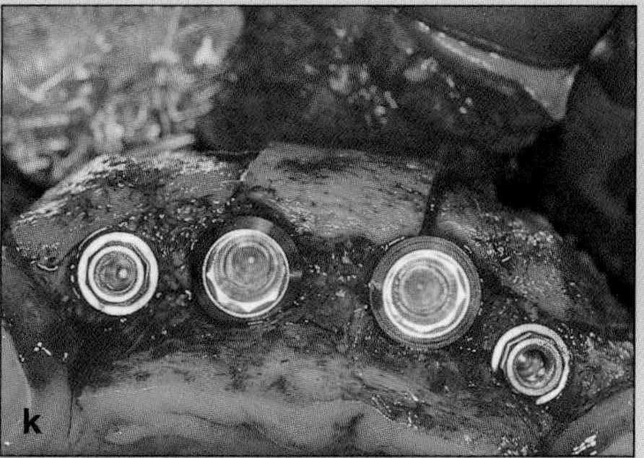
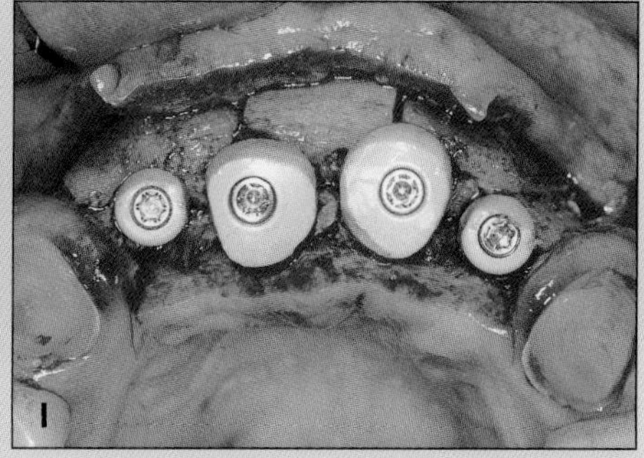

Figs 7-12j to 7-12l Access flap retracted for removal of fixation screws and placement of four nonsubmerged implants (Straumann USA). Narrow-neck implants were used in the lateral incisor positions. Excellent bone graft volume yield was obtained at the maxillary midline. This was facilitated by the use of the VIP-CT flap, which provides additional circulation for bone graft healing.

Fig 7-12m Four-month postoperative view following implant placement. Customizable healing abutments (Peek, Straumann USA) have supported the soft tissues, and there is positive soft tissue architecture.

Fig 7-12n Restorative abutments in place 4 months after implant placement. Note that vertical soft tissue augmentation afforded by the VIP-CT flap performed in conjunction with bone graft reconstruction has resulted in the restoration of inter-implant papillae.

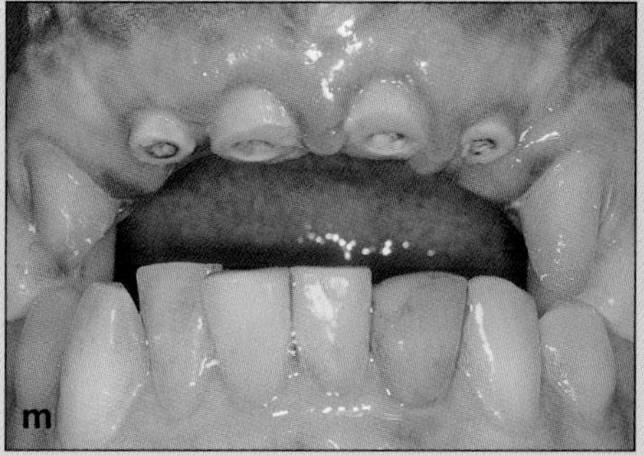
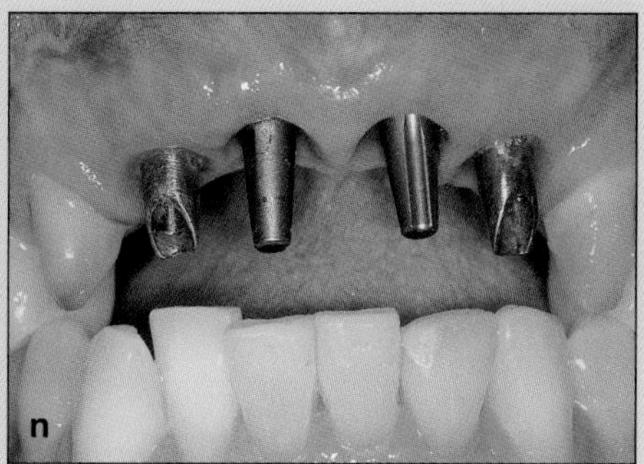

Fig 7-12o Radiographs taken 4 months after delivery of final restoration demonstrate stable crestal bone levels and anatomic placement of the implants. Although the underlying osseous architecture is flat, positive soft tissue architecture resulted from the use of the VIP-CT flaps, which provide the potential to increase tissue height or depth at anterior maxillary implant sites.

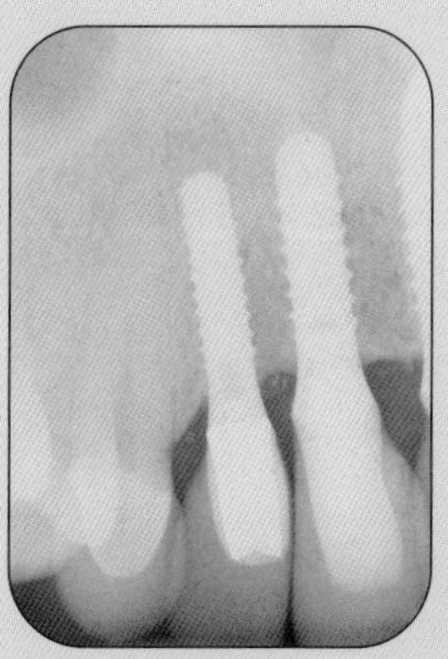
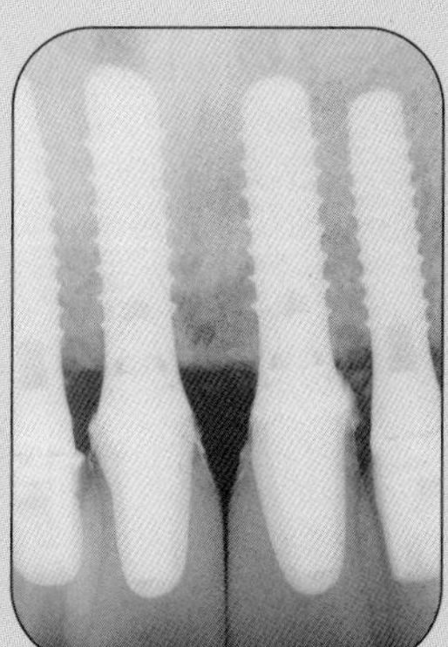
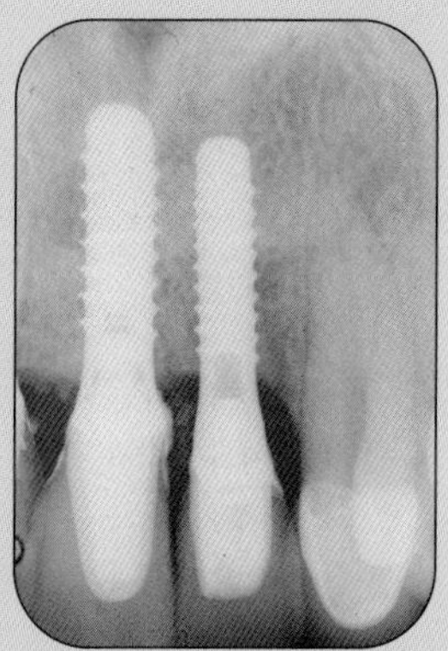

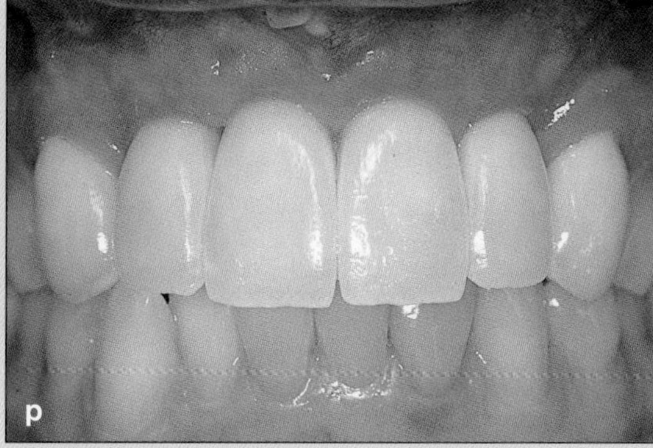
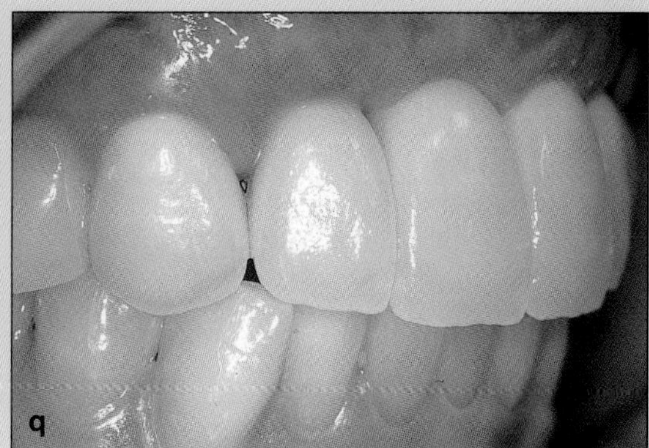

Figs 7-12p and 7-12q Final restoration 4 months after delivery. The inconspicuous appearance of the implant restoration was facilitated by the reconstruction of natural hard and soft tissue alveolar ridge anatomy. Vertical soft tissue augmentation obtained with the VIP-CT flaps was a key element to esthetic success in this case, which used four successive implants to support the restoration.

Hard and soft tissue site development aided by forced orthodontic eruption at a compromised adjacent tooth

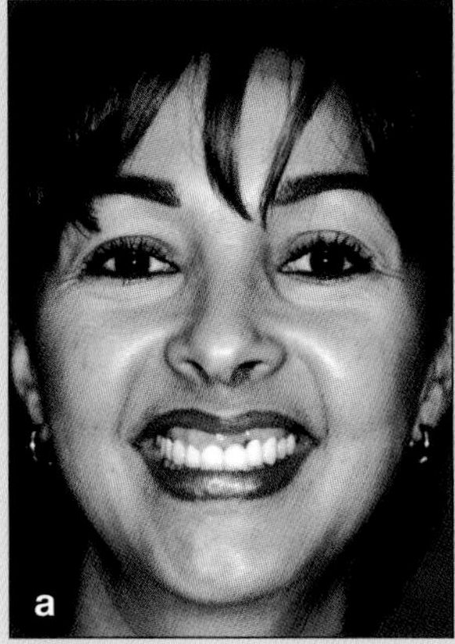

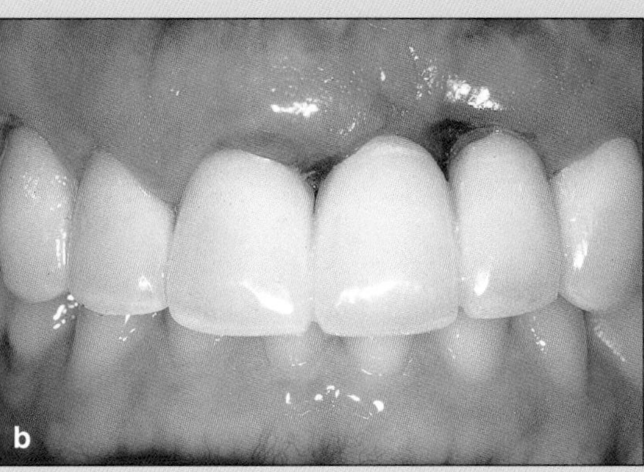

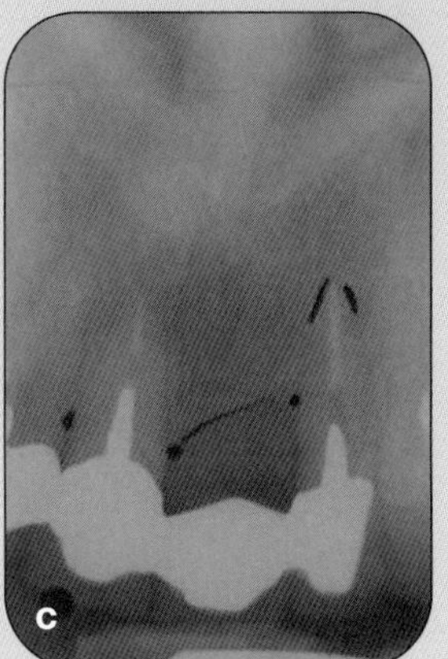

Figs 7-13a and 7-13b Facial and close-up views of left cental incisor implant site adjacent to lateral incisor with compromised crestal bone height. The treatment plan was to maintain the lateral incisor but improve the outcome of adjacent site-development procedures via forced orthodontic eruption of the lateral incisor and subsequently create a harmonious appearance via esthetic crown lengthening of adjacent dentition. A large-volume combination defect is evident at the left central incisor site.

Fig 7-13c Preoperative radiograph demonstrating compromised interdental bone height on the lateral incisor. A previous attempt to reconstruct the lost papilla was doomed to failure because of lack of underlying bone support.

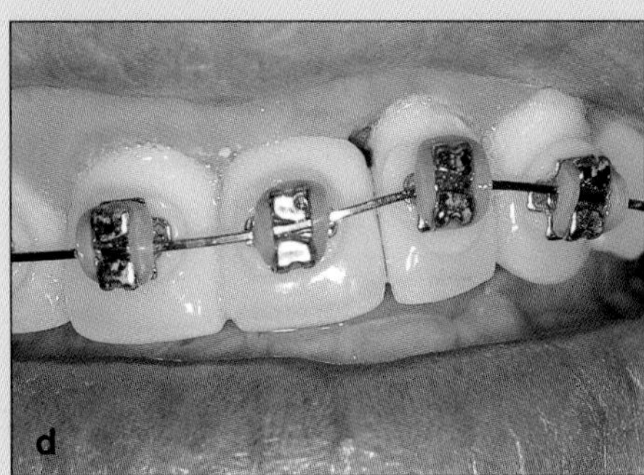

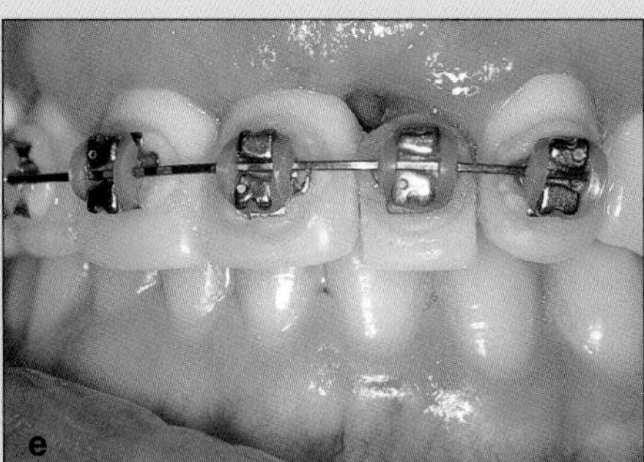

Figs 7-13d and 7-13e Following completion of forced orthodontic eruption, a stabilization period was allowed.

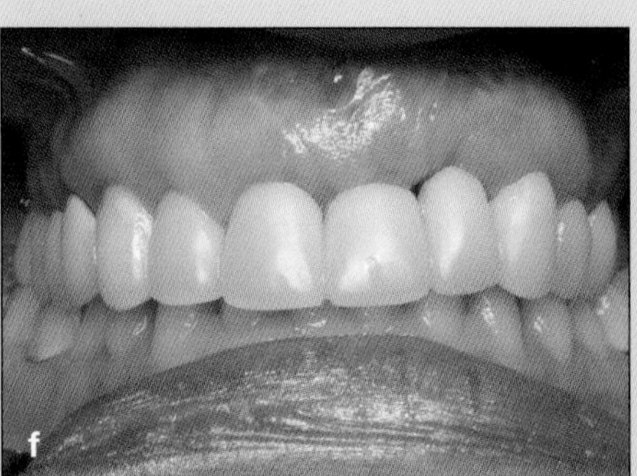

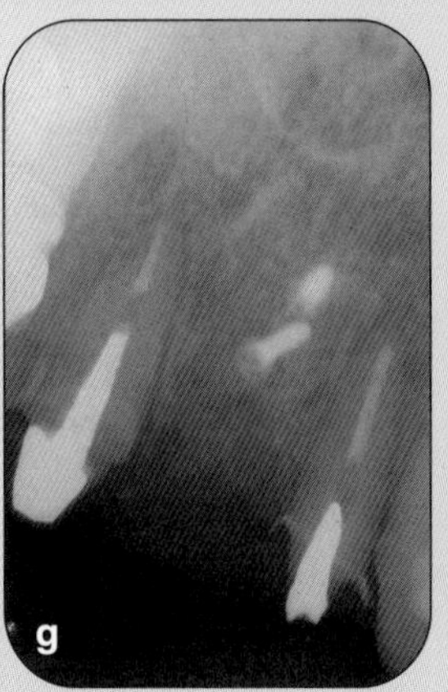

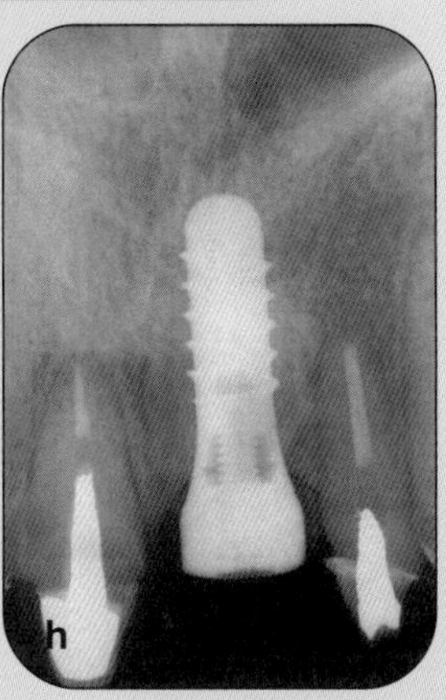

Fig 7-13f Simultaneous hard and soft tissue site development was performed with block bone grafting and a VIP-CT flap. Significant improvement was made in the ridge contours of the left central incisor implant site as well as in the lost papilla.

Figs 7-13g and 7-13h Radiographs following site development and implant placement. Note dramatic improvement of interdental bone height on the lateral incisor compared to pretreatment condition.

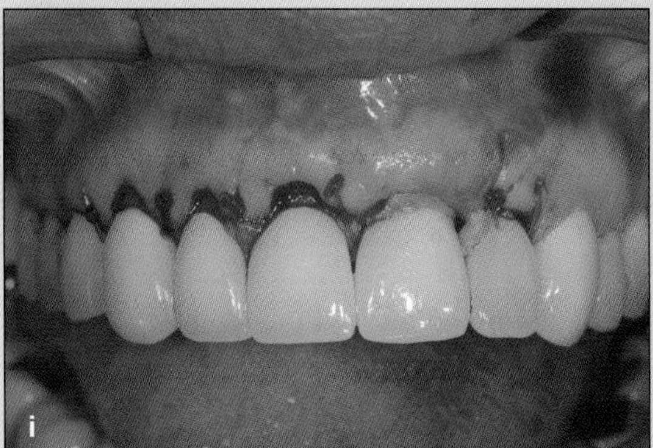

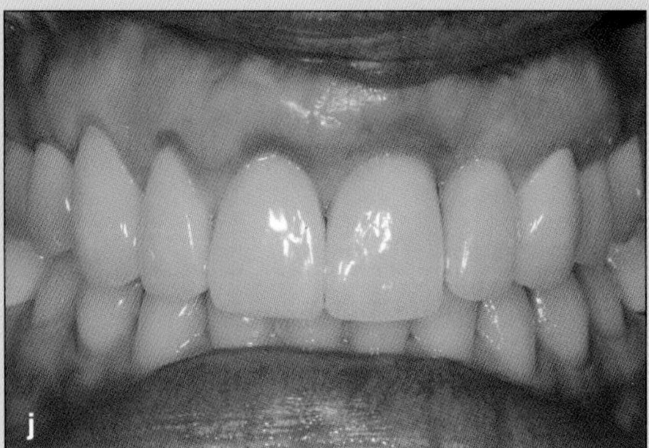

Fig 7-13i After allowing soft tissues to adapt around the implant provisional restoration, conservative esthetic crown lengthening was performed on selected adjacent dentition.

Fig 7-13j Pleasing gingival esthetics have been obtained with the exception of a small compromise owing to the patient's decision to maintain the lateral incisor instead of removing it and developing the site for an additional implant restoration. (Orthodontics and restorative dentistry by Dr Juan Diego Cardenas, Coral Gables, FL.)

Prosthetic Considerations for Enhancing Outcomes in Esthetic Implant Therapy

Interim provisional restorations

In esthetic implant therapy, close coordination with the restorative dentist increases the predictability of the results. Interim provisional restorations, which transmit micromotion to the implant site, have a negative effect on the volume yields from hard and soft tissue site-development procedures and, in certain instances, can contribute to failure of such grafts via the same mechanism attributed to implant failures. To avoid these deleterious effects, the author prefers to use toothborne interim provisional restorations whenever possible following esthetic implant site-development procedures and during the subsequent osseointegration period. Several types of toothborne provisional restorations are available to satisfy the needs of the patient, restorative dentist, and surgeon. One type that is especially useful in the immediate postoperative period is a modification of an Essex orthodontic retainer (Fig 7-14a). This interim provisional restoration is designed and fabricated to house either a tissue-supporting ovate pontic following tooth removal or an abbreviated pontic that accommodates swelling following hard and soft tissue site-development procedures. On occasion, the clinical crown of the extracted tooth is modified to serve as the pontic. This type of interim provisional restoration can be fabricated on the day of surgery and adjusted by the surgical team to ensure tissue support or stress-free healing at the surgical sites as needed. In-office fabrication of an Essex retainer requires the surgical or restorative team to obtain impressions to create a master cast as well as shade selection prior to the surgery procedure. The Essex interim provisional restoration is then conveniently fabricated using the MiniSTAR device (Great Lakes Orthodontics, Tonawanda, NY) (Fig 7-14b). Various thicknesses of Invisacryl or Biocryl (Great Lakes Orthodontics) translucent materials are available to suit the needs of individual cases. It is important to smooth and polish all of the edges after final trimming of the material. Alternatively, most dental laboratories can fabricate this type of provisional restoration in advance. In most cases, Essex interim provisional restorations are used only on a temporary basis until initial healing is achieved, after which they are replaced by a more definitive interim restoration fabricated by the restorative dentist. Nevertheless, on many occasions, patients have continued to use the Essex provisional restoration as their interim restoration until an implant-supported provisional restoration is delivered. Advantages of using modified Essex retainers as interim provisional restorations include excellent esthetics and phonetics and a relatively low cost. In addition, on-site fabrication by the surgical team eliminates the need to coordinate the surgical procedure with the restorative dentist, a convenience usually appreciated by most dentists and patients when a tooth must be removed on an urgent basis. A disadvantage of this type of interim restoration is the obvious difficulty of chewing when the appliance is worn. Patients must be informed of this drawback.

Another type of toothborne interim provisional restoration commonly used in esthetic implant therapy is the resin-bonded partial denture, which not only provides superior function and esthetics but also protects the underlying surgical site (Fig 7-15). This interim restoration can be designed to maintain the scalloped soft tissue architecture at the site and to support the adjacent interdental papillae. In the author's experience, this restoration is often used as a replacement for the Essex provisional restoration after initial healing following site-development or site-preservation procedures. The restorative team must evaluate whether an adequate amount of interocclusal space is available to accommodate this restoration and whether the occlusal scheme is favorable. Nevertheless, patients who are transitioned from an Essex type of provisional restoration to a resin-bonded partial denture are routinely instructed to keep their Essex as a back-up restoration should the resin bond fail. The author has experienced the best success when these resin-bonded interim provisional restorations are fabricated in the dental laboratory on an updated study cast taken approximately 6 weeks after hard and soft tissue site-development procedures.

Another option for supporting an interim provisional restoration in esthetic implant therapy is the strategic maintenance of certain natural tooth abutments ultimately planned for removal or for restoration (Fig 7-16). The teeth are maintained until a sufficient number of implants have achieved osseointegration, allowing a transition from an interim toothborne provisional restoration to an implant-supported provisional restoration. Subsequently, these teeth are either restored or removed depending on their long-term prognosis and the details of the treatment plan. Additional site-development procedures are then performed or additional implants are placed without concern for the deleterious effects of transmission of micromotion. The greatest advantage of this approach is the maintenance of a fixed prosthesis throughout the therapeutic sequence. One disadvantage of this approach is prolonged treatment time and an increase in the number

Interim provisional restorations: Modified Essex retainer

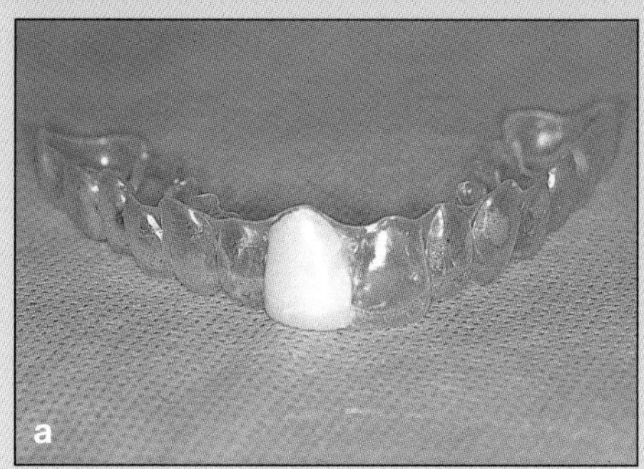

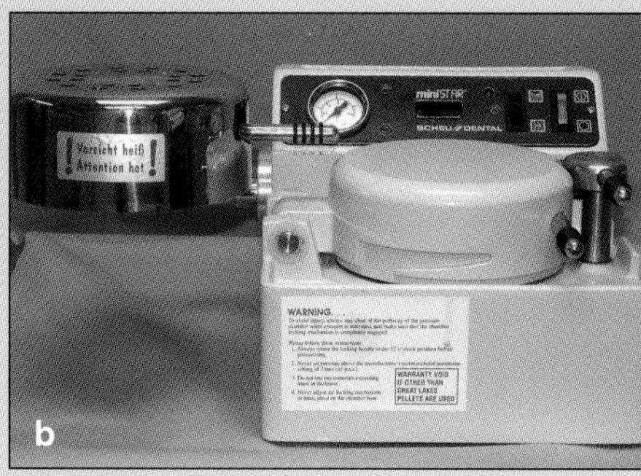

Fig 7-14a An Essex retainer that houses one or more pontics serves as a convenient interim provisional restoration that satisfies the immediate esthetic needs of a patient following the removal of a tooth.

Fig 7-14b The MiniSTAR device facilitates the fabrication of an Essex interim provisional restoration in the surgical office.

Interim provisional restorations: Resin-bonded fixed partial denture

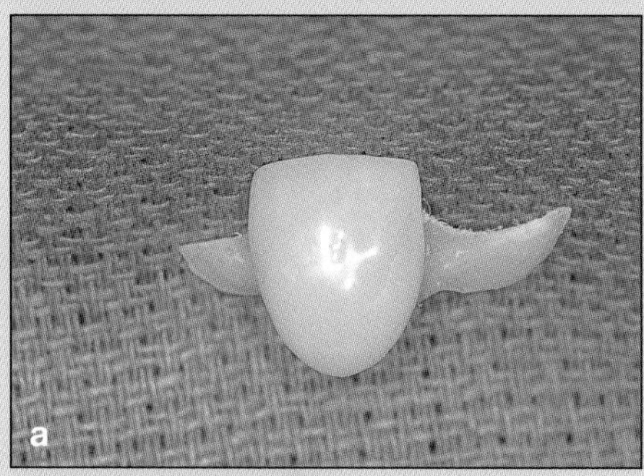

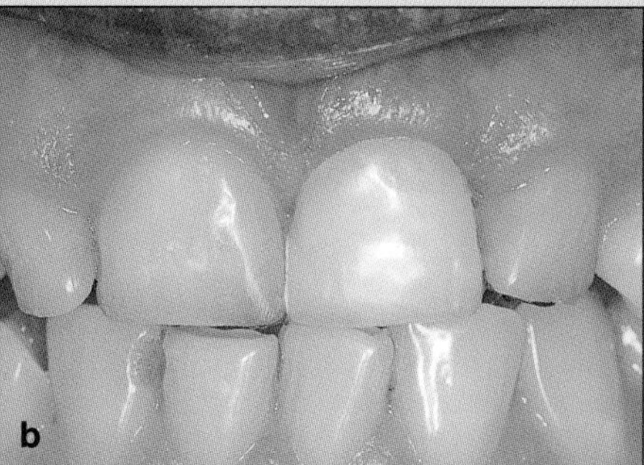

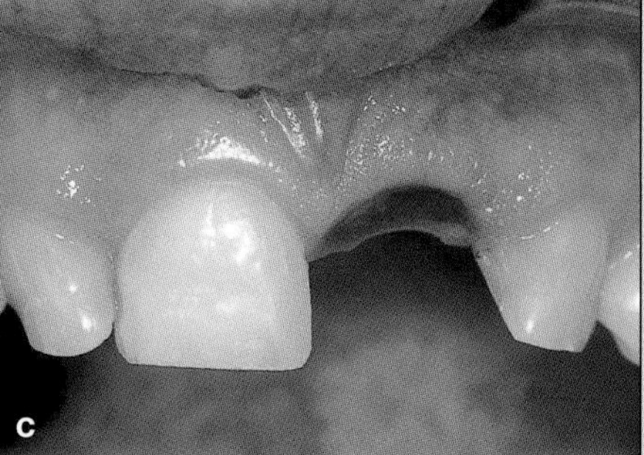

Figs 7-15a to 7-15c A resin-bonded fixed partial denture is an excellent means of providing an interim provisional restoration that supports the soft tissues and papillae at the site while avoiding transmission of micromotion.

Interim provisional restorations: Strategic use of natural abutments to support a toothborne interim provisional restoration

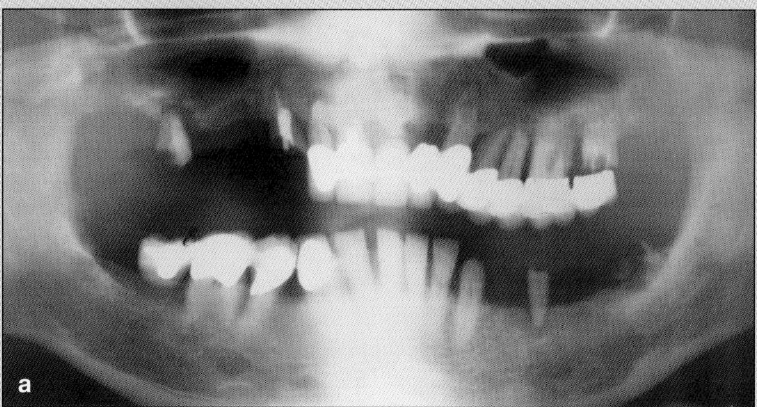

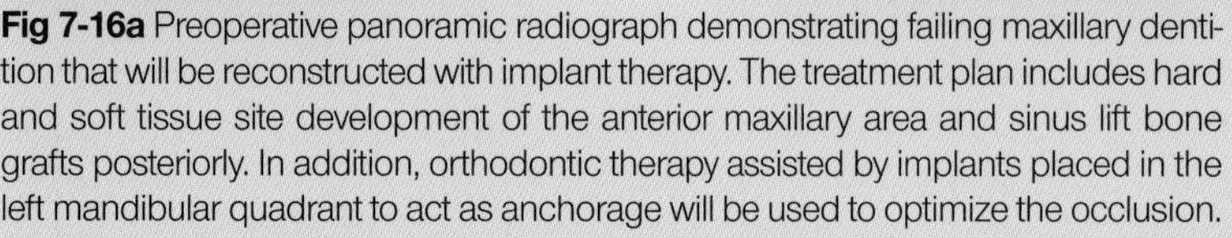

Fig 7-16a Preoperative panoramic radiograph demonstrating failing maxillary dentition that will be reconstructed with implant therapy. The treatment plan includes hard and soft tissue site development of the anterior maxillary area and sinus lift bone grafts posteriorly. In addition, orthodontic therapy assisted by implants placed in the left mandibular quadrant to act as anchorage will be used to optimize the occlusion.

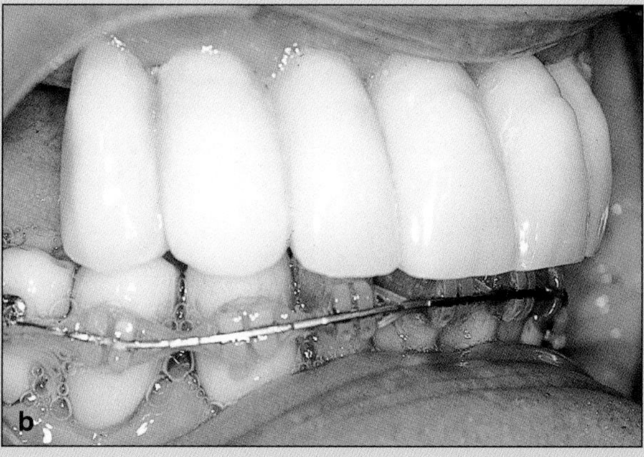

Fig 7-16b Clinical view (right side) of interim provisional restoration supported by three selected natural tooth abutments during the initial orthodontic and bone-grafting portion of the treatment.

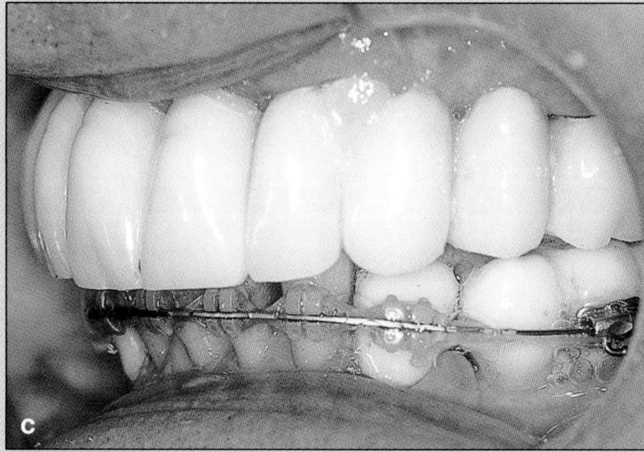

Fig 7-16c Clinical view (left side) of interim provisional restoration supported by three selected natural tooth abutments during the initial orthodontic and bone-grafting portion of the treatment.

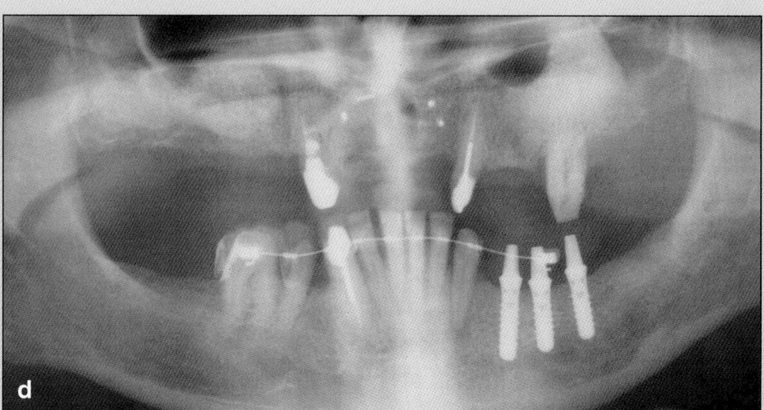

Fig 7-16d Panoramic radiograph following bone-grafting procedures. The left mandibular implants (Straumann USA) were used for orthodontic anchorage after an abbreviated (6-week) osseointegration period.

Figs 7-16e and 7-16f Four months after the bone-grafting procedures, the surgical guide and eight implants (3i) were placed in a nonsubmerged fashion. The surgical guide was supported by the retained natural abutments and provided precision guidance for osteotomy preparation. Two additional central incisor implants were placed in a submerged fashion.

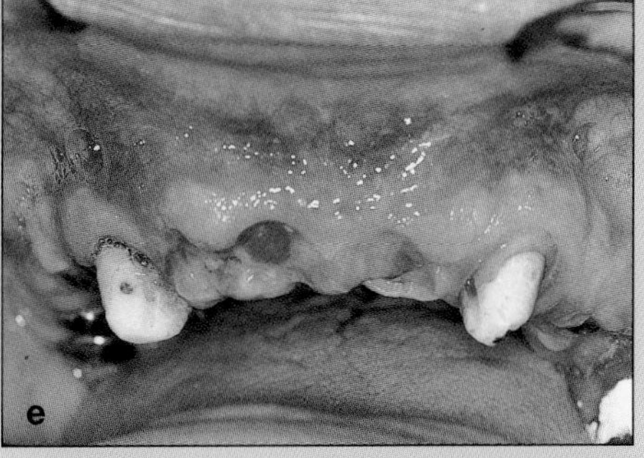

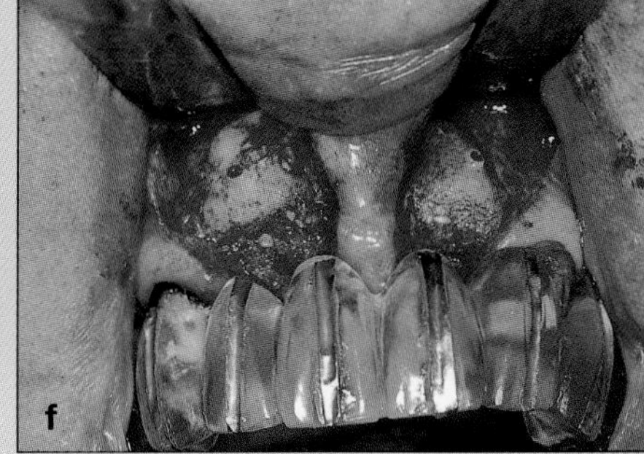

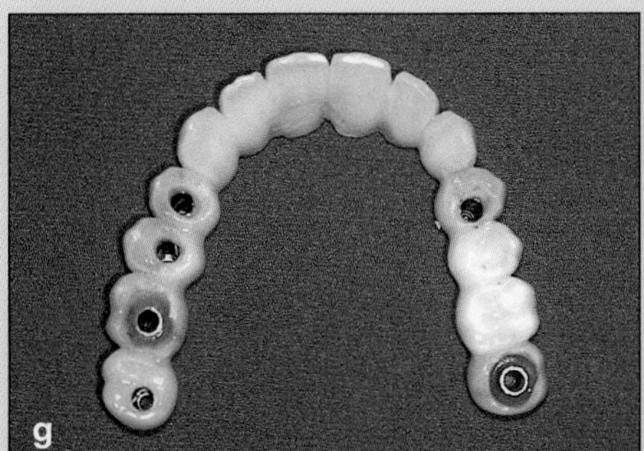

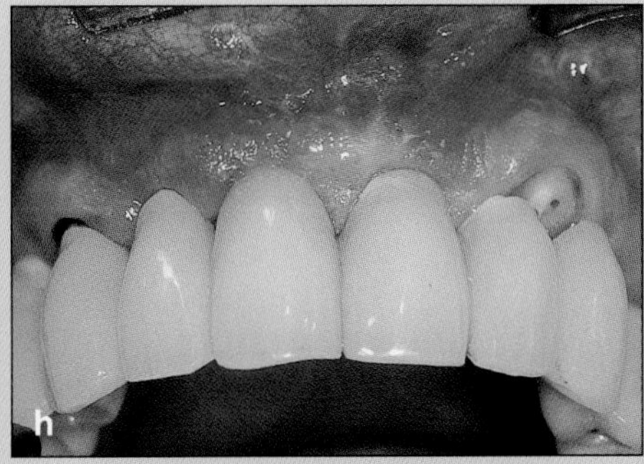

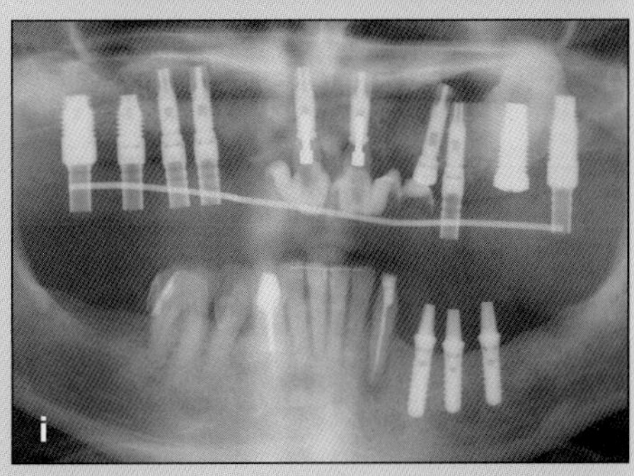

Figs 7-16g to 7-16i After the initial osseointegration period, an implant-supported provisional restoration was fabricated and delivered after the retained teeth were reduced to the gingival level. Note the malposed maxillary canine compared to the desired final position. The three retained teeth were removed and the left canine and molar were immediately replaced using the Bio-Col technique.

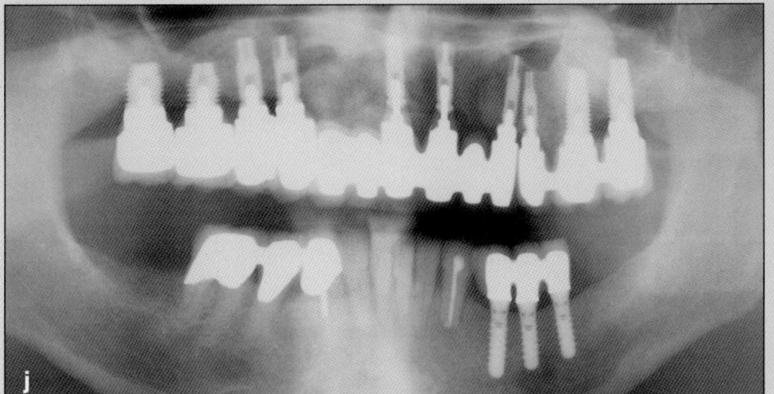

Fig 7-16j Panoramic radiograph after delivery of final restorations. Strategic retention of three teeth conveniently supported an interim fixed provisional restoration, thereby preventing the transmission of micromotion to bone graft and implant sites.

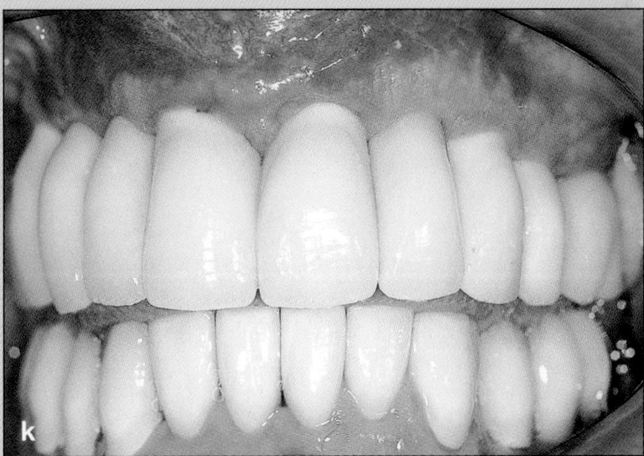

Fig 7-16k Final restoration in place. A comprehensive approach was required to reconstruct this severely compromised dentition. (Restoration by Dr Larry Grillo, Aventura, FL; orthodontics by Dr John Marchetto, Westin, FL.)

of follow-up visits to monitor any teeth that have a questionable prognosis. Failure to closely monitor these cases can lead to complications secondary to the inadvertent loading of the surgical site from loosening or shifting of the prosthesis secondary to occlusal forces.

When site-development procedures are necessary or implant placement is planned and none of the previous options is possible, immediate provisional implants may be used to support a fixed interim provisional restoration while hard or soft tissue grafts are healing or during osseointegration of simultaneously placed definitive implants (Fig 7-17). In most cases, these small-diameter provisional implants are placed adjacent to the definitive implants in a distribution that will allow the support of a fixed interim restoration until the definitive implants have achieved osseointegration, allowing transition to a fixed implant-supported provisional restoration. In most instances, removal of the provisional implants is a simple procedure performed under local anesthesia. In fact, in many instances the restorative dentist can remove the provisional implants at the appointment when the prosthesis is transitioned to the definitive implants. One disadvantage of using provisional implants is the need for frequent follow-up visits. The author recommends spacing these visits at 3-week intervals to monitor the stability of the interim prosthesis and the health of the bone and soft tissues around the provisional implants. In cases where it is not possible to place a sufficient number of immediate provisional implants to support a fixed interim restoration, these

Interim provisional restoration: Use of transitional implants to support an interim provisional restoration

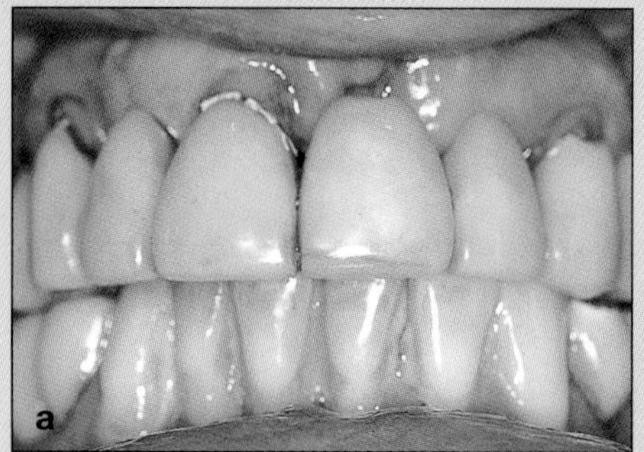

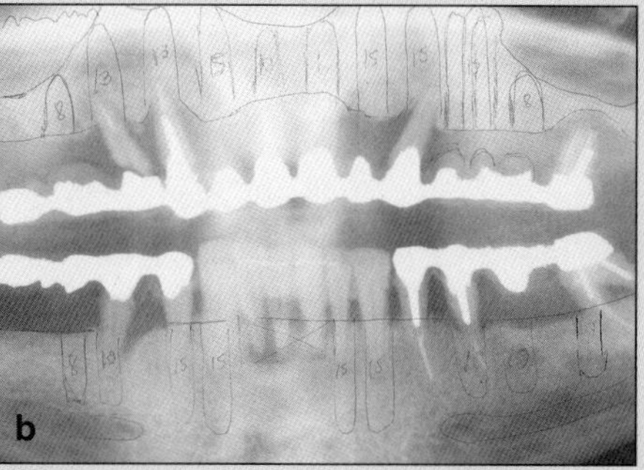

Figs 7-17a and 7-17b Preoperative clinical and radiographic views of failing maxillary and mandibular dentition despite intensive periodontal therapy. The patient's heavy smoking places this case in the high-risk category.

Fig 7-17c Immediate provisional implant system (Nobel Biocare) provides a convenient way to support an interim prosthesis.

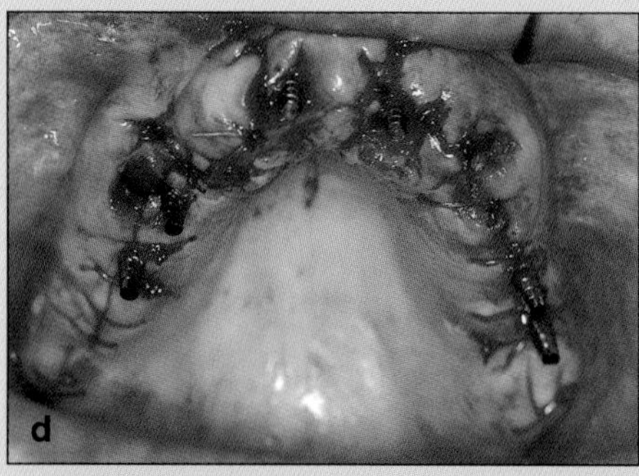

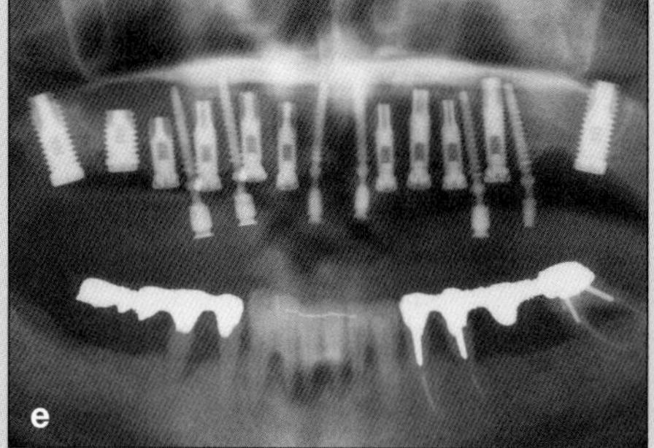

Figs 7-17d and 7-17e After the removal of remaining teeth and the placement of 11 submerged implants (3i), 6 provisional implants were placed so as to avoid jeopardizing the osseointegration of the permanent implants. Panoramic radiograph shows the positions of the provisional and permanent implants.

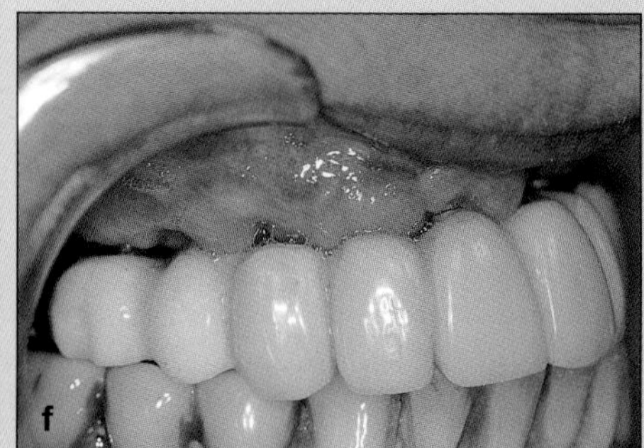

Fig 7-17f Fixed interim provisional restoration supported by the provisional implants.

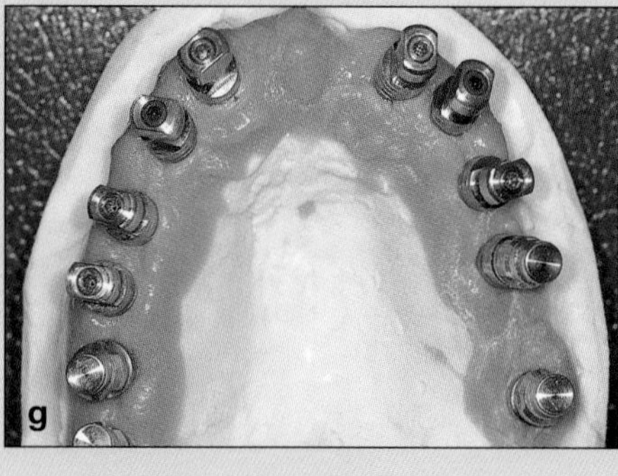

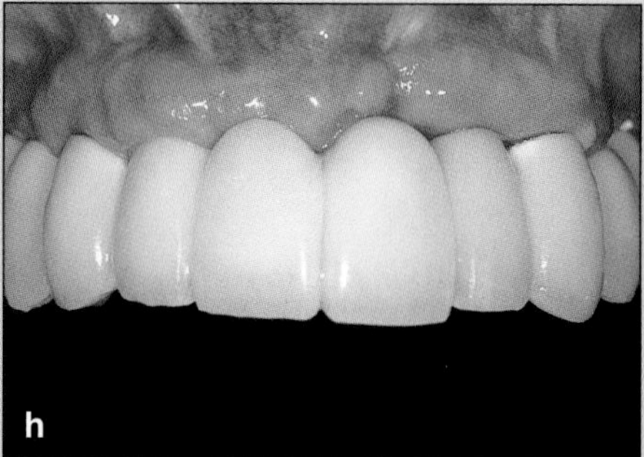

Fig 7-17g Final impression performed after successful osseointegration of permanent implants. The use of provisional implants provided a stress-free healing environment for the permanent implants, contributing to a successful outcome in this high-risk case.

Fig 7-17h The provisional implants were removed to allow try-in of the final restoration prior to final adjustments, glazing, and cementation. (Restoration by Dr Juan Diego Cardenas, Coral Gables, FL.)

interim implants can be used to stabilize a removable prosthesis, thereby reducing the possibility of transmucosal loading to the underlying surgical sites(s).

Prosthetic-guided soft tissue healing

Conceptually, the use of prosthetic-guided soft tissue healing to enhance esthetic outcomes in implant therapy involves the early introduction of prosthetic components (interim provisional restorations, tooth-form healing abutments, and implant-supported provisional restorations) at various stages of therapy that correspond to the cross-sectional anatomy of the lost tooth or the planned esthetic replacement at the gingival level. These components support and guide soft tissue healing following various surgical interventions and have tremendous influence on the final soft tissue architecture obtained at the implant site. As discussed in chapter 4, prosthetic-guided soft tissue healing techniques can be used to preserve existing soft tissue anatomy following tooth removal. This section describes prosthetic options available to the surgeon that provide a scaffold for guided healing of soft tissues immediately following implant emergence.

It is generally accepted that the morphology of blunted interdental papillae found between natural teeth can be consistently improved by manipulating the restorative contours of the adjacent teeth, provided there is sufficient interdental bone support underlying the col and papilla (see chapter 2). The author theorizes that the mechanism for this clinical observation is

Surgical indexing technique

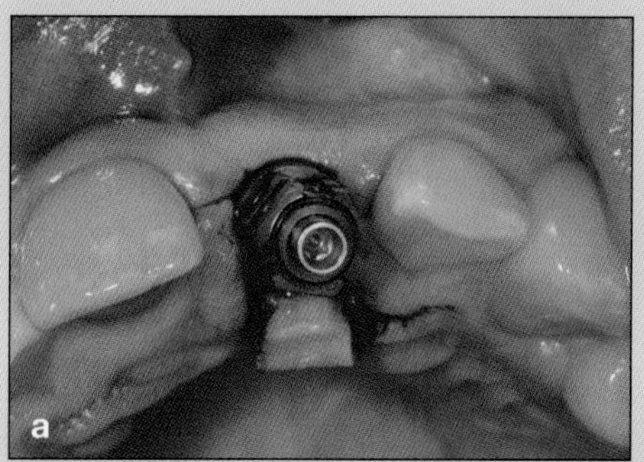

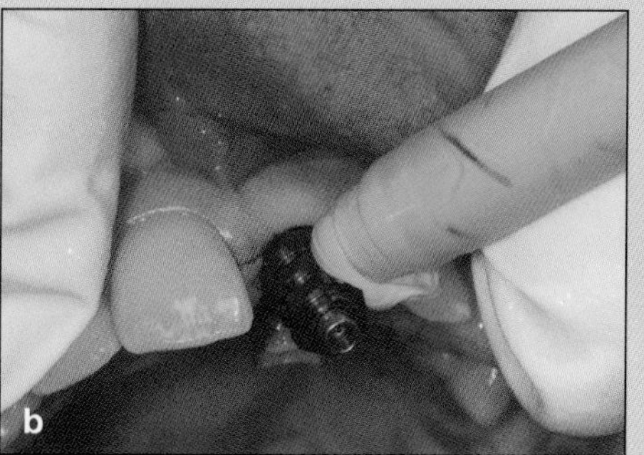

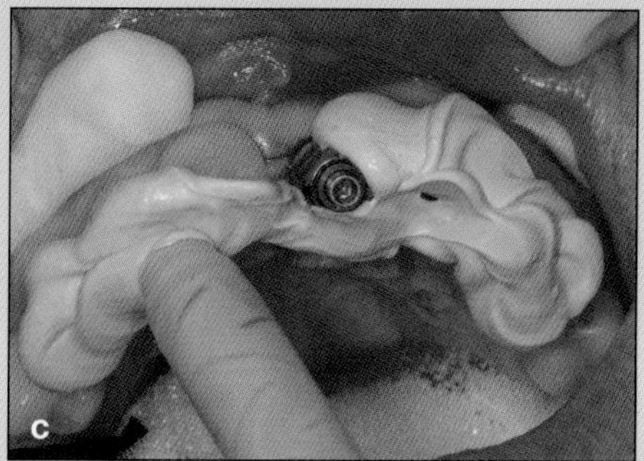

Fig 7-18a Following implant placement, a fixture-level impression coping (Straumann USA) is attached to the implant.

Figs 7-18b and 7-18c Blue Velvet impression material is used to register the position of the implant relative to that of the adjacent natural dentition.

Fig 7-18d The surgical index is used to create a working cast for fabrication of custom abutments or tooth-form healing abutments. First, a presurgical cast is altered by creating a receptor for an implant analog attached to the surgical index. Next, the index is seated on the cast and the analog is secured with quick-set plaster, rendering a working implant analog cast. A soft tissue mask can subsequently be added by taking a second impression after maturation of the soft tissues at the site.

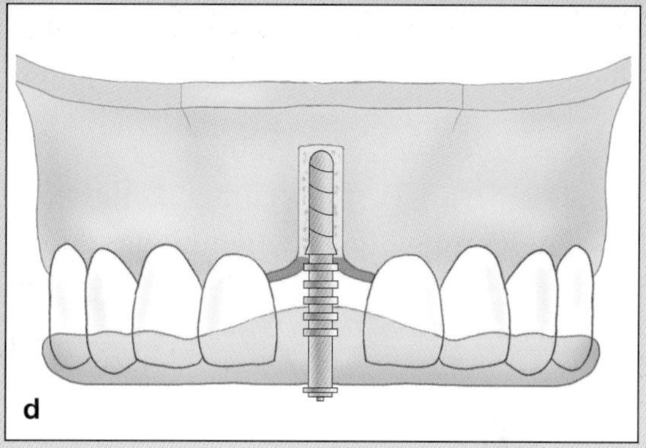

initiated by an inflammatory reaction that occurs in response to irritation caused by the changes in the restorative contours. The inflammatory response leads to vasodilation and edema within the papillae and ultimately to tissue regeneration via scarification. As discussed in chapter 1, the peri-implant soft tissues are characterized by a dense connective tissue scar and do not enjoy the benefit of a periodontal ligament and blood supply or the potential anastomotic connections between the periodontal ligament and supraperiosteal and intraosseous alveolar circulation. Therefore, the restorative dentist has only a limited opportunity and potential to influence the inter-implant papillae and the form of the peri-implant free marginal tissue. The early introduction of anatomically correct prosthetic elements takes advantage of the available healing dynamics and translates into optimal soft tissue contours and peri-implant soft tissue stability when compared with the loss of esthetic potential commonly experienced with the use of nonanatomic transmucosal elements. Although delaying the introduction of an anatomically correct prosthetic component until after soft tissue integration has occurred around a previously placed nonanatomic transmucosal component can eventually (12 to 18 months later) result in enhanced soft tissue contours at the site, this method lacks the practicality and does not provide the synergistic effects observed when guided soft tissue healing techniques are immediately used at the time of initial surgical intervention.

Custom abutments and provisional restorations

Delivery of custom abutments and provisional restorations immediately upon exposure of submerged implants is one method that can be used to initiate early guided soft tissue healing for enhanced esthetic soft tissue contours. At the time of implant placement, the surgeon must perform a surgical index (fixture-level impression) that is subsequently used to fabricate a working model upon which the abutment and provisional restoration are fabricated in the dental laboratory (Fig 7-18). The surgical index procedure involves attaching a specialized fixture-level impression coping to the implant and registering its three-dimensional position relative to the adjacent dentition. The author routinely uses fast-set Blue Velvet polyvinylsiloxane impression material (J. Morita, Irvine, CA) for this purpose. The material is injected around the index coping and over the incisal and occlusal surfaces of a sufficient number of adjacent teeth to provide an accurate index. The material is not injected into the surgical site. The surgeon dons a second set of sterile gloves to handle the impression gun. Once the index is complete, the second set of gloves is removed and the surgeon removes the index coping and attached impression material. An implant analog is attached to the Blue Velvet–impression coping complex and the combination is seated on an altered master cast fabricated from a full-arch impression taken prior to surgery. In order for the index to seat on the master cast, the edentulous site is prepared to receive the implant analog. Subsequent to seating the index, the analog is secured to the cast with quick-set plaster or acrylic resin. The result is a working model that contains a replica of the implant as recorded at the time of surgery. The working model should be fabricated within a few days to prevent any subsequent dimensional changes that might occur during prolonged storage of the index. Subsequently, the restorative dentist can impress the site to capture the soft tissue contours not initially registered by the surgical indexing. Approximately 3 months of healing following the last soft tissue surgical procedure are recommended prior to obtaining the impression for soft tissue model fabrication. The soft tissue model aids the laboratory technician in the placement of restorative margins at an appropriate depth on the custom abutment. In most instances, the laboratory either casts or mills a custom abutment that incorporates proximal rise to ensure that the restorative margins are located in the superficial aspect of the peri-implant sulcus circumferentially. In addition, the provisional restoration is fabricated with ideal contours to support and guide the healing of the peri-implant soft tissues immediately upon exposure of the submerged implant. In most instances, the surgeon then delivers the abutment and cements the provisional restoration at the second-stage surgery through a conservative approach as described in chapter 3. Significant occlusal adjustments or modifications to contours are rarely necessary. Nevertheless, the author recommends coordinating the exposure appointment with the restorative dentist, who should reserve time for the rare instance that significant modifications are needed. In the author's experience, the secondary impression used for soft tissue model fabrication discussed above virtually eliminates these problems. Another important consideration to discuss is the recommended timing and technique used by the restorative dentist for final impressions. In most situations, 2 to 3 months are allowed for the tissues to stabilize around the custom abutment and provisional restoration. In addition, this allows time for the restorative dentist to modify contours as needed to satisfy the patient's phonetic and esthetic demands.

There are two basic options for the final impression procedure. If a customized permanent abutment and provisional restoration were delivered upon implant exposure as described above, a direct impression is necessary at the site. Considering the dense connective tissue scar around the implant and the tenuous biologic seal mediated by hemidesmosomal attachments of the junctional epithelium, aggressive packing of cord is not recommended. In fact, even when the custom abutment is designed with proximal rise in the restorative margin, there is the possibility that the impression procedure may damage the peri-implant soft tissues, causing subsequent recession. A solution to this problem is to have the laboratory technician also fabricate a custom impression coping that captures the margins of the custom abutment. Provided that no marginal adjustments become necessary, the coping can be used to perform a minimally traumatic final impression. In the rare instances when the margins of the custom abutment must be modified, the author recommends that the restorative dentist remove the abutment, perform the adjustment, reline the custom impression coping to include the new margin, replace the abutment, and proceed with the final impression. Although this is rarely necessary, the author recommends that the surgeon initially secure the abutment with moderate torque force and that the restorative dentist apply the recommended final torque force to permanently secure the custom abutment immediately prior to final impression.

The second option for final impression is a fixture-level impression performed by the restorative dentist. This option is exercised when a one- or two-piece provisional abutment and restoration are fabricated on the index model and delivered by the surgeon upon implant exposure. The obvious advantage of this approach is that the final prosthesis is fabricated in the dental laboratory, ensuring excellent margins and decreasing chair time for the restorative dentist. The disadvantage of this approach can be the subsequent difficulty of delivering the final prosthesis at the fixture level. Trauma from this process can induce subsequent soft tissue recession in patients with a thin, scalloped periodontium. In the author's experience, these considerations become insignificant when an implant with an internal prosthetic connection is used since this greatly facilitates delivery of the custom abutment.

In summary, the use of custom abutments and provisional restorations at esthetic implant sites requires that the surgeon perform a surgical index procedure at the time of implant placement and subsequently deliver the prosthetic components at implant exposure. Although these techniques are very useful for enhancing esthetic outcomes through guided soft tissue healing, they require significant coordination with the restorative dentist and laboratory technician. There is also additional expense and chair time involved for the surgeon. Nevertheless, the enhanced esthetic result and the significant convenience realized by the patient warrant this approach in esthetic implant therapy (Figs 7-19 and 7-20).

Guided soft tissue healing via custom abutments and provisional restorations

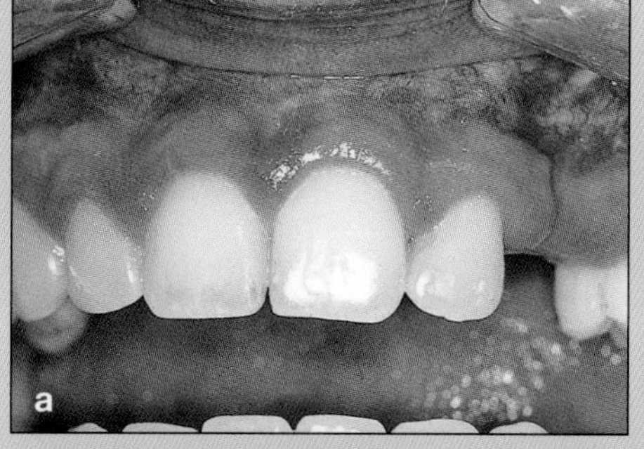

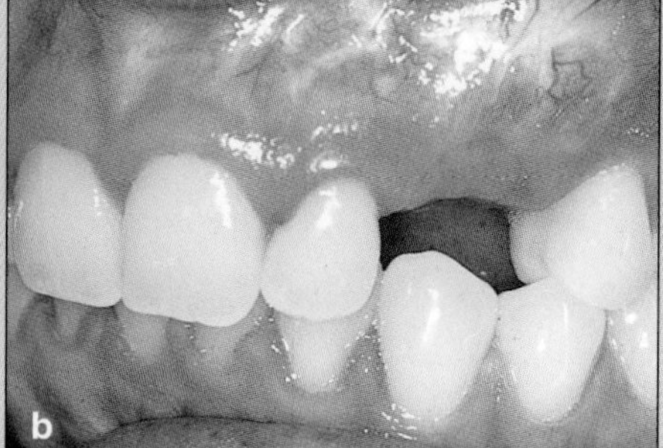

Fig 7-19a Preoperative view of maxillary canine implant site with large-volume combination hard and soft tissue esthetic ridge defects.

Fig 7-19b View of canine site 4 months following restoration of hard and soft tissue alveolar ridge contours.

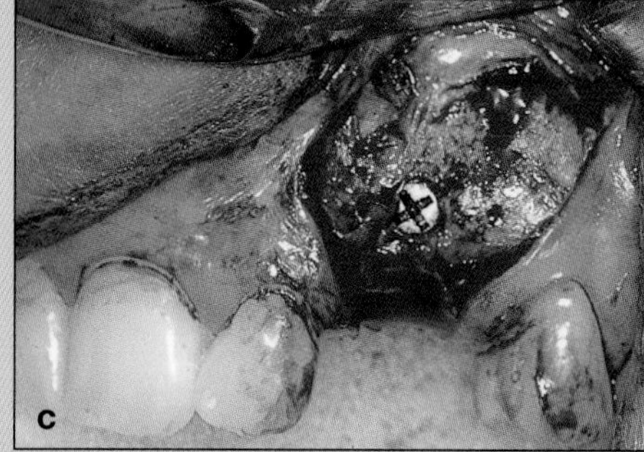

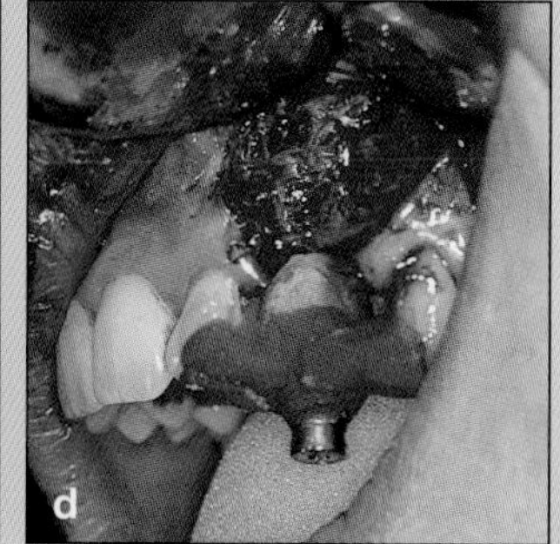

Fig 7-19c Access flap for implant placement preserves adjacent papilla and col tissues.

Fig 7-19d After placement of implant, a fixture-level impression coping is attached and the fixture position is registered relative to adjacent teeth.

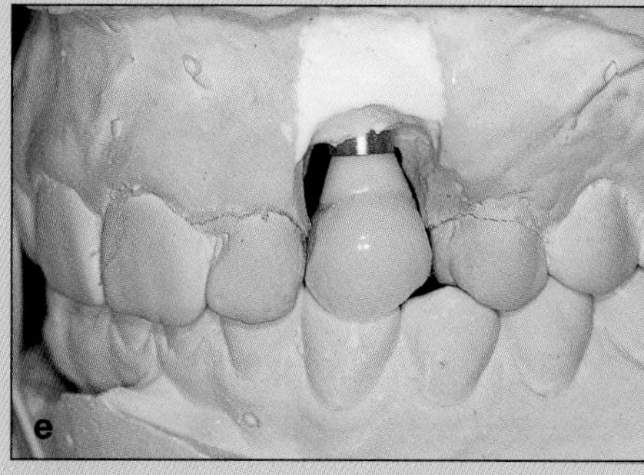

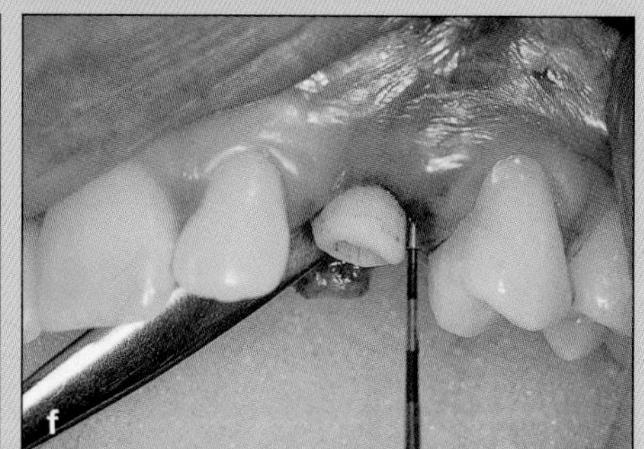

Fig 7-19e Implant analog cast fabricated by restorative dentist with customized ceramic abutment and provisional restoration.

Fig 7-19f Palatal peninsula flap used for abutment connection.

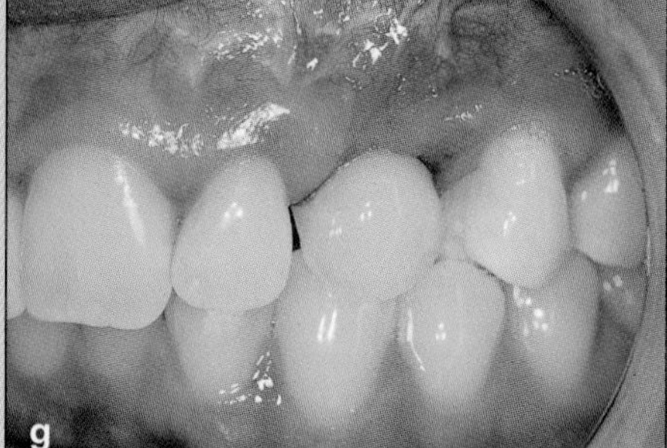

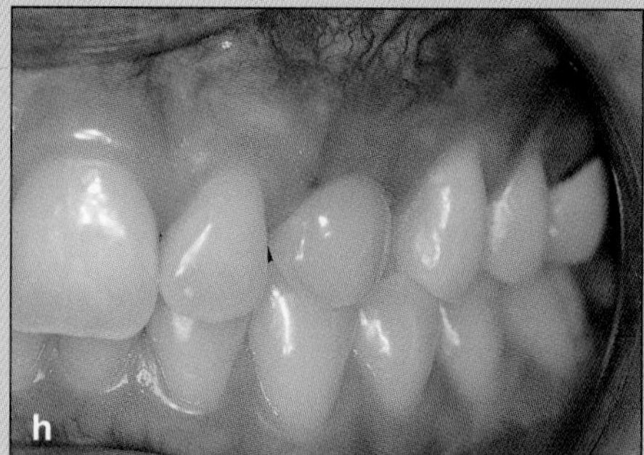

Figs 7-19g and 7-19h Guided tissue healing. The unesthetic soft tissue profile at the time of cementation of the provisional restoration improves dramatically during the 6-week provisional period. The contours of the provisional restoration have a tremendous influence on the final soft tissue architecture.

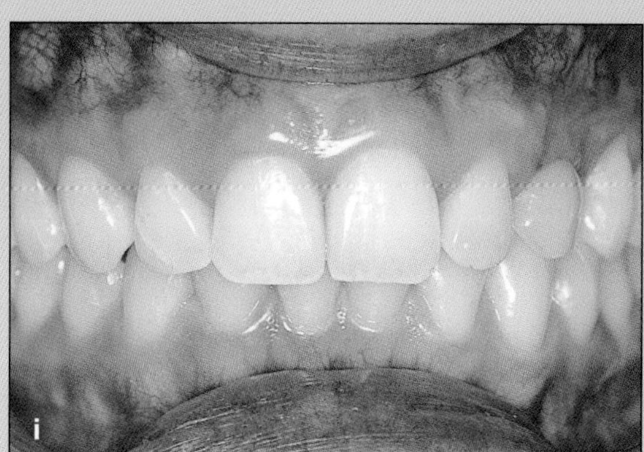

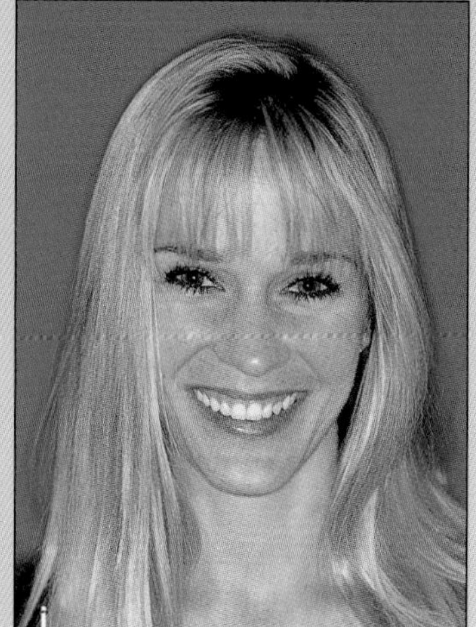

Figs 7-19i and 7-19j Final intraoral and facial views. The implant restoration is in harmony with the adjacent dentition, and the patient's smile is unencumbered. (Restoration by Dr Larry Grillo, Aventura, FL.)

Guided soft tissue healing via custom abutments and provisional restorations

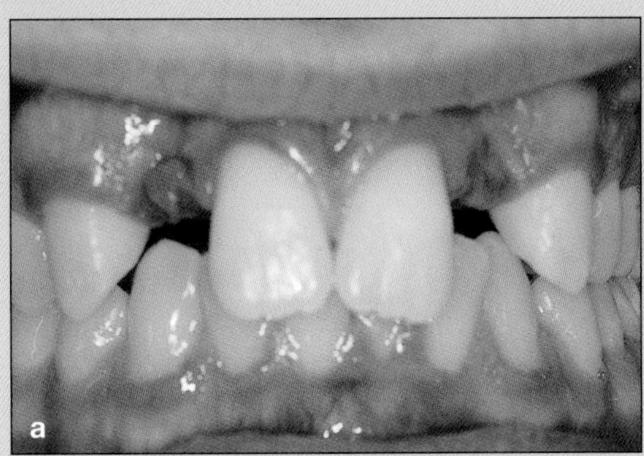

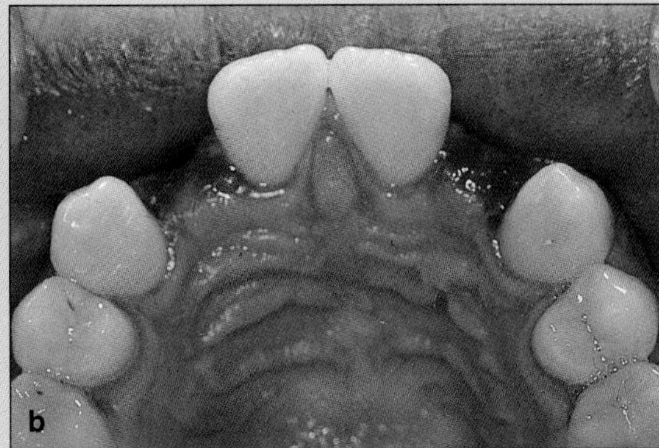

Figs 7-20a and 7-20b Preoperative view of congenitally missing lateral incisor implant sites with small-volume soft tissue esthetic ridge defects in a patient with a thin, scalloped periodontium previously restored with a fixed partial denture.

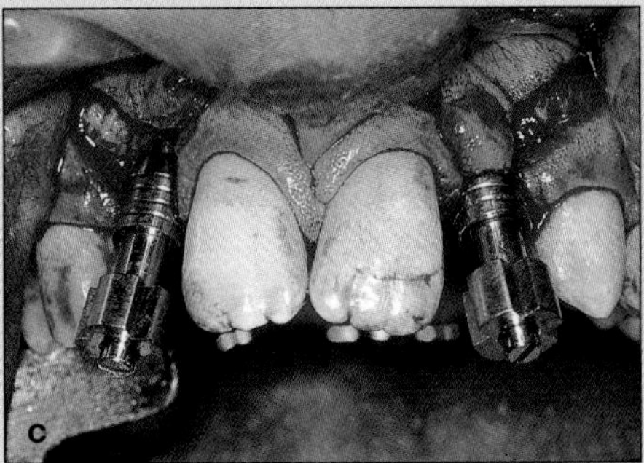

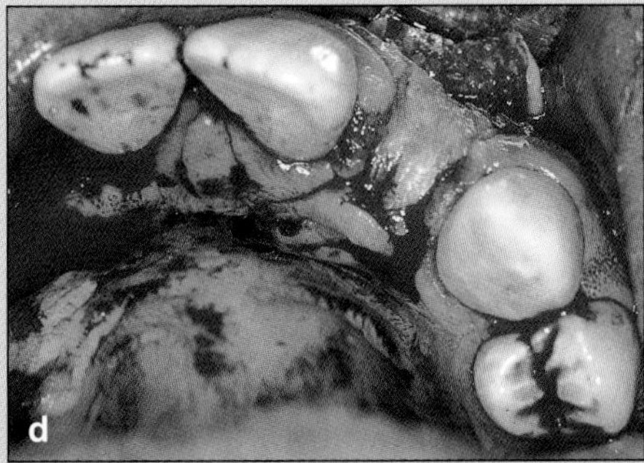

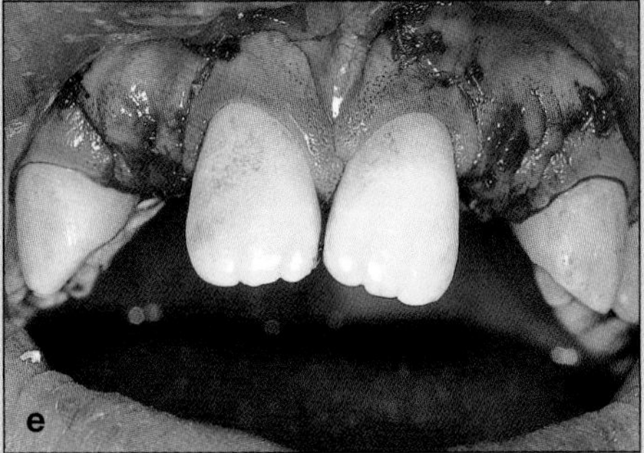

Figs 7-20c to 7-20e After implant placement (Nobel Biocare) via a papilla-sparing approach, surgical indexing is performed followed by subepithelial connective tissue grafting. The grafts are secured over the enlarged periosteal recipient sites provided by the buccal and palatal alveolar ridge. Tension-free primary closure is obtained.

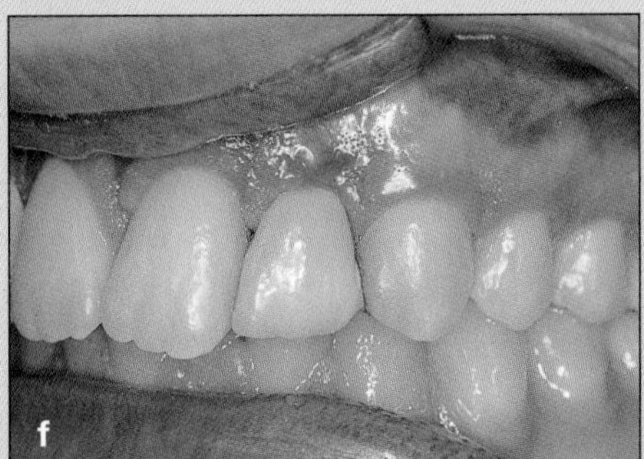

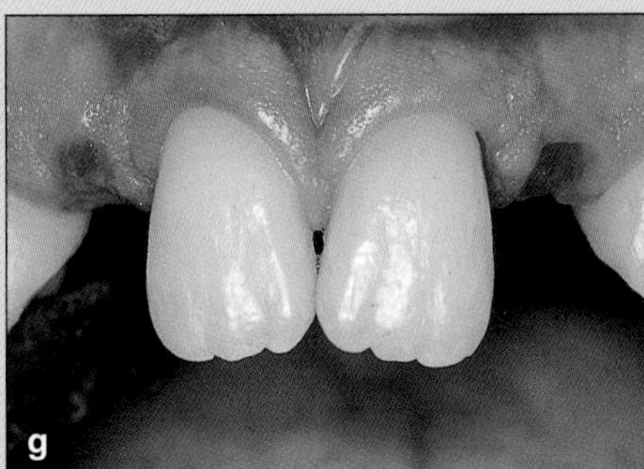

Fig 7-20f The patient's fixed partial denture has been modified to provide support to the adjacent papilla and then rebonded.

Fig 7-20g Three-month postoperative view demonstrates inconspicuous soft tissue reconstruction.

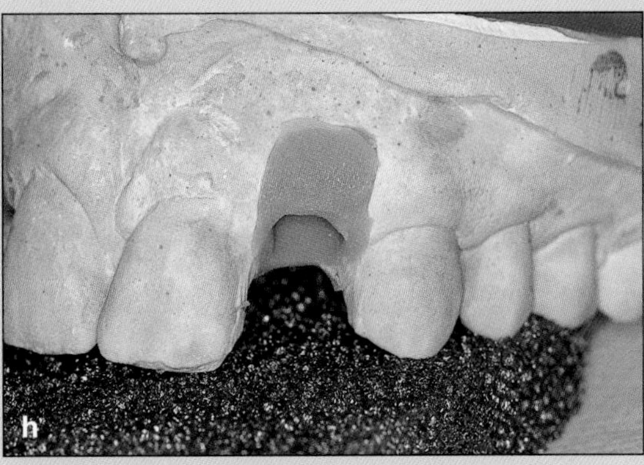

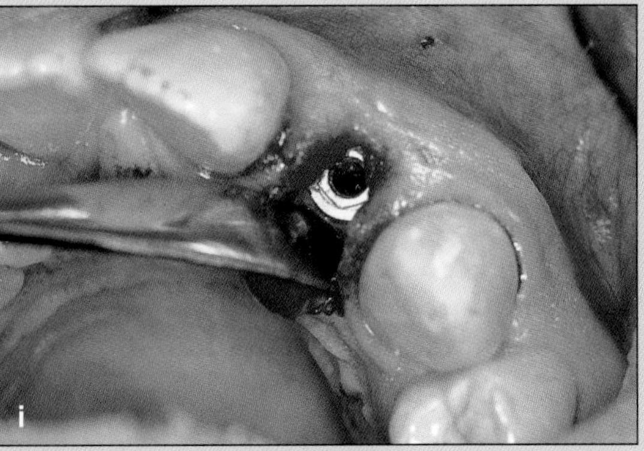

Figs 7-20h and 7-20i Prior to abutment connection, the restorative dentist removed the provisional fixed partial denture and took a second impression in order to add a soft tissue mask to the implant analog cast prior to fabrication of custom abutments and provisional restorations for delivery at second-stage surgery.

Figs 7-20j and 7-20k Palatal peninsula flaps used for delivery of custom abutments and provisional restorations at second-stage surgery. Note that the adjacent papillae appear to be deficient.

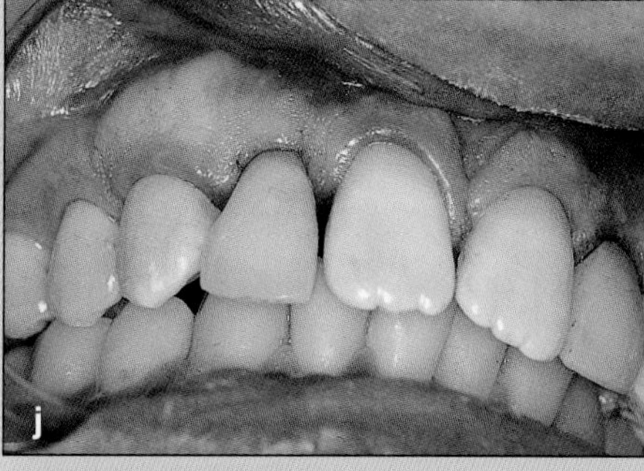

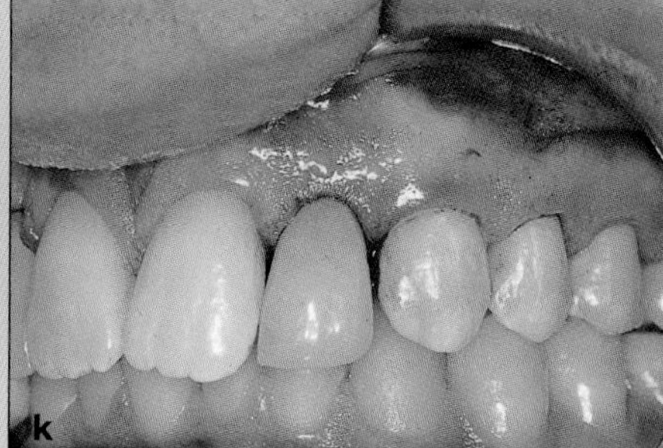

Figs 7-20l and 7-20m Two months following abutment connection, the adjacent papillae are completely recovered via the guided soft tissue healing initiated by the early introduction of properly contoured provisional restorations. A period of 2 to 3 months is allowed for the development of a stable suclus prior to final restoration.

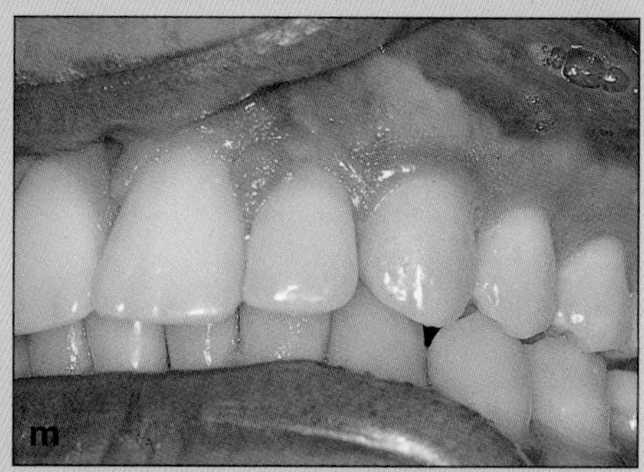

Figs 7-20n and 7-20o View of final restorations 2 weeks after delivery. Note that the contours of the final restoration duplicated those of the provisional restorations.

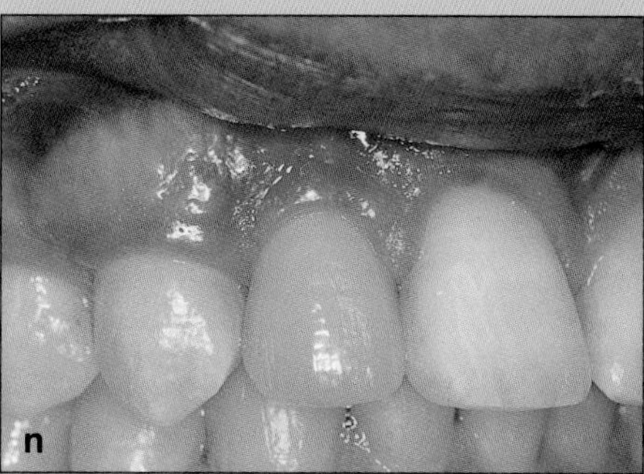

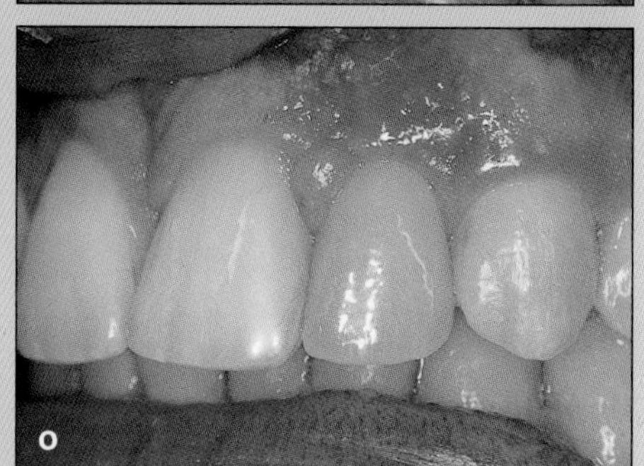

Figs 7-20p and 7-20q Radiographs taken 2 years following delivery of final restorations. Note the maintenance of interdental bone levels on the adjacent teeth.

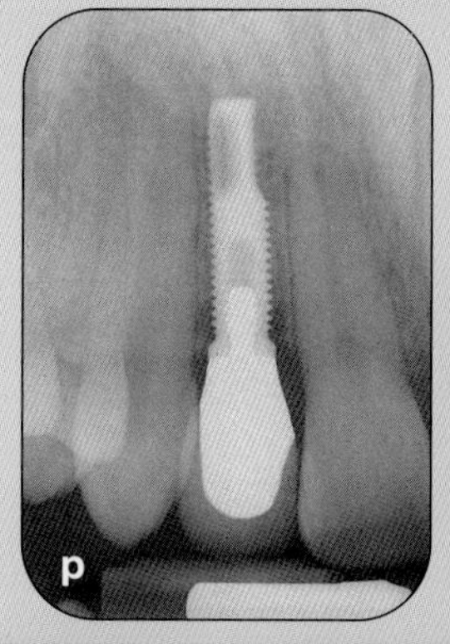

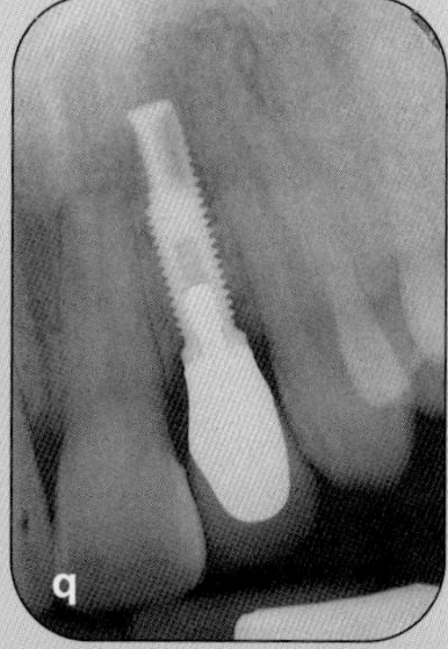

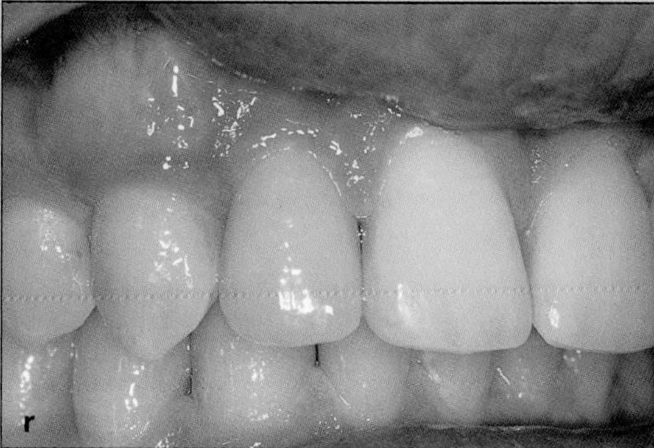

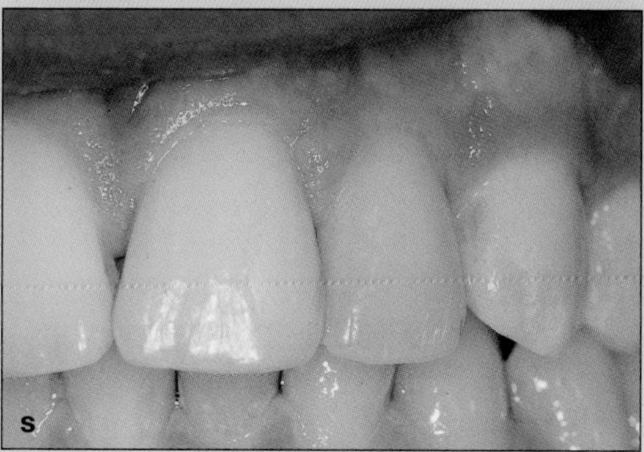

Figs 7-20r and 7-20s Two years after delivery of the final restorations, the implant restorations are inconspicuous and gingival esthetics are excellent. The soft tissue grafts have matured, and the overlying tissues have become keratinized and now blend with the adjacent tissues. (Restoration by Dr Cecil Abraham, Miami, FL.)

Guided soft tissue healing via custom tooth-form healing abutments

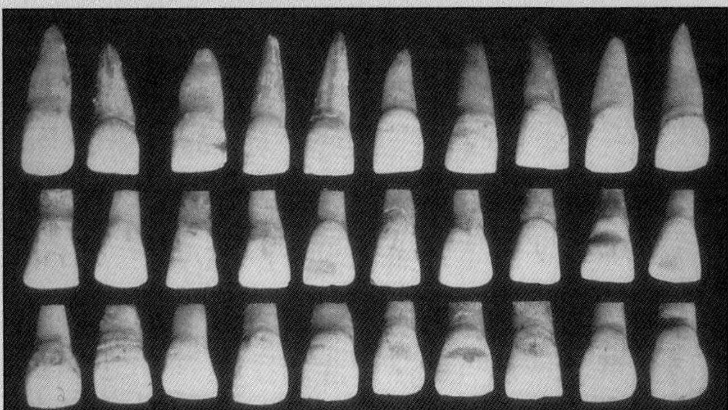

Fig 7-21a This photograph, taken from a 1916 textbook by George W. Clapp entitled *Prosthetic Articulation*, shows a group of central incisors of similar morphology. Nonetheless, there is tremendous individual variation in both their sizes and their shapes. For this reason, the use of custom "tooth-form" healing abutments upon implant emergence will improve esthetic results in certain cases.

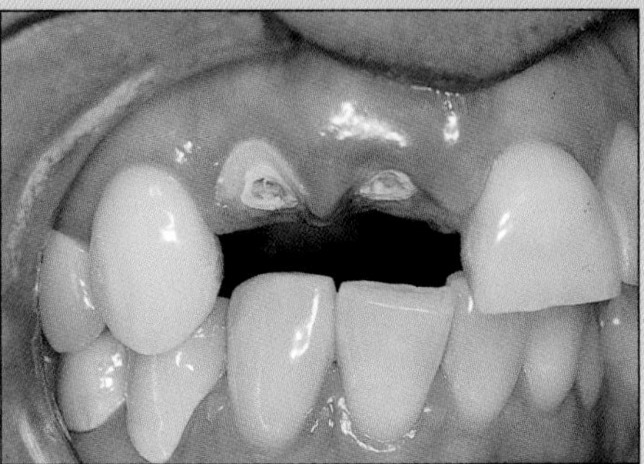

Fig 7-21b Customized Protec healing abutments (Friadent) that duplicated the cross-sectional anatomy of the cervical portions of the incisor teeth were delivered following tooth removal and immediate implant placement. The interdental papilla and surrounding soft tissues are supported and the scalloped soft tissue architecture has been preserved.

Custom tooth-form healing abutments

Another prosthetic technique used by the surgeon to initiate early guided soft tissue healing involves the use of custom "tooth-form" healing abutments. These anatomically shaped healing abutments closely approximate the cross-sectional anatomy of the lost tooth or the planned replacement at the gingival level. Since every anterior maxillary tooth is unique, prefabricated components are unlikely to yield an ideal result in terms of tissue support and guided soft tissue healing in every instance (Fig 7-21). Although prefabricated anatomically shaped healing abutments have proven useful for enhancing esthetic soft tissue contours in many cases, the use of custom tooth-form healing abutments will yield superior soft tissue results in certain instances. Custom tooth-form healing abutments can be fabricated in the laboratory from a surgical index, as described above, and subsequently delivered at implant exposure, or they can be fabricated on a working cast in preparation for nonsubmerged implant placement. This process involves laboratory modification of a prefabricated prosthetic component to approximate the cross-sectional anatomy of the proposed final restoration.

To start, a diagnostic waxup of the final restoration is performed and a surgical guide is fabricated. The laboratory technician alters the study cast, assumes ideal implant placement by the surgeon, and secures an implant analog in the altered cast according to the surgical guide. A modifiable stock prosthetic component is then secured to the analog, and a tooth-form healing abutment is customized for that site. The technician can use the contralateral tooth, when present, as a guide for accurate reproduction of contours. The surgeon then delivers the custom healing abutment immediately upon placement of the nonsubmerged implant. Minor chairside modifications are sometimes necessary.

Alternatively, the surgeon can modify a stock prosthetic component to create a custom tooth-form healing abutment for immediate use at the time of submerged implant exposure or nonsubmerged implant placement (Figs 7-22 to 7-24). When fabricated chairside, a prefabricated component is modified either by adding acrylic resin or by reducing, shaping, and polishing an oversized cylindrical stock component. While the goal is to closely approximate the cross-sectional form of the lost tooth or planned final restoration at the site, doing so can be very time consuming. A practical approach used by the author is to modify a stock component to match the mesiodistal width of the proposed replacement tooth and undercontour the facial aspect of the custom healing abutment. This provides support and guidance for the adjacent papillae while allowing excess soft tissues to collapse over the facial aspect, thereby preventing recession. The mesiodistal dimension of the contralateral tooth, if present, is measured with a Castro-Viejo caliper, and the dimensions are transferred to the modified healing abutment. The surgeon must have appropriate equipment

Chairside fabrication of a custom tooth-form healing abutment

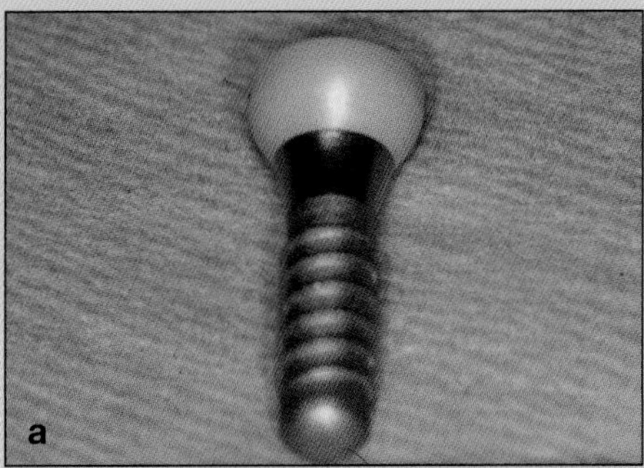

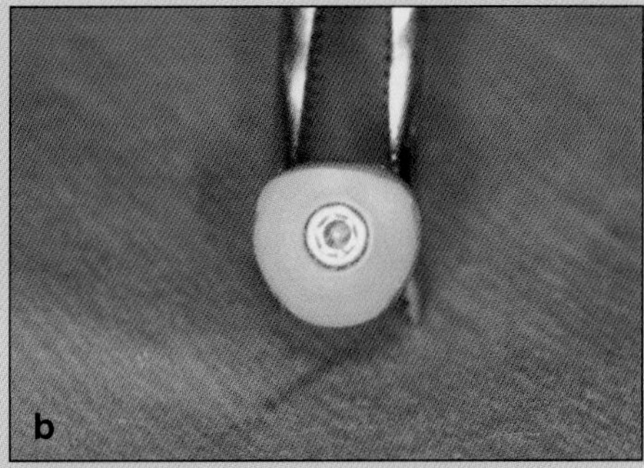

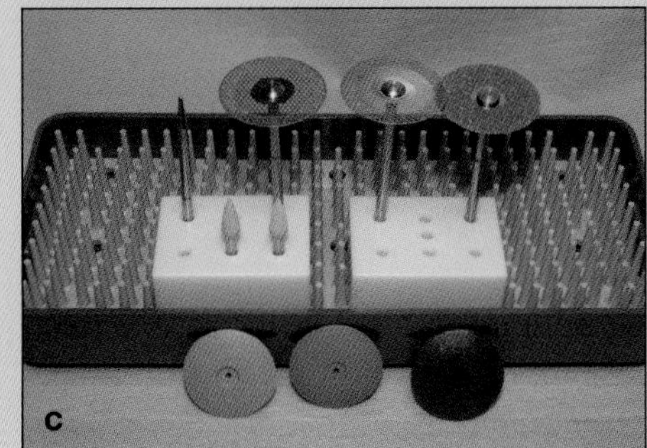

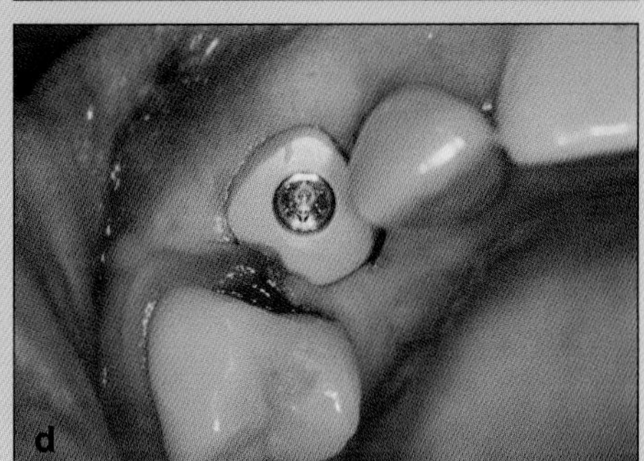

Fig 7-22a Customizable Peek healing abutment attached to an implant replica or analog for chairside customization.

Fig 7-22b Shaping the abutment to match the mesiodistal dimension of the lost tooth and incorporating a labial bevel to prevent recession of the buccal tissues is the most practical and time-efficient method to provide guided soft tissue healing and support to adjacent papillae or inter-implant tissues when multiple implants are placed in areas of esthetic concern.

Fig 7-22c Typical rotary instrumentation needed to shape and polish a custom tooth-form healing abutment upon implant emergence.

Fig 7-22d Customized Peek abutment provides immediate anatomic support for the tissues surrounding a nonsubmerged implant placed in the maxillary canine position. Note the support of the adjacent papillae and the reduced buccal contour and labial bevel, which prevent recession of the soft tissues in the area critical for esthetic emergence of the restoration.

Guided soft tissue healing via custom tooth-form healing abutments

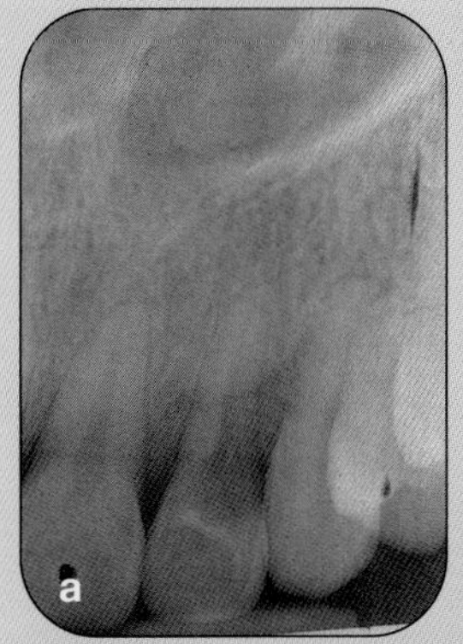

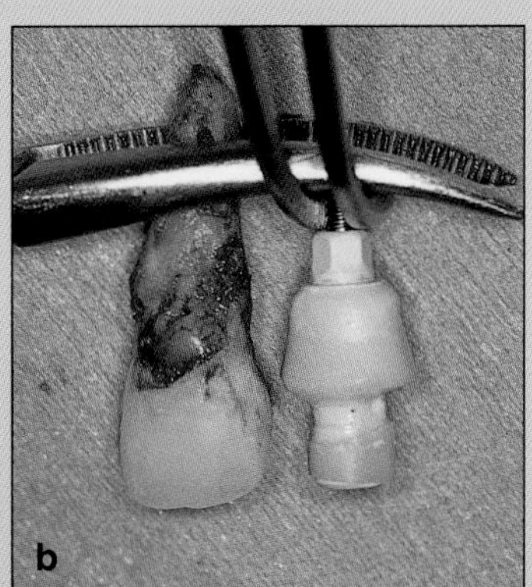

Fig 7-23a Preoperative radiograph of a lateral incisor that is failing secondary to resorption.

Fig 7-23b Following tooth removal, a customized Protec healing abutment (Friadent) was shaped and polished to duplicate the cervical contours of the extracted lateral incisor.

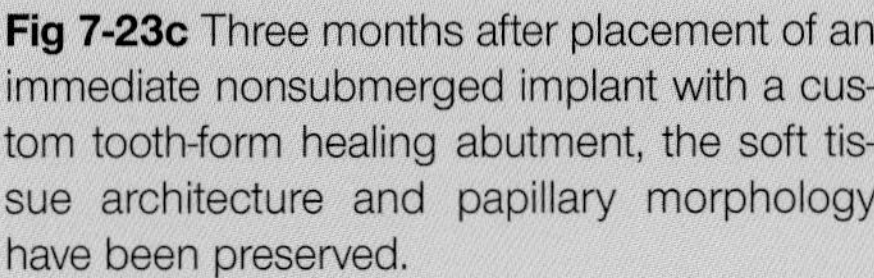

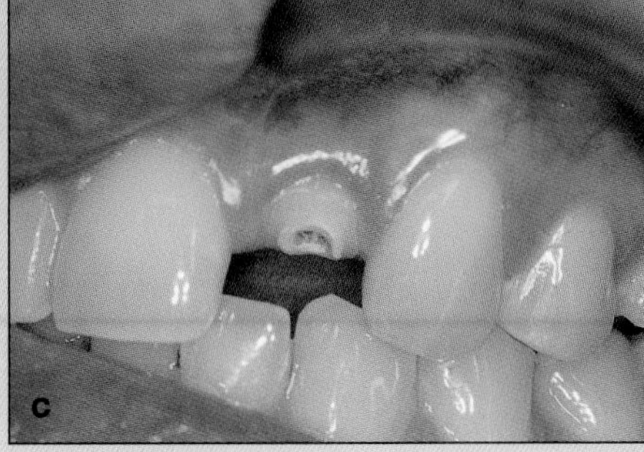

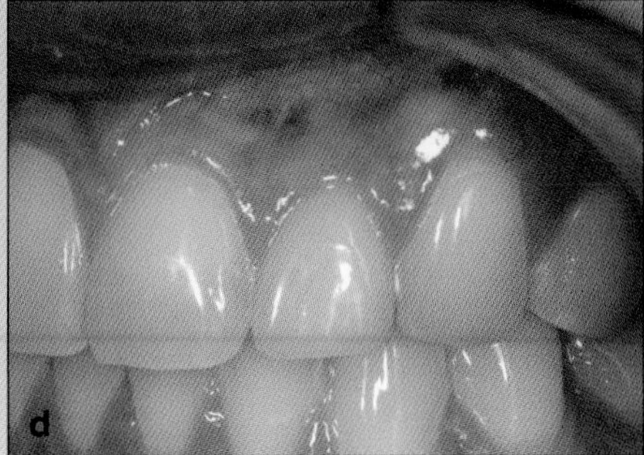

Fig 7-23c Three months after placement of an immediate nonsubmerged implant with a custom tooth-form healing abutment, the soft tissue architecture and papillary morphology have been preserved.

Fig 7-23d Final restoration 1 year after delivery. The implant restoration is inconspicuous, and natural gingival esthetics have been preserved. (Restoration by Dr Faustino Garcia, Coral Gables, FL.)

Guided soft tissue healing via custom tooth-form healing abutments

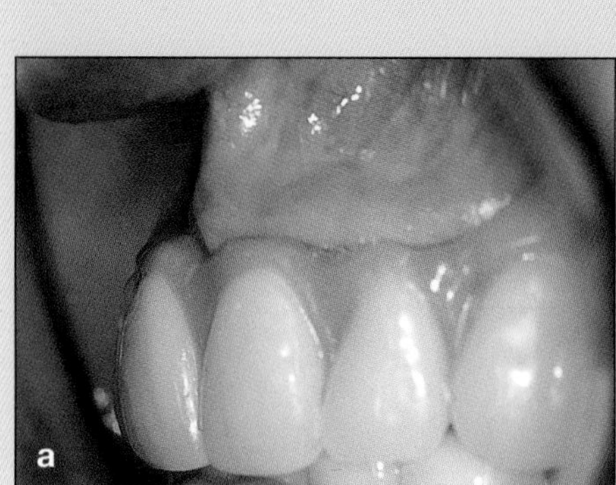
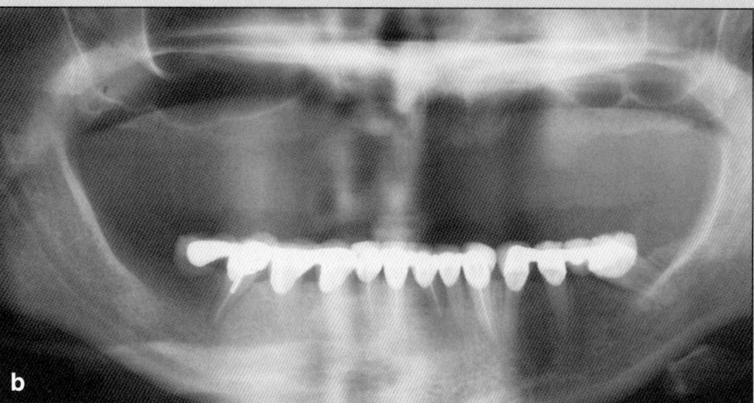

Figs 7-24a and 7-24b Preoperative views of atrophic maxilla with a maxillary denture that has functioned for more than 20 years against natural mandibular dentition. Note the advanced atrophy in the premaxillary region.

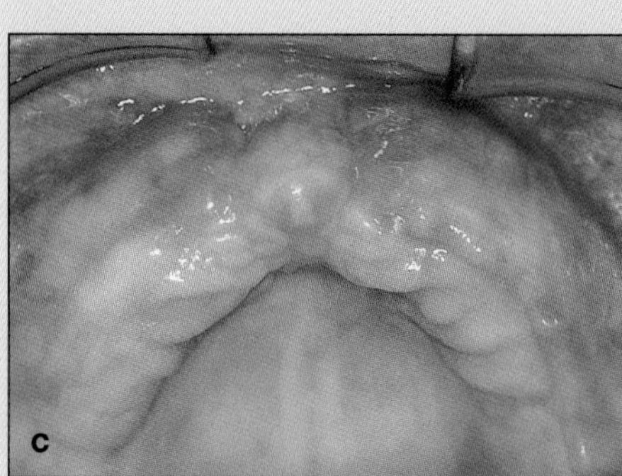
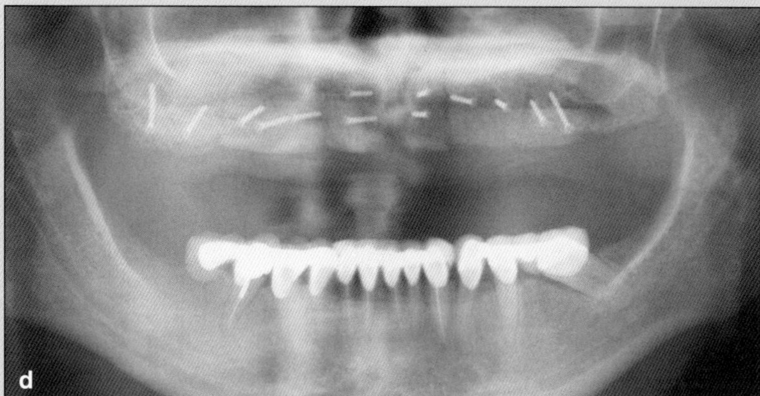

Figs 7-24c and 7-24d Bone graft reconstruction included bilateral sinus lift bone grafting with a mixture of autogenous cancellous bone and Bio-Oss and eight corticocancellous block grafts harvested from the ilium to reconstruct the thickness, volume, and arch form. Adequate alveolar ridge thickness and maintenance of the vestibular depth were achieved via a paramidline flap design as described in chapter 2. Excellent bone graft consolidation is visible on the 3-month postoperative panoramic radiograph.

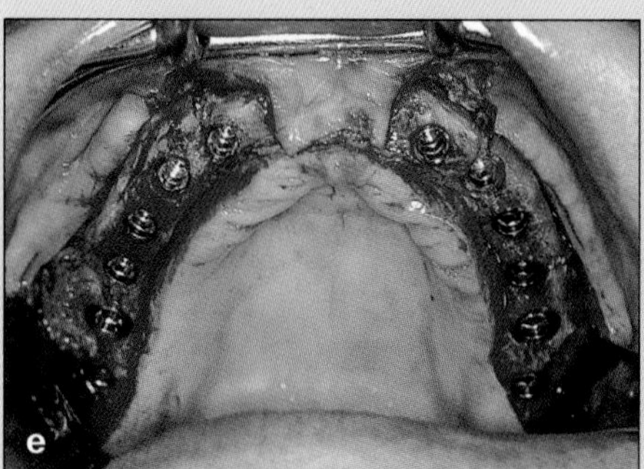
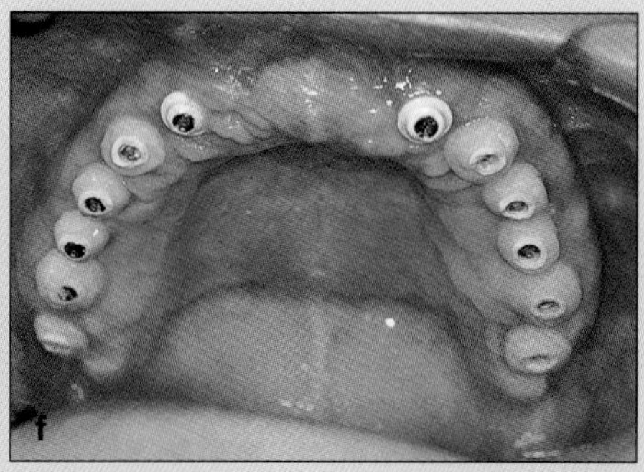

Fig 7-24e Four months after hard tissue site development, a paramidline approach was again used for access to remove the fixation screw and for placement of 12 diameter-appropriate implants (Frialit; Dentsply). A partial-thickness flap was elevated at the midline, and VIP-CT flaps were performed with coronal advancement of the cover flap. Custom Protec abutments were shaped, and afterward esthetic soft tissue closure was obtained.

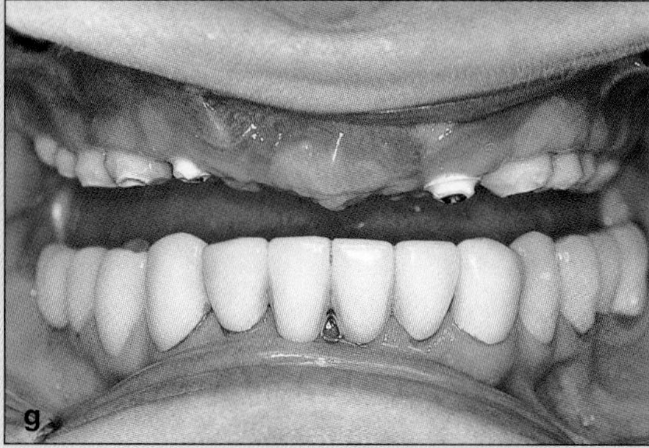

Figs 7-24f and 7-24g Four months after implant placement, guided soft tissue healing has resulted in positive soft tissue architecture. Also note the vertical soft tissue augmentation of the premaxillary area afforded by the VIP-CT flaps.

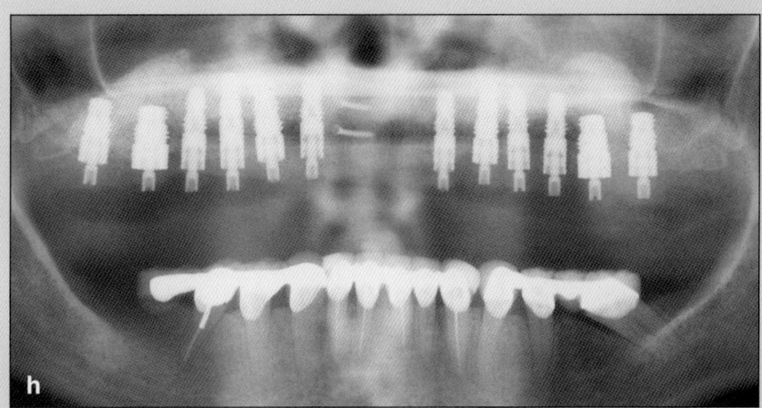

Fig 7-24h Panoramic radiograph taken 4 months after implant placement.

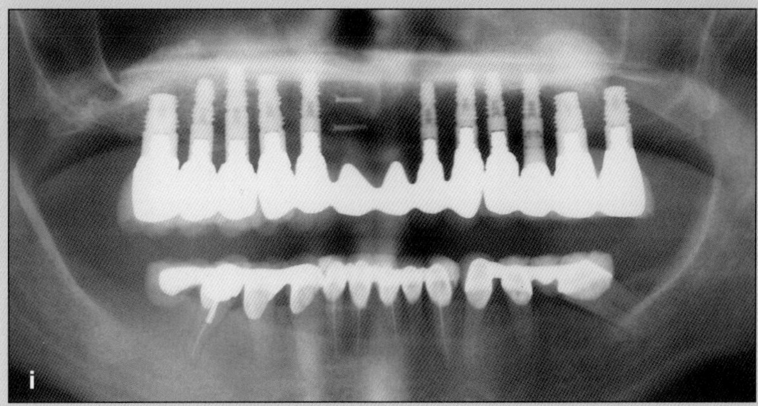

Fig 7-24i Panoramic radiograph taken 1 year after delivery of final restorations. Note that the implant-supported fixed partial denture with central incisor pontics was planned to provide the lip support desired by the patient.

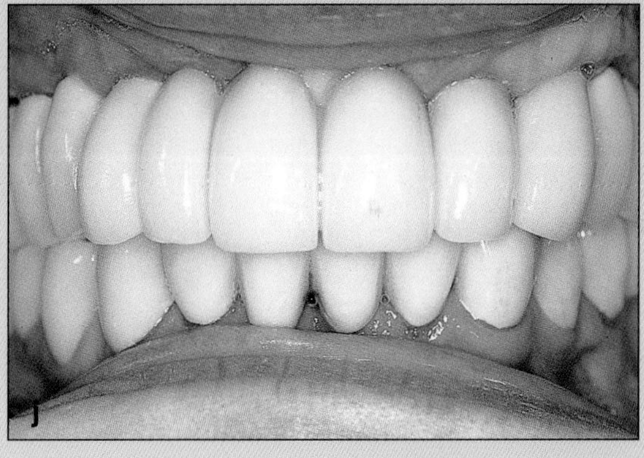

Fig 7-24j Final restoration 1 year after delivery demonstrates harmonious dental proportions. Early employment of guided soft tissue healing via custom tooth-form healing abutments, along with use of VIP-CT flaps at the central incisor pontic sites, resulted in a stable peri-implant soft tissue environment with adequate soft tissue volume for an esthetic restoration in this severely resorbed maxillary case. (Restoration by Dr Beatriz Fraga-Davidson, Miami, FL.)

to shape and polish the custom tooth-form healing abutment prior to its delivery. In addition, the process is facilitated when the surgeon attaches the modifiable abutment to an implant analog during the chairside fabrication process (see Fig 7-22a). In the author's experience, this chairside approach is easily accomplished and yields excellent results but requires additional chair time when compared with previously described laboratory techniques.

In summary, the use of custom tooth-form healing abutments is a practical approach for early initiation of prosthetic-guided soft tissue healing. This approach requires less time and expense than the use of custom abutments and provisional restorations, as described above. The author finds the use of custom tooth-form healing abutments to be especially useful when one-piece nonsubmerged implants are used. In these instances, the soft tissues are allowed adequate time for maturation, and any soft tissue recession that occurs is easily detected and corrected prior to the prosthetic phase. The restorative dentist can easily remove and replace the custom tooth-form abutment during impression procedures, thus facilitating the prosthetic management of the patient. As previously noted, provisional restorations must be designed to avoid unwanted loading of custom tooth-form healing abutments.

Guided soft tissue healing via anatomic abutments

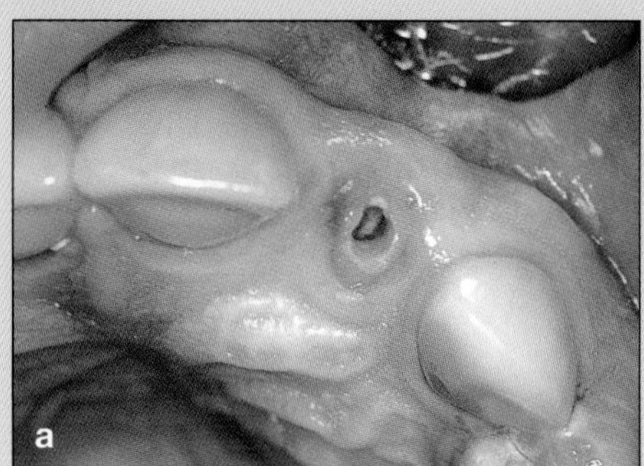
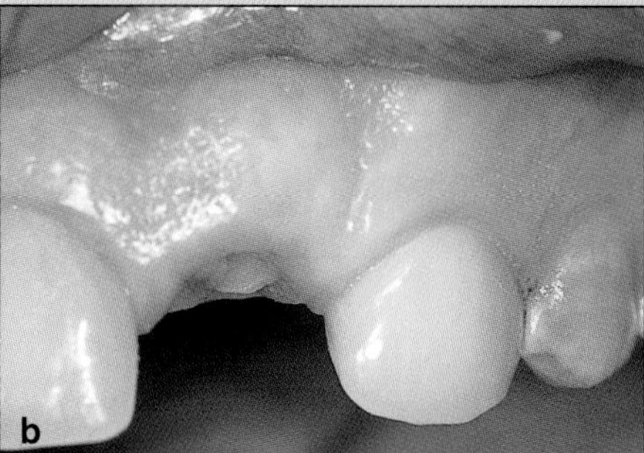

Figs 7-25a and 7-25b Preoperative views of fractured lateral incisor.

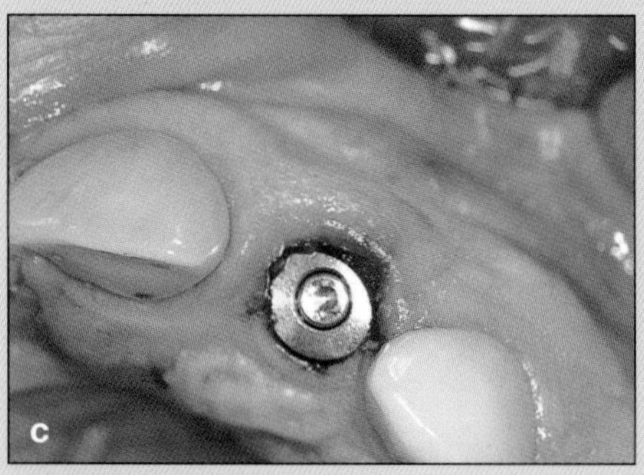
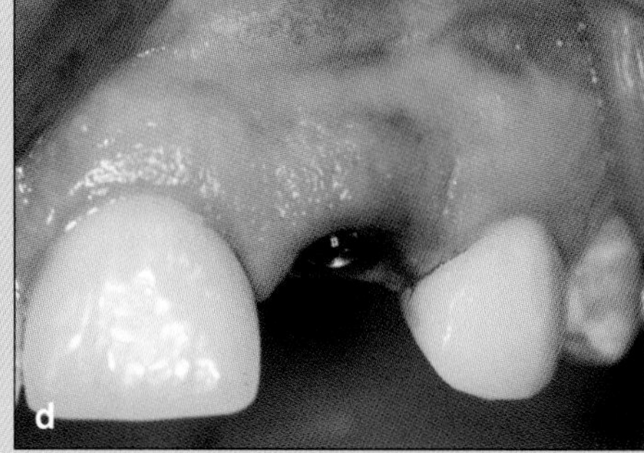

Figs 7-25c and 7-25d After tooth removal, a nonsubmerged implant was placed with the Bio-Col technique. A prefabricated machined titanium anatomic abutment with a labial bevel (Straumann USA) was used to support the adjacent papillae and prevent recession of the buccal tissues. Note the maintenance of scalloped soft tissue architecture afforded by guided tissue healing around the anatomic abutment.

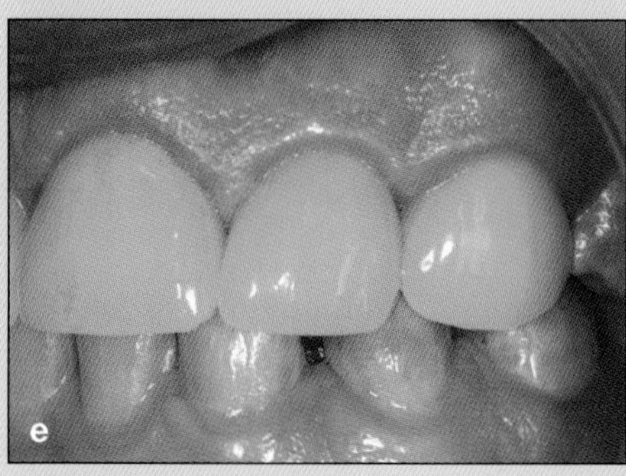
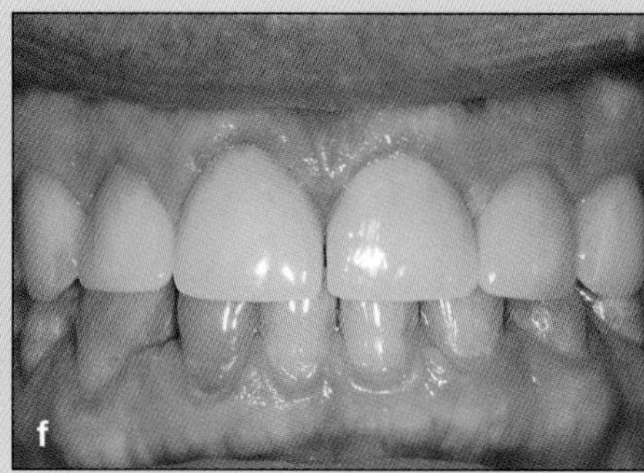

Figs 7-25e and 7-25f Final restoration 6 months after delivery demonstrates a natural appearance in harmony with the adjacent dentition. Papillae have been properly supported and buccal soft tissue recession was prevented by the use of a size-appropriate anatomic healing abutment. (Restoration by Dr Robert Sterling, Miami, FL.)

Anatomic healing abutments

Although custom tooth-form healing abutments are beneficial when a tooth with an unusual size or shape is being replaced in an area of esthetic concern, prefabricated anatomic healing abutments provide similar benefits for a large number of cases. The most important consideration in their use in an esthetic area is to avoid introducing excessive labial contouring, which can result in soft tissue recession. Furthermore, when an anatomic abutment is too small to adequately support adjacent papillae or inter-implant tissues, the loss of scalloped soft tissue architecture may not be recoverable. Similarly, when an anatomic abutment is too large, it can embarrass the circulation to the adjacent papillae or inter-implant soft tissues, leading to loss of tissue volume, which can be irreversible. Instead, an anatomic healing abutment that closely approximates the mesiodistal dimension of the tooth that is being replaced and that incorporates a labial bevel, thus preventing recession of the buccal soft tissues, is ideal (Fig 7-25).

Surgical Considerations for Enhancing Outcomes in Esthetic Implant Therapy

Cosmetic laser soft tissue resurfacing and sculpting

When multiple site-development procedures are necessary to prepare a site for esthetic implant replacement, significant soft tissue scarring or surface irregularities can result. This is especially evident in patients who have a thick, flat periodontium, as described in chapter 2. In addition, the natural scalloped soft tissue architecture may be lost or altered. Although such situations are traditionally managed with rotary instrumentation, laser-assisted soft tissue sculpting and resurfacing represents an innovative approach that offers the advantage of finely controlled tissue sculpting and the ability for uniform resurfacing of an area at a defined tissue depth, thus providing the surgeon with a tool for restoring scalloped soft tissue architecture and improving incision line esthetics. While many laser options exist, the author uses a CO_2 laser with a ceramic tip set at 2 watts of power in superpulse mode (Fig 7-26a). The procedure requires a minimal amount of instrumentation and may be performed quickly (Fig 7-26b). Patients experience little discomfort and generally are immediately able to resume normal diet and activities.

When sculpting procedures are necessary, they should be delayed until after appropriate soft tissue support has been achieved via a properly contoured provisional restoration or a custom tooth-form healing abutment, as previously discussed. The laser is used in a brush-stroke fashion to sculpt the tissues until the desired architecture is re-established. Sculpting and resurfacing of peri-implant soft tissues are usually performed after an appropriate time has been allotted for soft tissue maturation (2 to 3 months following the final soft tissue procedure). When resurfacing scarred and uneven incision lines, the best results are obtained when the tip of the laser handpiece is kept in focus and repeatedly passed across the incision in a perpendicular fashion. Subsequently, the laser is passed parallel to the incision in the peri-incisional area, avoiding a 1- to 2-mm area surrounding the incision line. This is repeated until the incision line area becomes flat. Next, laser resurfacing is performed over adjacent normal gingival and mucosal tissues to obtain a blending effect between the surgical site and the adjacent area. This greatly contributes to an inconspicuous appearance at the implant site. After each pass with the laser, a cotton swab or small gauze sponge moistened in saline is used to remove the char layer created by the laser. This prevents overheating and damaging of the soft tissues in the area and allows the surgeon to visually assess the depth of tissue removal following each pass of the laser.The surgeon must be careful to avoid removing too much tissue at one time. In most instances, the author makes two thorough passes over the entire area after initially completing the revision of displeasing incision lines. The area is re-evaluated after several months for additional laser surgery. The surgeon should inform patients that in some cases the red discoloration that results from the laser surgery might persist in the area for several months following the procedure and reassure them that the tissue will eventually regain a healthy and esthetically pleasing appearance (Figs 7-26c to 7-26l).

Creating harmony with cosmetic periodontal surgery

Despite the high degree of success obtained with site-development techniques used to restore deficient hard and soft tissue anatomy at esthetic implant sites, there are instances when cosmetic periodontal surgery is indicated to harmonize the implant restorations with the surrounding natural dentition. When indicated, cosmetic periodontal surgery techniques can be used in implant therapy to correct uneven gingival margins between implant restorations and the adjacent natural dentition, thus contributing to establishment of a pleasing gingival appearance and harmonious dental proportions. Esthetic crown lengthening and root-/abutment-coverage procedures are commonly used for this purpose. As discussed in chapter 2, to take advantage of the potential benefits of cosmetic periodontal surgery, the implant surgeon must have a good understanding of smile esthetics and must be able to visualize the final esthetic result desired. Patients also must be educated about any particular limitations associated with their case and the possibilities of overcoming these limitations by employing adjunctive procedures such as esthetic crown-lengthening, root-coverage, and cosmetic dental procedures. As a general rule, sequencing of cosmetic surgical procedures is most predictable when the soft tissues around the emerging implants have reached maturity. Nevertheless, there are many instances where the experienced surgeon may proceed with cosmetic periodontal procedures prior to final emergence of implant restorations. The following cases (Figs 7-27 to 7-29) demonstrate the application and sequencing of cosmetic periodontal surgery to create harmony between the implant restorations and the adjacent dentition.

Enhancing outcomes in esthetic implant therapy: Cosmetic laser soft tissue sculpting and resurfacing

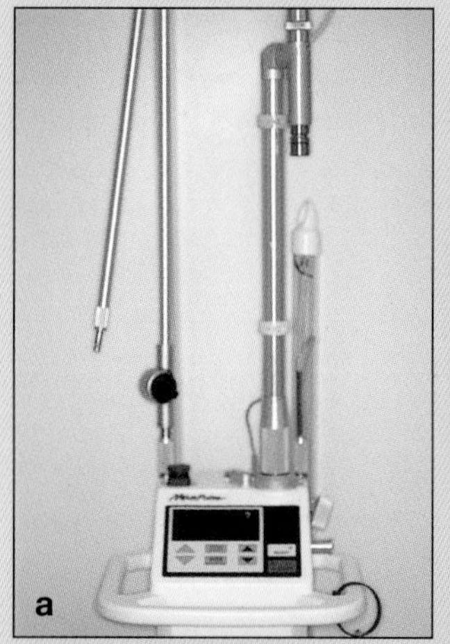

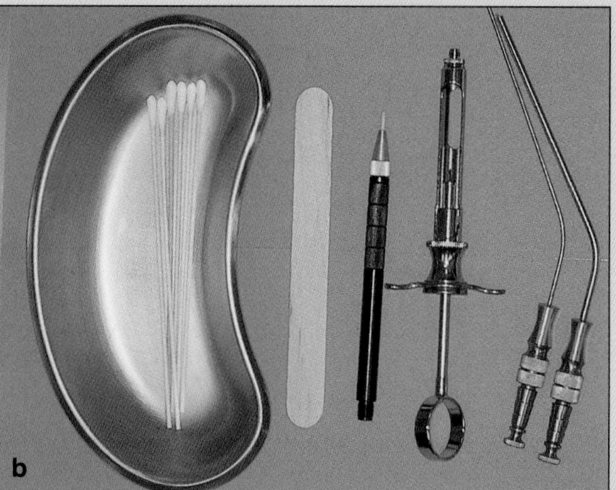

Fig 7-26a CO_2 laser used for sculpting soft tissues following soft tissue augmentation to recreate natural scalloped soft tissue architecture and resurfacing to improve cosmesis of scarred incision lines and create a uniform surface that blends with the adjacent soft tissues.

Fig 7-26b Instrumentation for laser procedure.

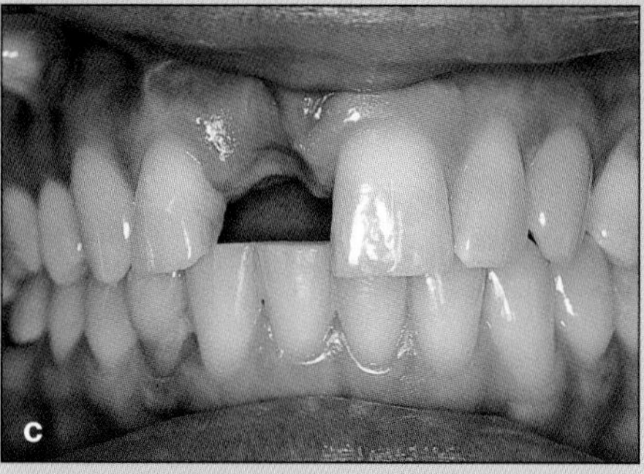

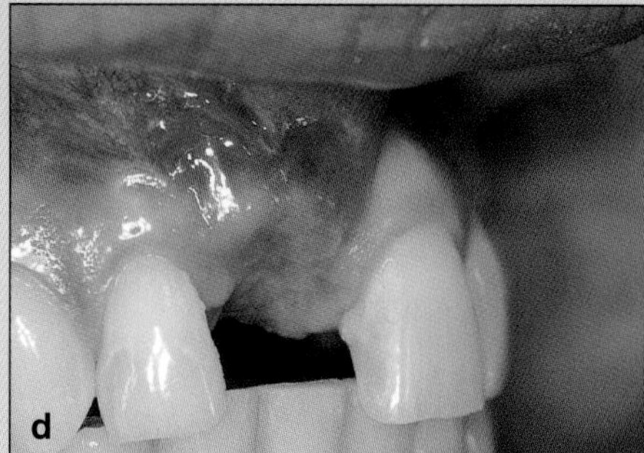

Fig 7-26c Central incisor site with large-volume combination hard and soft tissue ridge defect.

Fig 7-26d Four months following simultaneous hard and soft tissue site development with block bone grafting and a VIP-CT flap, moderate soft tissue scarring is visible. Nonsubmerged implant placement is planned.

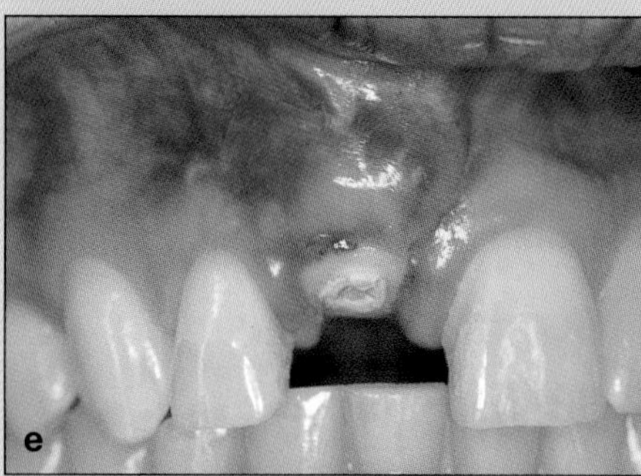

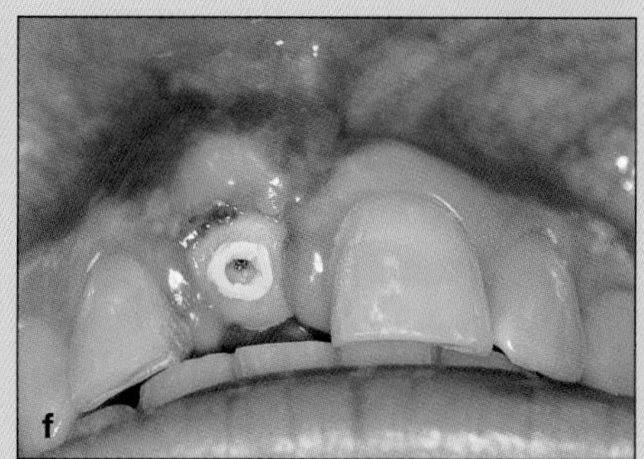

Figs 7-26e and 7-26f Four months after nonsubmerged implant placement, soft tissue scarring has been exacerbated. Laser soft tissue sculpting was performed with multiple passes made at 2 watts in superpulse mode with a ceramic tip to debulk the excess soft tissues provided by the VIP-CT flap and to improve incision line cosmesis prior to provisionalization.

Fig 7-26g Six weeks after the laser procedure, the provisional restoration was delivered and soft tissues were re-evaluated for a second laser procedure. Although the tissue contours and appearance were greatly improved, laser soft tissue resurfacing was indicated to create a blending effect between the soft tissues at the implant site and the adjacent soft tissues.

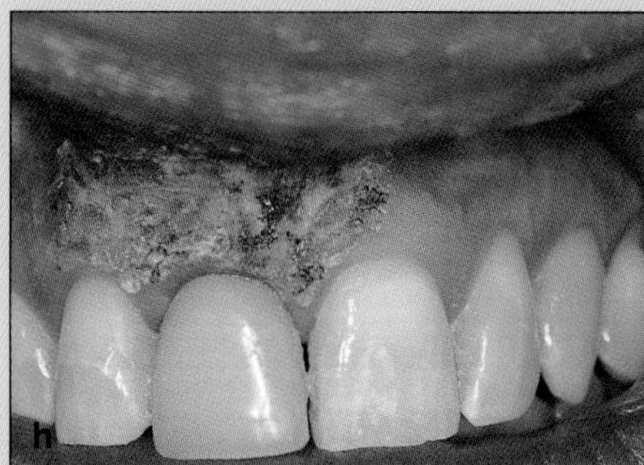

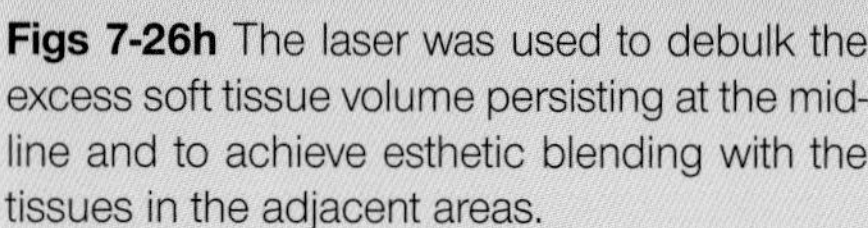

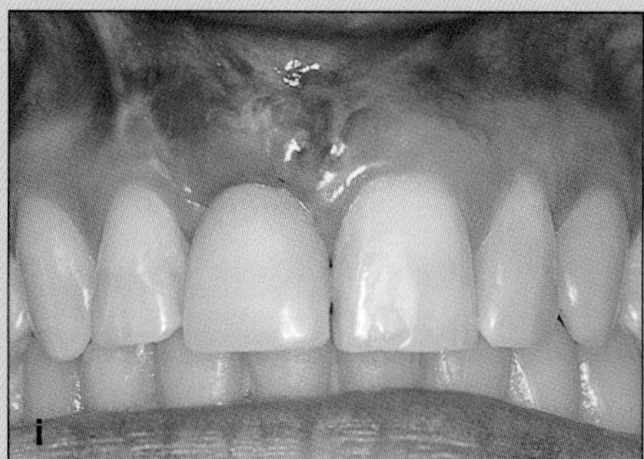

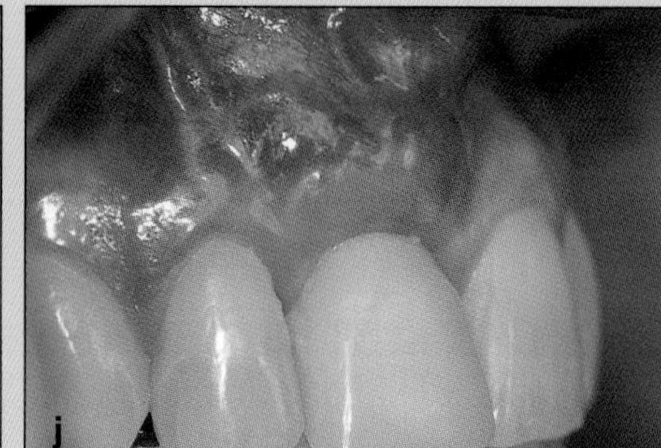

Figs 7-26h The laser was used to debulk the excess soft tissue volume persisting at the midline and to achieve esthetic blending with the tissues in the adjacent areas.

Figs 7-26i and 7-26j The second laser soft tissue procedure successfully removed the surface irregularities and achieved blending of the soft tissues with the adjacent areas. The red discoloration of the treated area usually persists for several months.

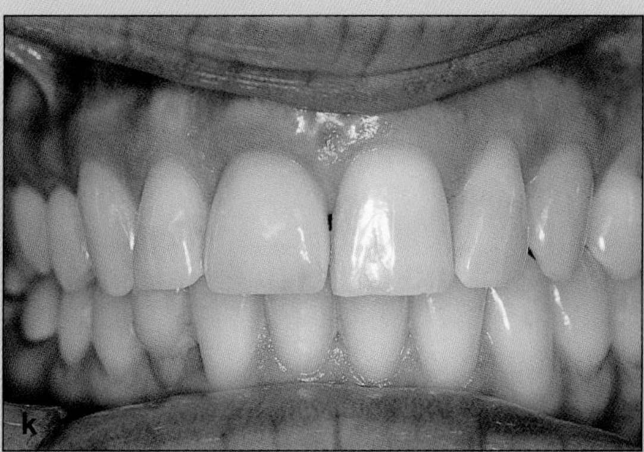
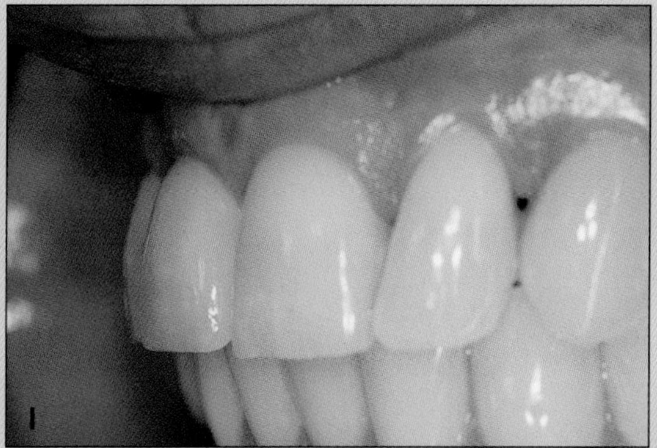

Figs 7-26k and 7-26l One year after delivery of the final restoration, the implant restoration and soft tissues at the site are inconspicuous. The red discoloration of the gingival tissues that can persist following soft tissue grafting and laser procedures has faded. (Restoration by Dr Iris Cruz, Miami, FL.)

Enhancing outcomes in esthetic implant therapy: Creating harmony with cosmetic periodontal surgery

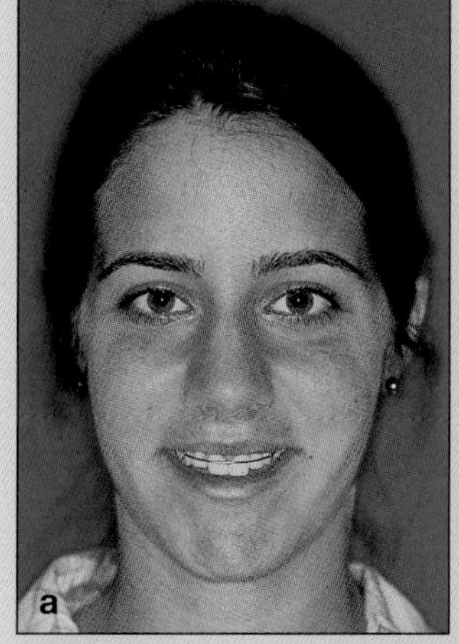
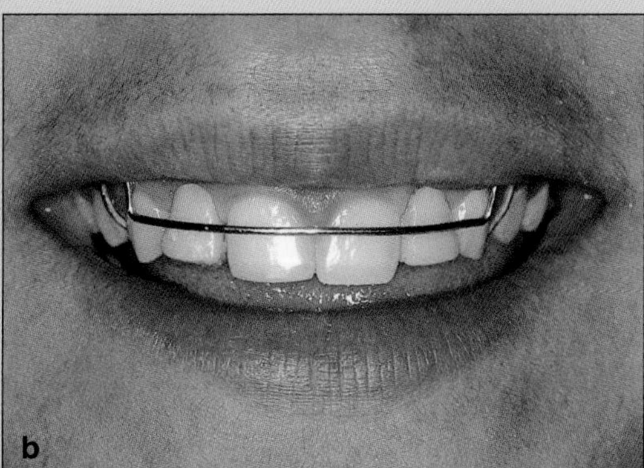
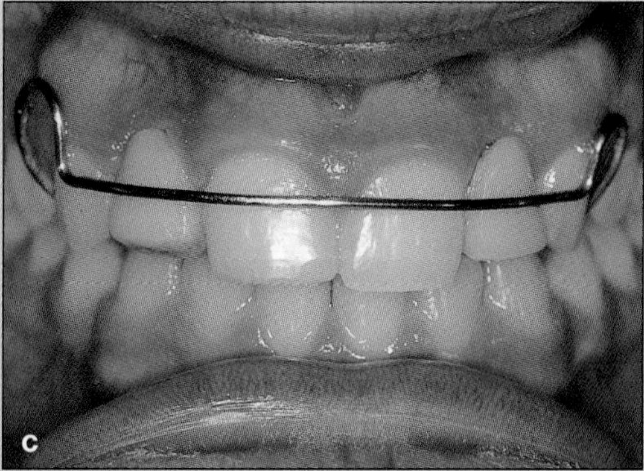

Figs 7-27a to 7-27c Pretreatment facial, animated smile, and intraoral views of patient with congenitally missing lateral incisor teeth following completion of orthodontic therapy. The incisal plane morphology, gingival pattern, intrinsic proportions of visible maxillary dentition, and asymmetry of central incisors all detract from smile esthetics.

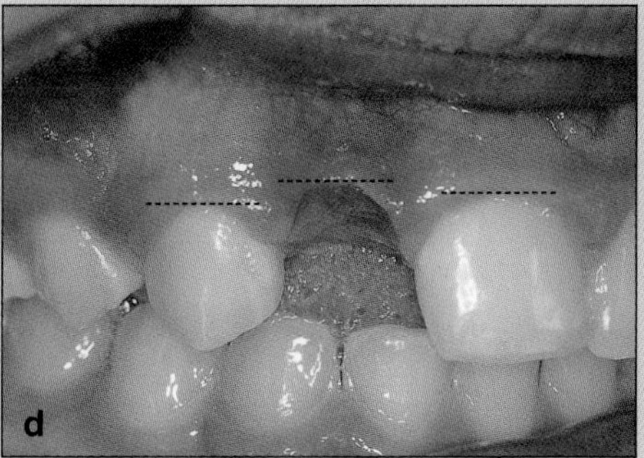
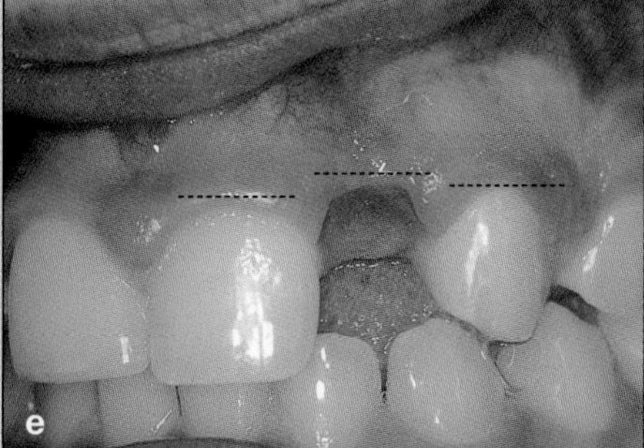
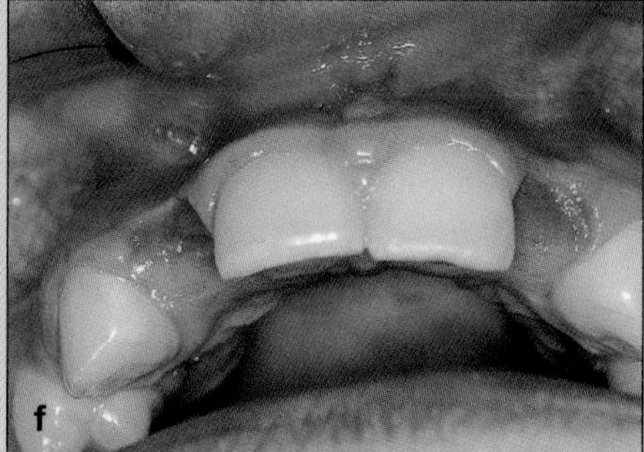

Figs 7-27d to 7-27f Frontal and occlusal views of implant sites with small-volume soft tissue esthetic ridge defects. Note lack of full clinical crown exposure of adjacent natural dentition and unesthetic gingival pattern *(dotted lines)*. Soft tissue grafting at implant sites and esthetic crown lengthening are indicated to create harmony between implant restorations and adjacent natural dentition.

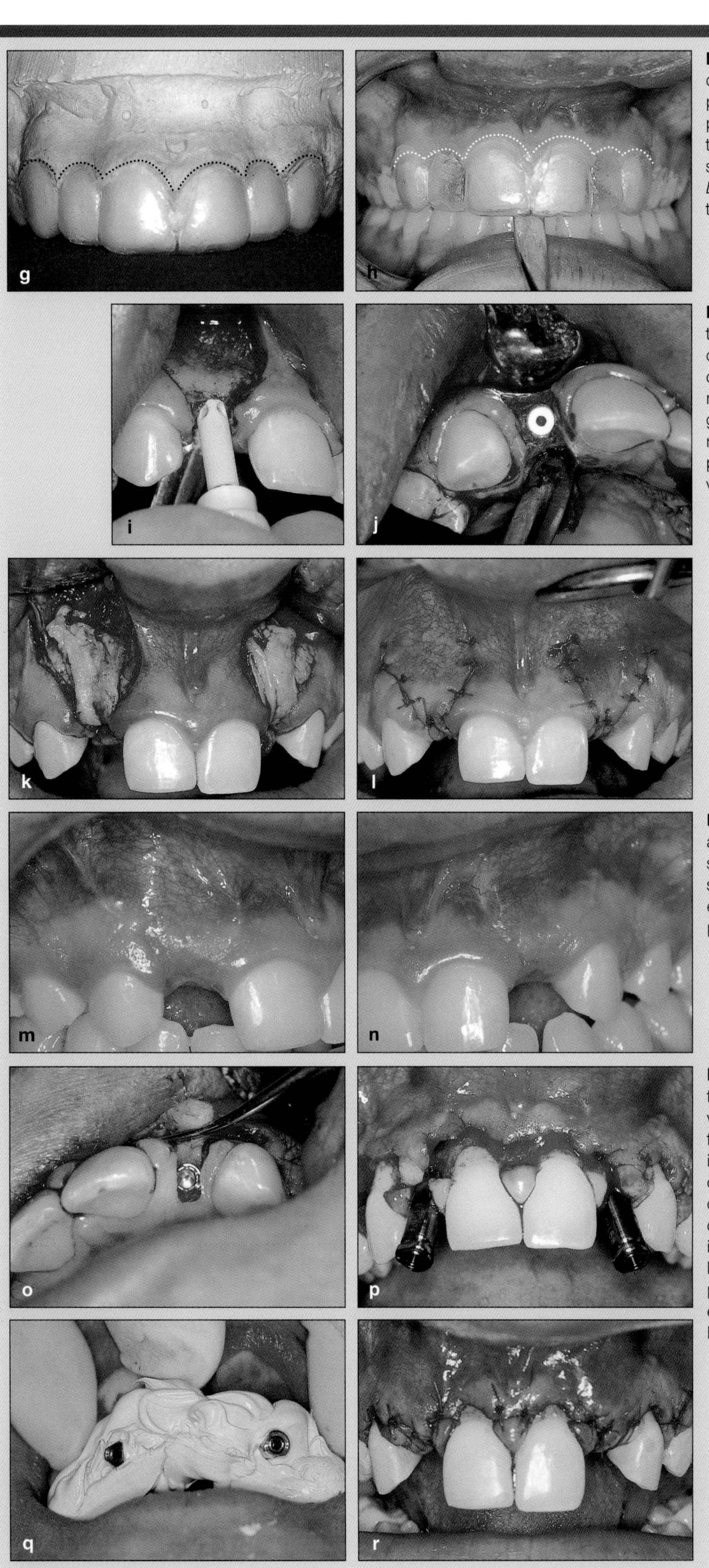

Figs 7-27g and 7-27h A diagnostic waxup of desired final result with harmonious dental proportions and esthetic gingival pattern was performed by the restorative dentist and used to create a template for subsequent soft tissue grafting and esthetic crown lengthening. *Dotted lines* indicate correction needed to establish an esthetic gingival appearance.

Figs 7-27i to 7-27l Full-thickness–partial-thickness curvilinear-beveled flap provides access for placement of small-diameter Spline cylinder implants (Centerpulse Dental) with simultaneous subeptithelial connective tissue grafting. The grafts were secured to the periosteal recipient sites on the buccal and palatal alveolar ridge. Tension-free coronal advancement was obtained.

Figs 7-27m and 7-27n Two-month postoperative view demonstrates inconspicuous incision line cosmesis and successful reconstruction of the small-volume soft tissue esthetic ridge defects simultaneous with implant placement.

Figs 7-27o to 7-27r Modified papilla-sparing flap design for esthetic crown lengthening with buccal peninsula flaps provided access for simultaneous surgical indexing of cylinder implants. Knowledge of peri-implant and periodontal soft tissue anatomy allows for modification of standard approaches when unusual case scenarios present. In this case, surgical indexing was delayed until after initial stabilization of the cylinder implant and was planned to be performed synchronous with esthetic crown lengthening, which required hard and soft tissue resection.

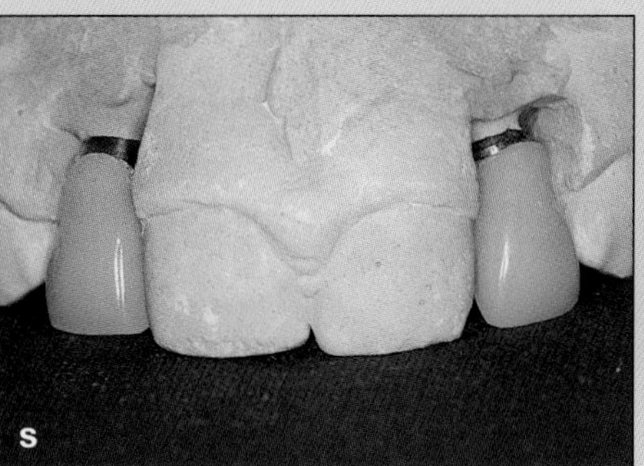

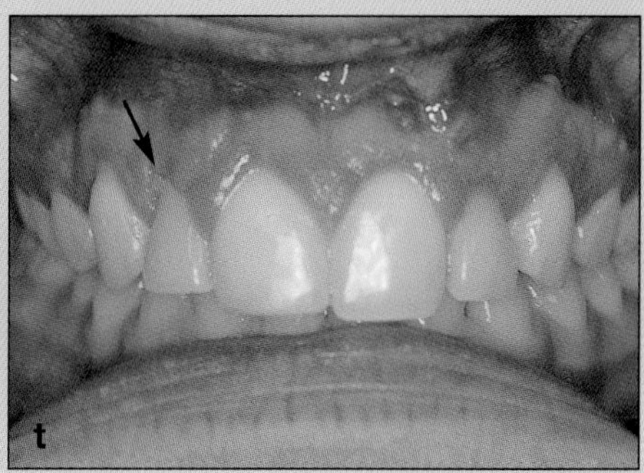

Fig 7-27s Implant analogue cast with custom abutments and provisional restorations fabricated from the surgical index. The fixture depth was determined relative to the proposed gingival margins of adjacent dentition after esthetic crown lengthening. The abutments and provisional restorations were delivered 2 months following the esthetic crown lengthening procedure.

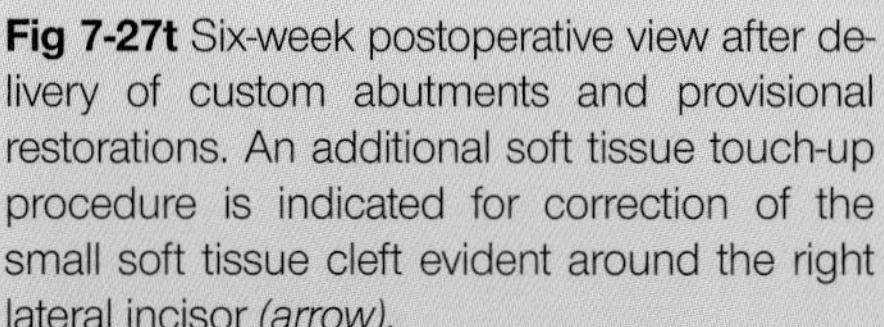

Fig 7-27t Six-week postoperative view after delivery of custom abutments and provisional restorations. An additional soft tissue touch-up procedure is indicated for correction of the small soft tissue cleft evident around the right lateral incisor *(arrow)*.

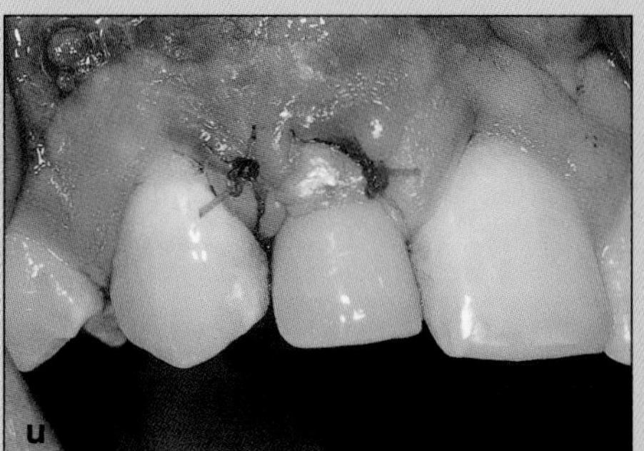

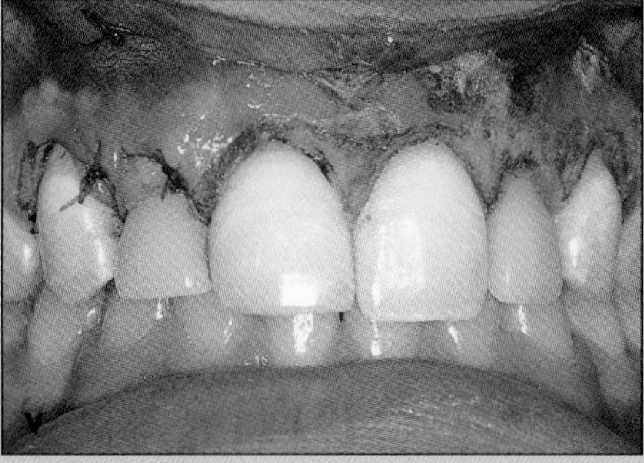

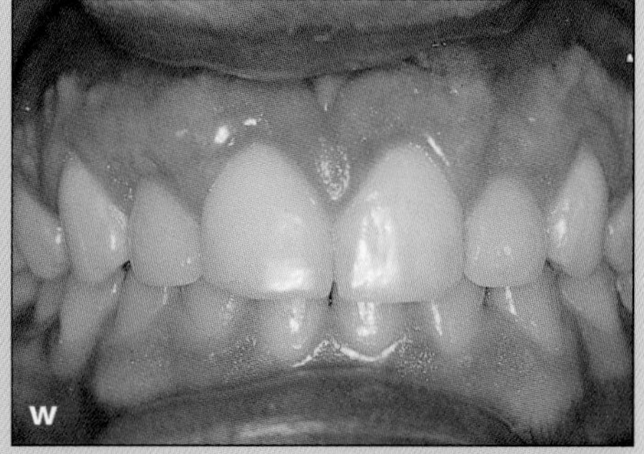

Figs 7-27u to 7-27w A subepithelial connective tissue graft performed via a closed recipient site successfully corrected the gingival defect at the right lateral incisor site. Additional laser soft tissue sculpting and resurfacing further refined the bulbous papillary morphology.

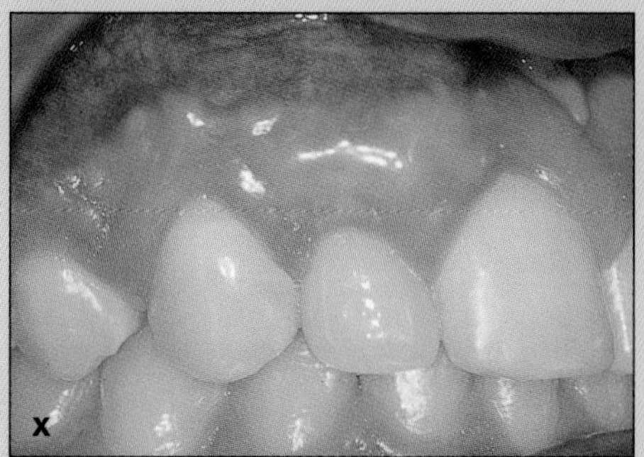

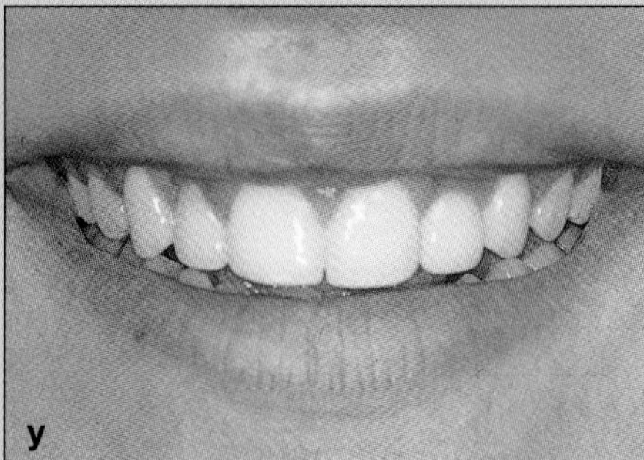

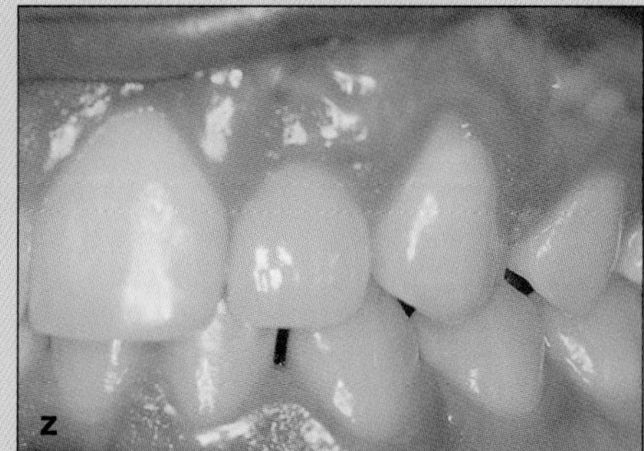

Figs 7-27x to 7-27z Intraoral and animated smile views following delivery of final restorations and minor esthetic enameloplasty of adjacent dentition. Note the improvement in gingival appearance, dental proportions, and smile esthetics as compared to pretreatment conditions. Although the sinuous gingival pattern appears somewhat exaggerated on intraoral views, the lip position during animation demonstrates that appropriate gingival levels were obtained to maximize smile esthetics.

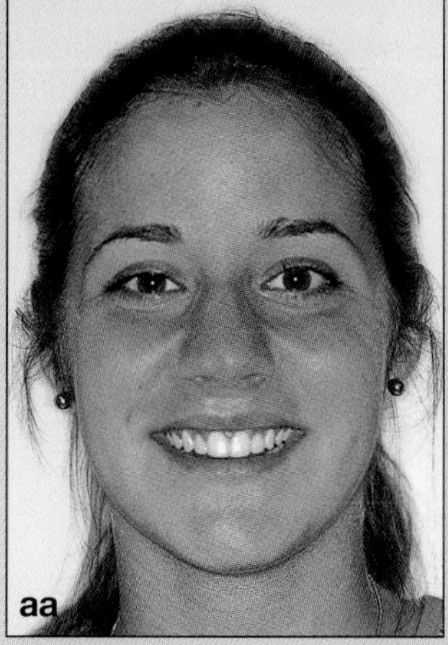

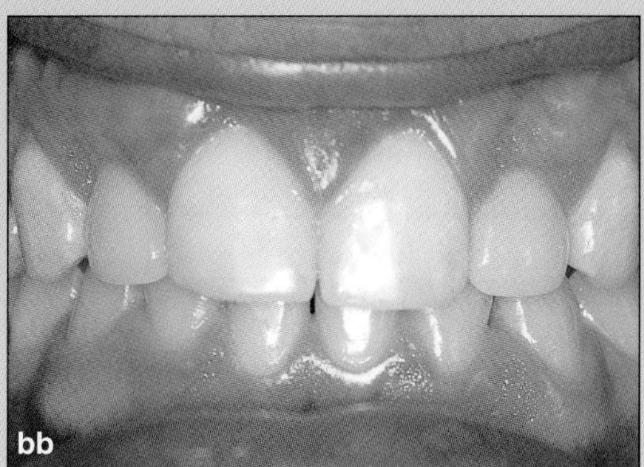

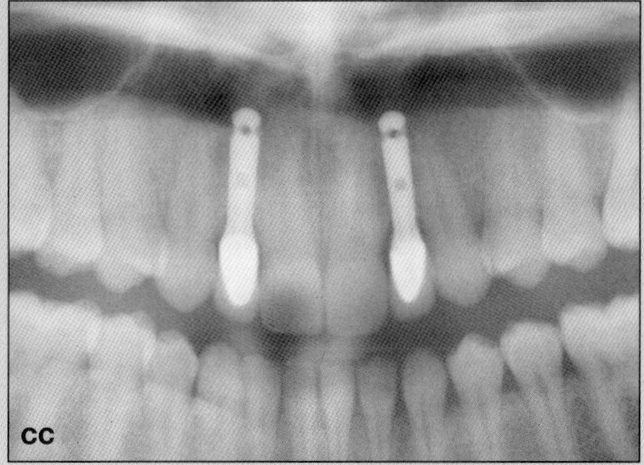

Figs 7-27aa to 7-27cc One-year post-restoration facial view, relaxed smile view, and panoramic radiograph. Improved smile esthetics were obtained by incorporating cosmetic periodontal surgery techniques with soft tissue grafting at lateral incisor sites. Implant restorations are harmonious with the adjacent dentition. Panoramic radiograph demonstrates harmonious implant restorations with stable osseous levels. (Restorative dentistry by Dr Jose Abadin, Coral Gables, FL.)

Enhancing outcomes in esthetic implant therapy: Creating harmony with cosmetic periodontal surgery

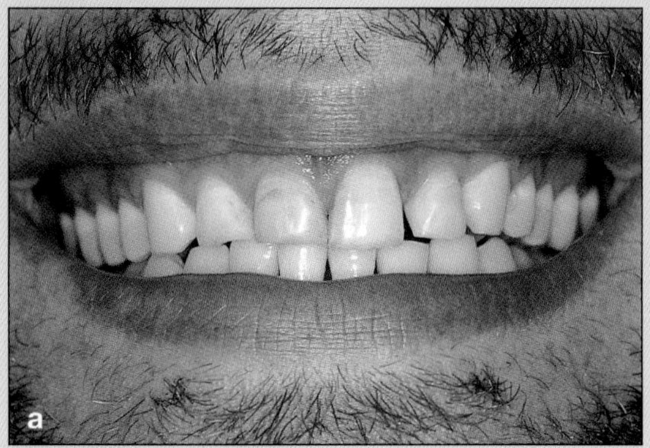

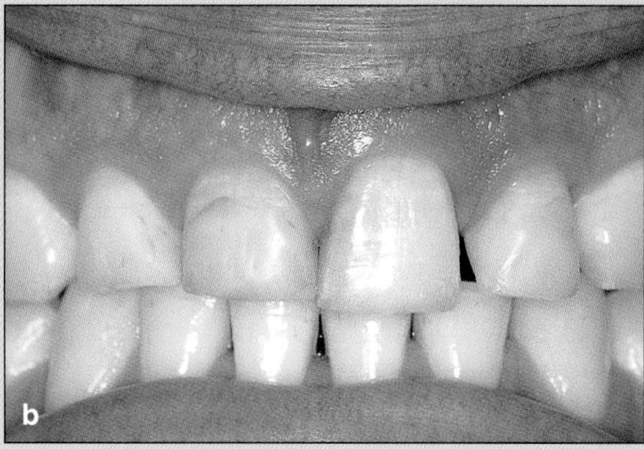

Figs 7-28a and 7-28b Preoperative animated smile and intraoral views of failing maxillary left central incisor. Elements that detract from the patient's smile include flat incisal plane, asymmetry between central incisors, diastema between left central and lateral incisors, unesthetic gingival arch pattern on the right side, and lack of progressive medial tipping of the anterior dentition.

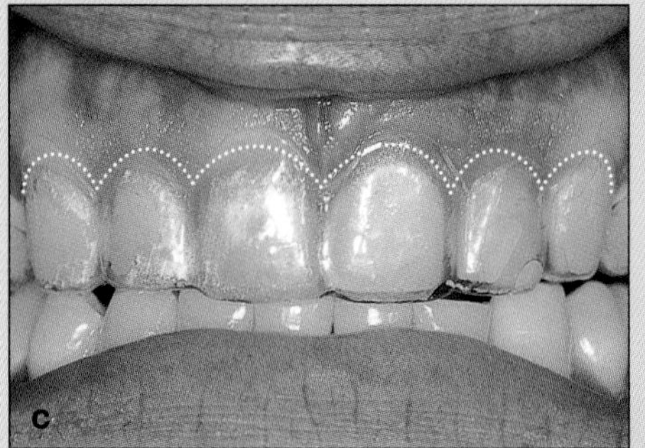

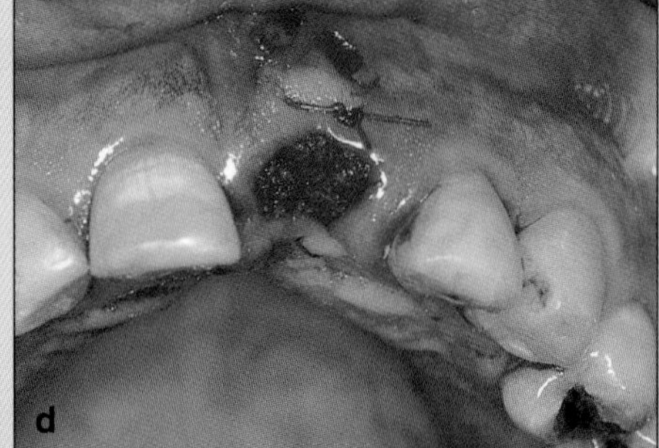

Fig 7-28c A diagnostic waxup of the desired final result with harmonious dental proportions and esthetic gingival pattern was performed by the restorative dentist and used to create a template for subsequent soft tissue grafting and esthetic crown lengthening. *Dotted white line* indicates correction needed to establish an esthetic gingival appearance.

Fig 7-28d The Bio-Col technique was performed after the central incisor was removed in preparation for delayed implant placement.

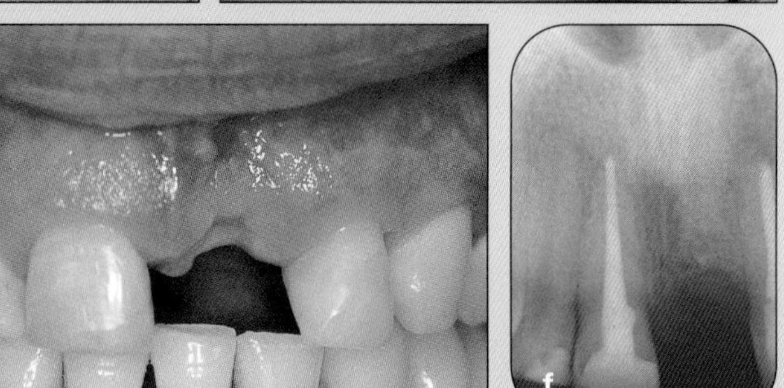

Fig 7-28e Three months after tooth removal, a small-volume combination esthetic ridge defect became evident.

Fig 7-28f Postoperative radiograph following tooth removal. Note grafted socket.

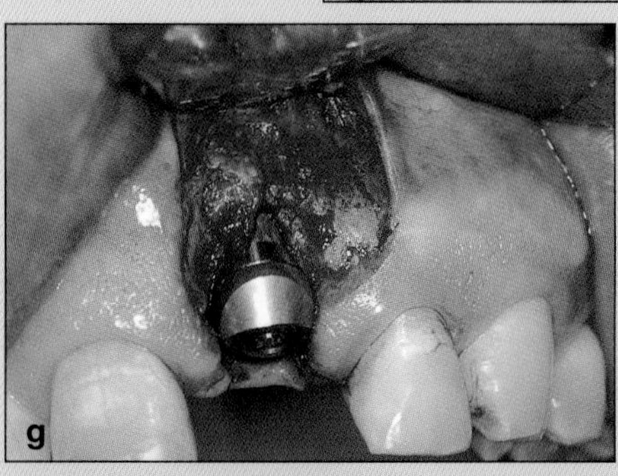

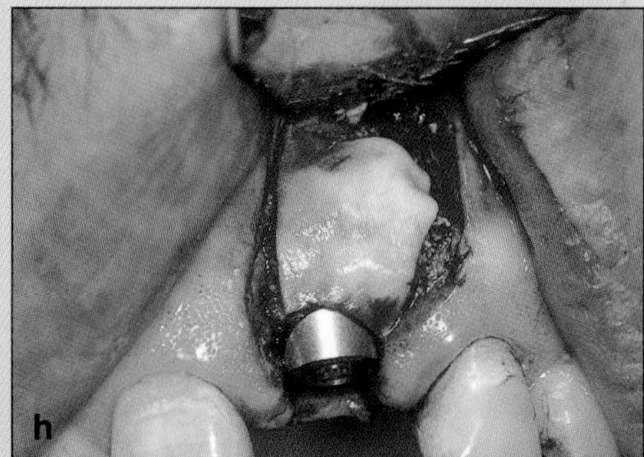

Figs 7-28g to 7-28i A nonsubmerged implant (Straumann USA) was placed at ideal depth, with consideration given to subsequent crown extension of natural tooth abutments. An unexpected osseous defect occurred at the buccal ridge crest. Because the defect was well within the alveolar housing, a decision was made to perform a guided bone regeneration procedure, despite the attending esthetic risks.

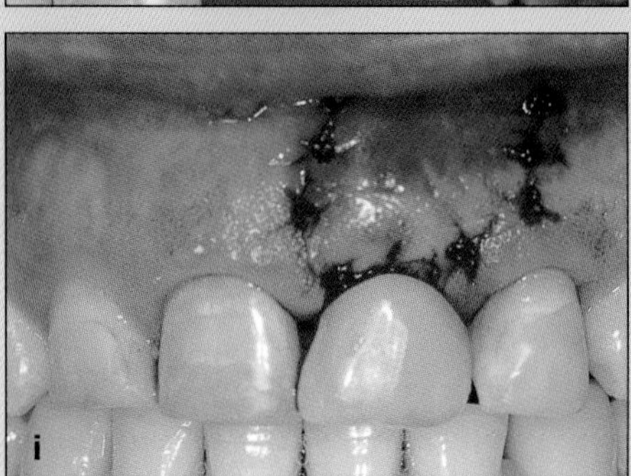

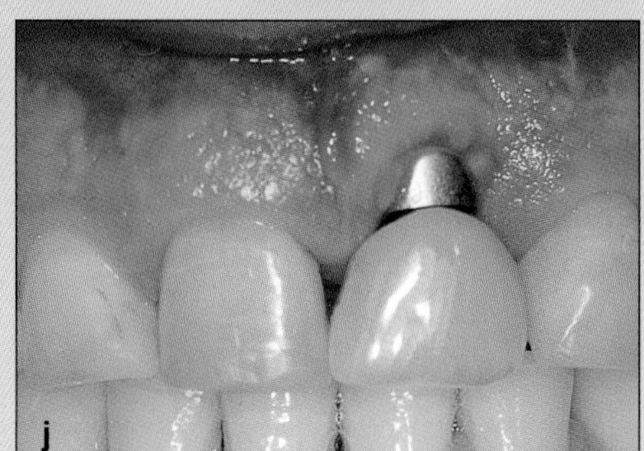

Fig 7-28j Four-month postoperative view demonstrates the soft tissue recession that commonly occurs following a guided bone regeneration procedure involving the buccal crest of the ridge in the anterior maxillary area.

Figs 7-28k to 7-28m The healing abutment was removed, and surgical indexing was performed. A smaller healing abutment was placed, after which a subepithelial connective tissue graft was performed via a closed recipient site. A custom provisional restoration was delivered 3 months later. Note the esthetic emergence of the provisional restoration. Tissues were allowed to stabilize for an additional 3 months prior to proceeding with the planned esthetic crown extension at the adjacent dentition.

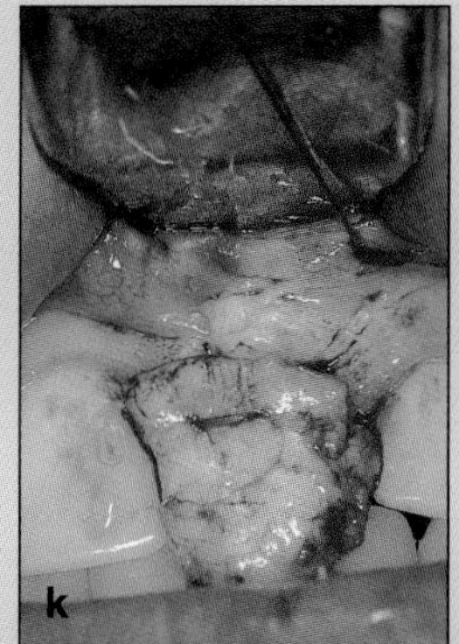

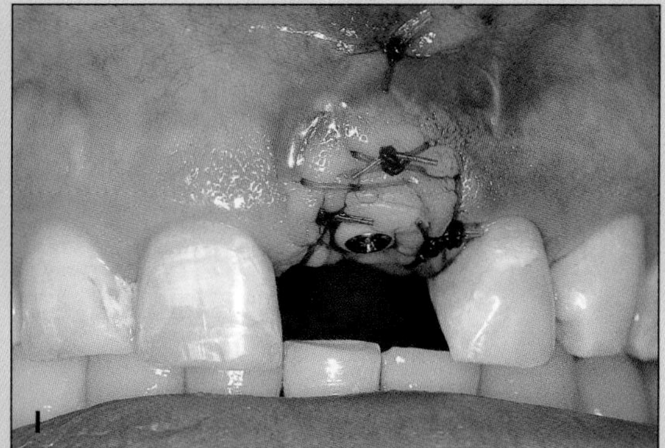

Fig 7-28n Radiograph taken 3 months after delivery of implant provisional.

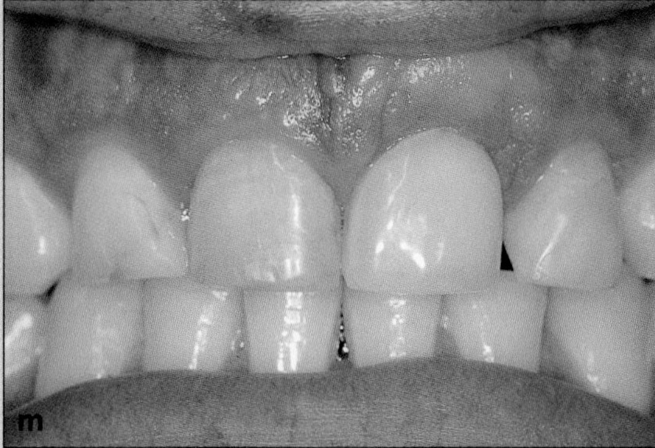

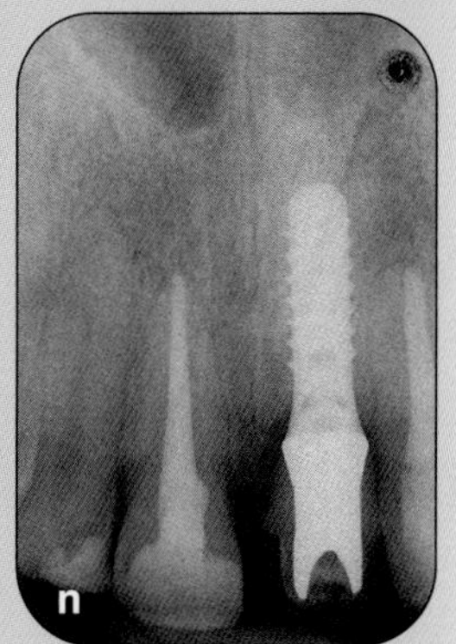

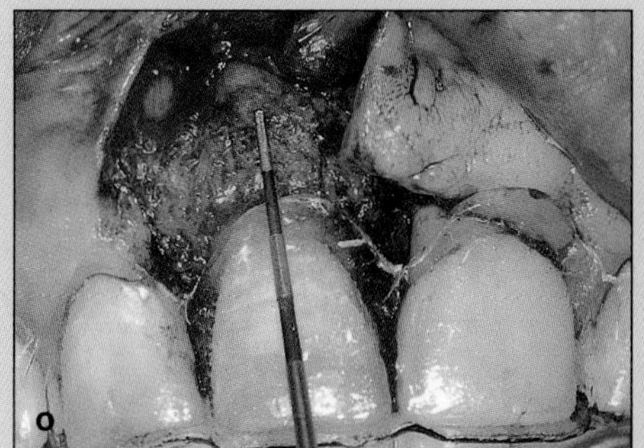

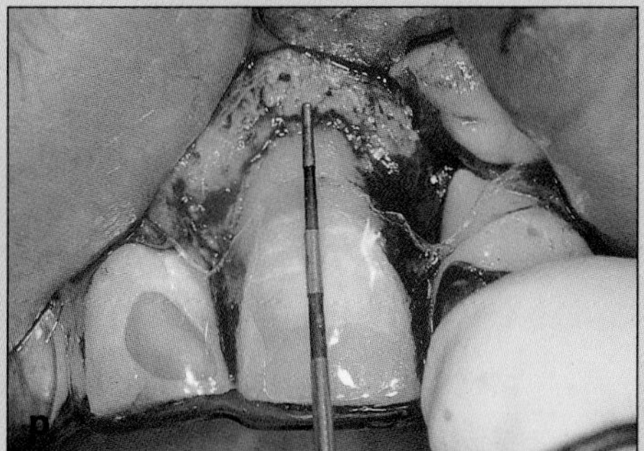

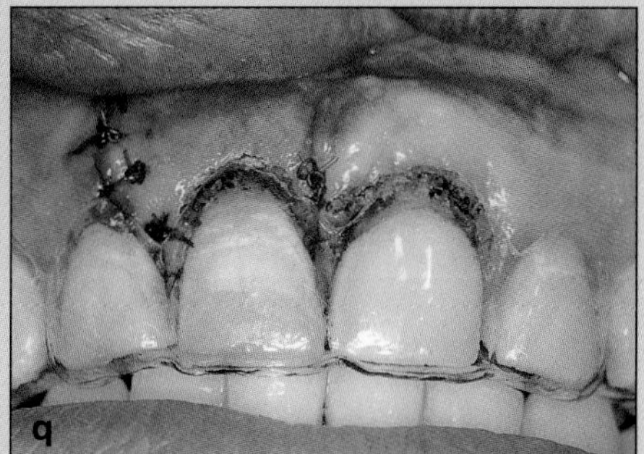

Figs 7-28o to 7-28q Esthetic crown lengthening, with osseous and soft tissue resection, performed on the right central incisor. Papillae elevation was necessary to prepare the central incisor and establish adequate biologic width in preparation for a full-coverage restoration. A CO_2 laser was used for simultaneous soft tissue sculpting. Tissue levels were verified with the surgical guide.

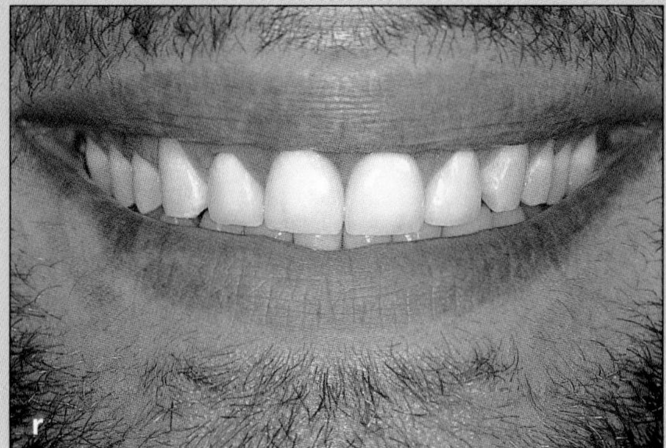

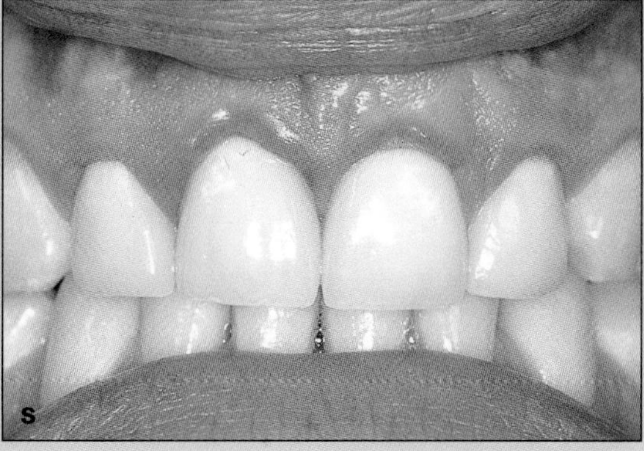

Figs 7-28r and 7-28s One year after delivery of final restorations, incisal plane correction is evident, symmetry has been established between the central incisors, and harmonious tooth proportions coexist with a pleasing gingival appearance. Use of cosmetic periodontal therapy has created harmony between the implant restoration and the adjacent natural teeth and eliminated those elements that detracted from this patient's smile. The unexpected osseous defect, corrected with a guided bone regeneration procedure at the time of implant placement, necessitated a subsequent soft tissue graft and extension of the healing period to ensure stable soft tissue levels prior to restoration. (Cosmetic and restorative dentistry by Dr Stephen Parr, Coconut Grove, FL.)

Enhancing outcomes in esthetic implant therapy: Creating harmony with cosmetic periodontal surgery

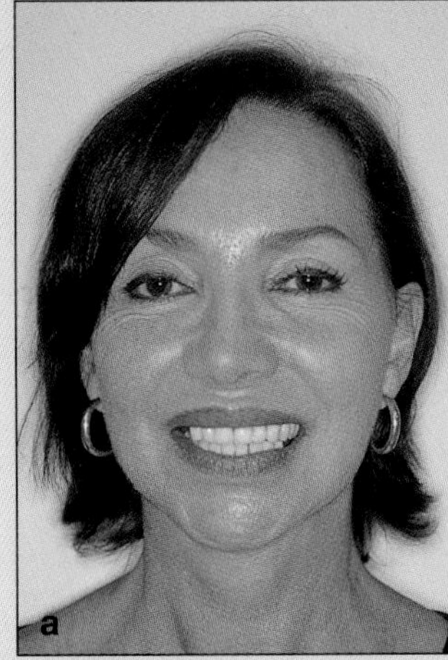
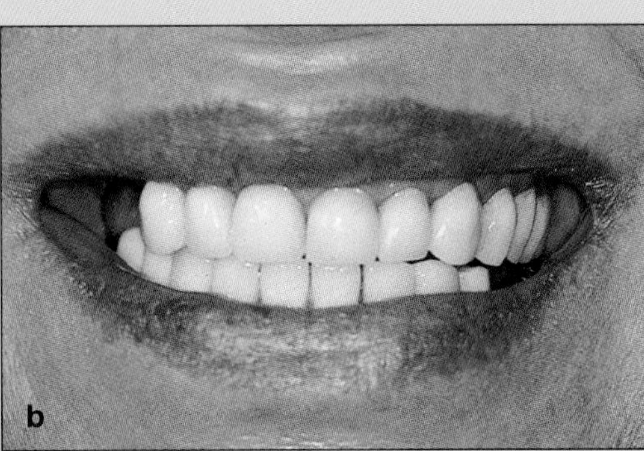
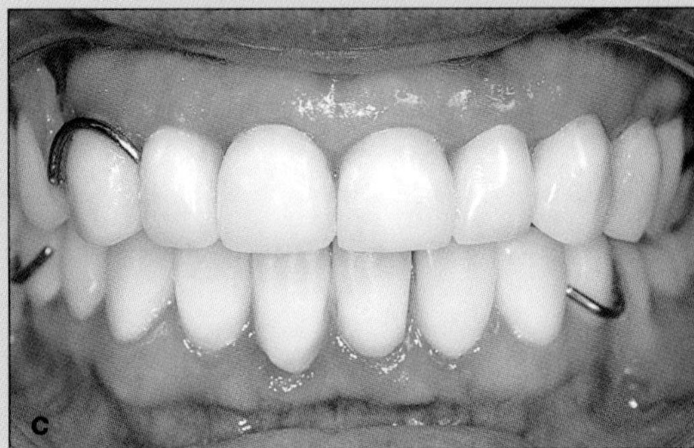

Figs 7-29a to 7-29c Pretreatment animated facial view, relaxed smile view, and intraoral view with removable partial denture restorations in place. The treatment plan included implant replacements for maxillary right and bilateral mandibular posterior quadrants in conjunction with replacement of fixed prosthesis on the natural dentition. The flat incisal plane, unesthetic dental proportions and relationships, and noncoincidence of incisal and occlusal planes all detract from smile esthetics. Soft tissue recession and inadequate soft tissue thickness are evident around the mandibular incisors.

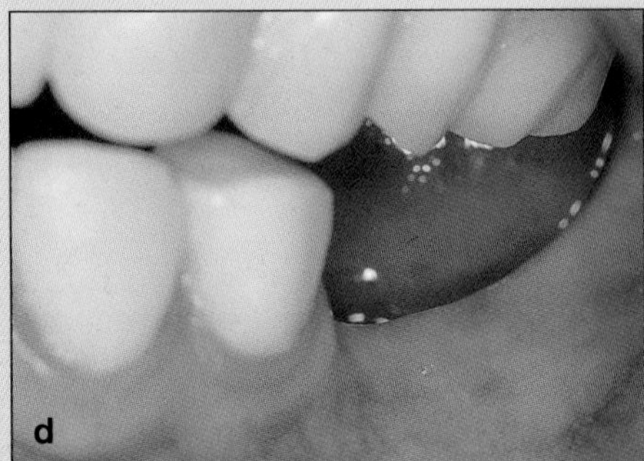

Fig 7-29d View of mandibular left quadrant with small-volume hard tissue defect to be restored with particulate bone graft–guided bone regeneration procedure that will be performed simultaneous with implant placment.

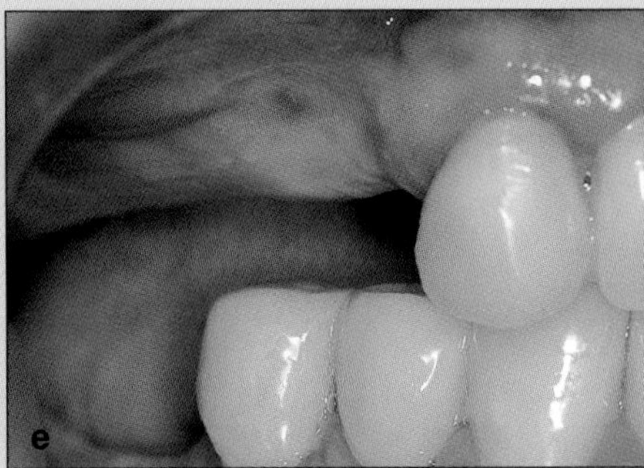

Fig 7-29e View of maxillary right quadrant with inadequate bone volume due to sinus pneumatization. This will be corrected with sinus lift bone grafting prior to implant placement.

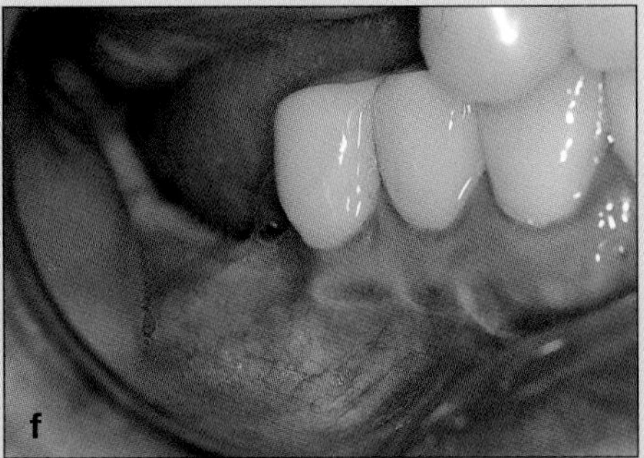

Fig 7-29f View of mandibular right posterior quadrant with large-volume hard tissue defect that will be corrected with block bone grafting prior to implant placement.

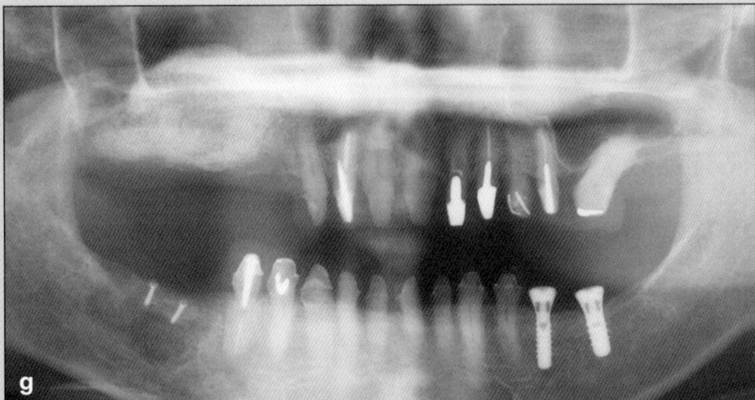

Fig 7-29g Postsurgical panoramic radiograph taken 3 months after sinus lift bone grafting of maxillary right quadrant, block bone grafting of mandibular right quadrant, and simultaneous particulate bone graft–guided bone regeneration procedure with nonsubmerged implant placement (Straumann USA).

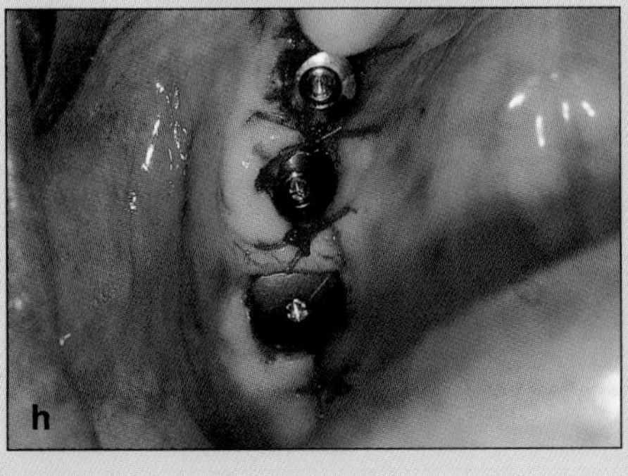
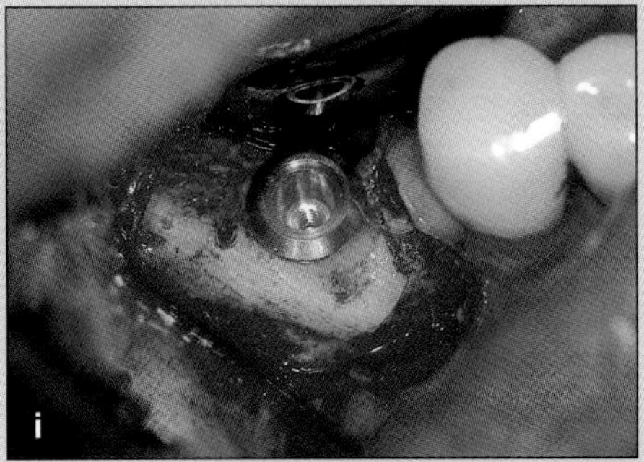

Figs 7-29h and 7-29i Four months after bone grafting, three nonsubmerged implants were placed in the maxillary right quadrant and the papilla-regeneration maneuver was used to obtain buccal soft tissue augmentation and positive gingival architecture around the maxillary implants. At the same time, a wide-neck implant was placed in the mandibular right quadrant, where excellent osseous reconstruction was evident.

Figs 7-29j to 7-29m Four months after implant placement in the maxillary and mandibular right posterior quadrants and 8 months after implant placement in the mandibular left quadrant, stable soft tissue levels have been obtained. Note the positive gingival architecture around the emerging maxillary implants and the adequate band of attached tissue around the mandibular implants.

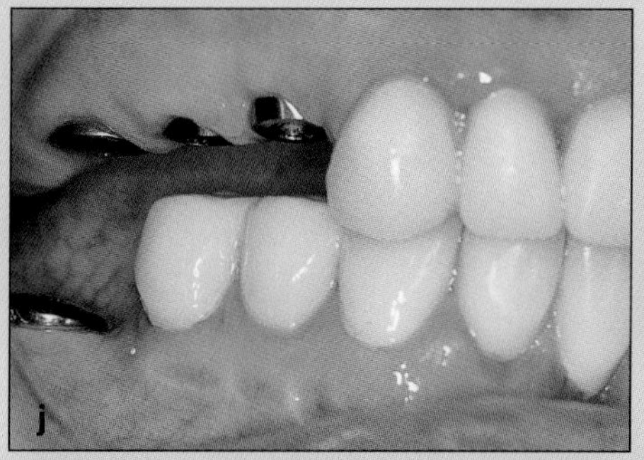

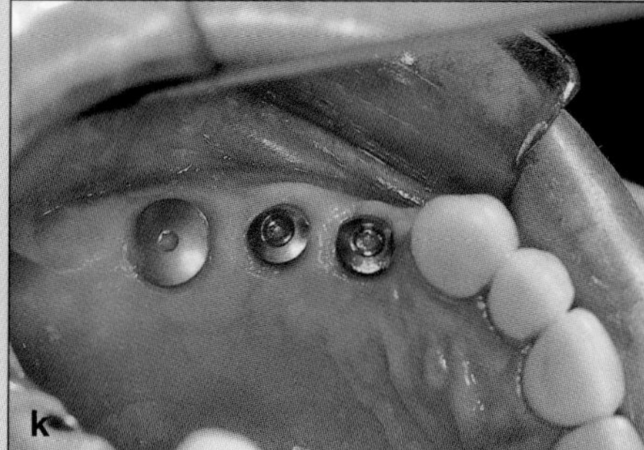

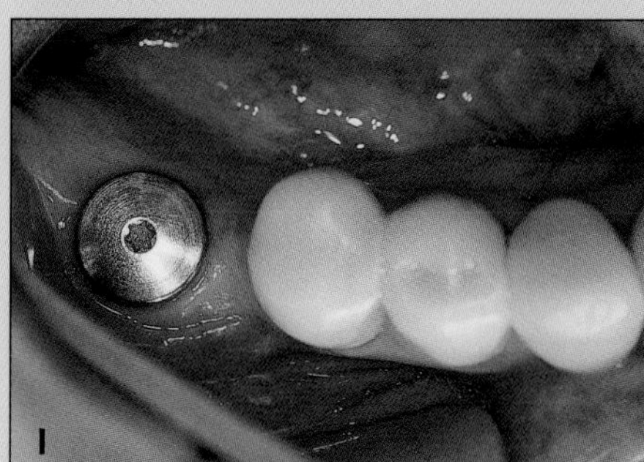

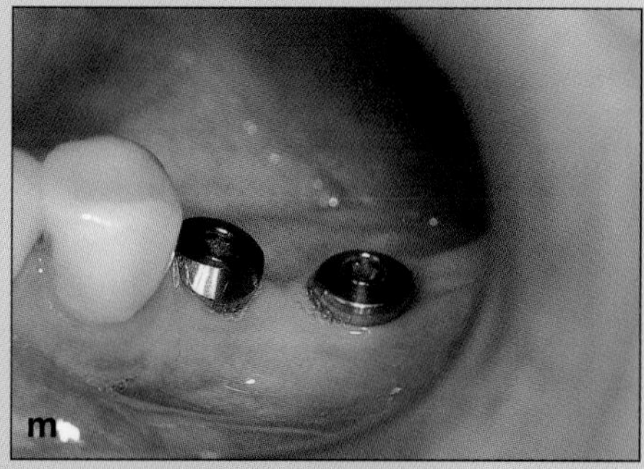

Fig 7-29n Panoramic radiograph taken prior to prosthetic restoration demonstrates stable osseous levels and successful maintenance of bone graft volume in each quadrant.

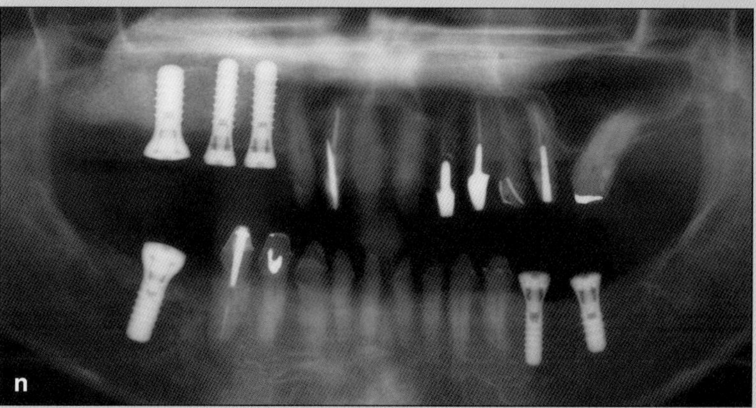

Figs 7-29o and 7-29p After implant provisional restorations were delivered, esthetic crown lengthening was performed from the right maxillary canine to the left second premolar. In addition, a subepithelial connective tissue graft was performed to increase the width and thickness of the attached tissue in the mandibular anterior area.

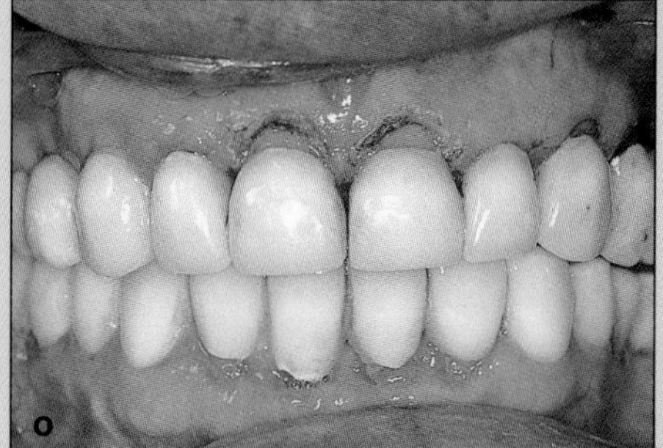

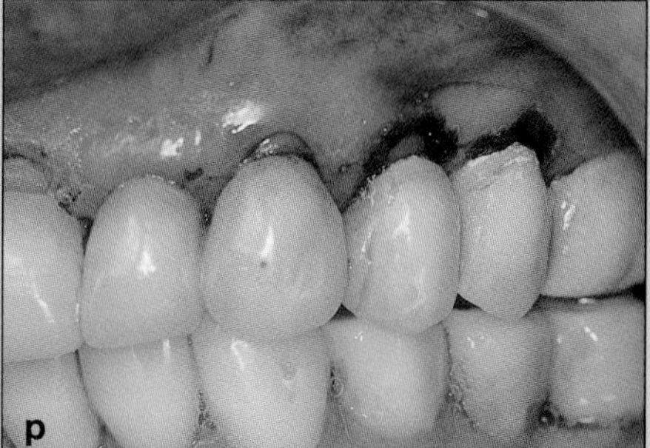

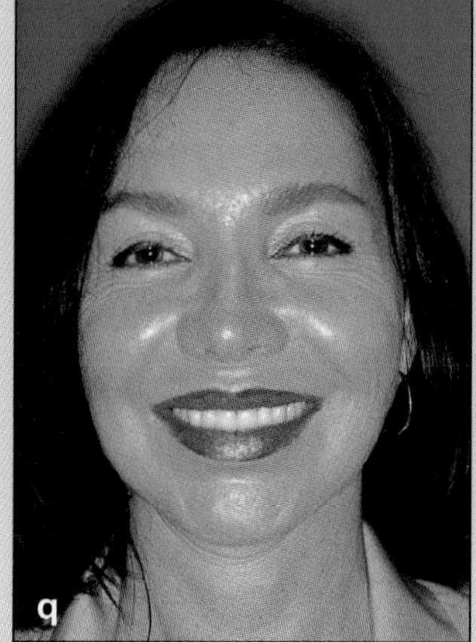

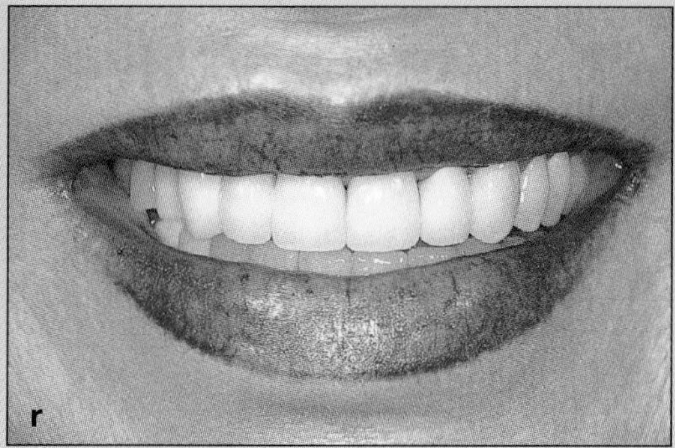

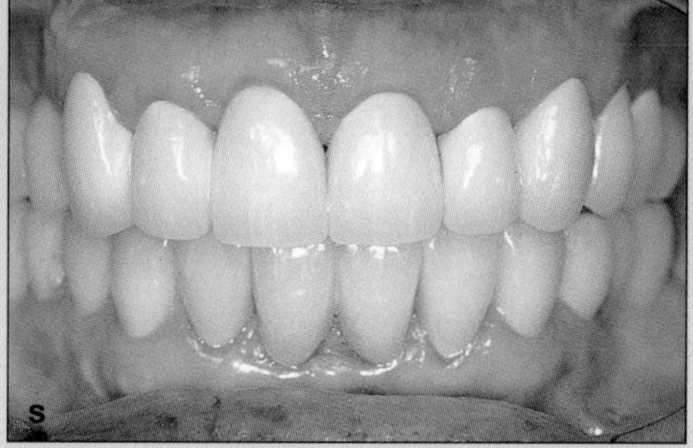

Figs 7-29q to 7-29s Final restorations 1 year after delivery. Note the improved incisal plane, occlusal plane, dental proportions and relationships, gingival health and esthetics, and the full-volume smile without visible voids in the buccal corridor upon full animation created by hard and soft tissue implant site development, esthetic peri-implant soft tissue management, cosmetic periodontal surgery, and cosmetic and reconstructive dentistry, all guided by initial visualization of the final result by the implant team and communication of the possibilities to the patient. Note also the return of periodontal soft tissue health around the mandibular incisors. (Restorative dentistry by Dr Jack Cohn, Miami, FL.)

Use of Platelet-Rich Plasma (PRP) to Enhance Outcomes in Implant Therapy

General considerations

In recent years, the use of PRP has become a practical and effective tool to enhance wound healing in implant therapy. Procurement and processing of PRP within the outpatient dental environment is now simple and safe for patients and auxiliary personnel. FDA-approved devices that automate the sequestration and concentration of platelets have streamlined the process, enabling the implant surgeon to provide PRP as an adjunct to wound healing in various clinical scenarios related to implant therapy. In addition to providing biologically active blood components (fibrin, fibronectin, vitronectin) to enhance cell mobility, PRP is a potential source of growth factors (PDGF, TGF-beta), which theoretically affect nearly all wound-healing mechanisms.

From a practical standpoint, office acquisition, processing, and delivery are simple procedures. Standard phlebotomy techniques are used to draw 20 to 120 mL of blood (depending on whether single or multiple sites are to be treated) into a syringe preloaded with a defined amount of anticoagulant (citrate phosphate dextrose) and air (Fig 7-30a). Subsequently, the air bubble is used to gently mix the anticoagulant with the blood, and the mixture is injected into a processing module and placed into an automated device that sequesters and concentrates the platelets (Figs 7-30b and 7-30c). The processing separates the platelets from the plasma, which is drawn off. A defined amount of plasma is then used to re-suspend the platelets, resulting in nonactivated PRP solution that is still anticoagulated (Figs 7-30d and 7-30e). In general, 3 to 4 mL of PRP solution is sufficient for use at multiple surgical sites where hard or soft tissue grafts are performed. Approximately 1 mL of nonactivated PRP solution is used to moisten hard or soft tissue grafts during storage. The remainder of the solution is loaded into a dual-syringe delivery gun (Harvest Technologies) (Fig 7-30f) that houses the nonactivated PRP solution in one syringe and thrombin and calcium chloride solution in the other syringe. As the surgeon pushes the plunger, the coagulant is mixed with the nonactivated PRP solution to cause the formation of a PRP blood clot. As a result, platelets are activated and growth factors are released. The average working time before the clot forms is 60 to 90 seconds. After this, manipulation of the PRP clot at the surgical site may be detrimental, since fibrin cross linking may be disrupted and the natural scaffold for cell mobility within the wound may be harmed.

The use of PRP in implant therapy to provide adhesive and tensile strength for wound stabilization and sealing is of critical importance to osseointegration itself. It is recognized that attachment and stabilization of the blood clot to the surface of a dental implant facilitates the migration of bone cells to the implant surface, resulting in contact osteogenesis, a process that ultimately determines the percentage of bone-to-implant contact. In addition, the growth factors contained within PRP theoretically provide an enhanced rate of maturation of bone and periodontal soft tissues. This information forms the basis for the clinical rationale for use of PRP to enhance wound healing and clinical outcomes in implant therapy. Some of the common clinical procedures that may benefit from the use of PRP include alveolar ridge preservation in preparation for delayed implant placement or in conjunction with immediate implant placement (as demonstrated in chapter 4), hard and soft tissue grafting, and immediate-load implant therapy. Furthermore, the use of PRP as a strategy to enhance the rate of maturation and volume yields from hard and soft tissue grafting is an extremely important consideration in esthetic implant therapy, where small differences in volume yields can result in the need for secondary grafting procedures or the acceptance of esthetic compromises due to contour defects in areas critical for prosthetic emergence.

When PRP is used in implant therapy, the clinician must recognize its significant technique sensitivity, which can have a profound effect on the outcomes observed. The venipuncture technique and blood draw must be performed in a fashion that avoids activation of the platelets. Use of a relatively large-bore needle and minimizing negative pressure on the syringe will usually accomplish this. Use of an automated device, which simplifies the sequestration of the platelets and careful suspension of these platelets in a defined amount of plasma, determines the quality (platelet concentration) of PRP solution that is obtained (see Fig 7-30e). In general, a fivefold increase in the patient's baseline platelet count is desired in order to realize the documented positive effects that platelet-derived growth factors have on hard and soft tissue healing. Overdilution of the platelets by suspension in an excessive amount of platelet-poor plasma may result in a reduction of the theoretical wound-healing capacity compared to that provided by the patient's own natural blood clot. The author recommends individualizing the amount of platelet-poor plasma used to suspend the sequestered platelets according to the size of the surgical site or graft. This will avoid unnecessary overdilution of the growth factors at the site. The emphasis is on the quality of the PRP solution, not

Use of platelet rich plasma to enhance outcomes in implant therapy

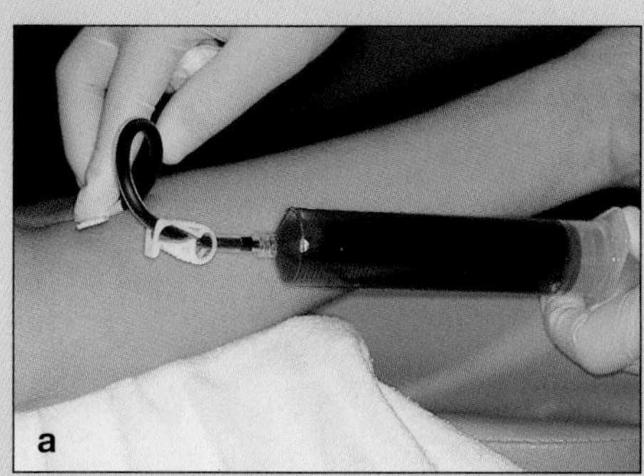

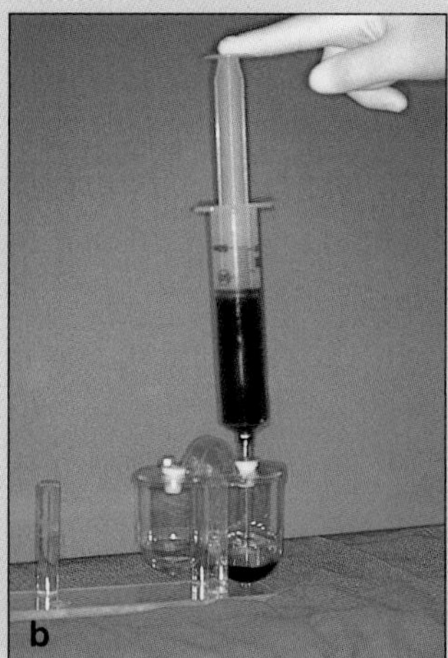

Fig 7-30a Standard phlebotomy technique is used to draw as little as 20 mL and up to 120 mL of blood, yielding between 2.0 and 6.0 mL of PRP solution. On average 1.0 mL of PRP is sufficient for a single site requiring a hard or soft tissue graft, and 3.0 mL is required for the average sinus lift bone graft procedure.

Figs 7-30b and 7-30c The blood is injected into the appropriate processing module and processed in an automated device (Harvest Technologies, Boston, MA) for approximately 12 minutes.

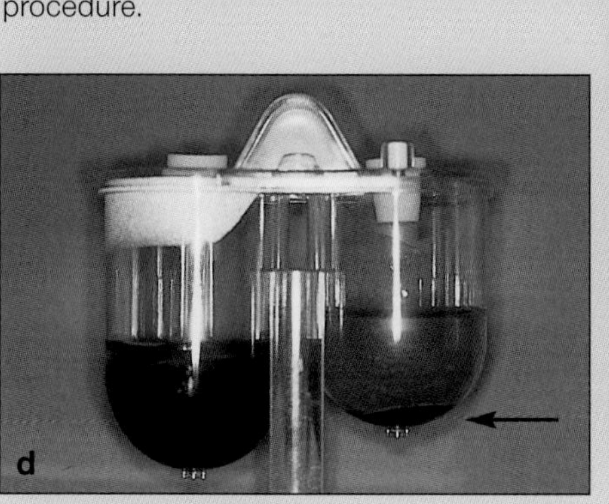

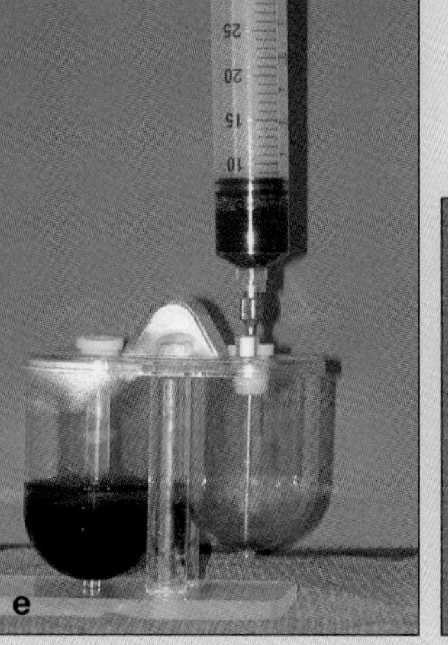

Figs 7-30d and 7-30e The sequestered platelets visible at the bottom of the processing module *(arrow)* are prepared for clinical use by first drawing off and then adding back a defined amount (1 to 3 mL, depending on the volume of the initial blood draw) of platelet-poor plasma to create the nonactivated PRP solution. The smaller volume of platelet-poor plasma used improves the concentration (quality) of the PRP solution.

Fig 7-30f A dual-syringe delivery gun mixes the PRP solution with calcium chloride and thrombin to activate platelets directly upon application to the site.

the quantity. Furthermore, even after delivery of the PRP solution to the graft or surgical site, dilution of growth factors can easily occur secondary to the use of irrigation fluids, additional local anesthetic injections, or the indiscriminate use of platelet-poor plasma at the site.

Hard tissue considerations

Enhancing osseointegration

When PRP is used to enhance the osseointegration of an implant placed in an immediate or delayed approach, the process can be as simple as delivering the activated PRP solution into the socket or osteotomy preparation as the implant is delivered to full sink depth. The goal is to ensure that the growth factor–enriched blood clot and its fibrin network occupy any voids between the implant and the socket or osteotomy walls. The resultant PRP blood clot with activated platelets should be absorbed and stabilized to both the implant surface and the osseous preparation in order to facilitate the migration of osteocompetent cells to the implant surface. Application of activated PRP directly to the implant surface prior to placement may not give the desired results since the PRP blood clot may be disrupted or pulled away from the implant surface during fixture placement. Furthermore, attachment and stabilization of the PRP blood clot to the walls of the osseous preparation may not occur since there is a limitation imposed by the rate at which the PRP blood clot forms after it is activated.

Use of PRP to enhance outcomes in implant therapy: Hard tissue considerations (block and particulate bone grafting)

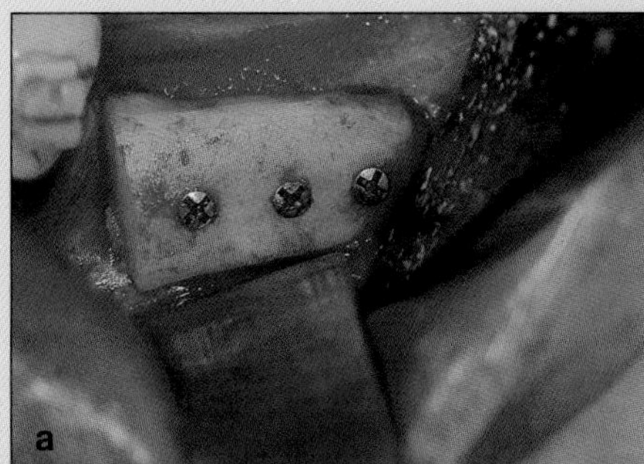

Fig 7-31a Once they are harvested, corticocancellous block and particulate cancellous bone grafts are stored in nonactivated PRP solution. Subsequently, rigid fixation screws are used to adapt the block graft at the prepared recipient site.

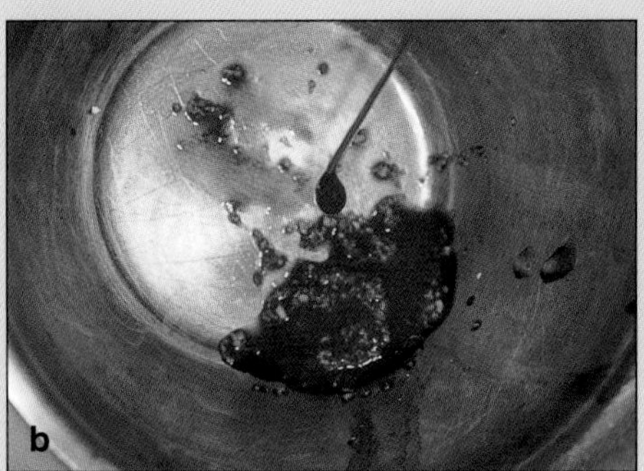

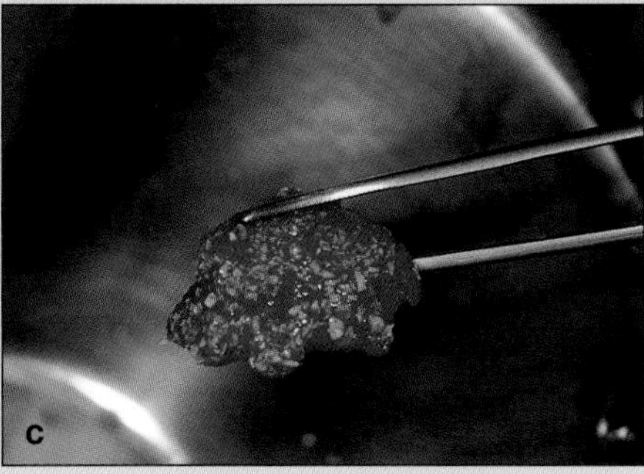

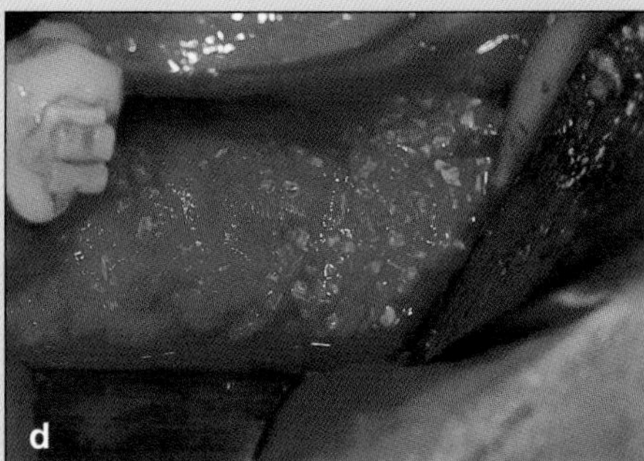

Figs 7-31b to 7-31d A xenograft is added to the particulate bone graft immediately preceding delivery to the recipient site. The mixture is moistened with activated PRP solution to create a moldable bone graft that is easily transferred and condensed at the recipient site.

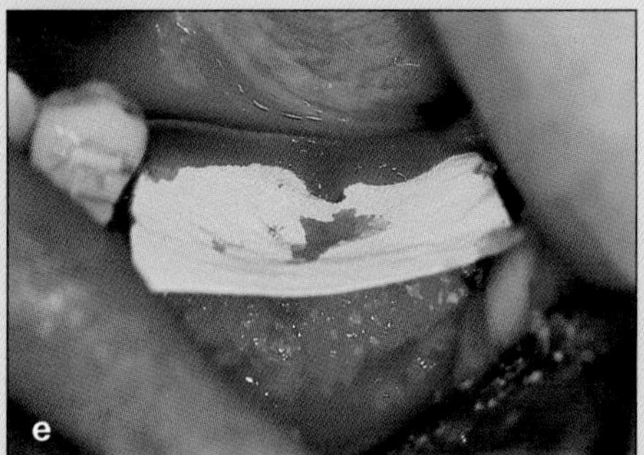

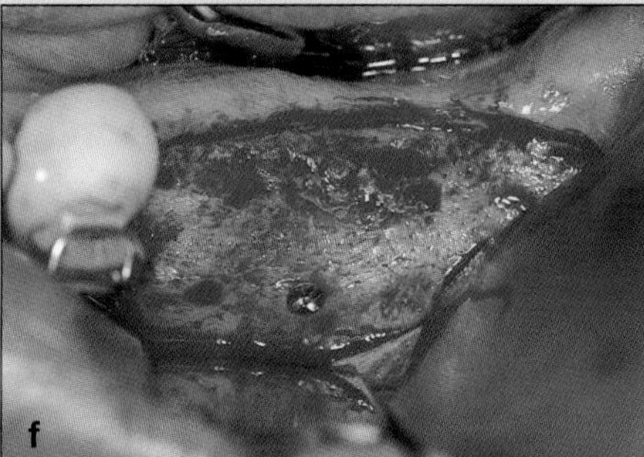

Fig 7-31e Additional activated PRP solution is used at the site to ensure that an intact fibrin network is present throughout the graft for optimal cellular conduction. An absorbable collagen membrane (Bio-Gide) is then adapted over the graft and becomes stabilized by absorbing the PRP solution.

Fig 7-31f Upon re-entry to the site for implant placement 4 months following bone graft procedures, advanced healing of the bone graft is evidenced by an inability to distinguish the Bio-Oss particles and the almost completely submerged fixation screws. This clinical observation is attributed to improved cellular conduction within the bone graft as well as the theoretical effects of the growth factors contained in PRP.

Alveolar ridge preservation

When particulate bone grafts are part of the immediate placement protocol (Bio-Col technique) to occupy the voids between the implant body and the socket wall, mixing the xenograft material (Bio-Oss) with PRP provides the technical advantage of facilitating the delivery of the graft material to the site. Once the PRP-graft mixture is delivered and condensed at the site, a few drops of additional activated PRP solution should be injected into the graft area to ensure saturation of the implant body, graft material, and socket wall as well as to re-establish the fibrin network within the graft that is disrupted during graft delivery and condensation. Alternatively, the graft material can be delivered and condensed as described in chapter 4 and the activated PRP solution subsequently delivered to the area to saturate the site.

Autogenous bone grafts

When autogenous particulate cancellous bone grafts are used for hard tissue grafting in implant therapy, it is recommended that the autogenous bone be moistened in nonactivated PRP prior to delivery to the site to allow for theoretical "uptake" of growth factors by the viable bone cells. Ideally, the bone should be transferred to a plastic container immediately following harvest and enough nonactivated PRP solution should be added to ensure that the graft is moistened in the solution. As previously discussed, although the graft is moistened in nonactivated PRP solution, a small degree of activation of the solution is usually observed in and around the graft. Theoretically, this allows for initial uptake of the growth factors released by the activated platelets to the viable bone cells within the graft. If a xenograft is to be used as a graft expander, the soaking of the autogenous bone is accomplished prior to mixing with the xenograft material. In either case, once the graft has been moistened in nonactivated PRP solution, it can be carried directly to the recipient site and activated by topical application of activated PRP solution. Alternatively, it can be activated in a separate container and quickly transferred and condensed at the recipient site before the final application of activated PRP is performed (Fig 7-31).

Corticocancellous bone grafts for onlay-type alveolar ridge augmentations are stored in a similar fashion after the cancellous portion of the graft is moistened with nonactivated PRP solution. After rigid fixation of corticocancellous block grafts at the previously prepared recipient sites, particulate bone grafts are combined with activated PRP and delivered and condensed into any voids between the recipient site and the secured bone block, as previously discussed. A few drops of activated PRP solution are then used to moisten the surface of the composite bone graft, and an absorbable collagen membrane is draped over the graft. The membrane is stabilized by absorbing the activated PRP solution at the site. Use of activated PRP solution provides the technical advantage of facilitating the placement and fixation of the resorbable collagen membrane during surgery, contributing to optimal guided bone regeneration (Fig 7-32).

Soft tissue considerations

When soft tissue grafting is performed to augment soft tissue volume, to obtain root or abutment coverage, or to improve soft tissue quality at an implant site, use of PRP provides significant technical and clinical advantages. Donor tissues are moistened in nonactivated PRP prior to delivery and immobilization at the recipient site (Fig 7-33). The rationale for moistening a free soft tissue graft with a few drops of nonactivated PRP solution is based on the observation that surface activation of the solution probably occurs as a result of contact with topical tissue thromboplastin. When onlay soft tissue grafting is performed, activated PRP solution is then injected over the surface of the immobilized graft as a growth factor–enriched "wound dressing." When an interpositional graft is performed, activated PRP solution is injected between the graft and cover flap after graft immobilization, and excess solution is quickly expelled by applying pressure over the site before securing the cover tissue. Again, the activated PRP solution is then applied topically as a wound dressing. PRP may also be used at donor sites to enhance healing and minimize complications (Fig 7-34). When root-coverage procedures are performed, cellular adhesion molecules contained in PRP (fibronectin, vitronectin) are acceptable to the root surface, thus aiding in initial adherence and attachment of the donor tissue to the exposed root surface. Application of activated PRP solution to a soft tissue graft prior to its immobilization at the recipient site is contraindicated and should be avoided; this may cause graft sloughing in the same fashion that a thick blood clot placed between a soft tissue graft and its recipient site impairs initial plasmatic diffusion and ultimately revascularization of any oral soft tissue grafts.

Clinical observations of enhanced outcomes with the use of PRP in implant therapy

When used according to the specific procedures described above, PRP has enhanced clinical outcomes in many clinical situations. Observations include enhanced maturation of particulate bone grafts consisting of Bio-Oss and autologous cancellous bone (see Figs 7-31, 7-32, and 7-34) or Bio-Oss alone upon reentry of previously grafted sites and via evaluation of serial radiographs. In addition, histologic samples obtained from particulate bone grafts were consistent with clinical impressions of an enhanced rate of maturation demonstrating increased density and greater quantities of viable bone than expected. These clinical observations by the author are attributed to enhanced osteoconduction within the bone grafts as well as the theoretical contribution of growth factors contained in the PRP. Healing of soft tissue flaps (Fig 7-35; see also Fig 7-32) and free soft tissue grafts (Fig 7-36; see also Fig 7-34) was also enhanced, and increased volume yields were observed from interpositional soft tissue grafts and consistently less retraction of coronally advanced flaps performed as part of implant-site development. Based on the author's initial 42-month clinical experience, the use of PRP as a wound-healing adjunct in implant therapy is warranted. The implant surgeon should realize that the use of PRP according to the principles and protocol presented above does not compensate for poor surgical technique or allow the surgeon to ignore basic surgical principles. Although early clinical observations are positive, additional studies must be conducted in order to scientifically document the benefits of using PRP in implant therapy and to guide the clinician in case selection.

Hard tissue considerations (block and particulate bone grafting)

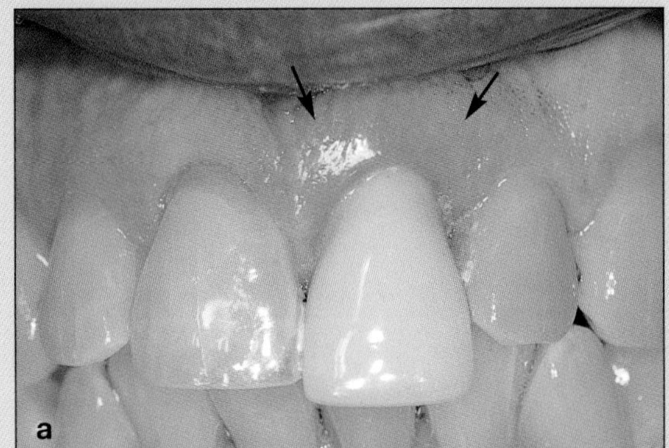
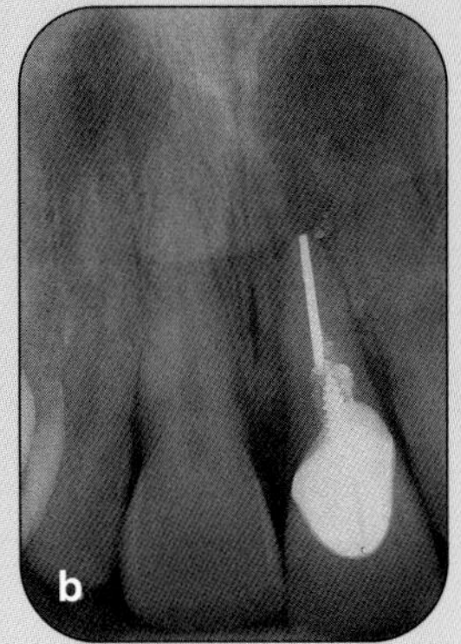

Figs 7-32a and 7-32b Clinical and radiographic views of failing left central incisor compromised by a history of traumatic injury and endodontic therapy. Note the soft tissue edema *(arrows)* associated with tooth mobility and buccal plate dehiscence. This will result in a soft tissue esthetic ridge defect after tooth removal despite application of a site-preservation technique or use of PRP.

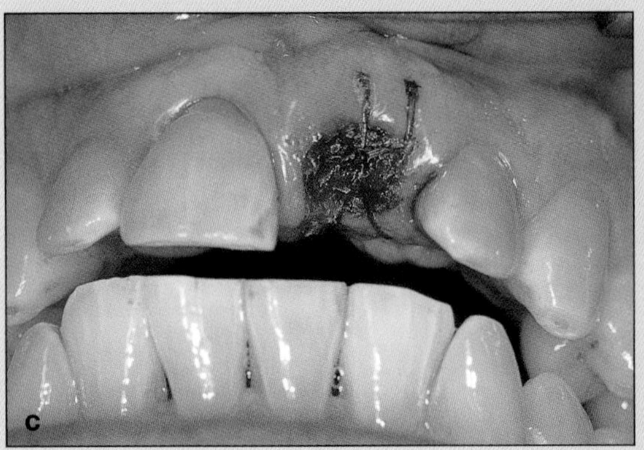
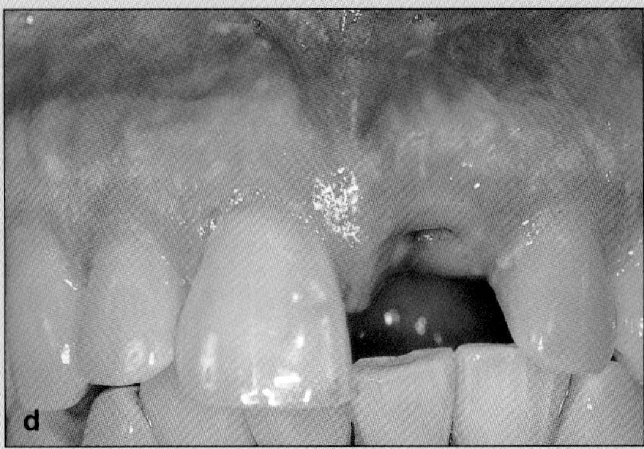
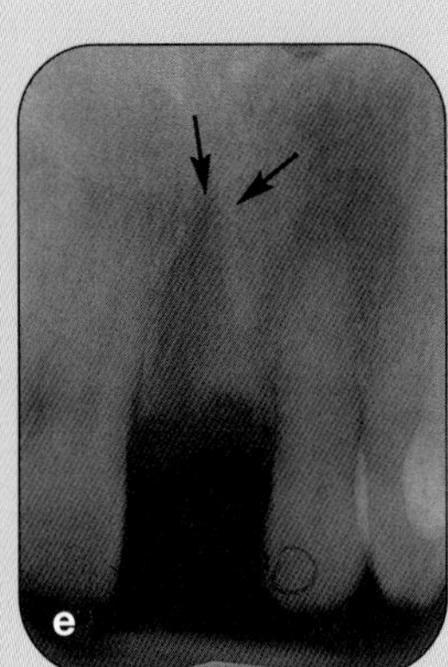

Figs 7-32c to 7-32e Following tooth removal, the Bio-Col technique was used to prevent collapse of the soft tissues at the site in preparation for block bone graft reconstruction of the ridge defect of unfavorable morphology. Very little bleeding was observed at the time of tooth removal. A large-volume combination defect became evident 3 months later. Incomplete incorporation of the Bio-Oss graft was evident on the 3-month postoperative radiograph *(arrows).*

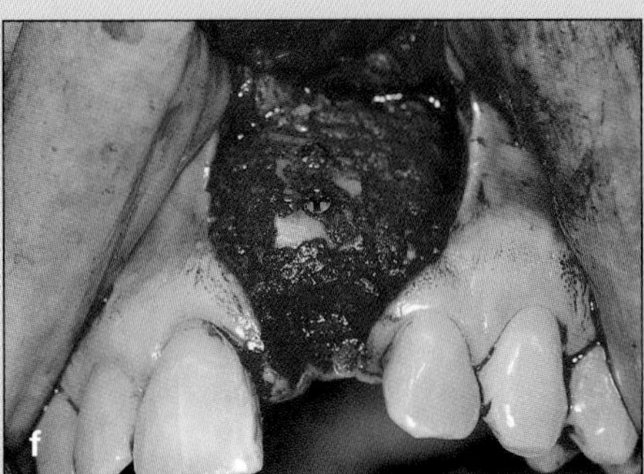

Fig 7-32f Access to site obtained with a curvilinear-beveled flap. Particulate bone graft moistened with activated PRP solution delivered to and condensed around a corticocancellous block graft previously secured at the prepared recipient site. The block and particulate grafts were moistened with non-activated PRP solution prior to delivery.

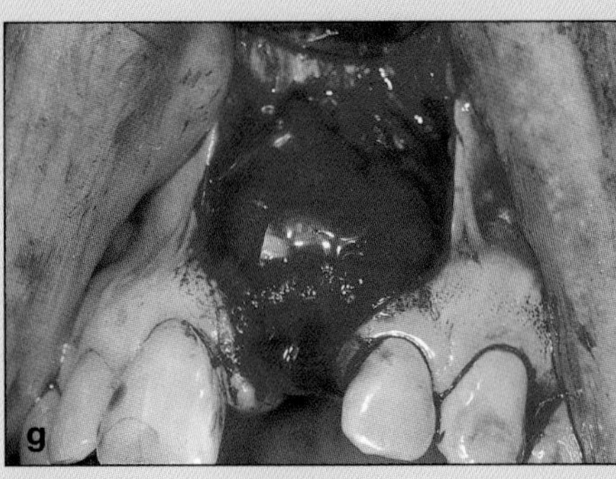
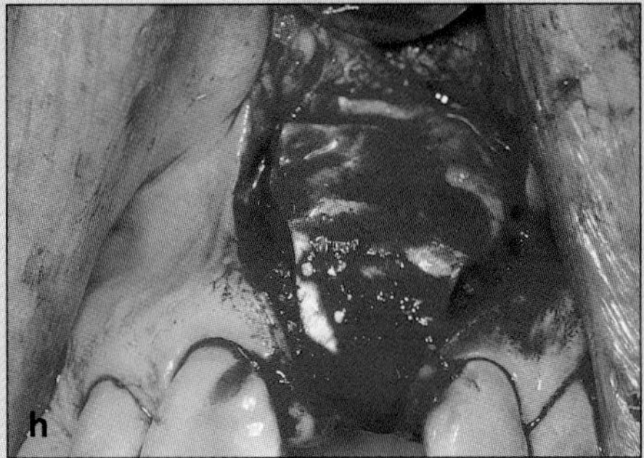
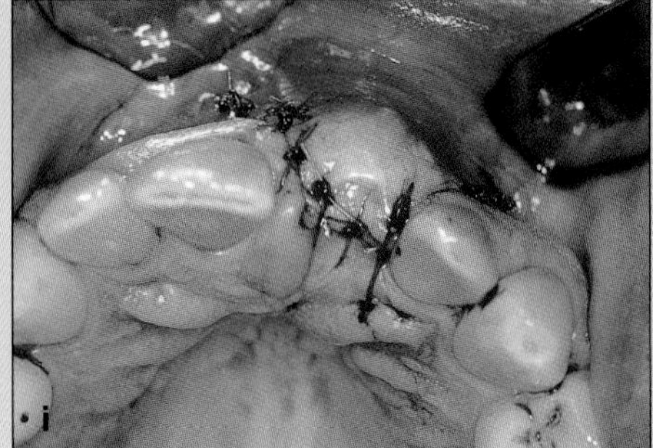

Figs 7-32g to 7-32i Additional activated PRP solution is applied and an absorbable collagen membrane is stabilized at the site by absorbing excess PRP solution, after which tension-free closure of the soft tissues is obtained.

Fig 7-32j Postoperative radiograph demonstrating bone graft fixation at the site.

Fig 7-32k Four-month postoperative view of site demonstrating excellent soft tissue healing. Enhanced soft tissue healing is observed with the use of PRP.

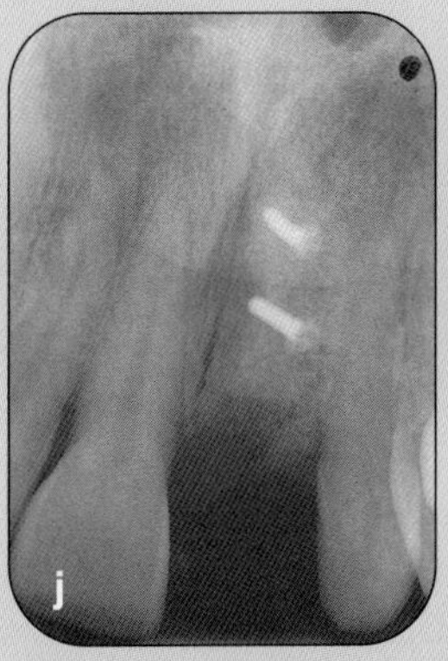

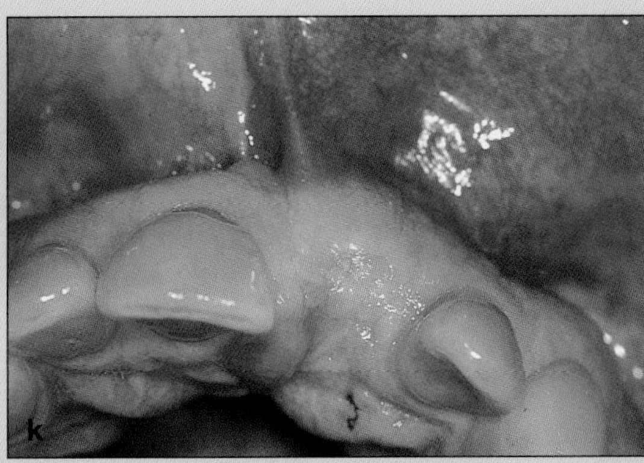

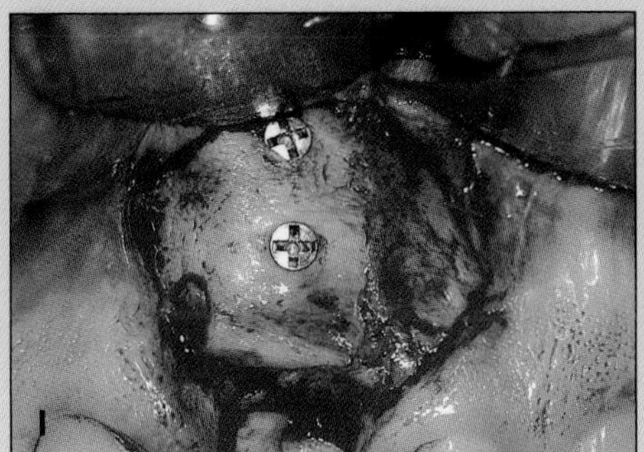

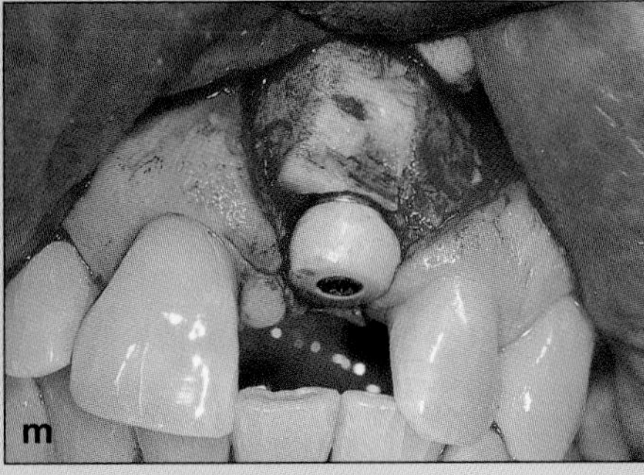

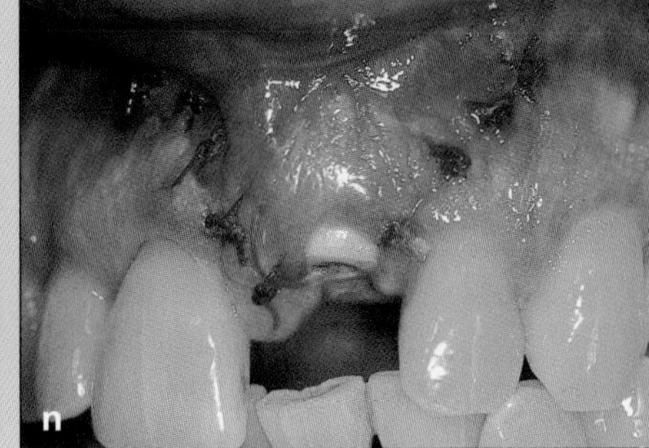

Figs 7-32l to 7-32n Upon re-entry for implant placement 4 months after bone grafting, clinical observation of advanced healing of the block and surrounding particulate bone grafts was observed. The block bone graft cannot be discerned from the surrounding particulate graft. Bio-Oss particles are not readily discernible within the particulate graft. Revascularization of the block graft is evidenced by its bleeding surface. A nonsubmerged implant with a custom tooth-form healing abutment (Peek) was placed, and tension-free soft tissue closure was obtained.

Figs 7-32o and 7-32p Eight-week postoperative clinical and radiographic views demonstrate stable hard and soft tissues at the site.

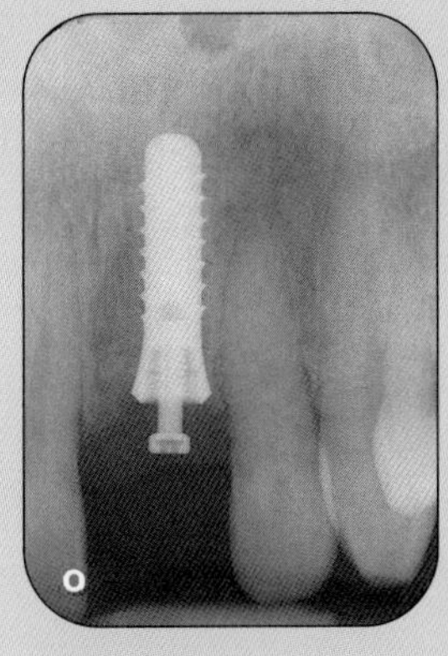

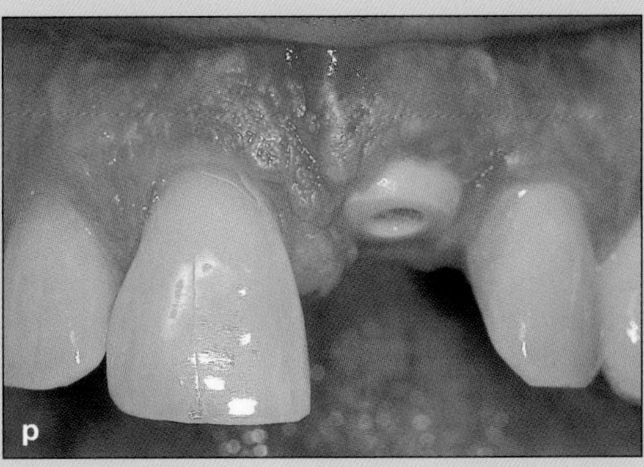

Figs 7-32q and 7-32r One-year post-restoration clinical and radiographic views of implant restoration demonstrate a stable and esthetically acceptable restoration. The loss of soft tissue volume around the implant restoration was associated with the pre-existing soft tissue edema secondary to tooth mobility observed prior to tooth removal. In this particular case, the patient declined the subepithelial connective tissue graft that was needed to idealize the gingival level. This highlights the fact that the enhanced wound healing observed with the use of PRP does not eliminate the need to follow surgical principles and standard treatment protocols for site development, as presented in this chapter. (Restorative dentistry by Dr Bob Cuckler, Homestead, FL.)

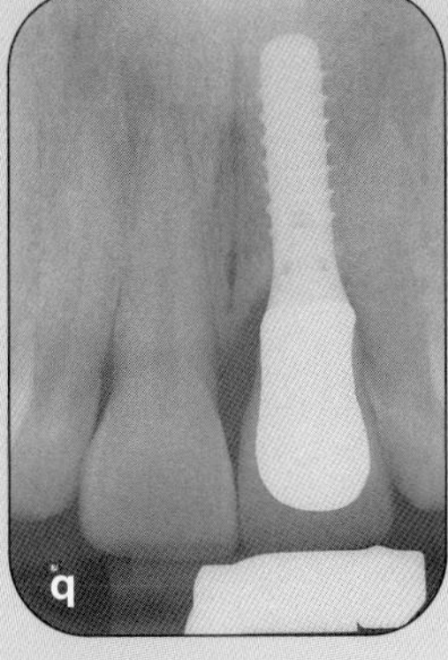

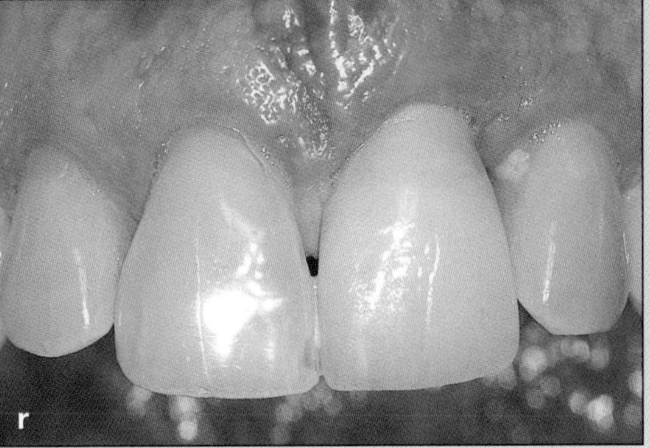

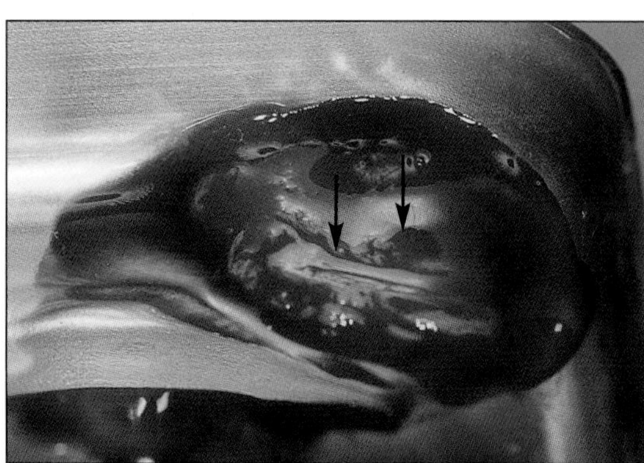

Fig 7-33 To take advantage of the theoretical effect of growth factors, free soft tissue grafts are moistened and stored in nonactivated PRP solution prior to their immobilization at the recipient site. Surface activation of the PRP solution usually is observed in the form of a thin coating of activated PRP on the surface of the graft *(arrows)*. This superficial activation of platelets may result from contact with tissue thromboplastin, thereby releasing growth factors.

Use of PRP to enhance outcomes in implant therapy: Soft tissue considerations

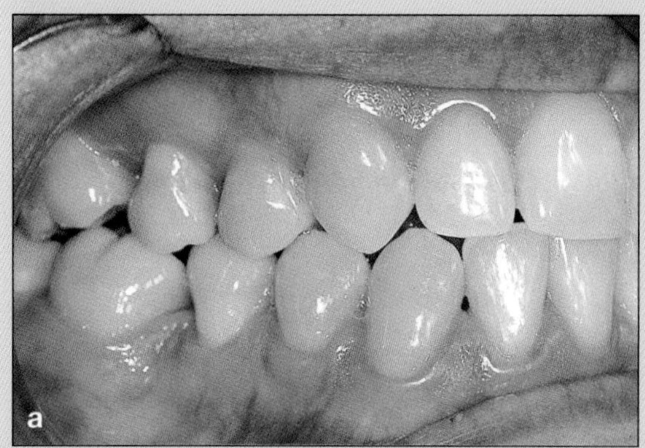

Fig 7-34a Preoperative view of recession defects involving the mandibular premolars and first molar. The prominence of the mesial root of the molar and the loss of interdental hard and soft tissue on the mesial and distal aspects of the second premolar are limitations to complete root coverage.

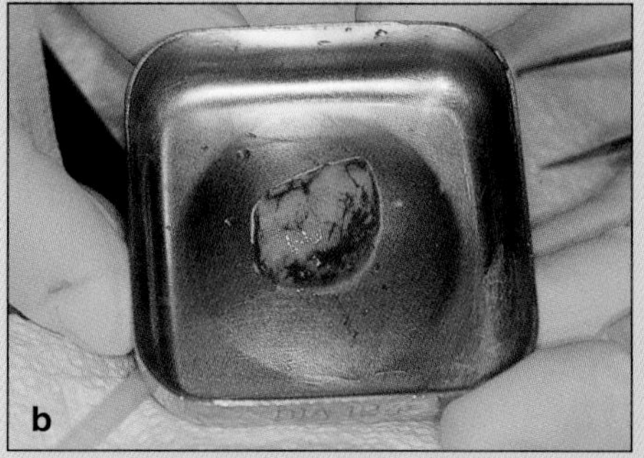

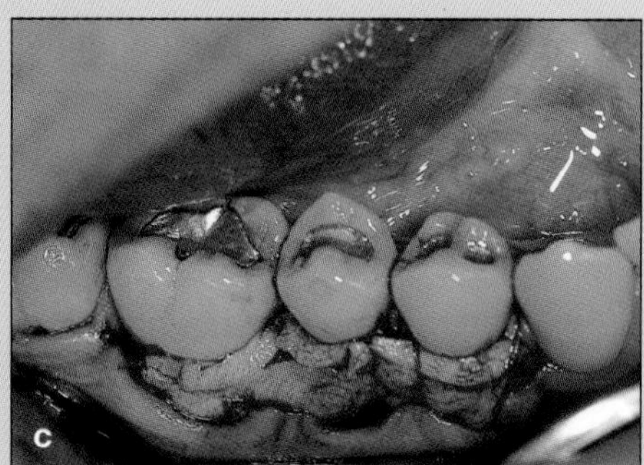

Figs 7-34b and 7-34c After recipient-site preparation, subepithelial grafts are moistened in nonactivated PRP solution prior to delivery and immobilization at the recipient site.

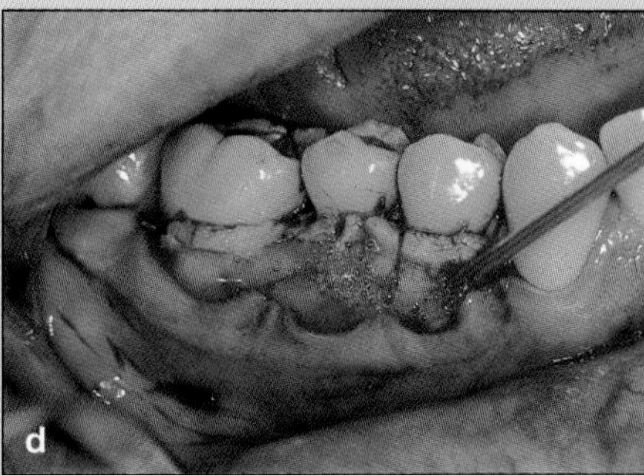

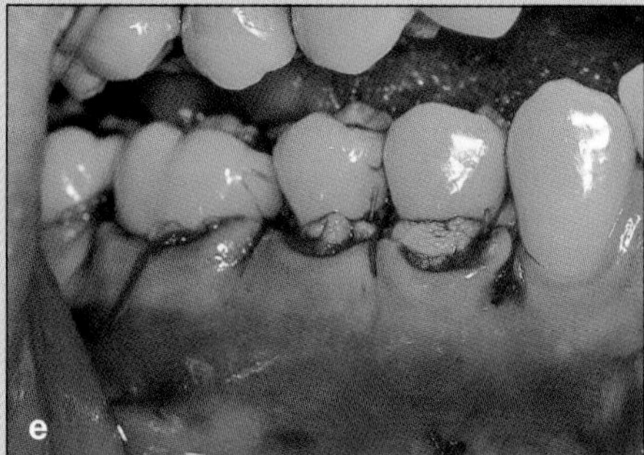

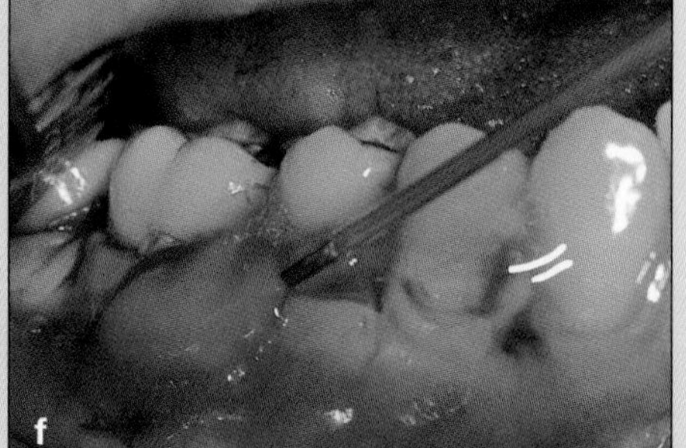

Figs 7-34d to 7-34f Next, a few drops of activated PRP solution are applied between the surface of the graft and the cover tissue, and pressure is immediately applied to expel any excess solution, thereby avoiding the formation of a thick clot between the graft and cover tissue. The cover tissue is secured with sutures, and activated PRP solution is applied topically as a growth factor–enriched wound dressing. A wound-sealing effect is achieved.

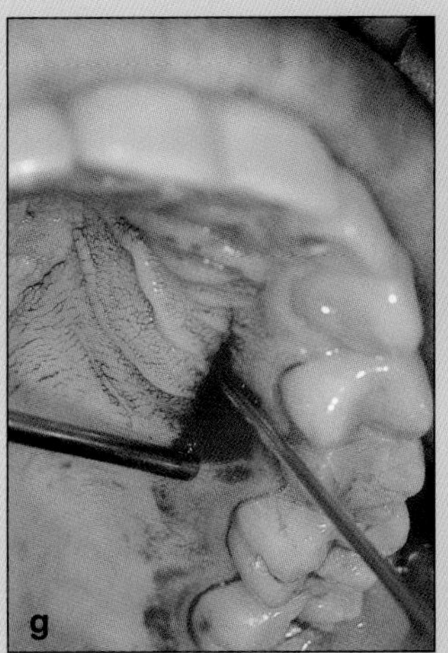
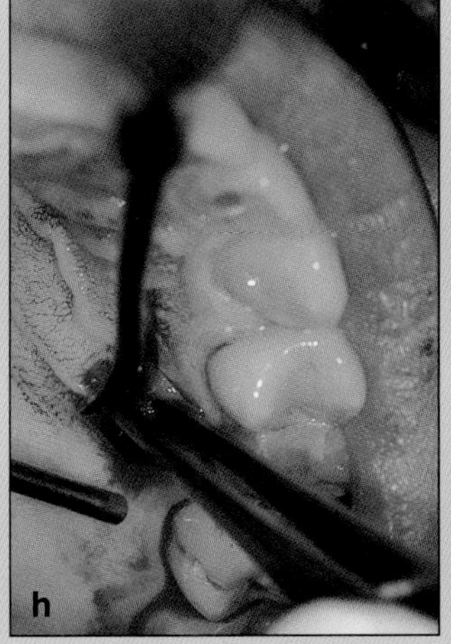
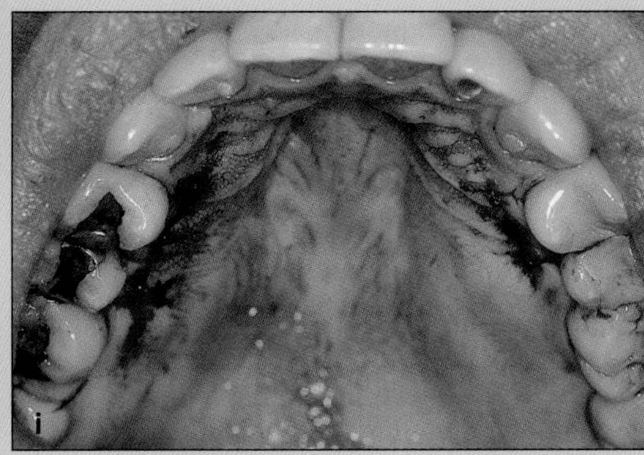

Figs 7-34g to 7-34i In this case, the remaining PRP solution was injected into the left palatal donor site. An absorbable collagen dressing was then immediately inserted, pressure was applied, and primary closure was obtained. The other donor site was treated in the same fashion except that PRP was not used.

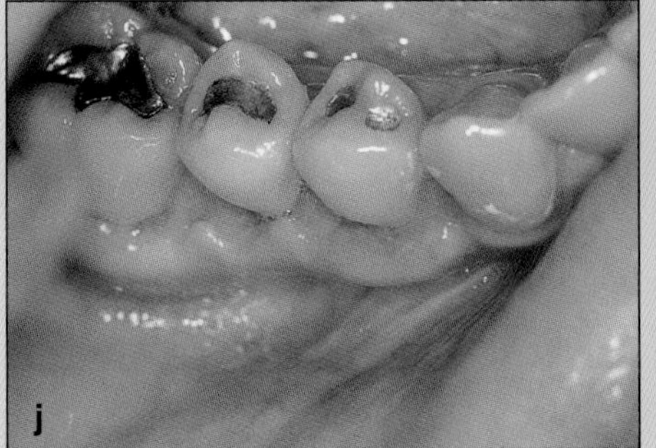
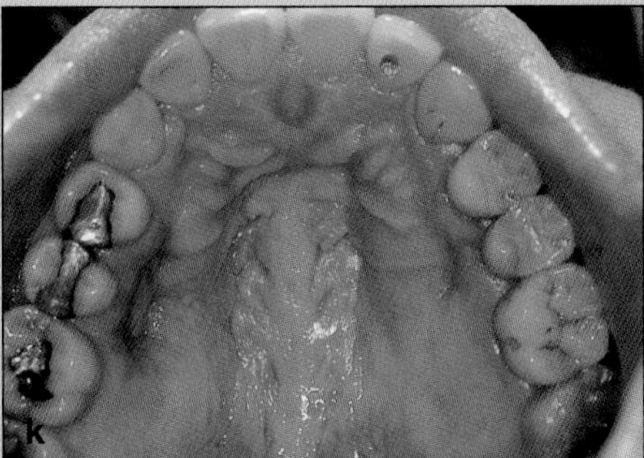
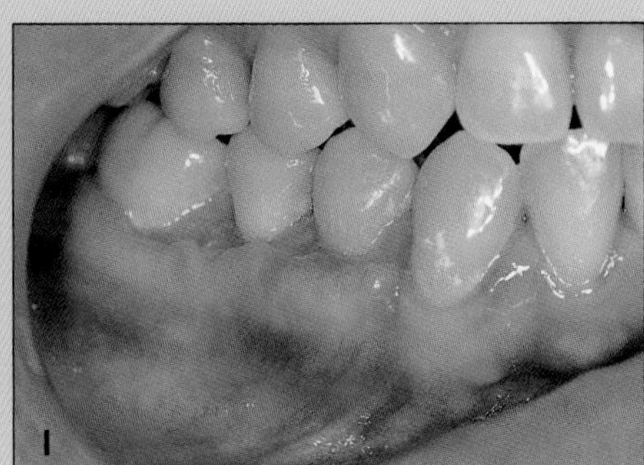

Figs 7-34j and 7-34k Ten-day postoperative view of donor sites demonstrates improved healing at the donor site where PRP was used.

Fig 7-34l Ten-day postoperative view of recipient site demonstrates accelerated graft incorporation and healing of the cover tissues.

Use of PRP to enhance outcomes in implant therapy: Soft tissue considerations

Figs 7-35a and 7-35b Upon exposure of submerged implants (Osteotite; 3i) placed 4 months earlier with sinus lift bone grafting, temporary healing abutments were secured and lateral advancement and papilla-regeneration maneuvers were performed to improve the volume of soft tissue in the buccal corridor and to create positive gingival architecture around the implants. PRP was injected under the flaps and in and around the emerging healing abutments after sutures were secured.

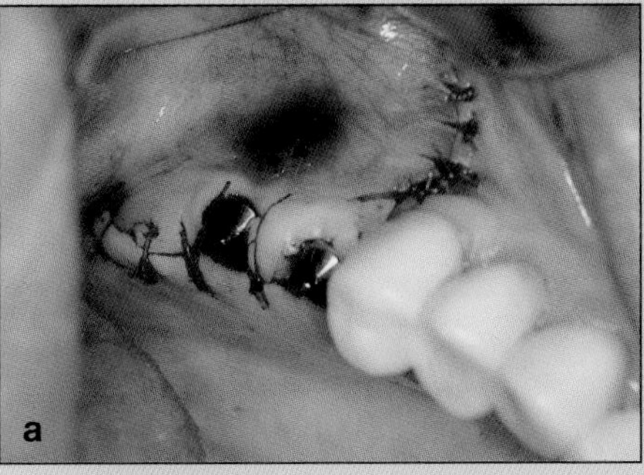
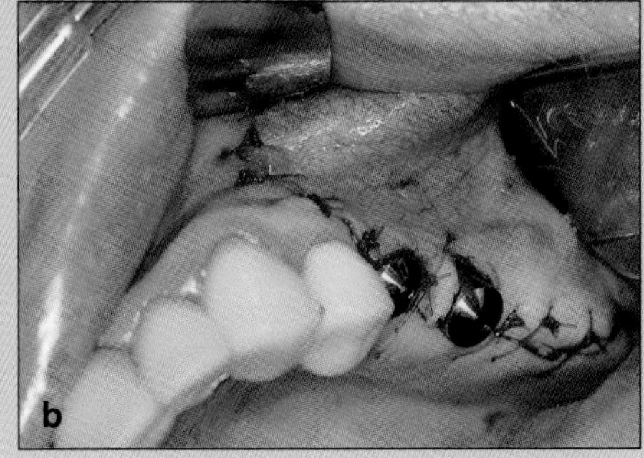

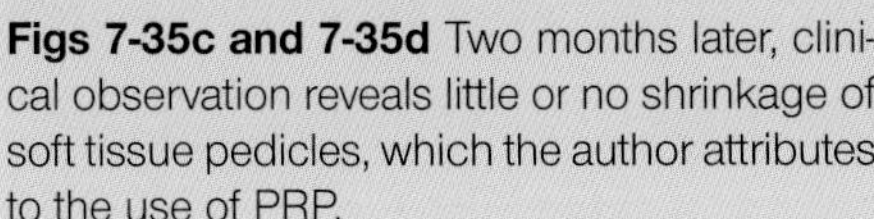

Figs 7-35c and 7-35d Two months later, clinical observation reveals little or no shrinkage of soft tissue pedicles, which the author attributes to the use of PRP.

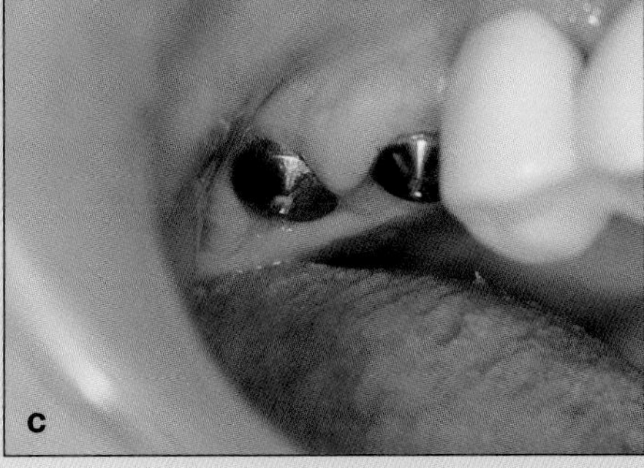
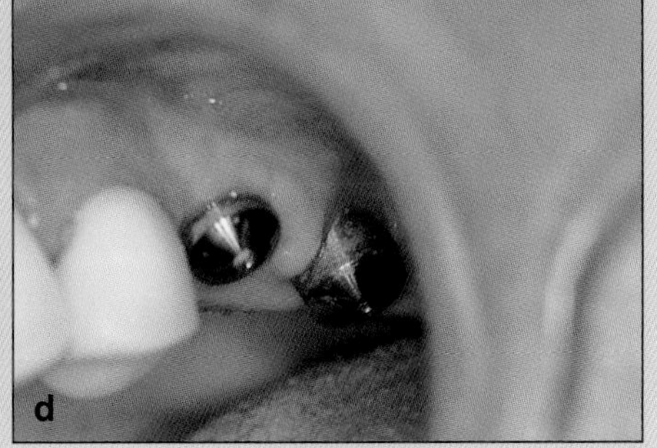

Use of PRP to enhance outcomes in implant therapy: Hard and soft tissue considerations

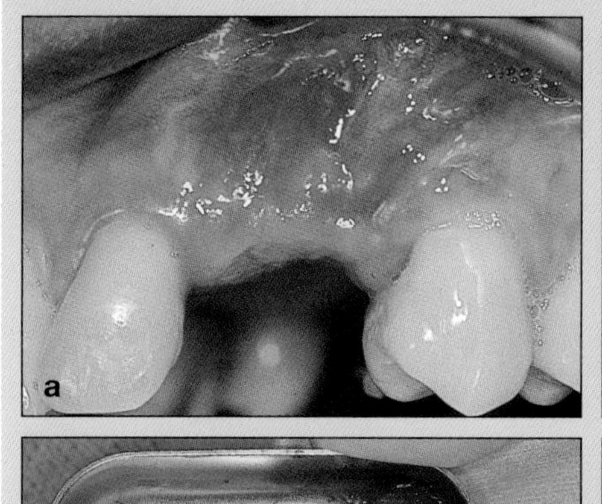

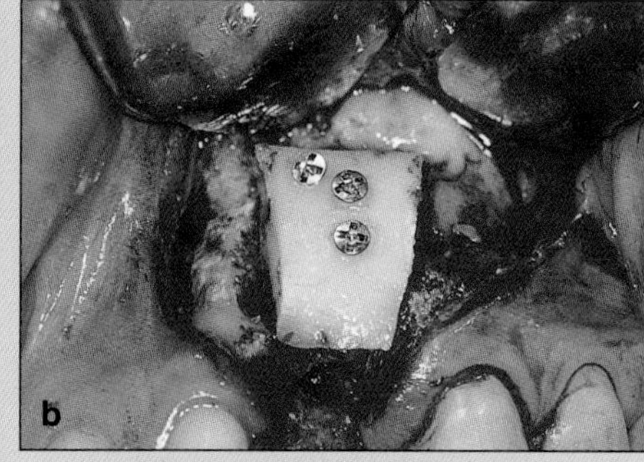

Fig 7-36a Preoperative view of compromised maxillary canine implant site after failed bone graft and implant. Note the large-volume combination hard and soft tissue esthetic ridge defect and chronic soft tissue inflammation at the site.

Fig 7-36b A corticocancellous block graft was secured at the prepared recipient site.

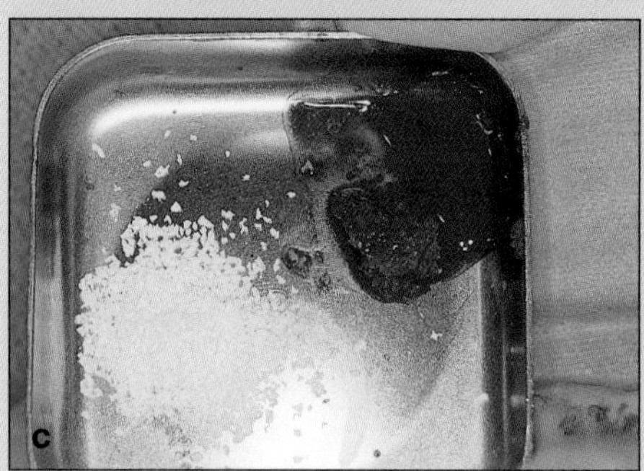

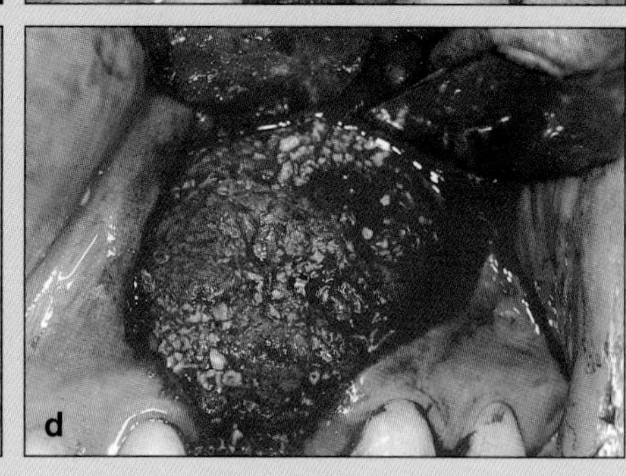

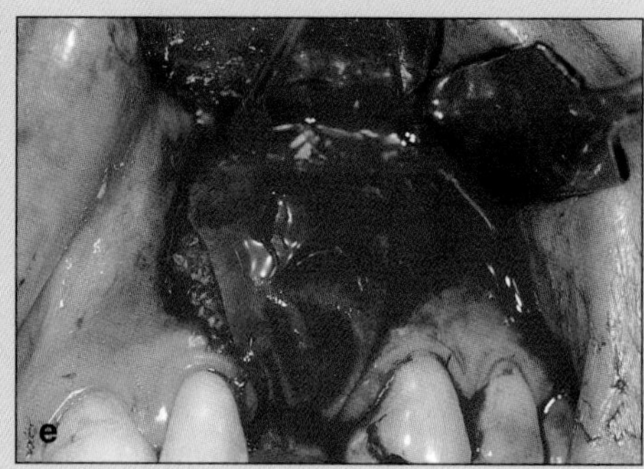

Figs 7-36c to 7-36e A mixture of Bio-Oss and autogenous cancellous bone previously stored in nonactivated PRP solution was moistened in activated PRP solution and delivered to the site. An absorbable collagen membrane was secured over the graft by absorbing additional activated PRP applied over the surface of the graft.

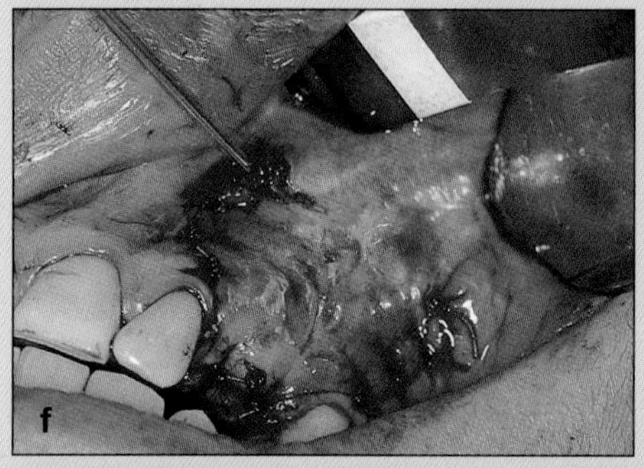

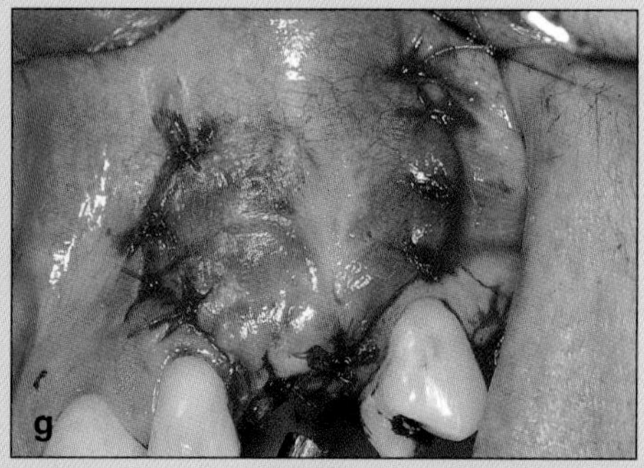

Figs 7-36f and 7-36g After tension-free soft tissue closure was obtained, a small amount of activated PRP solution was injected at the incision lines and pressure was immediately applied to expel any excess solution and to aid in hemostasis. Note that a thin layer of clotted PRP has sealed the incisions. A wound-sealing effect is achieved when PRP is used in this fashion.

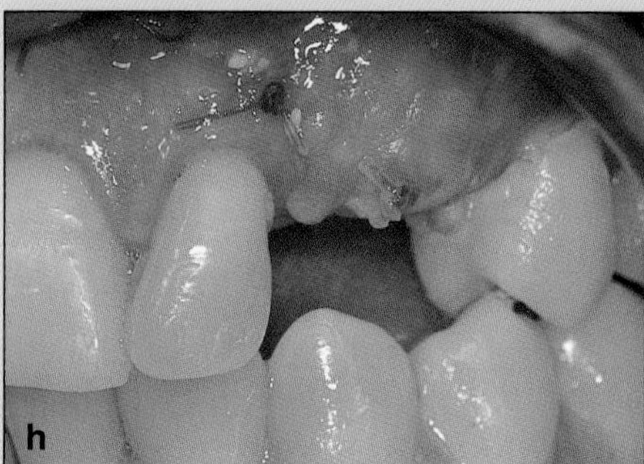

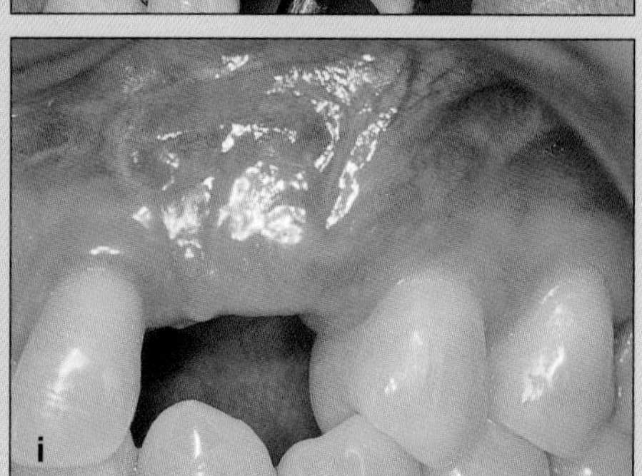

Fig 7-36h One-week postoperative view. Clinical observation of accelerated soft tissue healing is evident with negligible flap retraction.

Fig 7-36i Four-month postoperative view demonstrates negligible soft tissue shrinkage and resolution of soft tissue inflammation.

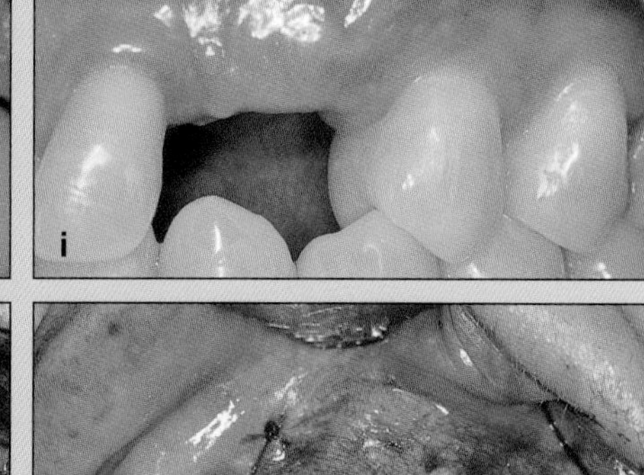

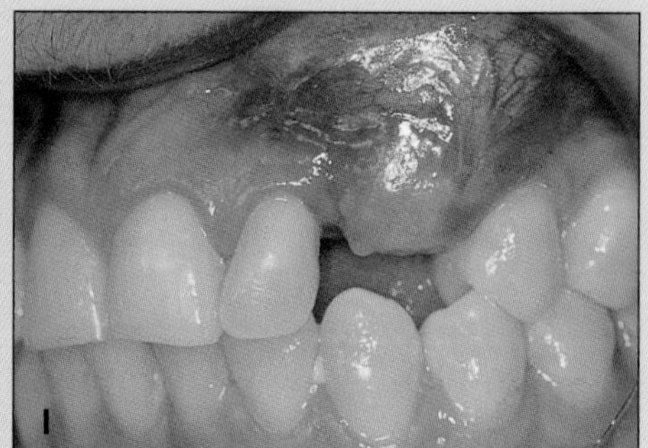

Figs 7-36j and 7-36k The site was re-entered 4 months after bone grafting for implant placement and subepithelial grafting to offset loss of soft tissue volume that usually follows hard tissue site development. PRP was again used to enhance healing of the soft tissue graft.

Fig 7-36l Four months following implant placement and subepithelial connective tissue grafting, negligible shrinkage of the graft or retraction of the coronally advanced cover flap occurred, resulting in vertical soft tissue augmentation not usually realized via these techniques. This was attributed to the use of PRP with both hard and soft tissue site development at this previously compromised implant site.

Conceptual Framework for Esthetic Implant-Site Development

A conceptual framework for esthetic implant-site development aids the surgeon in the selection and sequencing of the necessary site-development procedures required in esthetic implant therapy. Once the regenerative potential of the site(s) has been determined and the volume and nature of the defect in need of reconstruction has been classified, the surgeon must select the appropriate procedures, properly sequence them, and closely coordinate the surgical and restorative care to achieve the desired result. In addition, the surgeon must be able to estimate the number of procedures and total treatment time required for this process. This information is then shared with the patient, and realistic expectations are established. The author finds it useful to conceptually divide esthetic implant-site development into three distinct phases: initial, intermediate, and final site development. The author views these as three distinct opportunities for surgical intervention aimed at preserving or restoring hard and soft tissue volume and architecture at the site. The information below describes each of these conceptual phases and discusses the procedures most commonly performed at each. When treating complex esthetic cases with pre-existing alveolar ridge defects, surgical treatment planning can be simplified by organizing the indicated procedures into the appropriate conceptual phases of implant-site development.

Esthetic site-development opportunities

Initial site development

Initial site development represents the opportunity to preserve or restore hard and soft tissue volume prior to implant placement. The procedures most commonly performed during initial site development include orthodontic therapy, alveolar ridge preservation with the Bio-Col technique, staged hard and soft tissue grafting, simultaneous hard and soft tissue grafting, and associated prosthetic management.

Orthodontic therapy is used in initial site development for optimization of tooth positions, rotations, and axial inclinations to enhance esthetics. In addition, forced orthodontic eruption is used to restore lost hard and soft tissue around a compromised tooth or teeth in preparation for restoration or eventual removal. Alveolar ridge preservation is used to prepare for delayed implant placement or to prevent collapse of the soft tissues into extraction sites with large buccal wall defects, which require subsequent bone grafting. The most common indication for soft tissue augmentation during initial site development is to counteract soft tissue shrinkage that predictably occurs following the correction of large-volume hard tissue defects. In addition, soft tissue grafts are sometimes required prior to bone-grafting procedures to gain adequate soft tissue quality and bulk to ensure the success of the hard tissue graft. Soft tissue augmentation is also indicated during initial site development whenever a large-volume soft tissue defect is identified prior to placement of a nonsubmerged implant in an esthetic area. Finally, large-volume combination defects are reconstructed either in stages or simultaneously with autogenous block grafts and the VIP-CT flap during the initial site-development phase. The goal of prosthetic management during initial site development is to provide an interim provisional restoration that allows adequate soft tissue support, function, and esthetics while avoiding the transmission of micromotion to the surgical sites.

Intermediate site development

Intermediate site development represents the opportunity to develop the site during the period beginning with submerged implant placement and extending through the osseointegration period. The procedures commonly employed in this phase of site development include the Bio-Col alveolar ridge preservation technique with immediate implant placement, particulate bone grafts for the correction of small-volume hard tissue defects, one or more subepithelial connective tissue grafts for the correction of small- and large-volume soft tissue defects, the VIP-CT flap for correction of large-volume soft tissue defects simultaneously with submerged implant placement, and associated prosthetic management. Surgical indexing is performed to facilitate the fabrication of customized prosthetic components subsequently delivered by the surgeon at implant exposure. The goal of prosthetic management during the intermediate site-development phase is essentially the same as during initial site development: to preserve soft tissues by providing support to the marginal tissues and adjacent interdental papillae. Interim provisional restorations are designed to provide acceptable function and esthetics while avoiding the transmission of micromotion at sites where soft tissue grafting or guided bone regeneration procedures were performed simultaneously with implant placement. Subsequent to initial osseointegration of the underlying implant or maturation of the augmented soft tissues, the provisional restoration can be modified to begin forming the final soft tissue architecture at the site.

Table 7-1 Site-development opportunities: Sequencing, timing, selection, and duration

Treatment period	Treatment timing	Procedures most commonly performed	Treatment duration
Initial site development	Prior to implant placement	Hard tissue grafting Soft tissue grafting Extraction-site management Prosthetic soft tissue management	Up to 12 months
Intermediate site development	Implant placement through osseointegration period	Hard tissue grafting Soft tissue grafting Extraction-site management Prosthetic soft tissue management	6 weeks to 9 months
Final site development	Transmucosal emergence of implant through final restoration	Abutment connection Prosthetic-guided soft tissue healing Soft tissue grafting Esthetic soft tissue resurfacing	Up to 4 months
Recall phase	Recall period	Soft tissue grafting Esthetic soft tissue resurfacing	Variable

Final site development

Final site development begins with transmucosal emergence of the implant and ends with delivery of the final restoration. The procedures most commonly employed during final site development include conservative exposure techniques associated with abutment connection, soft tissue grafting for the correction of small-volume soft tissue defects, prosthetic-guided soft tissue techniques, and laser soft tissue sculpting and resurfacing. Due to recipient-site limitations, only small-volume esthetic soft tissue defects or minor soft tissue irregularities should be routinely corrected in conjunction with abutment connection, as discussed in chapter 5. The surgeon should also realize that a nonsubmerged implant is always placed during final site development; therefore, as previously discussed, all site-development procedures other than correction of small-volume soft tissue defects should be performed prior to nonsubmerged implant placement in esthetic areas. Surgical exposure of submerged or semi-submerged implants in esthetic areas should be performed via a conservative U-shaped peninsula flap or tissue-punch technique, as discussed in chapter 3. Prosthetic management during this phase is aimed at the early introduction of anatomically correct prosthetic components to initiate guided soft tissue healing. Custom abutments and provisional restorations, anatomic healing abutments, and custom tooth-form healing abutments are used for this purpose. Finally, the CO_2 laser is used during final site development when precision sculpting and resurfacing of the soft tissues is needed to re-establish natural scalloped soft tissue architecture and eliminate surface irregularities that detract from esthetic soft tissue appearance.

Recall phase

Finally, additional site-development procedures are sometimes necessary after final restoration for correction of hard or soft tissue defects arising during the recall period. The most common soft tissue problem that develops during this period is soft tissue recession. Coverage of an exposed restorative margin or abutment surface and masking of any discoloration that can be seen through thin buccal tissues is generally managed with a subepithelial connective tissue graft secured in either a closed (pouch) recipient site or, in certain cases, underneath a coronally advanced flap. The choice of technique for recipient-site preparation will depend on the criteria discussed in chapter 5. Correction of soft tissue recession should be performed as soon as possible once it is detected. Failure to do so may jeopardize the potential to correct the resultant larger defect because of limitations in the recipient site. In these cases the implant may need to be resubmerged. The VIP-CT flap is the preferred method for resubmerging an implant to correct a large-volume recession defect. However, a subepithelial connective tissue graft can also be used to correct such a defect providing vestibular depth is adequate to gain sufficient coronal advancement of the cover flaps.

Case 1: Replacement of failing maxillary incisors with individual esthetic implant restorations

Case history

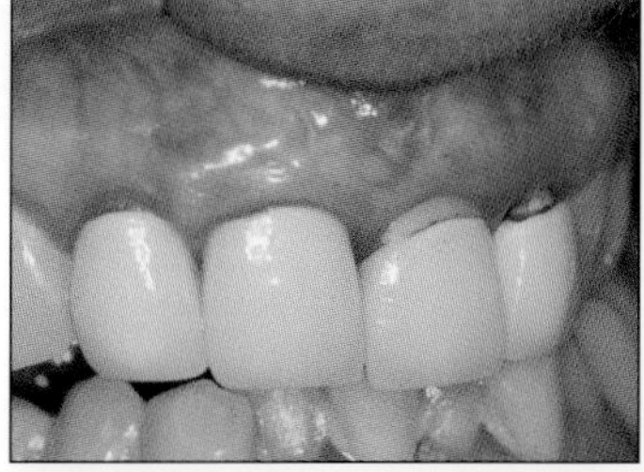
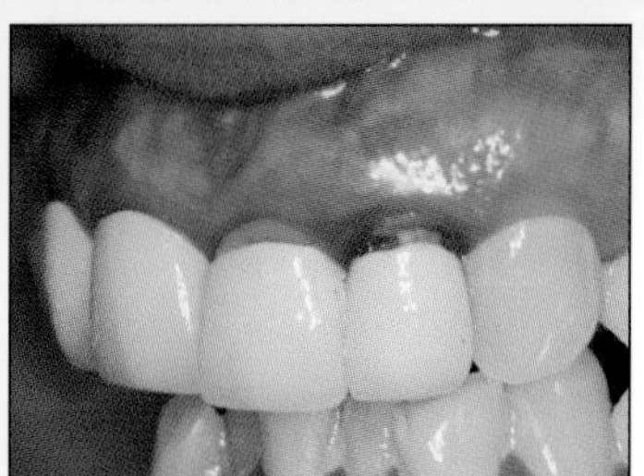
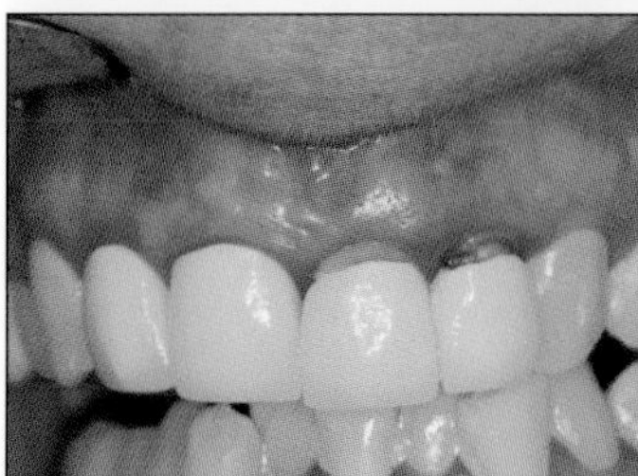
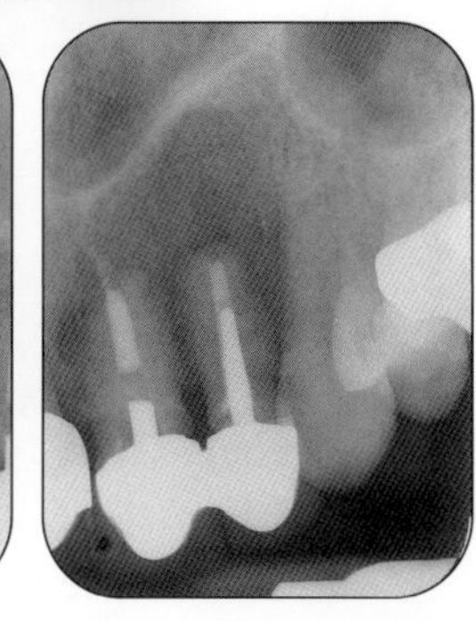

This 61-year-old patient presented with failing maxillary central and lateral incisors. Clinical evaluation revealed tooth mobility, soft tissue edema, and recurrent decay. The patient was concerned about her appearance and function during treatment as well as total treatment time. In addition, she desired individual restorations. The treatment plan was for removal of the four incisors using the Bio-Col technique in preparation for delayed implant placement or for further site development if osseous remodeling changes or soft tissue shrinkage was evident. Tooth removal was coordinated so as to immediately follow a visit where the restorative dentist reduced the failing teeth to a subgingival yet supraosseous level and fabricated a provisional fixed partial denture supported by the adjacent canine abutments with ovate pontic incisors.

Initial site development

3 months

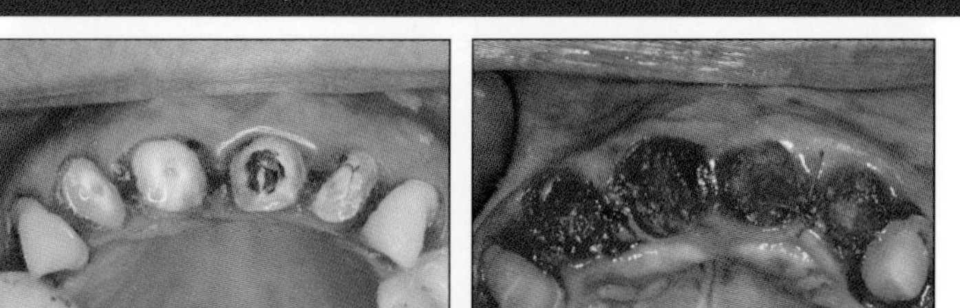

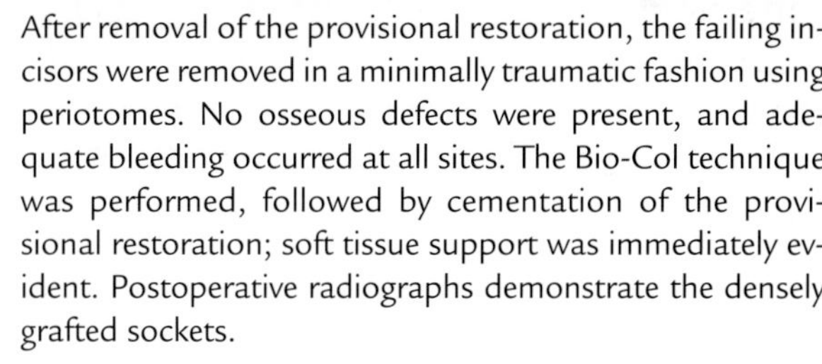

After removal of the provisional restoration, the failing incisors were removed in a minimally traumatic fashion using periotomes. No osseous defects were present, and adequate bleeding occurred at all sites. The Bio-Col technique was performed, followed by cementation of the provisional restoration; soft tissue support was immediately evident. Postoperative radiographs demonstrate the densely grafted sockets.

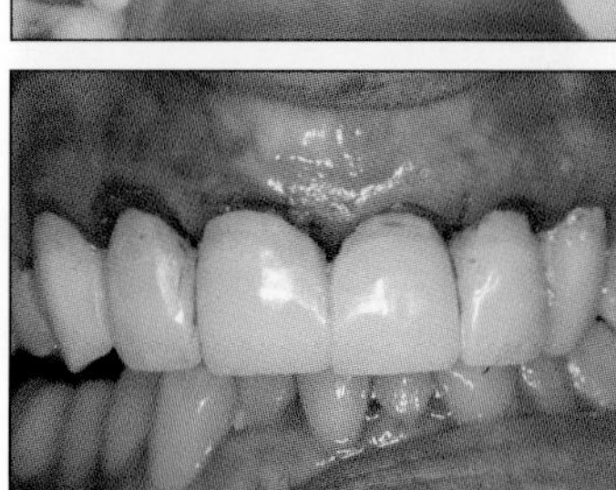
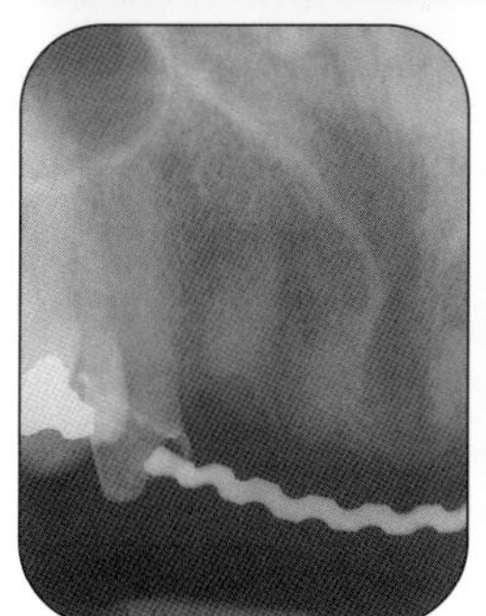
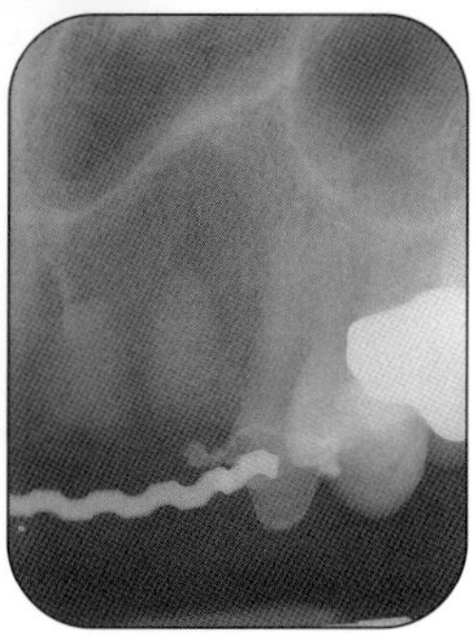

Intermediate site development 3 months

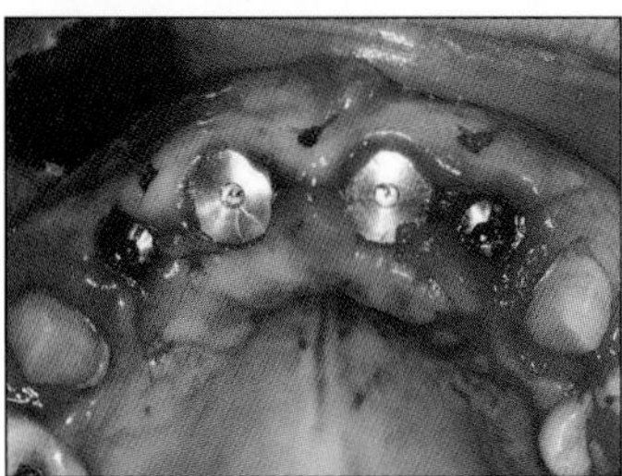
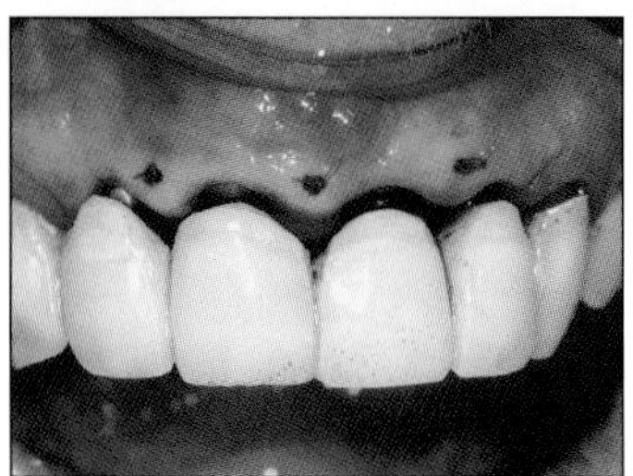
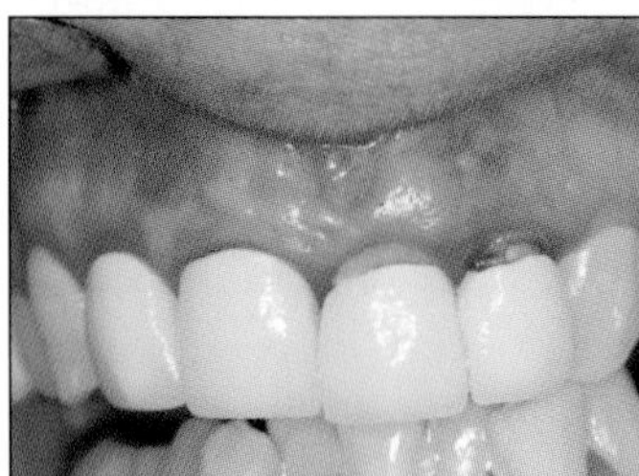
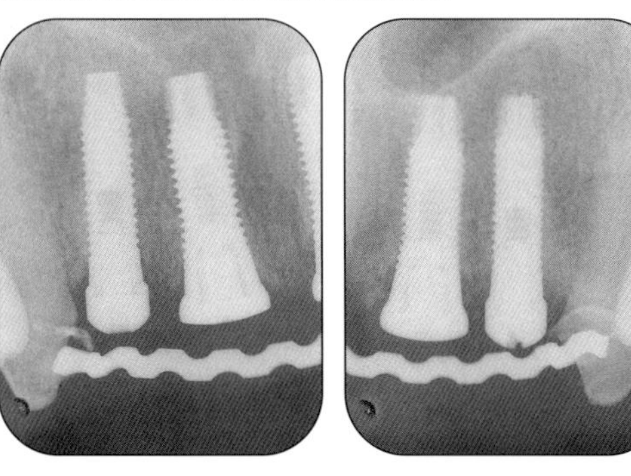

Three months following tooth removal, one-piece nonsubmerged implants and micro-mini implants were used to replace the central and lateral incisors, respectively. Healing abutments were immediately connected to the small-diameter hex-topped lateral incisor implants so that they were also placed in a non-submerged approach. No flap was elevated, and no incisions were made. Vertical mattress sutures were used in the inter-implant areas to tent up the papillary tissues prior to try-in, adjustment, and cementation of the provisional restoration. Radiographs taken 3 months after implant placement demonstrate further incorporation of the Bio-Oss grafts, evidence of osseointegration, and maintenance of adequate inter-implant bone width to support the overlying papillae.

Final site development 4 months

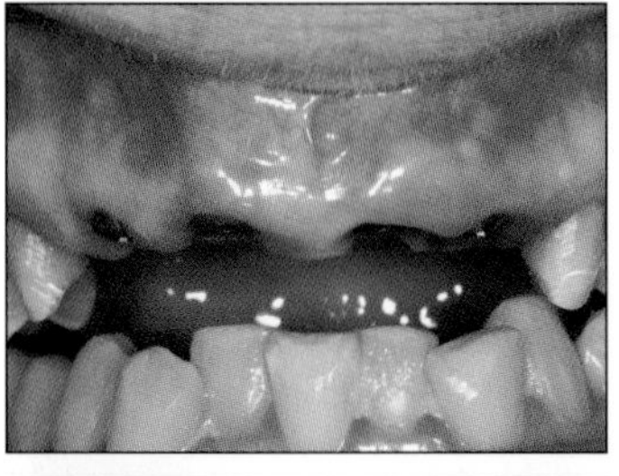
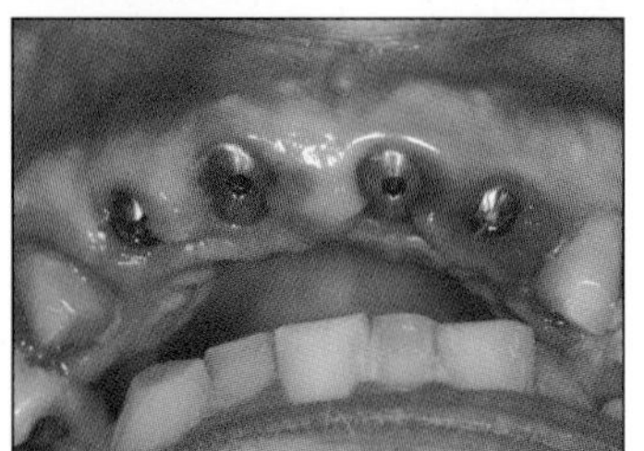
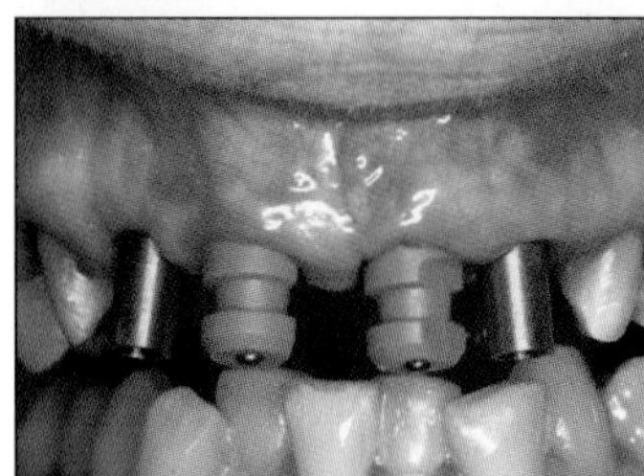
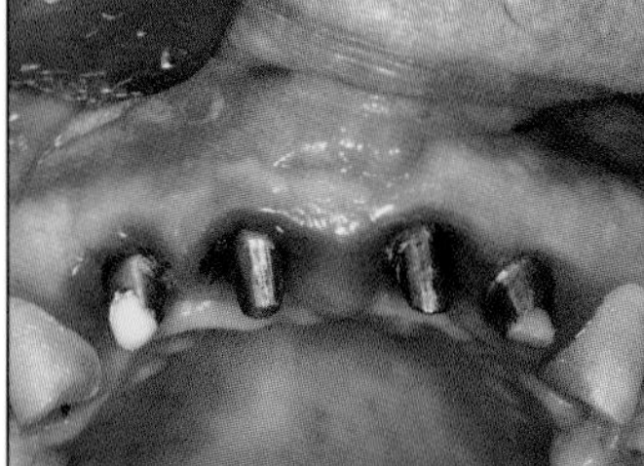
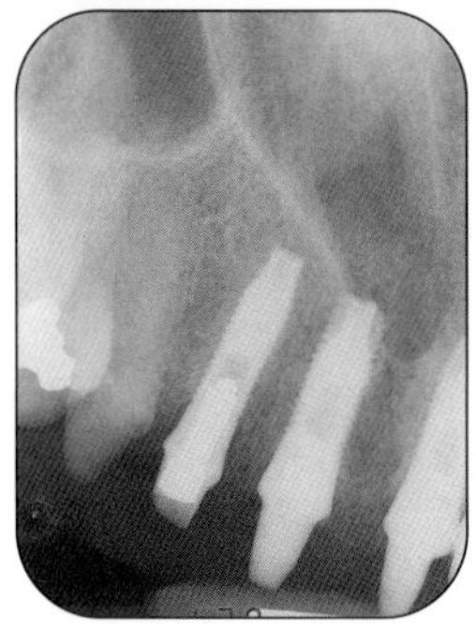
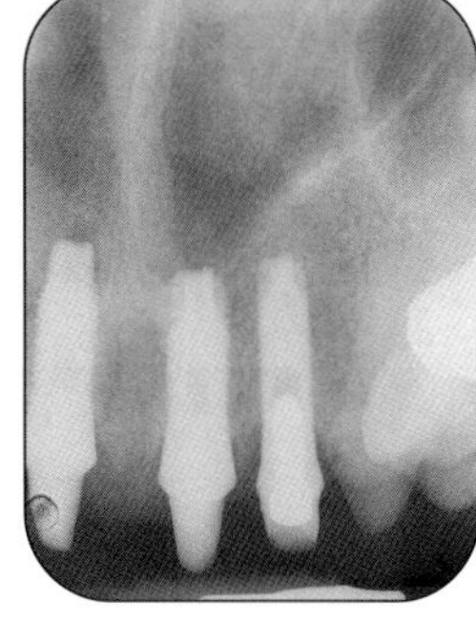
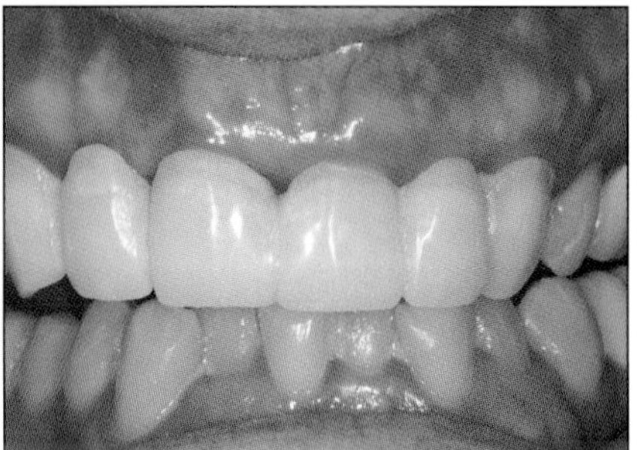

Three months following implant placement, the provisional fixed partial denture was removed and impressions were obtained. Subsequently, the provisional restoration was relined over the implant abutments, polished, and cemented. Four months were allowed for guided soft tissue healing and stabilization of the tissue levels in this case. During this time, the importance of oral hygiene was reinforced by the restorative dentist until all soft tissue inflammation was resolved.

Final result

Total: 10 months

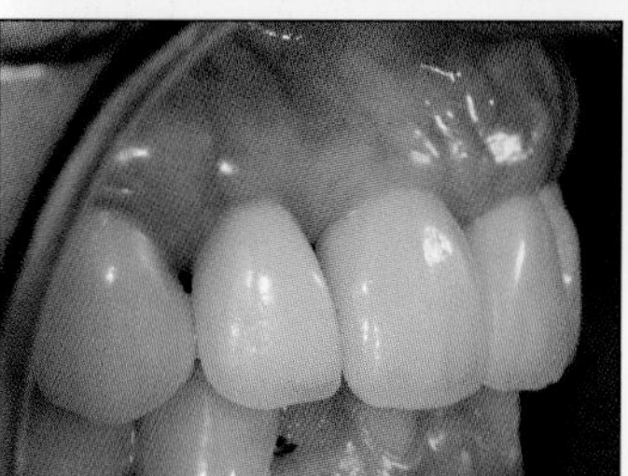
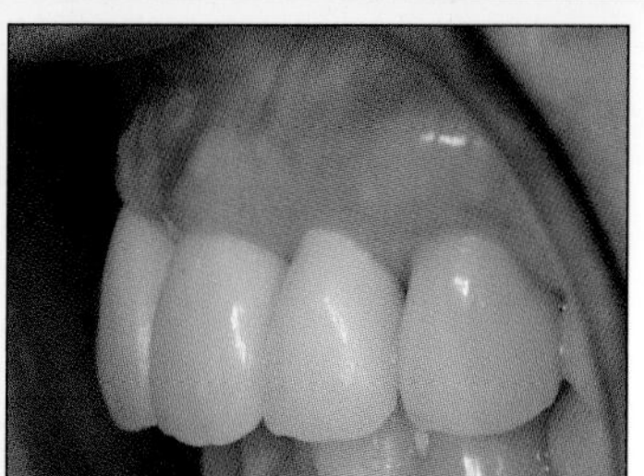
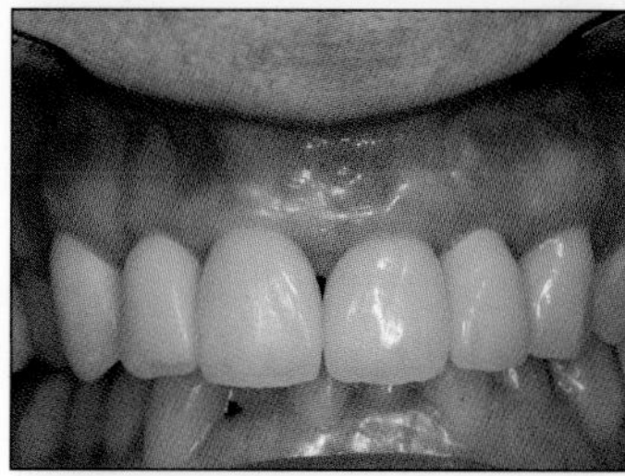
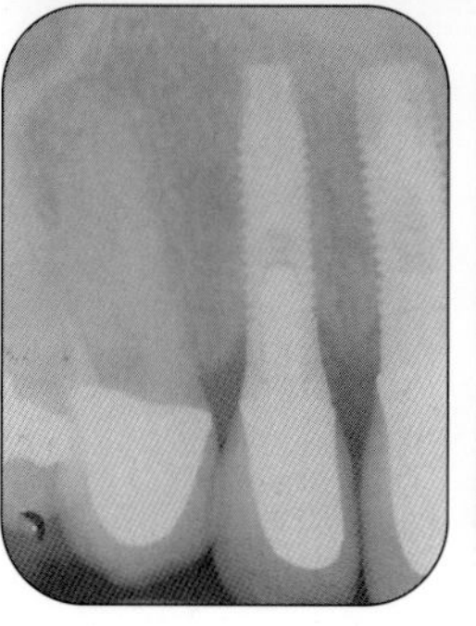
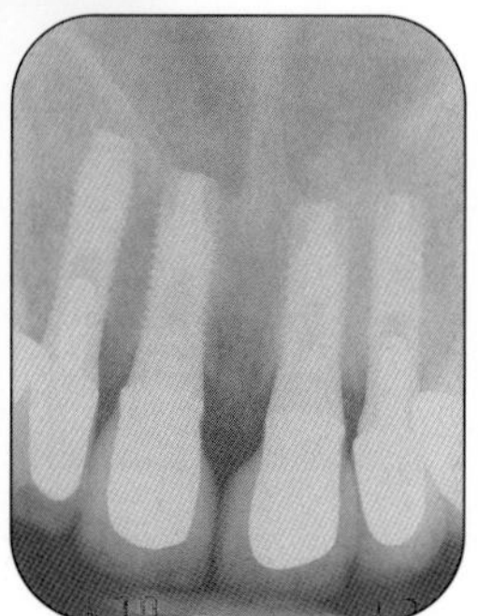
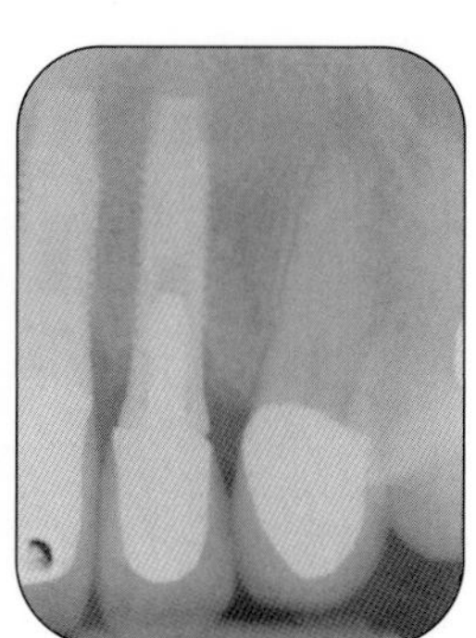

Two surgical procedures and a total treatment time of 10 months were required to replace the failing maxillary incisors with individual esthetic implant replacements. This case emphasizes the importance of close coordination between surgical and restorative care in the delivery of esthetic implant replacements. Prosthetic support for the soft tissues was scheduled prior to tooth removal and during the osseointegration period. Despite the use of a nonsubmerged approach, additional prosthetic refinements were accomplished after abutment connection and sufficient time for stabilization of the soft tissues was allowed. Persistent inflammation associated with inadequate oral hygiene was also managed through patient education in the final site-development phase, thereby delaying delivery of the final restorations. The clinical decision to delay implant placement was based on reducing the esthetic risk posed by tooth mobility and associated edema of the marginal gingival tissues even though immediate implant placement was feasible and consistent with the patient's desires. The final result demonstrates harmonious dental esthetics with a healthy, natural-looking gingival appearance. The postoperative radiographs demonstrate preservation of hard tissue anatomy at the sites. (Restoration by Dr Larry Stein, Miami, FL.)

Case 2: Staged reconstruction of large-volume combination esthetic ridge defect for replacment of maxillary canine

Case History

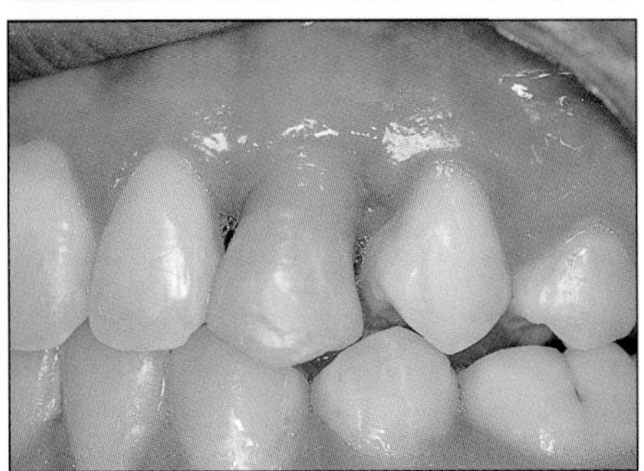

This 19-year-old patient presented with a failing maxillary canine and a compromised lateral incisor secondary to loss of supporting bone as a complicating factor resulting from previous orthodontic eruption of the impacted canine. Initial treatment plan included forced orthodontic eruption of the failing canine prior to its removal. Subsequent re-evaluation of the lateral incisor would determine whether it should be retained or removed prior to proceeding with hard and soft tissue site development, implant placement, and esthetic restoration.

Initial site development — 12 months

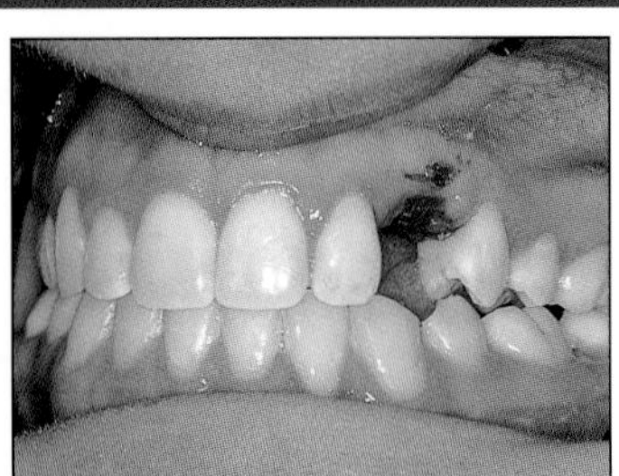

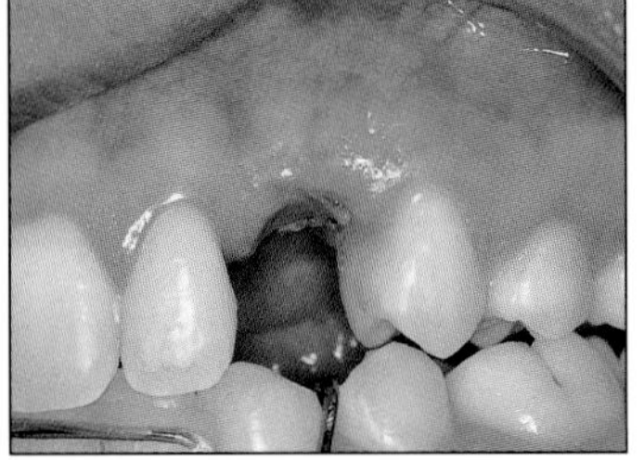

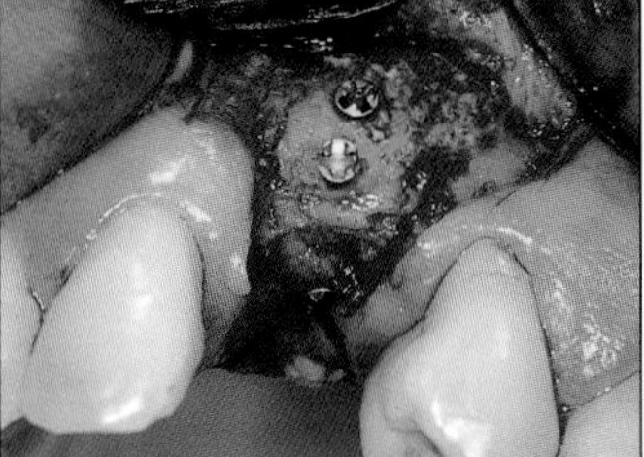

Initial site development included forced orthodontic eruption as a hard and soft tissue site-development technique. After 3 months of orthodontic eruption, an additional 2 months were allotted for stabilization of the tooth and maturation of the bone and soft tissues at the site prior to tooth removal. Mobility of the lateral incisor resolved, and interdental bone and soft tissue levels were greatly improved. As a result, a decision was made to retain the lateral incisor. The Bio-Col technique was performed in conjunction with removal of the canine to maintain the reconstructive soft tissue envelope in the presence of an unforeseeable buccal wall defect in preparation for subsequent hard and soft tissue site development. Three months were allotted for healing prior restoring missing hard tissue volume with autogenous block and particulate grafts. A curvilinear-beveled flap was used for access for autogenous block and particulate bone grafting performed to restore missing hard tissue anatomy at the recipient site previously improved by the orthodontic eruption of the canine. A period of 4 months was allotted for maturation of the graft.

Intermediate site development — 4 months

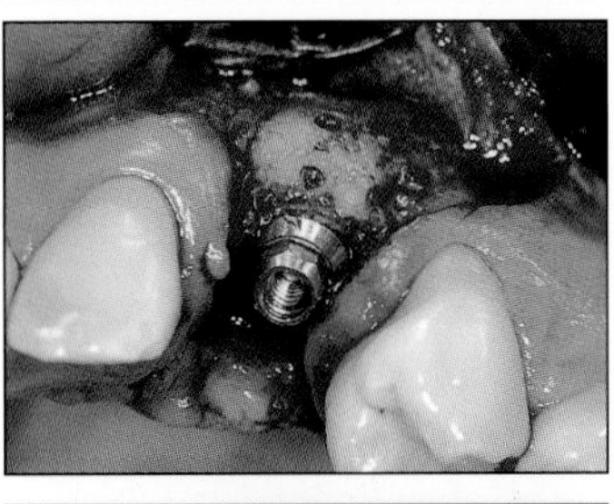

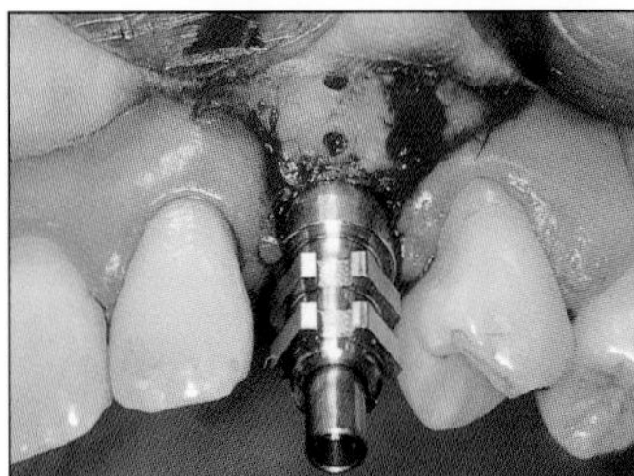

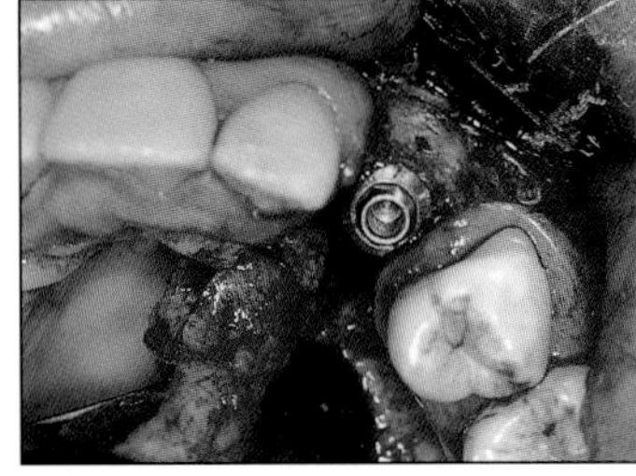

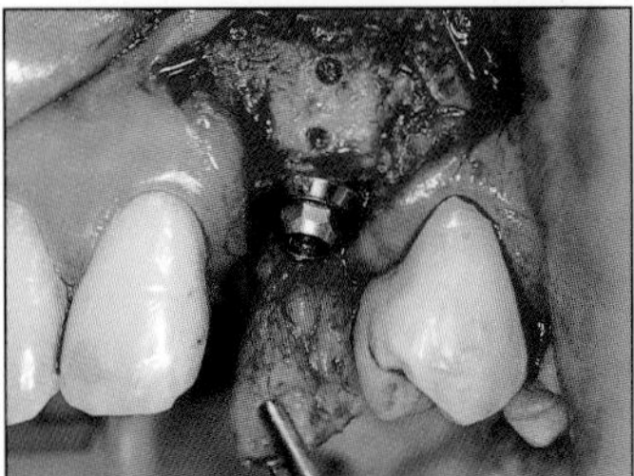

A full thickness–partial thickness curvilinear flap was used for access for placement of a one-piece nonsubmerged implant, and a surgical index was performed. Subsequently, a VIP-CT flap was developed at the adjacent palatal donor site, rotated over the neck of the implant, and secured to the periosteum at the periphery of the recipient site.

Intermediate site development *(continued)*

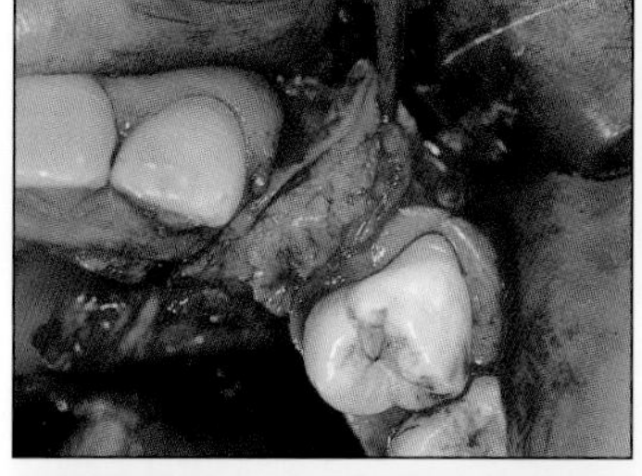
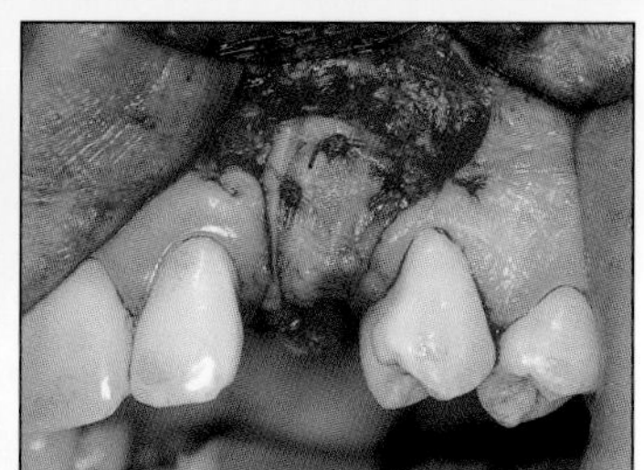
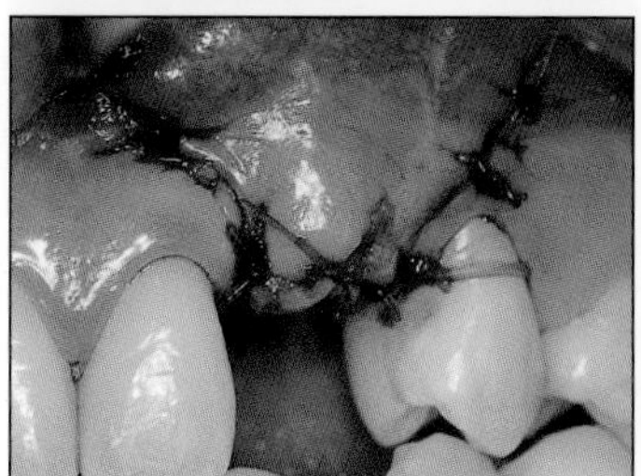
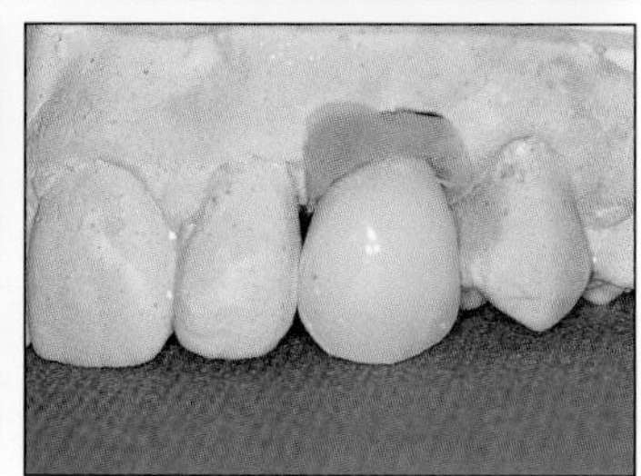

Coronal advancement of the access flap was facilitated by tension-releasing cutback incisions, and tension-free closure was accomplished. Submerging a one-piece implant that was designed to be placed in a nonsubmerged fashion with the VIP-CT flap effectively expanded the soft tissue envelope at the site. After 3 months of healing, an impression was taken of the site to enable an accurate soft tissue mask to be added to the implant-analog cast. Four months were allowed for osseointegration.

Final site development — 3 months

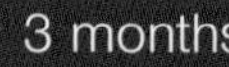

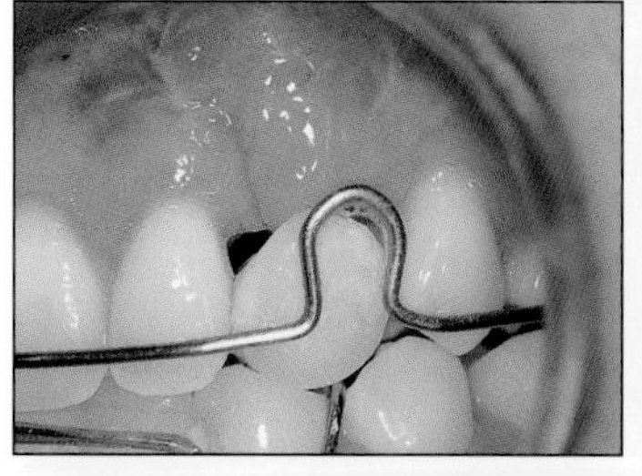
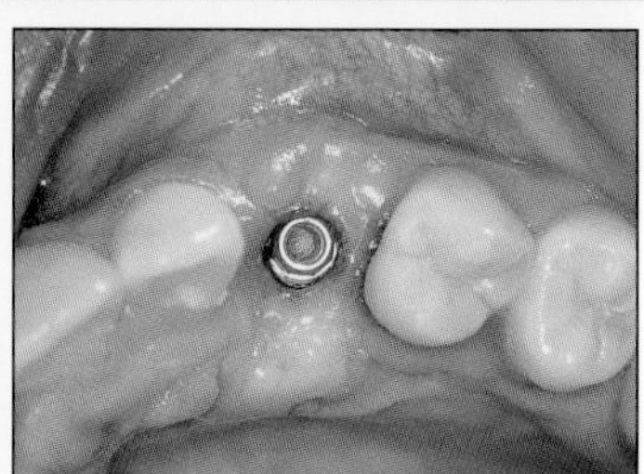
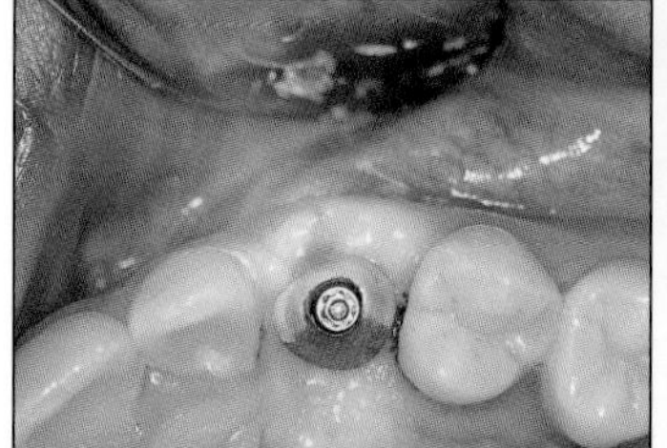
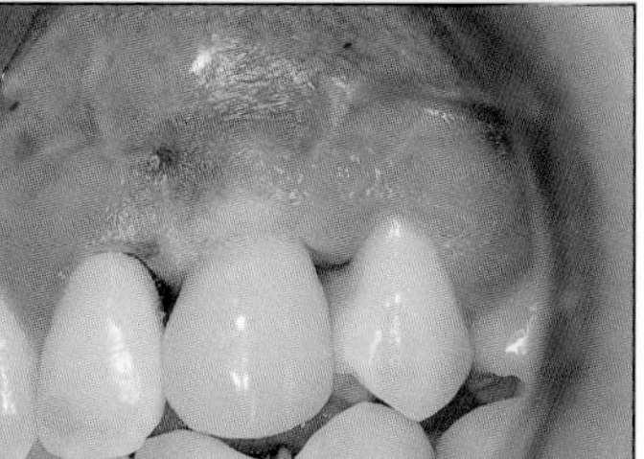

The implant was exposed through a conservative tissue-punch approach. A custom abutment and provisional restoration was delivered, and laser soft tissue resurfacing was performed to blend the soft tissue with the adjacent areas. An additional 3 months were allotted for guided soft tissue healing prior to final impression and delivery of the final restoration.

Final result — Total: 19 months

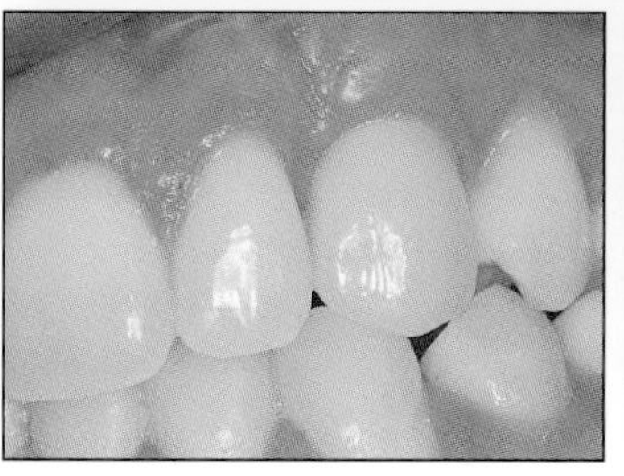
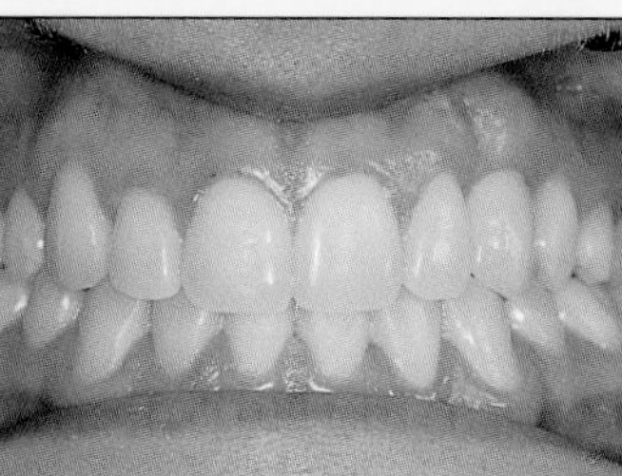

Total treatment time was 19 months. Close coordination with the restorative dentist and orthodontist was required for management of interim provisional restorations to avoid transmission of micromotion to the surgical sites. The final result was an inconspicuous implant replacement and the unexpected salvage of the adjacent compromised lateral incisor. Use of the VIP-CT flap to intentionally submerge the one-piece implant resulted in significant vertical soft tissue augmentation. (Orthodontics by Dr Idalia Lastra, Coral Gables, FL; restoration by Dr Aquiles Mas, Hialeah, FL.)

Case 3: Staged reconstruction of large-volume combination esthetic ridge defect for replacement of central incisor

Case history

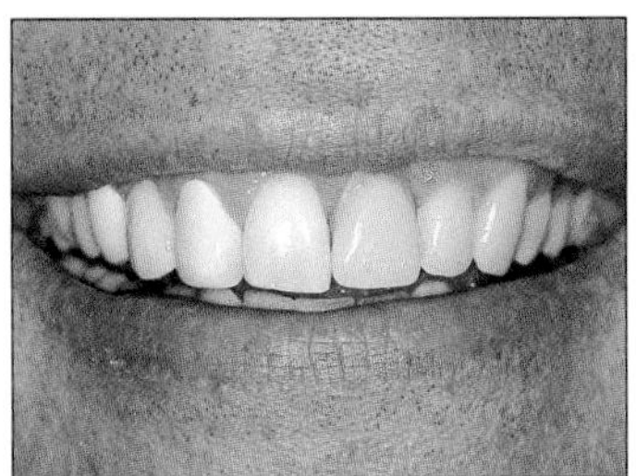
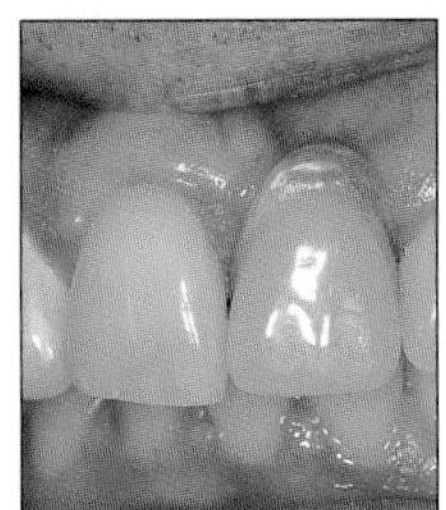
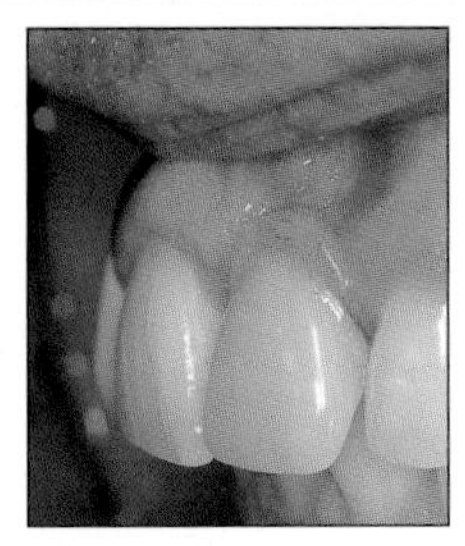
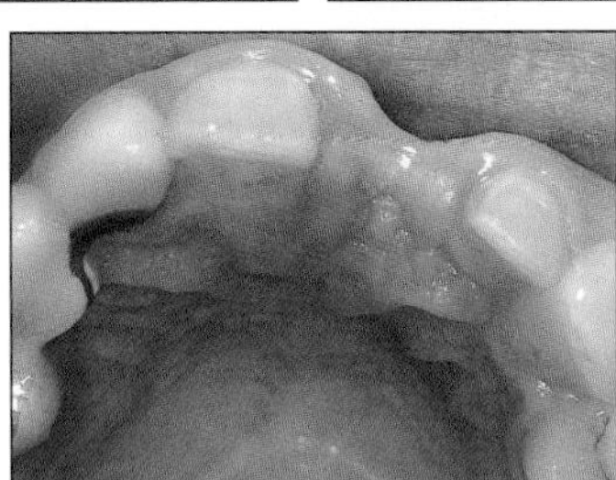

This 47-year-old male patient presented 3 months after his left central incisor was removed secondary to failed endodontic intervention. A large-volume combination hard and soft tissue esthetic ridge defect resulted. The patient demonstrated considerable gingival show in the relaxed smile position. His primary concerns included the ability to function and his appearance during the surgical phases of treatment. The current interim provisional restoration included a tissue-colored flange to camouflage the ridge defect. He also wanted to be assured that acceptable esthetics could be achieved with an implant restoration.

Initial site development

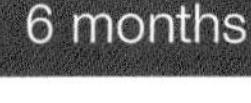
6 months

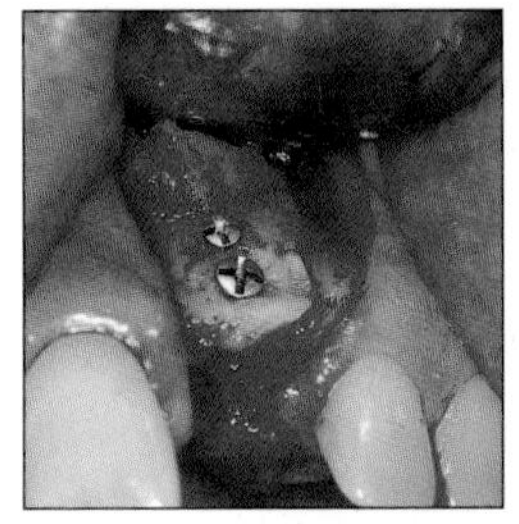
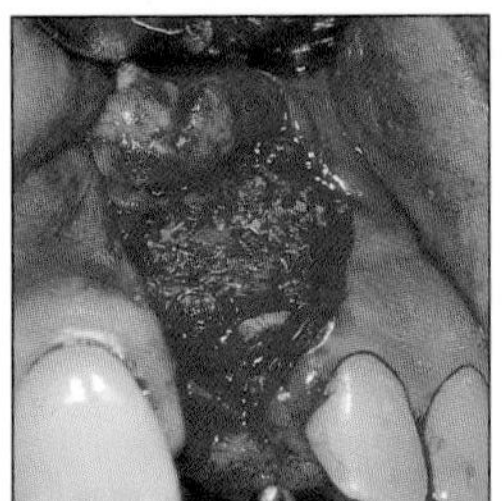
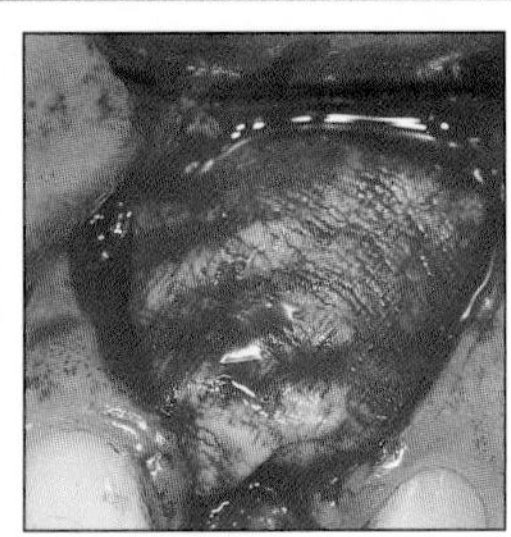
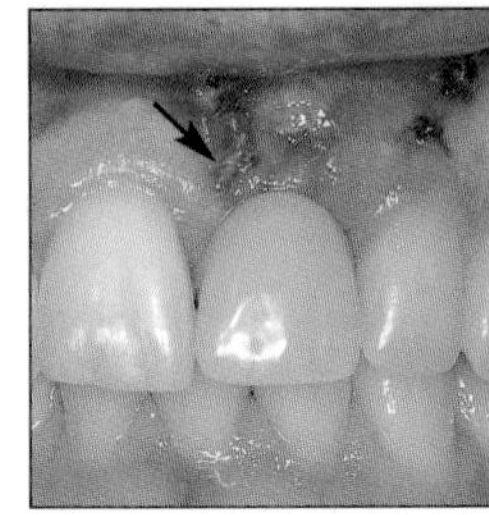
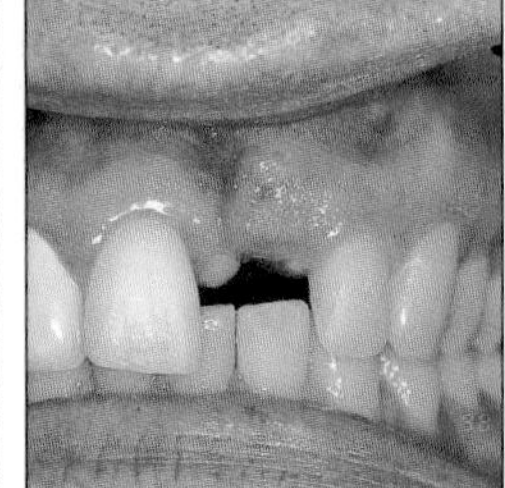

Block and particulate autogenous bone grafting performed via curvilinear-beveled access flap. An absorbable collagen membrane was stabilized by absorbing blood at the site, and tension-free closure was obtained. Dehiscence of the mesial wound margin *(arrow)*, attributed to transmission of micromotion to the area by the labial flange of the removable interim provisional restoration, was noted at the 10-day postoperative visit. The flange was completely removed, and afterward the site healed uneventfully. Nevertheless, while excellent hard tissue volume yield from the graft was obtained at the distal aspect of the site, diminished volume yield resulted at the mesial aspect of the site. Two additional months of healing were allowed in this case because of the early wound dehiscence.

Intermediate site development

6 months

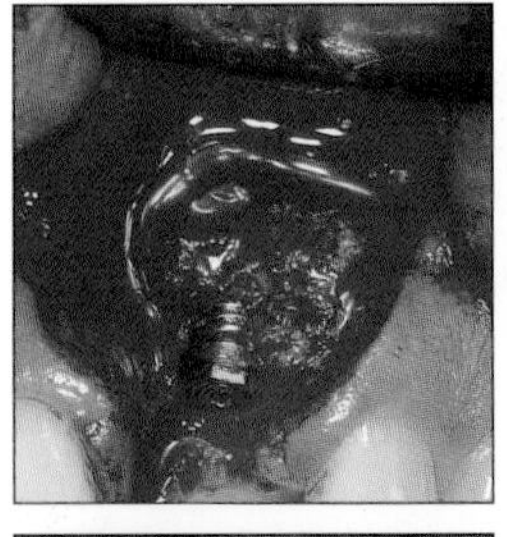
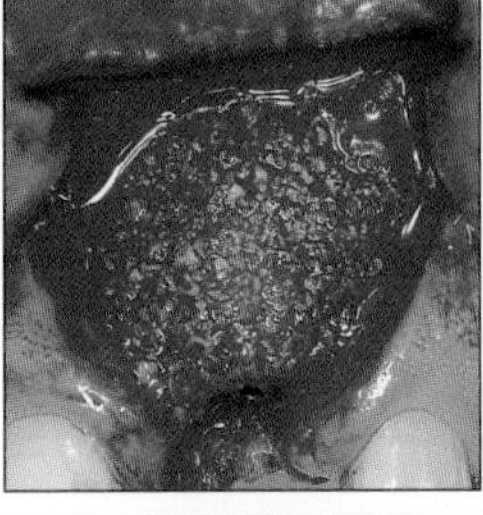
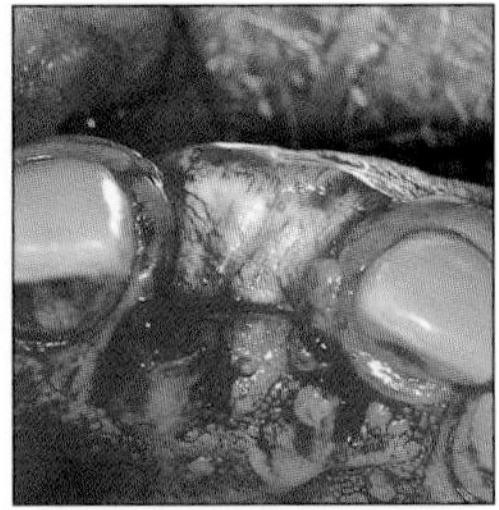
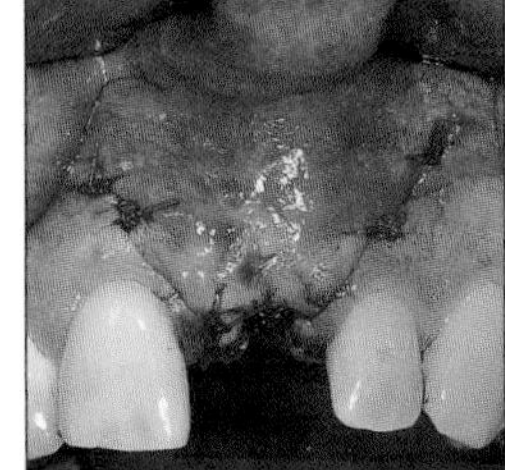
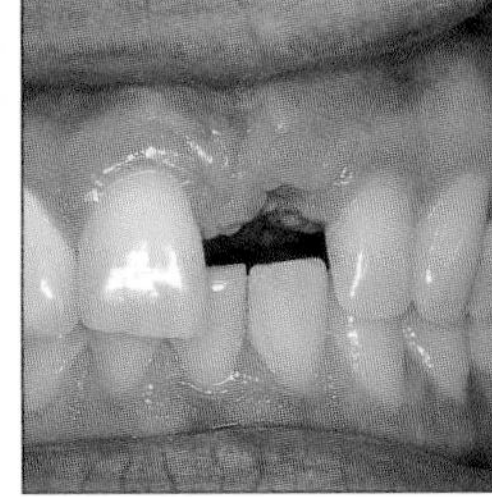
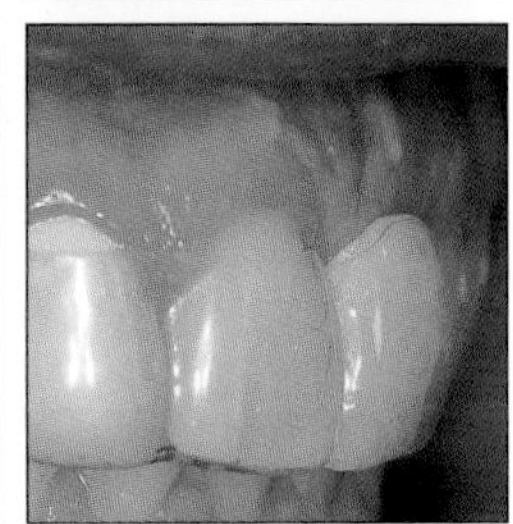

The site was re-entered 6 months after the bone graft procedure for additional grafting, which in this case was performed simultaneous with implant placement since exuberant bone graft healing was observed in those areas not adversely affected by the interim provisional, and ideal placement was feasible. A surgical index was performed prior to the additional bone grafting and guided bone regeneration procedures. An Essex provisional restoration was designed to prevent transmission of micromotion to the site. Six months were alloted for complete bone graft maturation and osseointegration of the implant. Although excellent volume yield resulted from the second bone graft, soft tissue shrinkage was evident at the site.

Intermediate site development

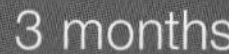

3 months

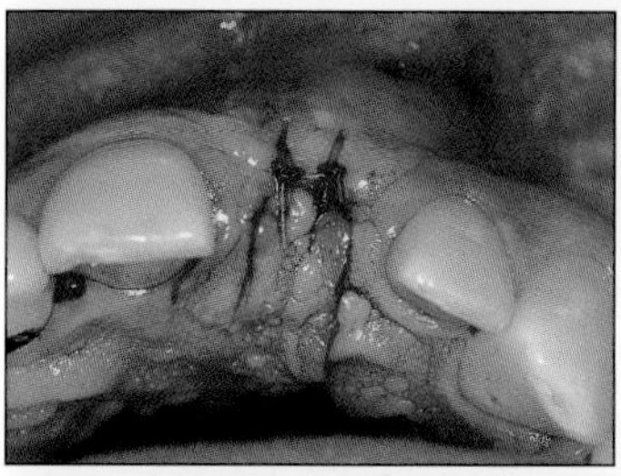
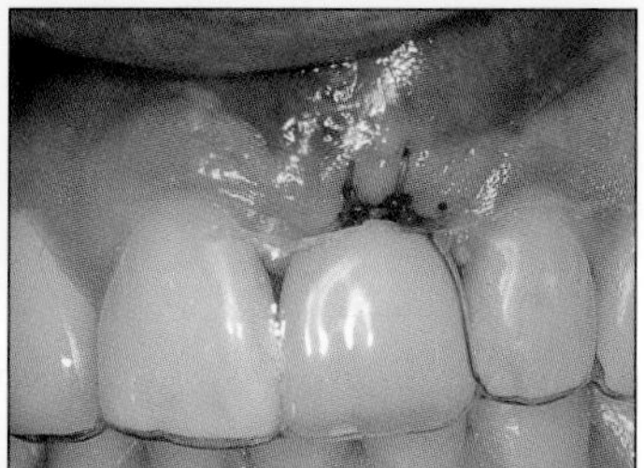
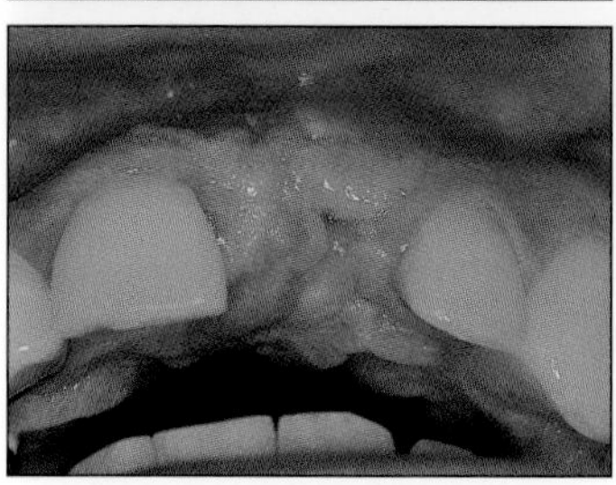
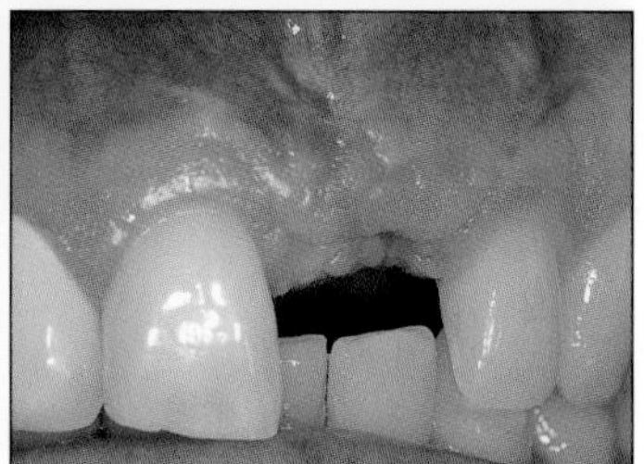

A palatal approach was used to perform a subepithelial connective tissue graft via a closed recipient site and interim provisional restoration managed to avoid micromotion during the 3-month healing allotted following the soft tissue grafting. Although the natural alveolar ridge contours were now completely restored, surface irregularities were present in the soft tissues.

Final site development

4 months

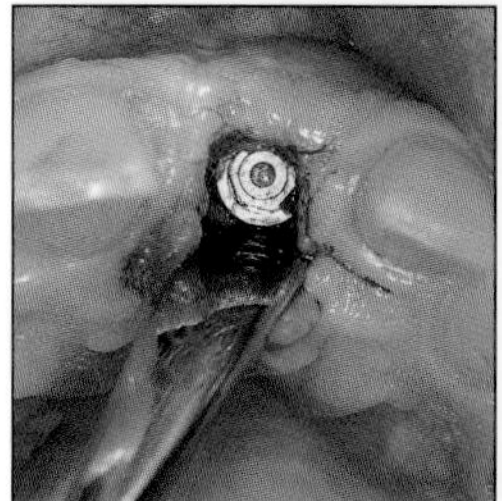
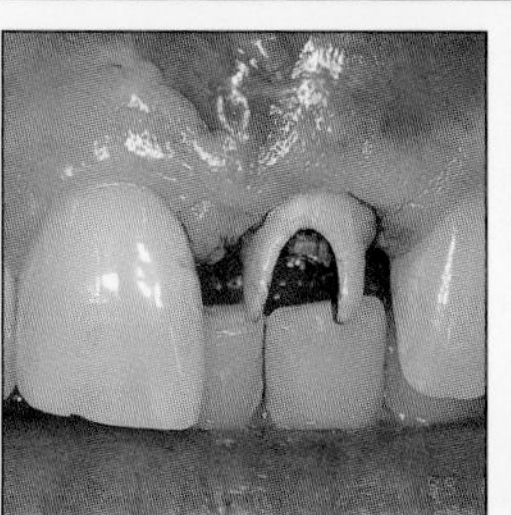
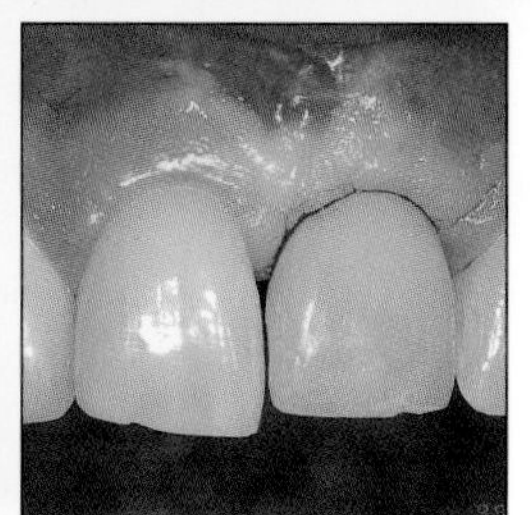
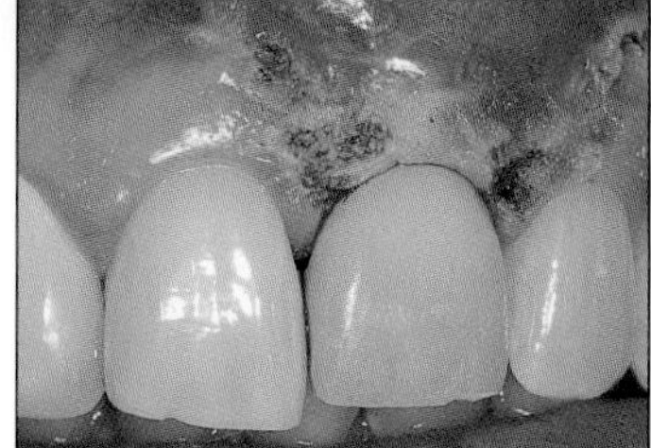
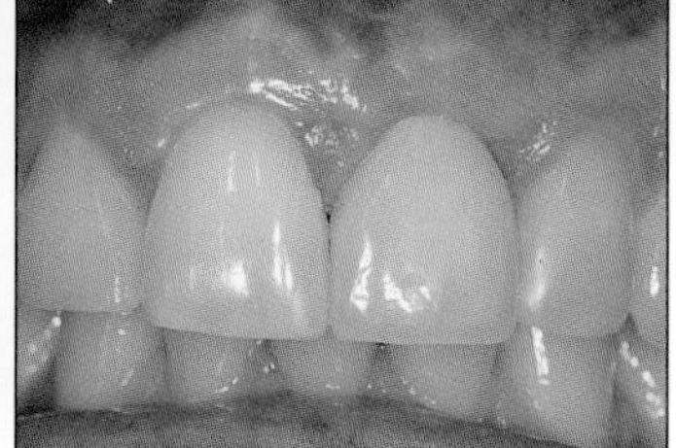

A palatal peninsula flap was used for conservative access for the delivery of a custom abutment and a provisional restoration, avoiding further scarring of the buccal soft tissues. Laser soft tissue resurfacing was performed to remove soft tissue surface irregularities and to blend the soft tissue appearance with the adjacent areas. The restorative dentist modified the contours of the provisional restoration at the beginning of final site development to provide the prosthetic-guided soft tissue healing necessary for optimal gingival esthetics.

Final result

Total: 19 months

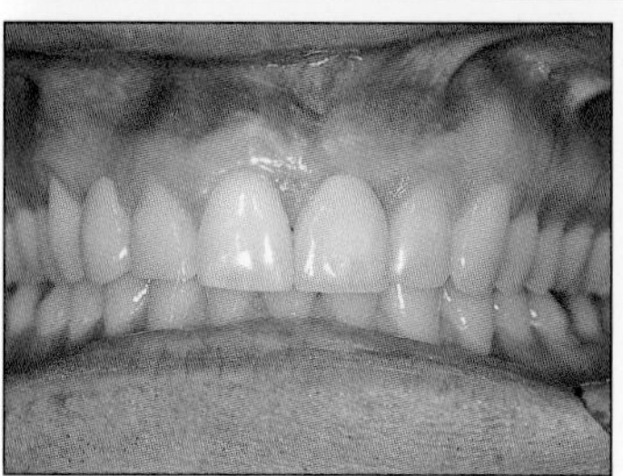
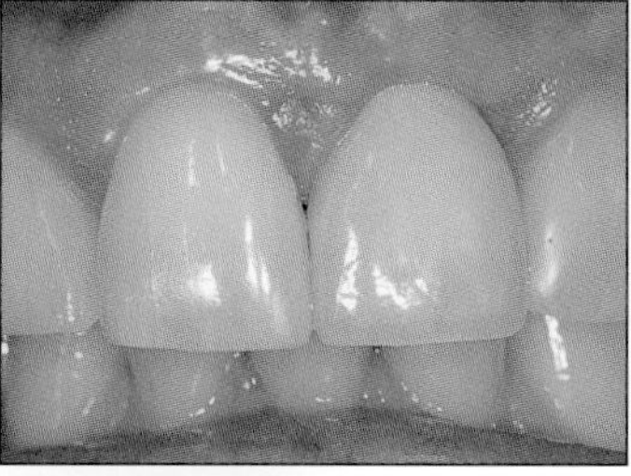
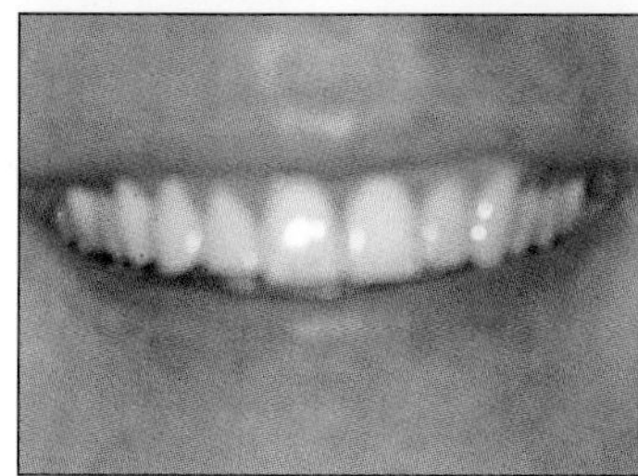

Reconstruction of this large-volume combination esthetic ridge defect required five surgical procedures and a total treatment time of 19 months. Close coordination with the restorative dentist, along with the patient's acceptance of a temporary esthetic compromise, was required for management of interim provisional restorations to avoid transmission of unwanted micromotion to the surgical sites, thus allowing complete restoration of missing alveolar ridge contours. A surgical index allowed the fabrication and delivery of a custom abutment and provisional restoration that provided prosthetic-guided soft tissue healing. The end result was an inconspicuous implant restoration in harmony with the adjacent dentition and a patient who could once again smile without hesitation. (Restoration by Dr Cecil Abraham, Miami, FL.)

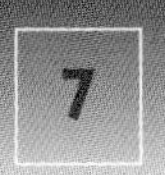

Case 4: Staged reconstruction of large-volume hard tissue esthetic ridge defect for replacement of lateral incisor

Case History

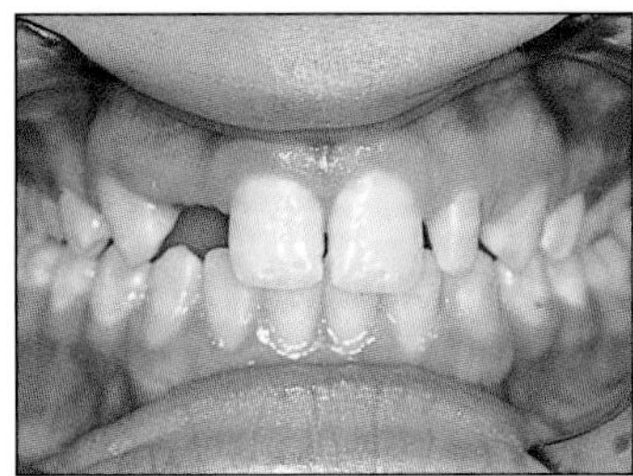
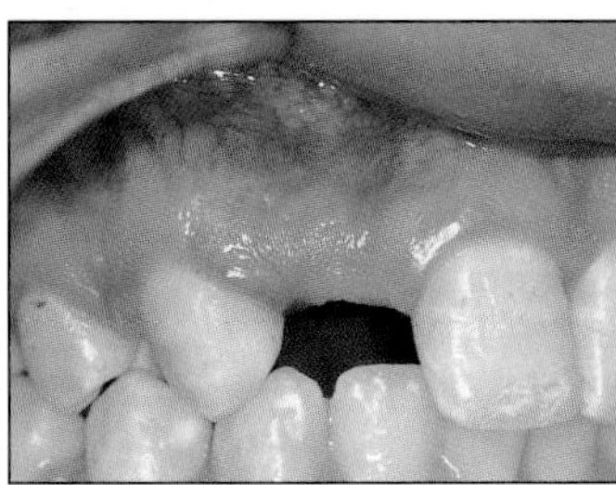
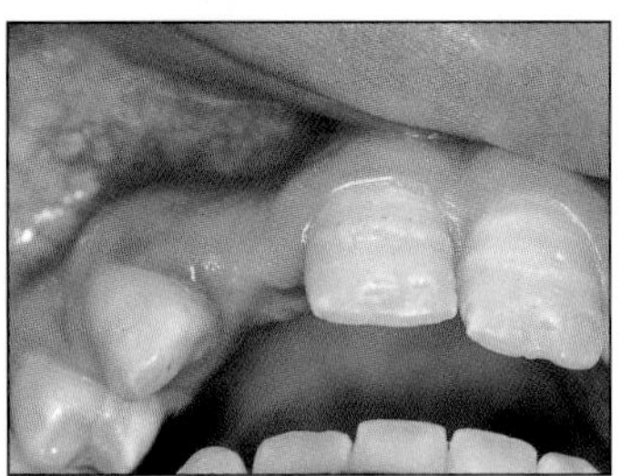

This 18-year-old patient presented for implant replacement of a missing lateral incisor. Pretreatment evaluation revealed a large-volume hard tissue esthetic ridge defect at the implant site as well as unesthetic dental proportions and relationships. The restorative dentist performed a diagnostic waxup that indicated the need for esthetic crown lengthening of adjacent teeth and cosmetic veneer restoration in order to achieve an esthetically pleasing result. Note that the osseous defect precludes ideal implant placement.

Initial site development — 4 months

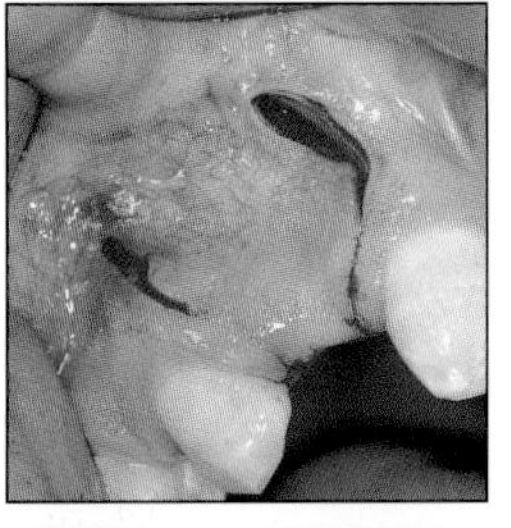
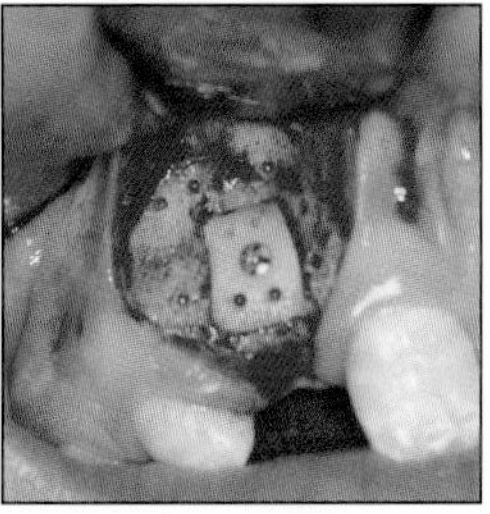
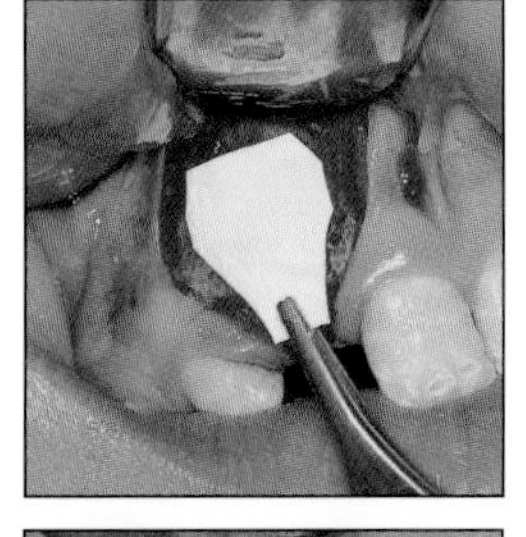
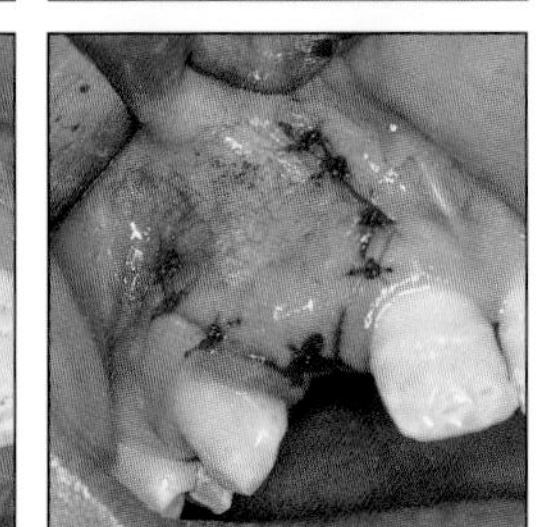

Curvilinear-beveled flap used for access for block and particulate bone grafting at the site. Tension-releasing cutback incisions ensured passive flap accommodation over the large-volume bone graft without embarrassing circulation to flap margins. Tension-free closure was obtained, and the interim provisional restoration managed to avoid transmission of micromotion to the surgical site. A 4-month period was allotted for bone graft healing.

Final site development

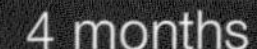

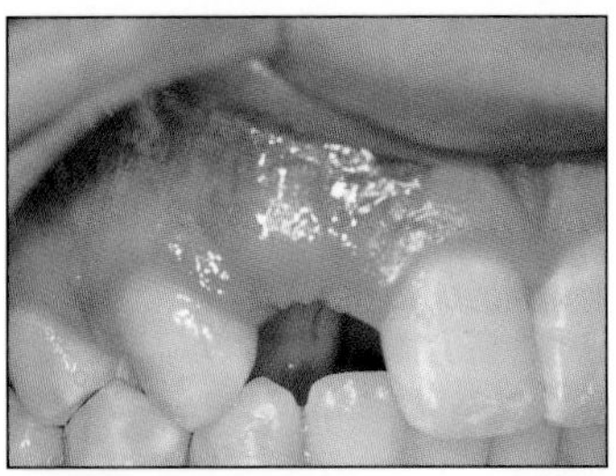
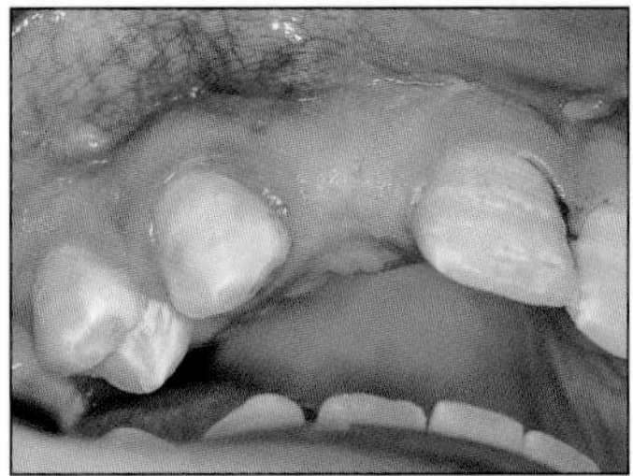
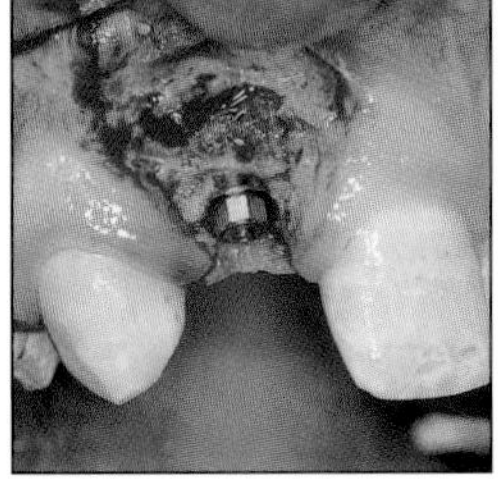
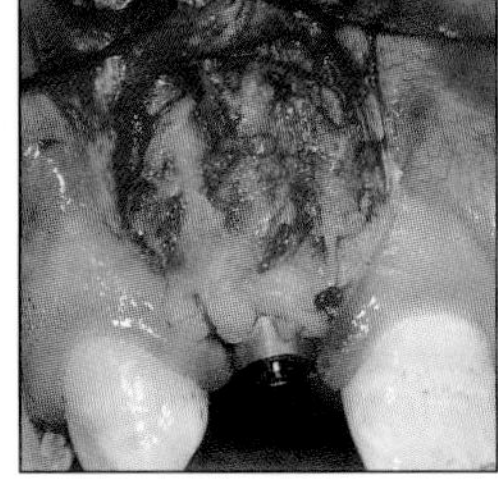
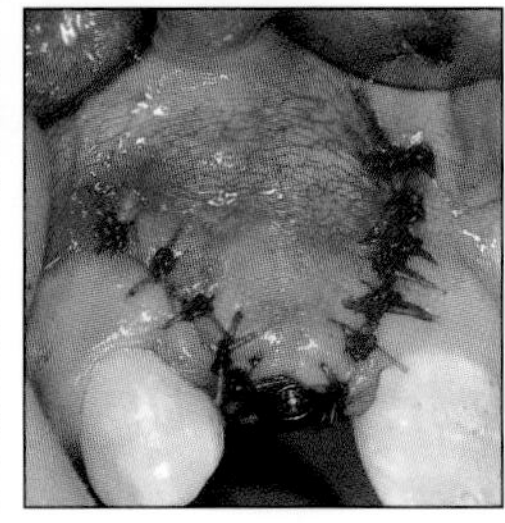

Four months after hard tissue site development, ideal alveolar ridge contours are apparent. Nevertheless, a subepithelial graft was performed simultaneous with nonsubmerged implant placement to offset the predictable loss of soft tissue volume that occurs following re-entry for removal of fixation screws and implant placement. A smaller-diameter, narrow-neck implant was necessary to maintain adequate thickness of adjacent interdental bone to support the overlying papillae. An anatomic healing abutment provided support for the surrounding tissues and adjacent interdental papillae, preventing their collapse. Furthermore, the additional soft tissue thickness provided by the graft improved the esthetic appearance of the soft tissues and their resistance to recession following subsequent intracrevicular prosthetic procedures.

Final site development — 7 months

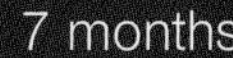

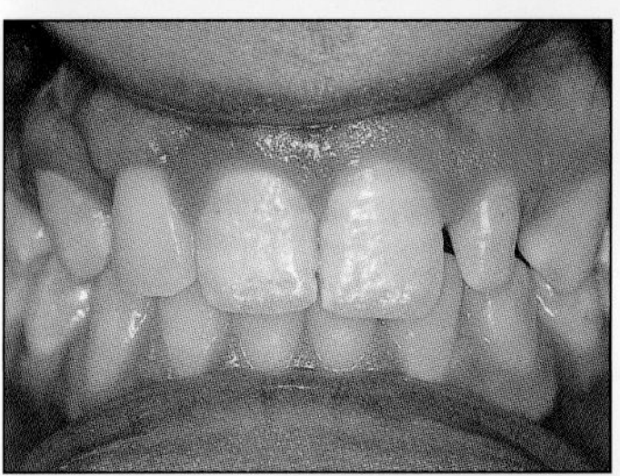

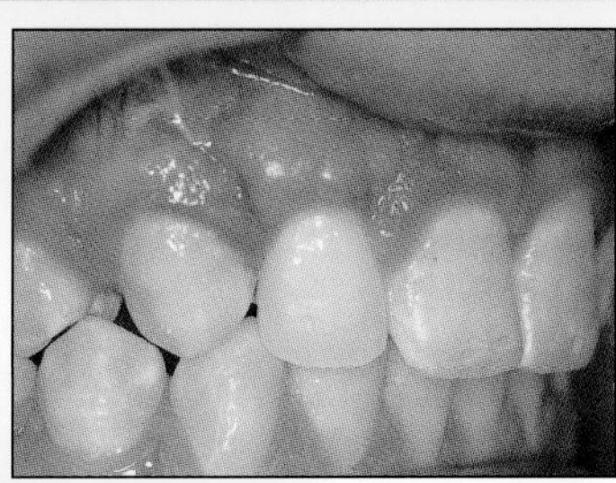

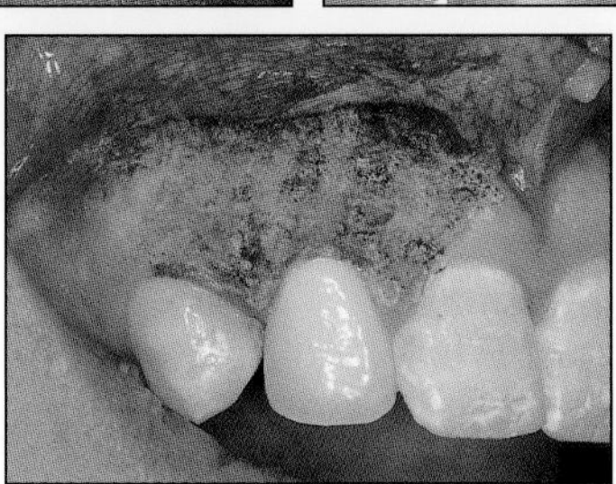

Three months were allowed for maturation of soft tissues and osseointegration of the implant at the site, after which time a provisional restoration was delivered and laser soft tissue resurfacing was used to obtain a blending of the soft tissue appearance with the adjacent areas. Two additional months were allotted for soft tissue healing and prosthetic-guided soft tissue healing. After stabilization of the soft tissues around the provisional implant restoration, esthetic crown lengthening was performed, and preparation of the adjacent teeth was accomplished with delivery of the interim restoration. Two months later, the final restorations were delivered.

Final result — Total: 15 months

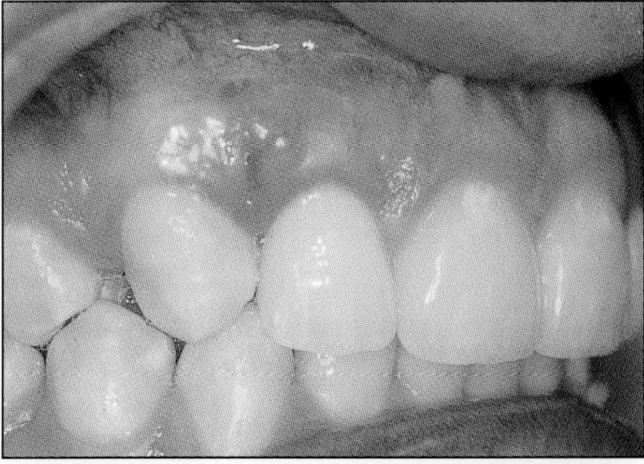

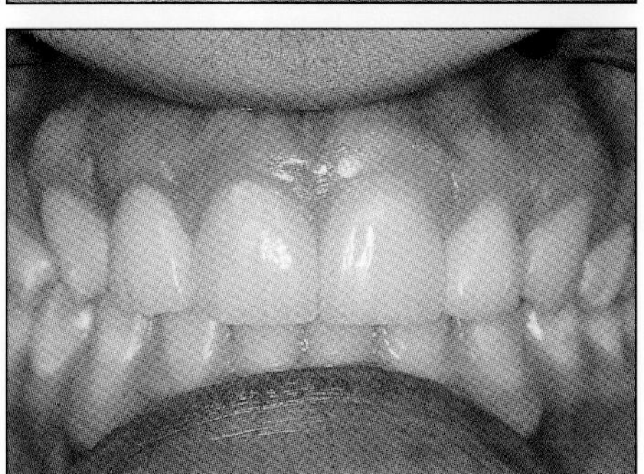

Reconstruction of this large-volume hard tissue esthetic ridge defect required two site-development procedures, a soft tissue refinement procedure, and cosmetic periodontal surgery on the adjacent dentition. The total treatment time was 15 months. Close coordination with the restorative dentist was required for management of interim provisional restorations to avoid transmission of unwanted micromotion to the surgical sites. In addition, communication of the proposed gingival margin positions of the adjacent canine and central incisor influenced fixture placement. An anatomic healing abutment and subsequent provisional implant restoration provided prosthetic-guided soft tissue healing. The end result was an inconspicuous implant restoration and greatly improved smile esthetics for this esthetics-conscious patient. (Restoration by Dr William R. Bronkan, Miami, FL.)

Case 5: Simultaneous reconstruction of large-volume combination esthetic ridge defect for replacement of four maxillary incisors

Case history

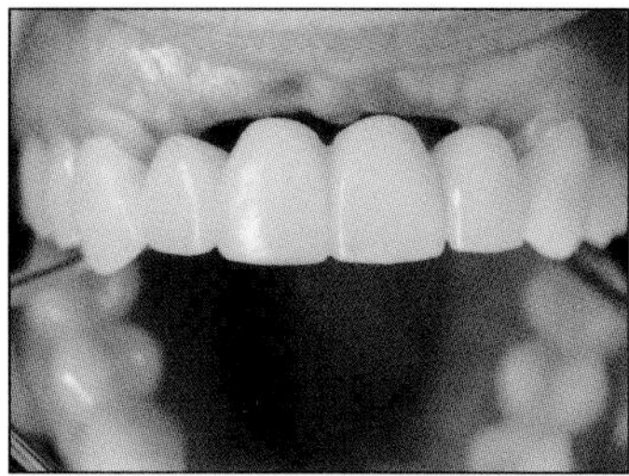

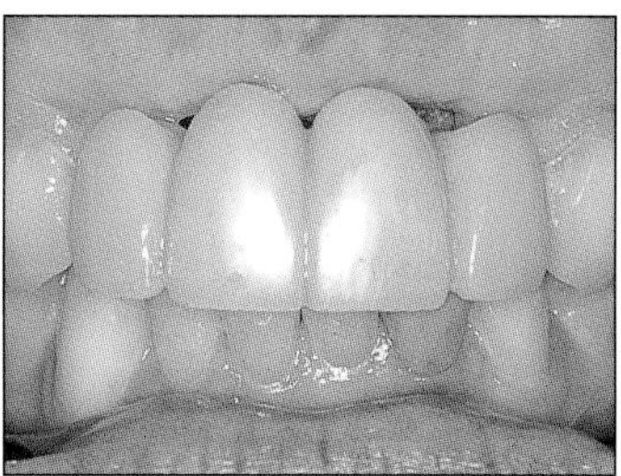

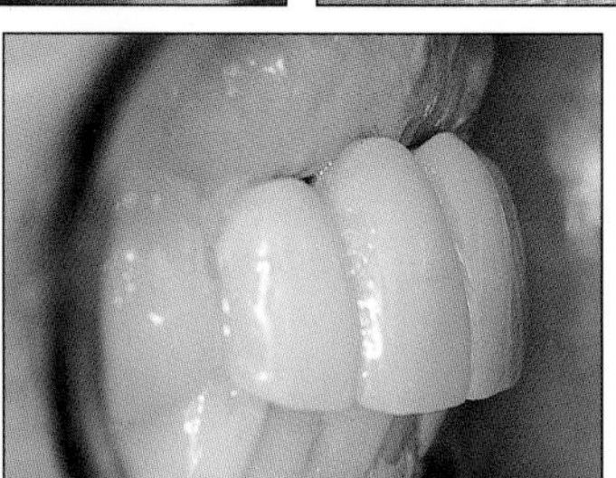

This 43-year-old female patient with a high smile line presented with large-volume combination esthetic ridge defects involving the maxillary central and lateral incisor implant sites. These sites were considered compromised in terms of regenerative potential secondary to a history of multiple interventions leading to tooth loss and failure of previous bone graft procedure performed several months earlier. The patient's primary concern was whether it was possible to replace the four missing maxillary incisors with inconspicuous implant restorations. She was also concerned about the number of procedures and total treatment time required. Prior to commencing with therapy, a diagnostic waxup was performed and a new interim provisional restoration was delivered in order to establish realistic expectations for the final result. Treatment plan included simultaneous hard and soft tissue site development followed by nonsubmerged implant placement with custom tooth-form healing abutments. Total treatment time was estimated to be 12 months.

Initial site development

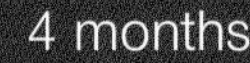

4 months

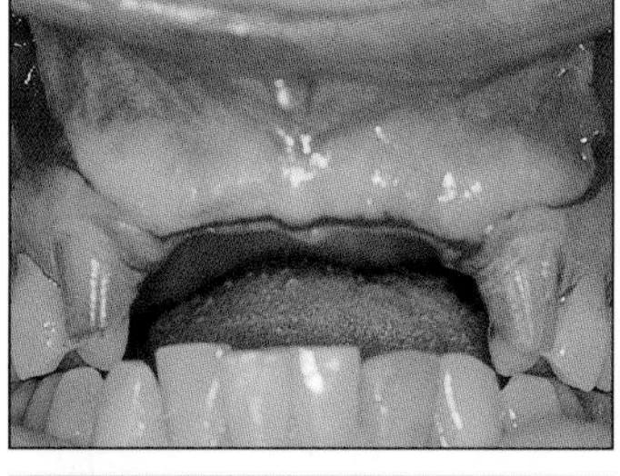

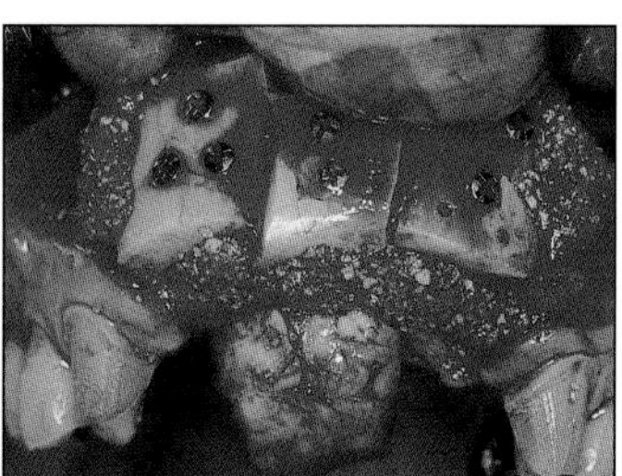

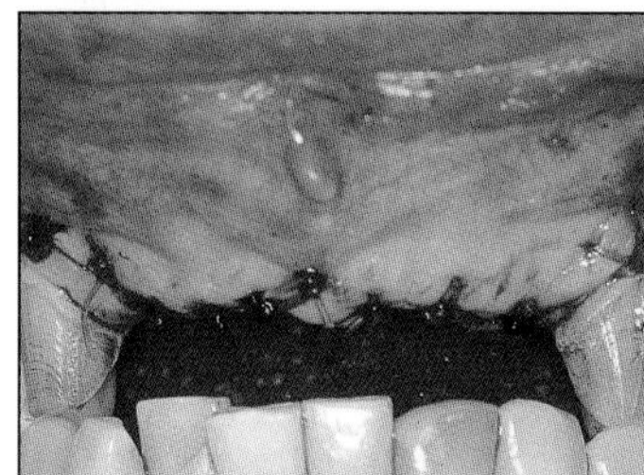

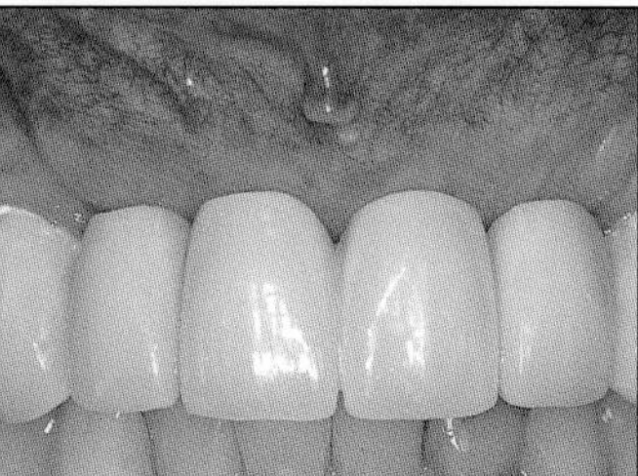

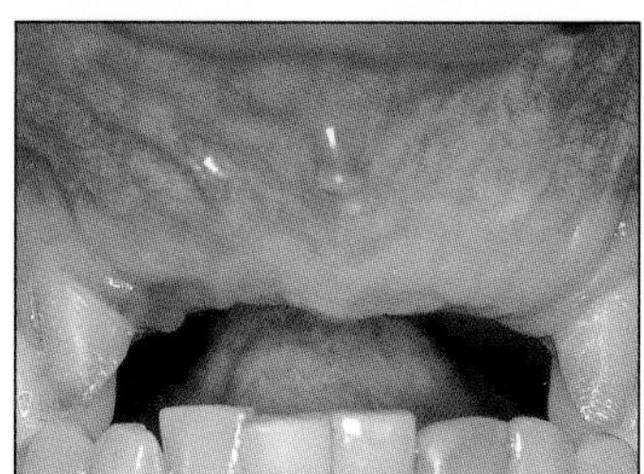

Exaggerated curvilinear-beveled incisions with tension-releasing cutback incisions outline the access flap for simultaneous hard and soft tissue site development. The vertical legs of the incisions were initiated over the second interdental area between the premolars bilaterally. De-epithelialization of the adjacent buccal attached tissues and the papillary and col areas was performed. Corticocancellous block grafts were harvested from the body of the mandible and secured at the site; bilateral VIP-CT flaps were then developed from within the palate bilaterally. A particulate bone graft, consisting of autogenous cancellous bone and Bio-Oss, was condensed around the periphery of the bone block bone grafts, and the VIP-CT flaps were secured over the bone grafts and interposed beneath the recipient site flap, which was coronally advanced to achieve tension-free closure. The provisional restoration was modified to avoid transmission of micromotion to the site during initial healing. Three months after surgery, a second provisional restoration was delivered. Removal of the provisional restoration revealed successful reconstruction of lost alveolar ridge contours with significant vertical soft tissue augmentation.

Final site development — 4 months

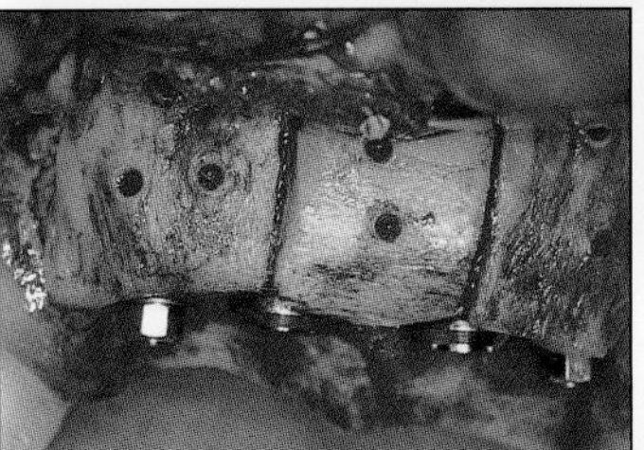
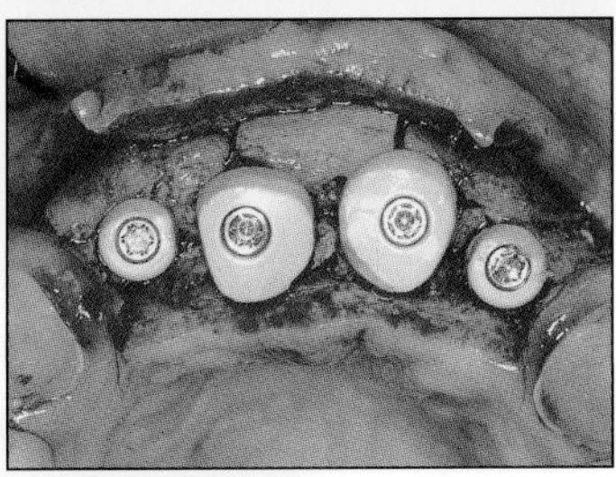
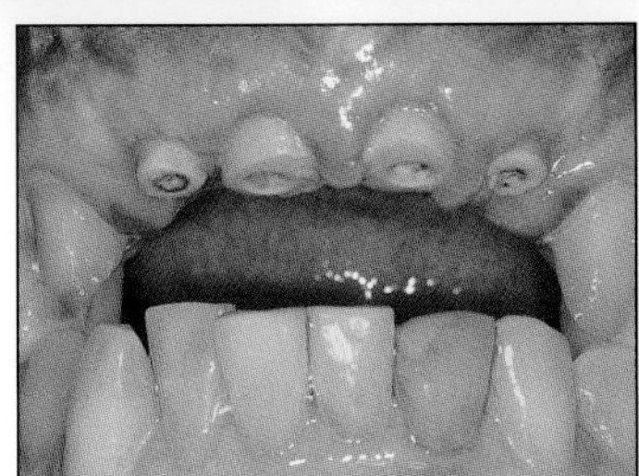

Four months after simultaneous hard and soft tissue site development, the site was re-entered for implant placement. The initial incision was retraced and bone graft fixation screws were removed. Four one-piece nonsubmerged implants were placed. Custom tooth-form healing abutments were shaped and polished chairside prior to their delivery. The thick soft tissues provided by the VIP-CT flaps allowed the use of the papilla regeneration maneuver to ensure adequate volume of inter-implant papillae. Scalloped soft tissue architecture was evident 4 months after implant placement. The early employment of guided soft tissue healing provided by the customizable healing abutments provided a synergistic effect with esthetic flap management at the time of nonsubmerged implant placement.

Final site development — 2 months

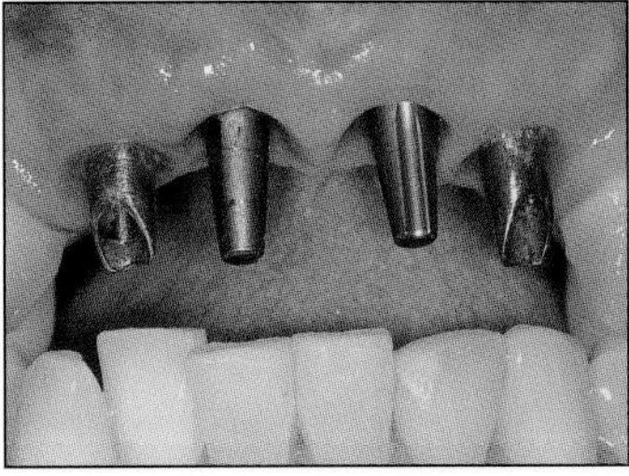
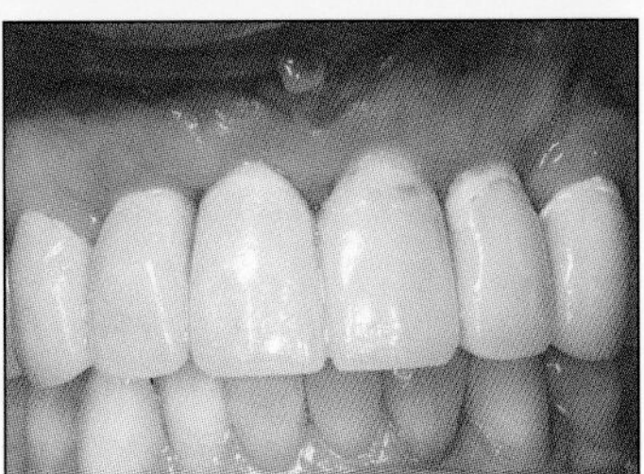

Stability and health of the peri-implant soft tissues facilitated the delivery of the restorative abutments and implant-supported provisional restoration. The nonsubmerged approach allotted sufficient time for the soft tissue integration and the development of a stable sulcus, providing a prosthetic-friendly environment and improving esthetic predictability of the final restoration.

Final result — Total: 10 months

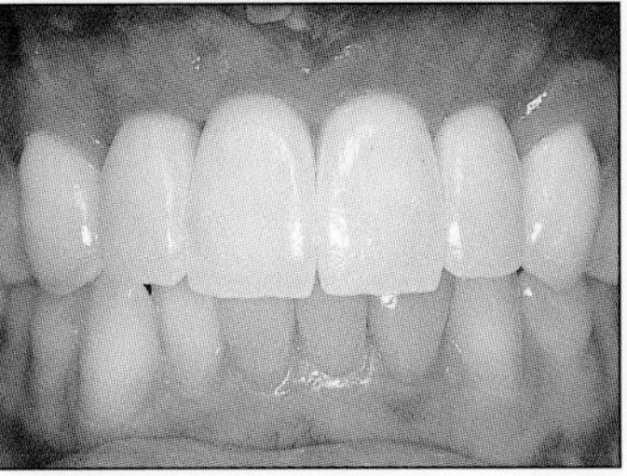
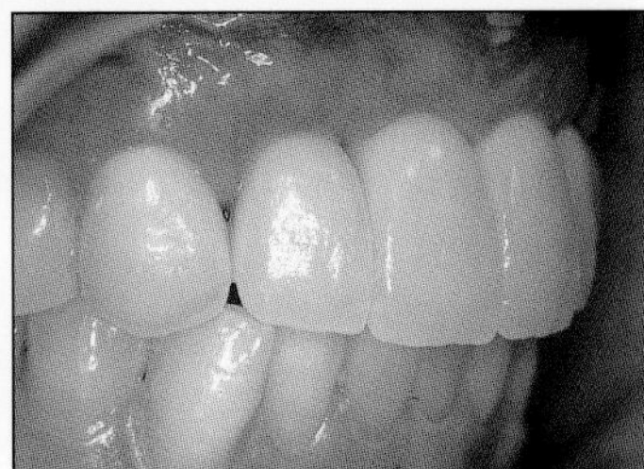
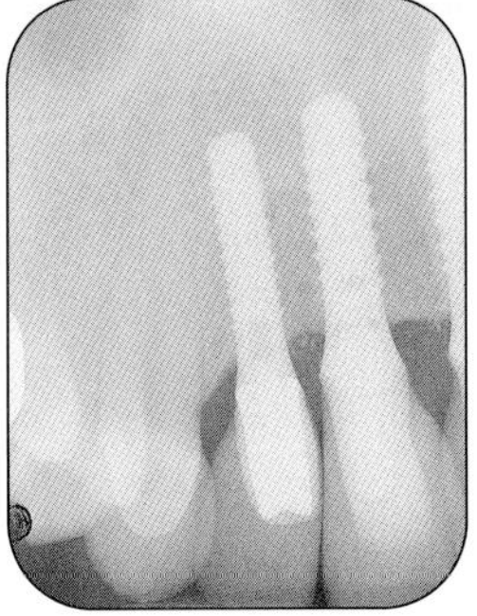
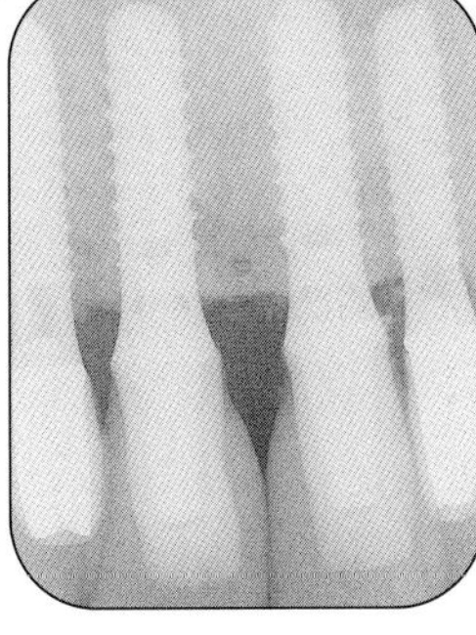
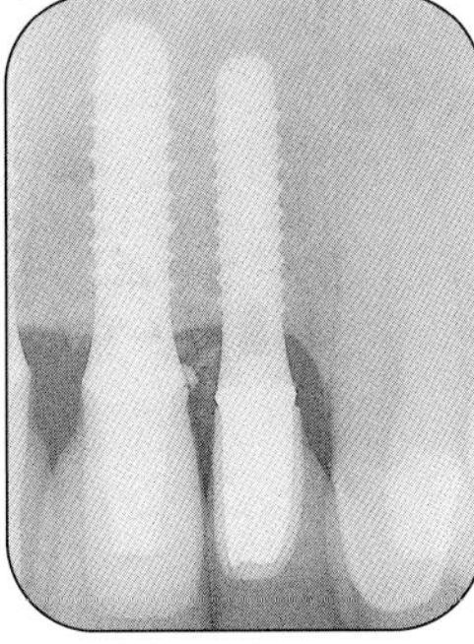

The final restorations are harmonious in appearance 4 months after delivery. Simultaneous reconstruction of missing hard and soft tissue alveolar ridge contours and subsequent use of a nonsubmerged implant approach with custom tooth form healing abutments allowed for esthetic restorative emergence and a pleasing gingival appearance with fewer procedures and reduced treatment time (10 months) when compared to conventional techniques and protocols. Despite the flat osseous anatomy evident on posttreatment radiographs, the use of the VIP-CT flaps provided the necessary vertical soft tissue augmentation in this case. (Restoration by Dr Juan Diego Cardenas, Miami, FL.)

Case 6: Reconstruction of small-volume soft tissue defects simultaneous with and subsequent to nonsubmerged implant placement

Case History

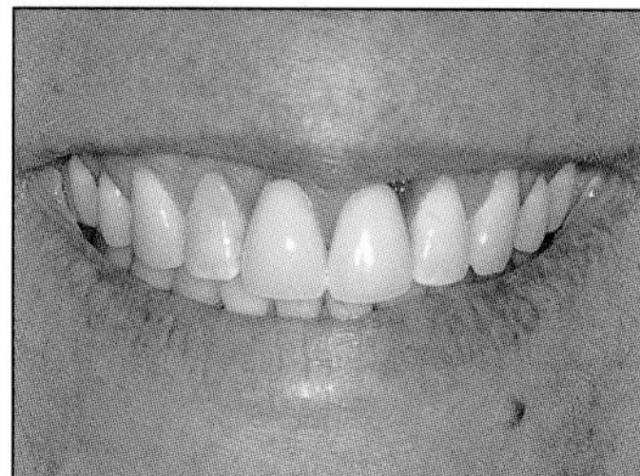
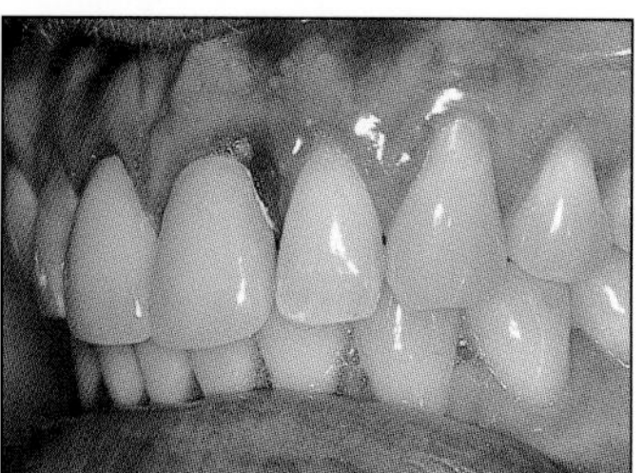
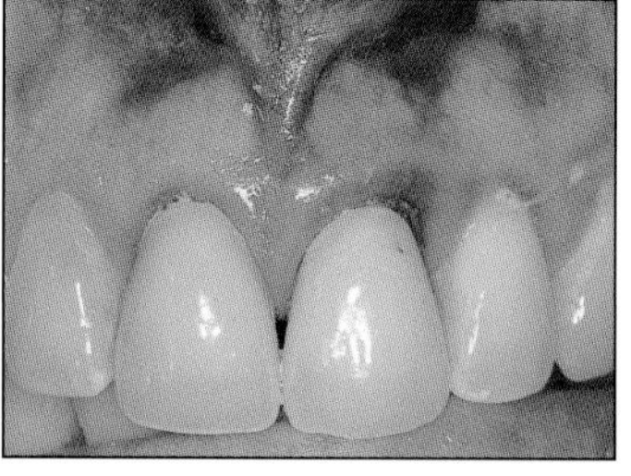

This 33-year-old female patient with a high smile line and generous gingival show in the relaxed smile position presented with failing maxillary central incisors, a thin, scalloped periodontium, and tissue edema associated with mobility of the left central incisor.

Initial site development — 3 months

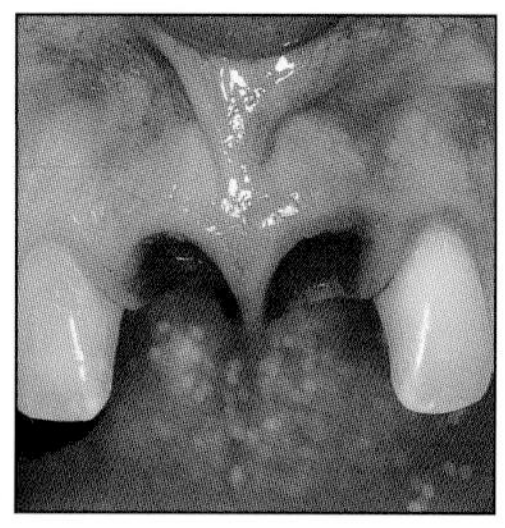
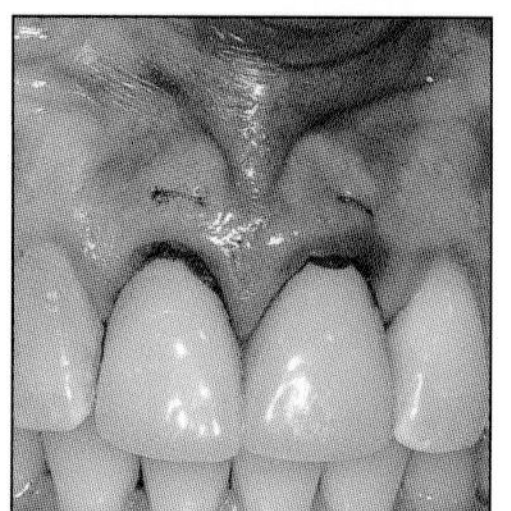
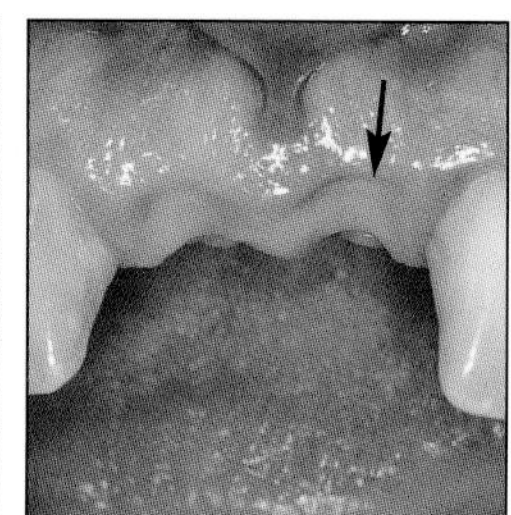

The Bio-Col technique was performed following tooth removal to minimize bone resorption and preserve soft tissue architecture at the sites. A small-volume soft tissue esthetic ridge defect was evident 3 months later in the area where soft tissue edema pre-existed around the mobile left central incisor *(arrow)*.

Final site development — 3 months

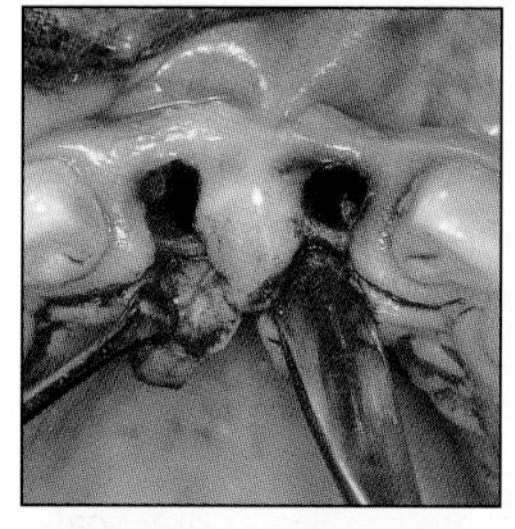
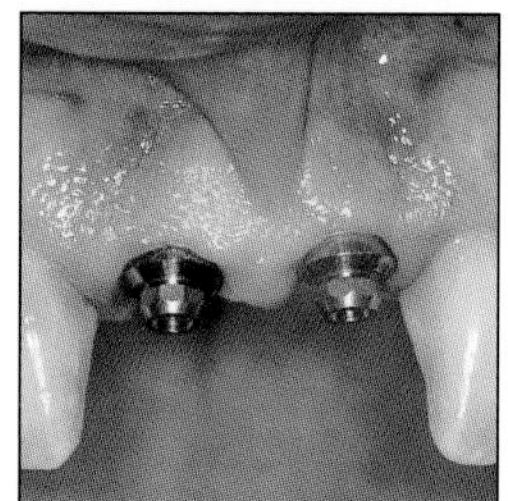
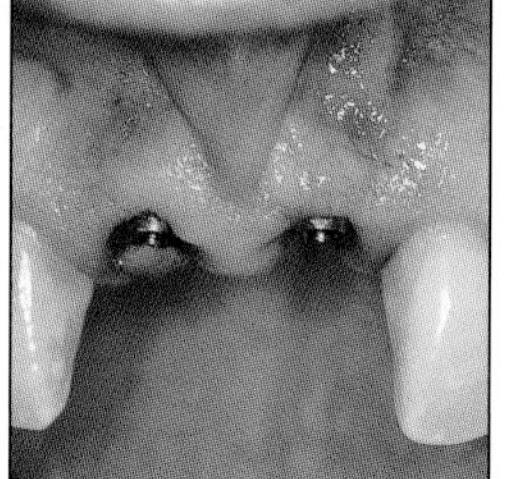

Palatal peninsula flaps were used to gain access for nonsubmerged implant placement. After performing surgical indexing, protective caps were placed and a subepithelial connective tissue graft was performed simultaneously to correct the small-volume soft tissue defect present at the left central incisor site.

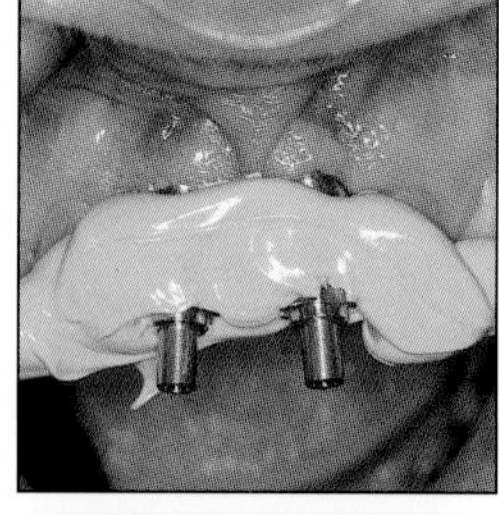
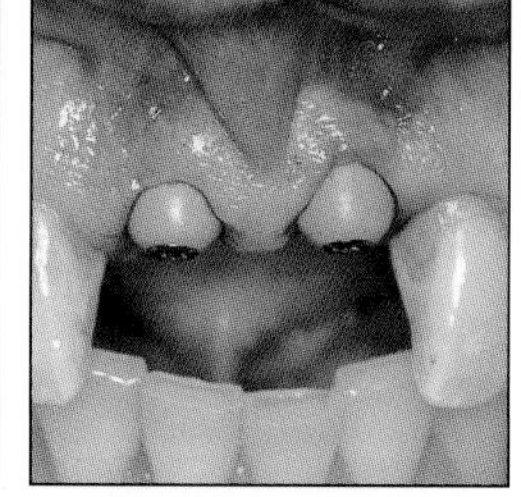
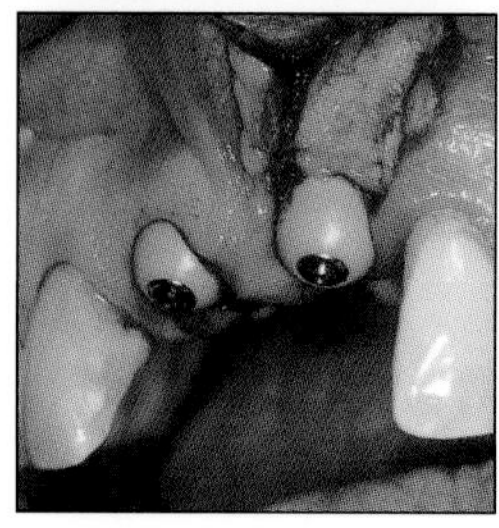
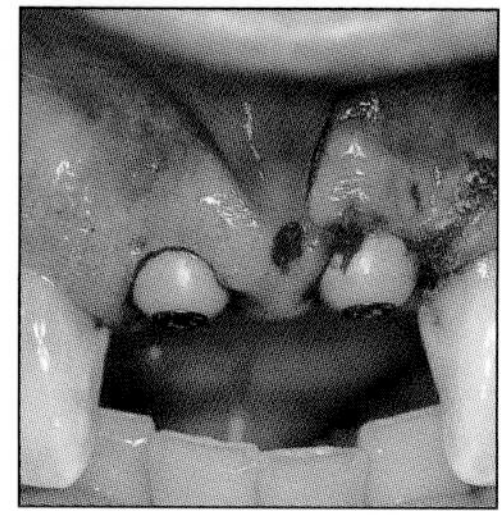

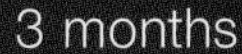

Final site development — 3 months

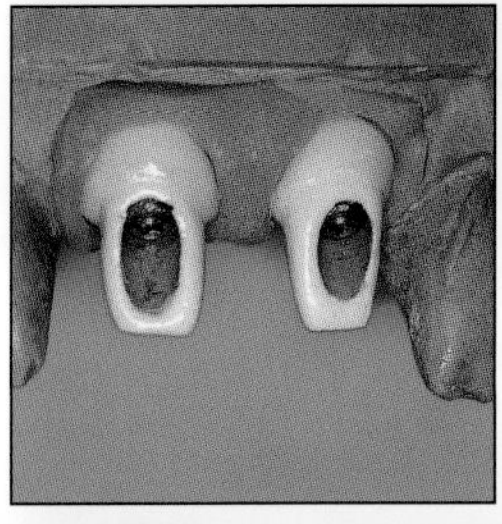
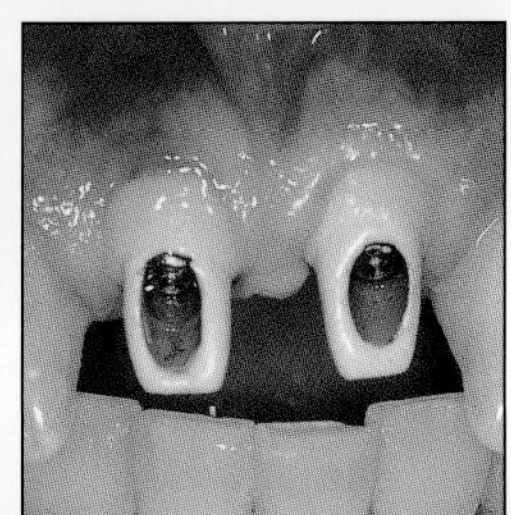
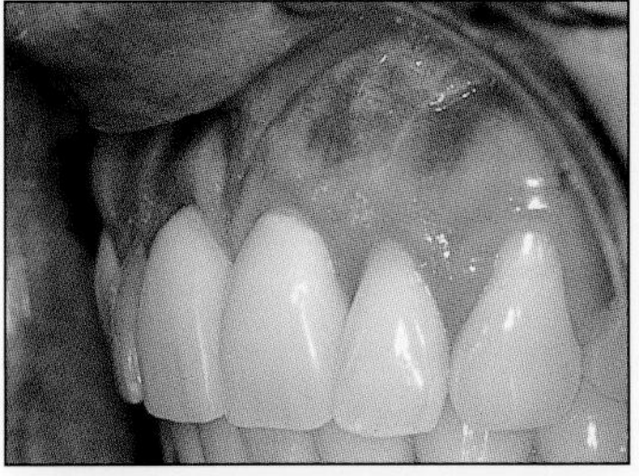
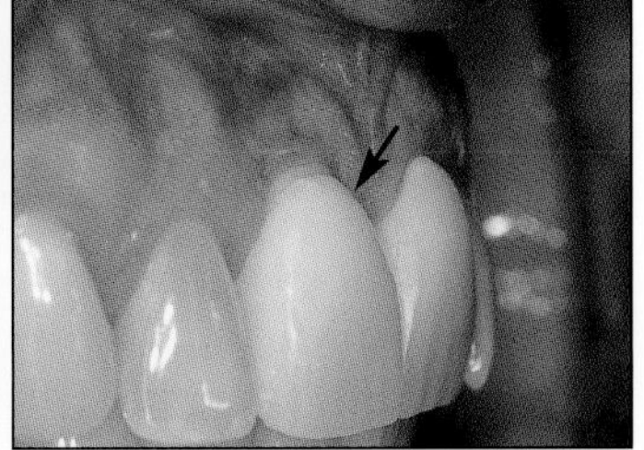
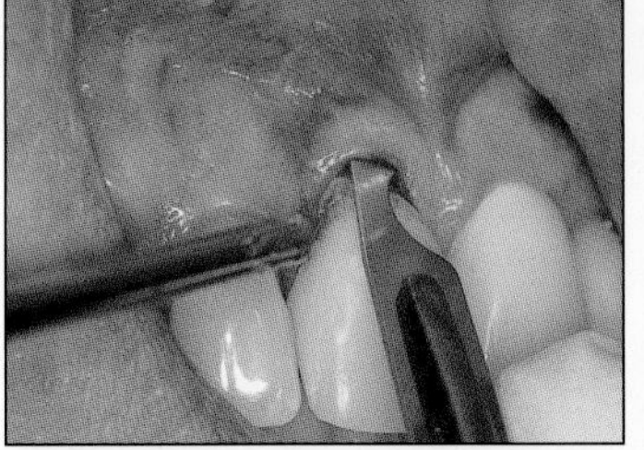
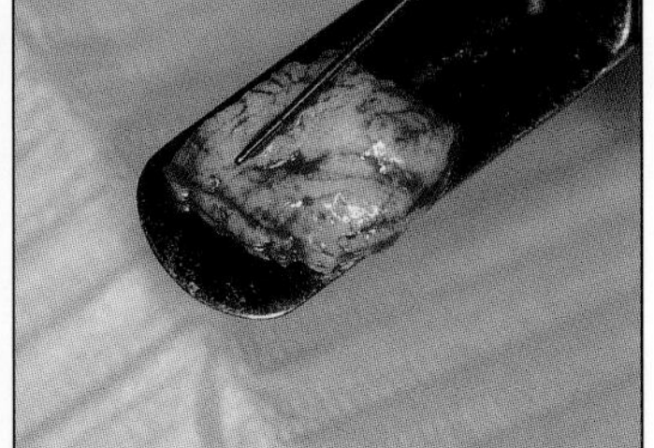
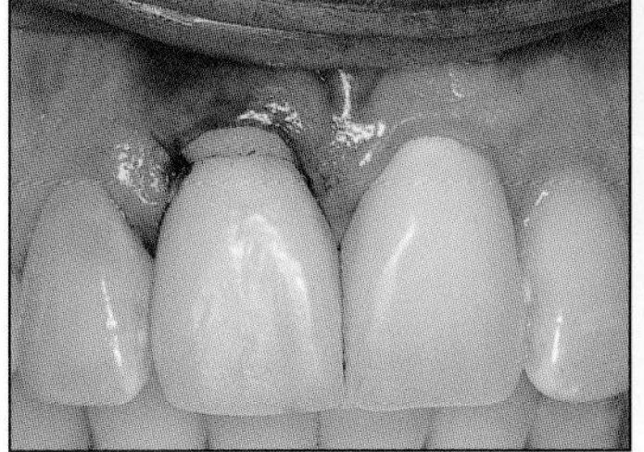
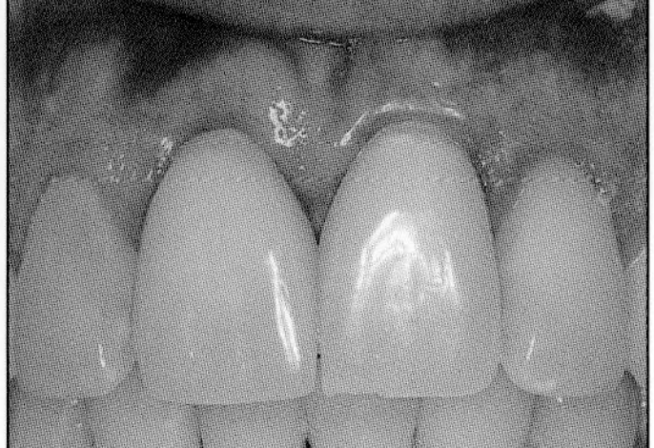

Three months after implant placement and soft tissue grafting of the left central incisor site, custom abutments and provisional restorations were delivered by the restorative dentist, who subsequently noticed that soft tissue recession at the right central incisor site occurred soon after abutment connection *(arrow)*. This response to surgical or prosthetic interventions is typical of the thin, scalloped periodontium. A second subepithelial connective tissue graft harvested from the same donor site yielded increased volume of good-quality connective tissue, which was used to correct the recession defect on the right central incisor via a closed recipient site. This resulted in symmetrical gingival levels on both central incisors.

Final result — Total: 9 months

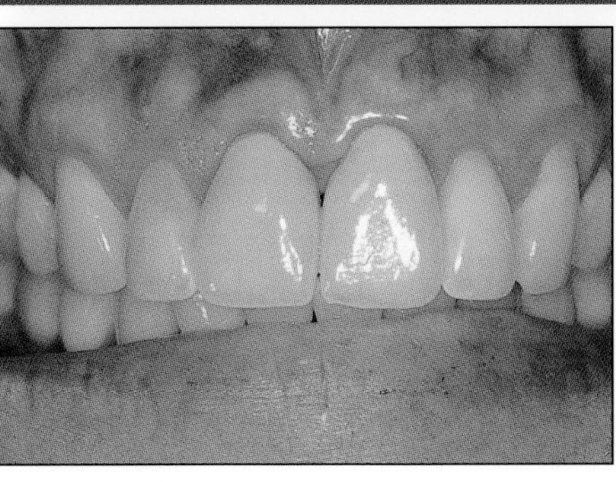

Three surgical procedures and a total treatment time of 9 months were necessary to replace the failing central incisors with esthetic implant restorations. This case emphasizes the need for prophylactic soft tissue grafting when esthetic implant replacements are desired in a patient with a thin, scalloped periodontium. Doing so on both sides simultaneous with implant placement in this case would have reduced the treatment time by 3 months. Use of custom abutments and provisional restorations provided prosthetic-guided soft tissue healing and allowed for tissue refinements prior to delivery of the final restoration. Peri-implant soft tissue health and stability resulted from the soft tissue grafting procedures. The final implant restorations are inconspicuously esthetic and harmonious with the adjacent dentition. (Restoration by Dr Larry Grillo, Aventura, FL.)

Case 7: Reconstruction of small-volume esthetic ridge defect simultaneous with submerged implant placement

Case History

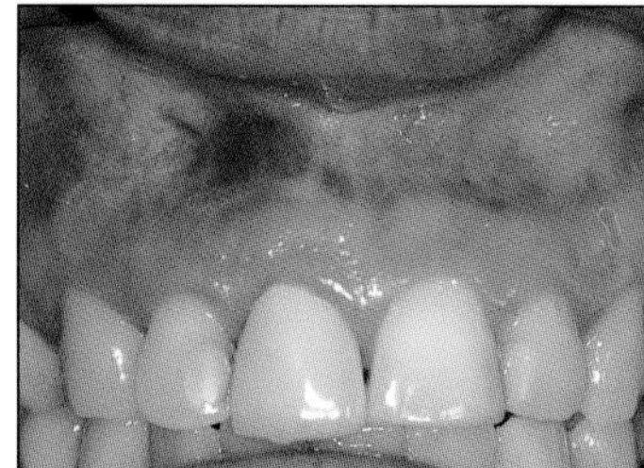

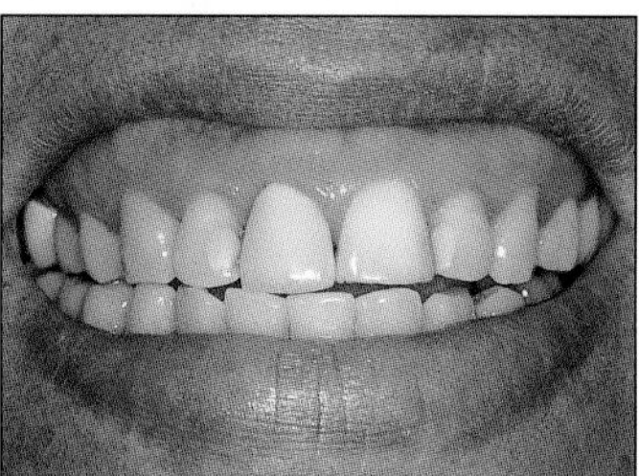

This 30-year-old female patient presented with a failing central incisor after surgical endodontics failed. The marginal tissue edema was associated with tooth mobility and was clearly demarcated from the adjacent healthy soft tissues. A soft tissue defect predictably results when this clinical scenario is encountered. Proceeding with immediate implant placement is associated with significant esthetic risk.

Initial site development 2 months

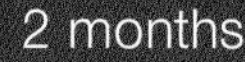

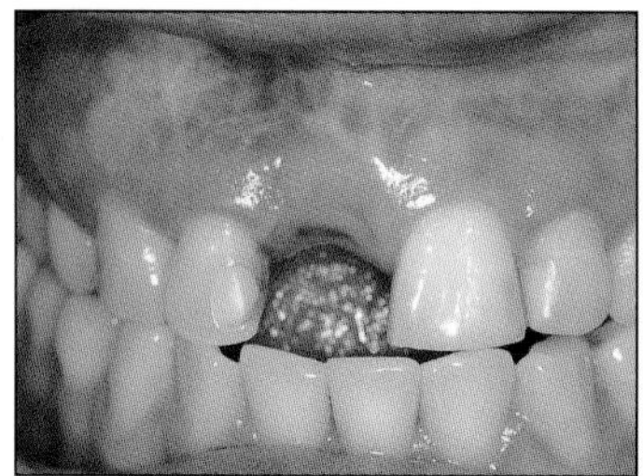

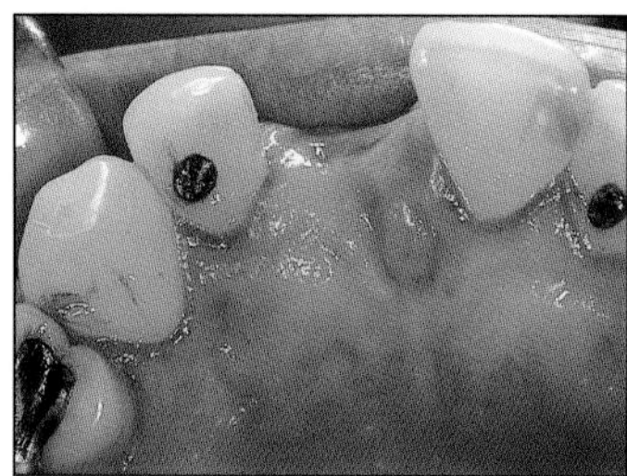

The Bio-Col alveolar ridge preservation technique was performed in conjunction with tooth removal. Nevertheless, a small-volume soft tissue esthetic ridge defect as expected was evident 2 months later.

Intermediate site development 3 months

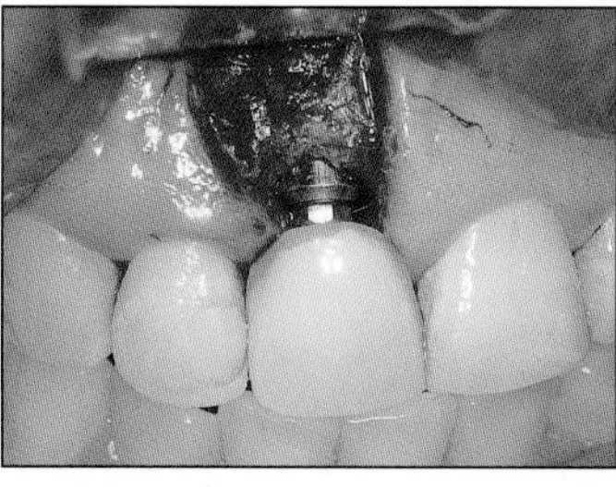

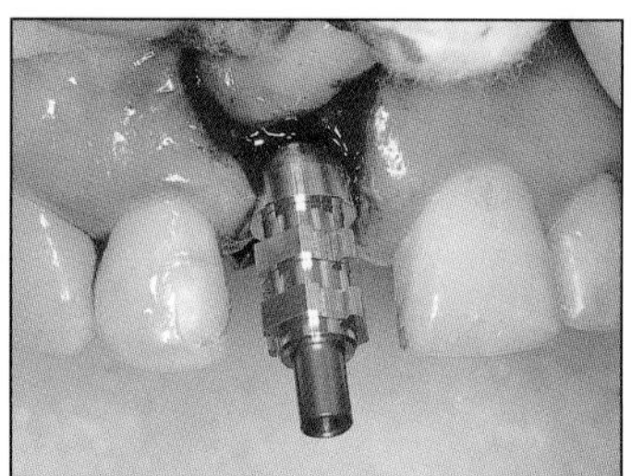

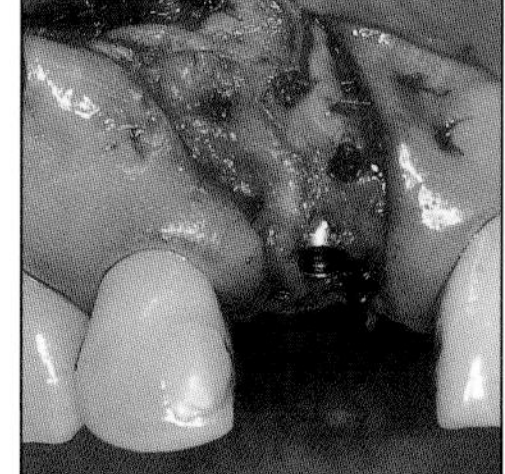

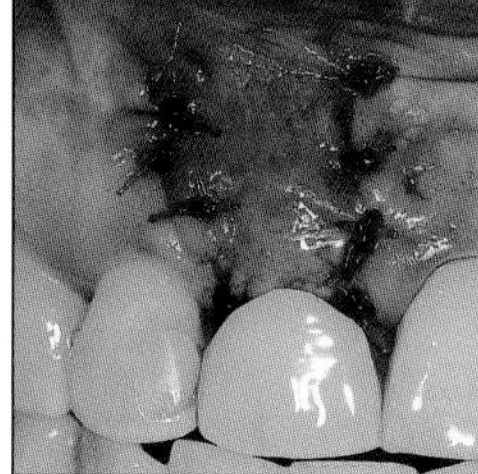

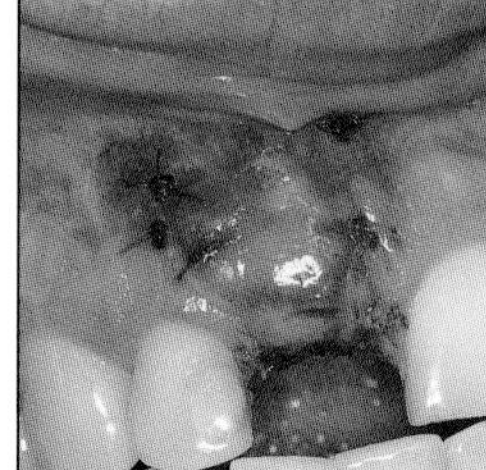

A subepithelial connective tissue graft was performed simultaneously with placement of a one-piece nonsubmerged implant. Surgical indexing preceded the soft tissue grafting procedure. Coronal advancement of the cover flap over the soft tissue graft and neck of the nonsubmerged implant effectively expanded the soft tissue envelope, providing vertical soft tissue augmentation in the area critical for prosthetic emergence. This was facilitated by abundant vestibular depth in the area. Although slight compromise to the flap margin was noted at the 1-week postoperative visit, soft tissue integrity was maintained.

Final site development — 2 months

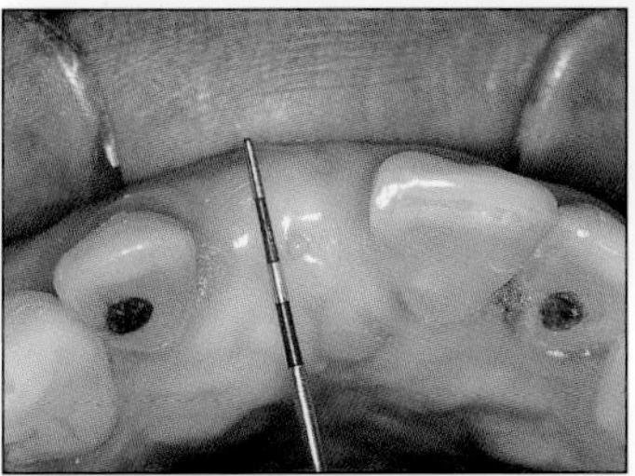
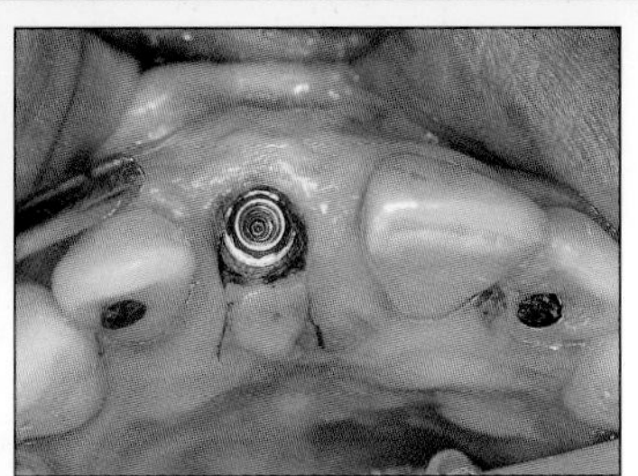
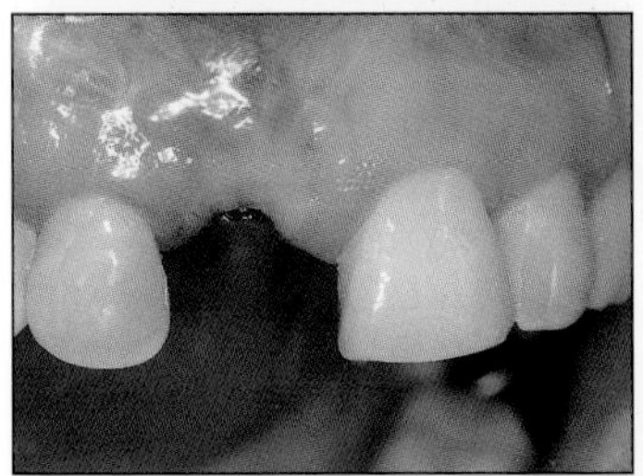
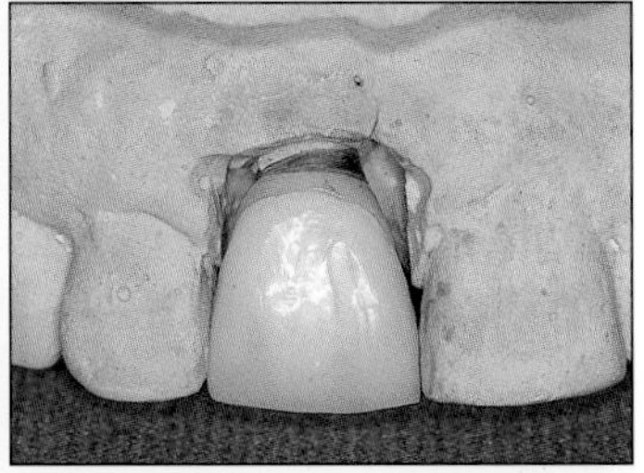
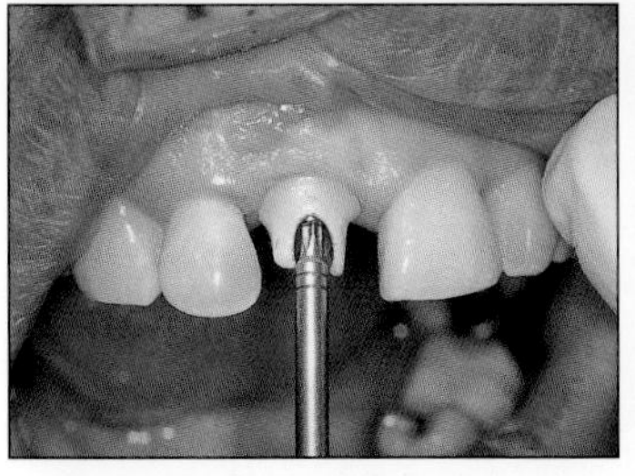
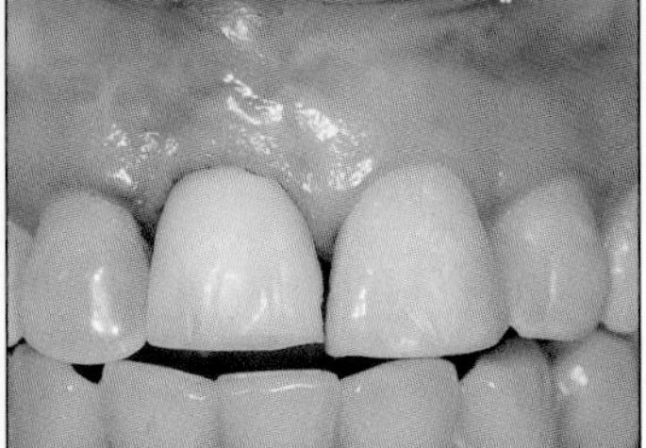

After 3 months, complete correction of the small-volume soft tissue defect was evident, and a conservative palatal peninsula flap was used to expose the implant. A custom healing abutment fabricated on an implant analog cast was delivered, and a provisional restoration was cemented, providing the necessary prosthetic-guided soft tissue healing to restore natural soft tissue architecture at the site. Six weeks were allotted prior to delivery of the final restoration.

Final result — Total: 7 months

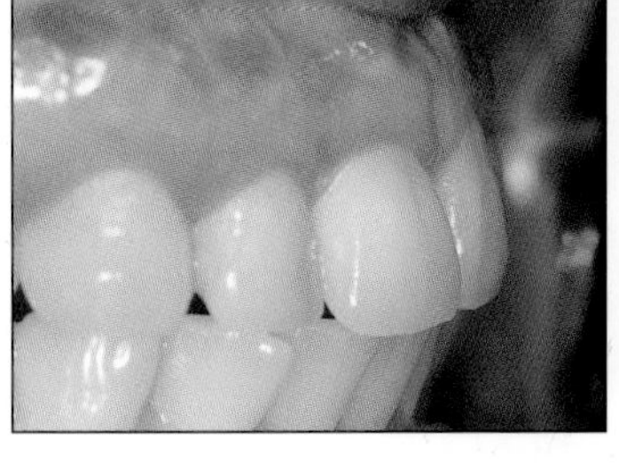
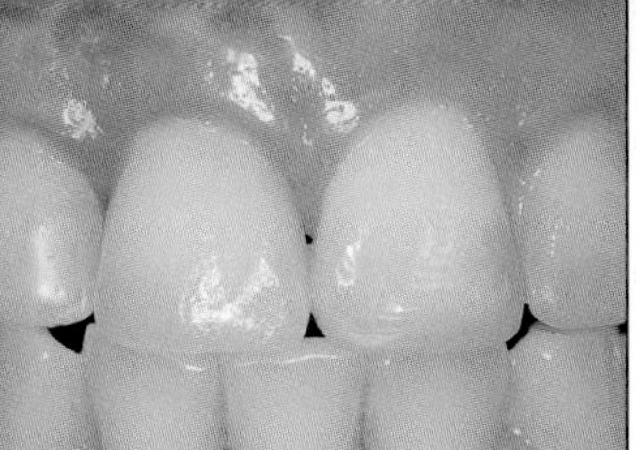

Three surgical procedures and a total treatment time of 7 months were required to successfully replace this failing central incisor with an esthetic implant restoration. The soft tissue edema associated with tooth mobility or, in certain instances, with chronic irritation from an ill-fitting restoration predictably leads to an esthetic soft tissue ridge defect despite the use of ridge preservation at the time of tooth removal. The surgical index procedure facilitated the fabrication of a custom abutment to provide prosthetic-guided soft tissue healing upon exposure of this implant, which was designed to be placed in a nonsubmerged fashion. A submerged approach was possible, however, because of the tissue elasticity provided by the abundant vestibular depth at the site. The final restoration is indistinguishable from the adjacent central incisor, and a pleasing gingival appearance was achieved. (Restoration by Dr Cathy Hamilton, Miami, FL.)

Case 8: Reconstruction of small-volume soft tissue esthetic ridge defect simultaneous with nonsubmerged implant placement

Case history

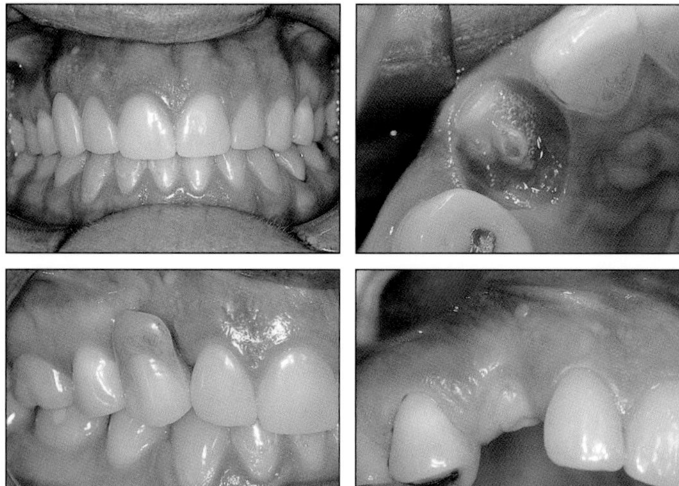

This 30-year-old female patient became frustrated when an implant placed immediately following removal of a fractured maxillary canine failed to achieve osseointegration. The failed implant was removed, and the Bio-Col technique was performed to prepare the site for delayed placement of a second implant. Three months later a small-volume soft tissue esthetic ridge defect was evident. The surgical plan included simultaneous subepithelial connective tissue grafting with nonsubmerged implant placement.

Final site development

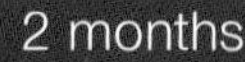

2 months

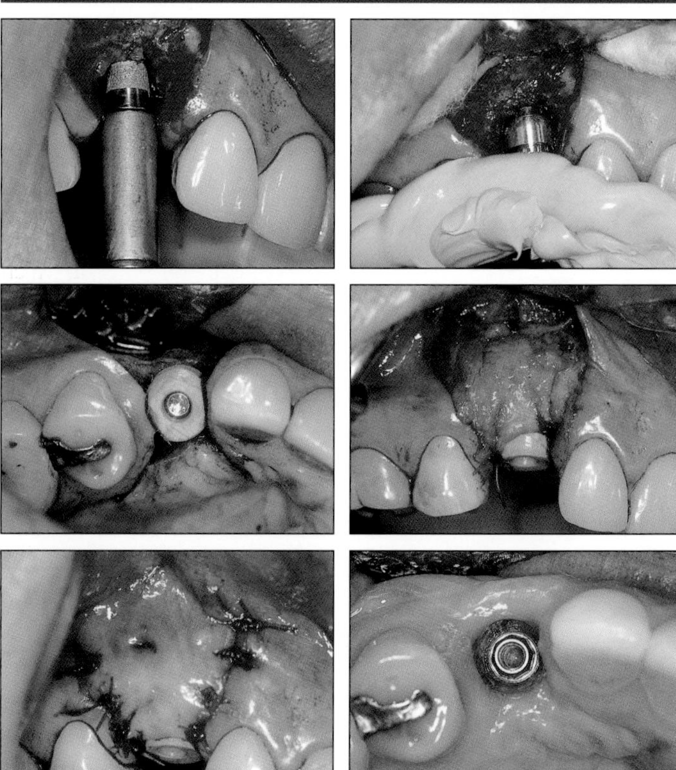

A full-thickness–partial-thickness curvilinear-beveled flap was used to provide access for implant placement and simultaneous soft tissue grafting. After placement of a one-piece nonsubmerged implant, a surgical index was performed, and a custom tooth-form healing abutment was shaped, polished, and delivered. This abutment was used as a scaffold for the connective tissue graft in a similar fashion that a denuded root structure physically supports the graft during root-coverage procedures. After securing the connective tissue graft with a sling suture passed around the healing abutment, the graft was secured to periosteum at the recipient site. The cover flap was coronally advanced, and tension-free closure was obtained. After 2 months of healing, osseointegration was confirmed, and correction of the soft tissue defect was evident.

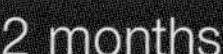

Final site development — 2 months

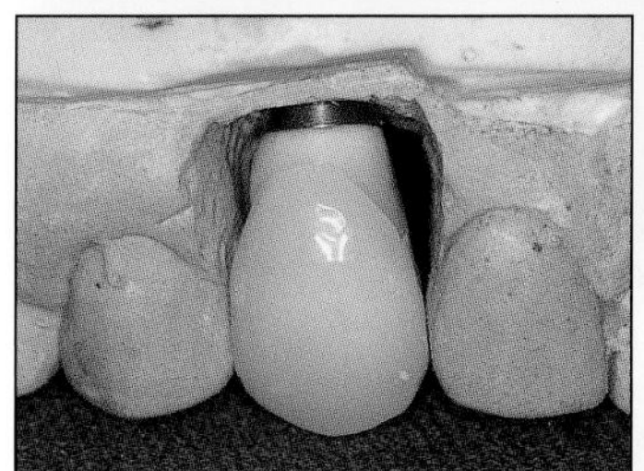

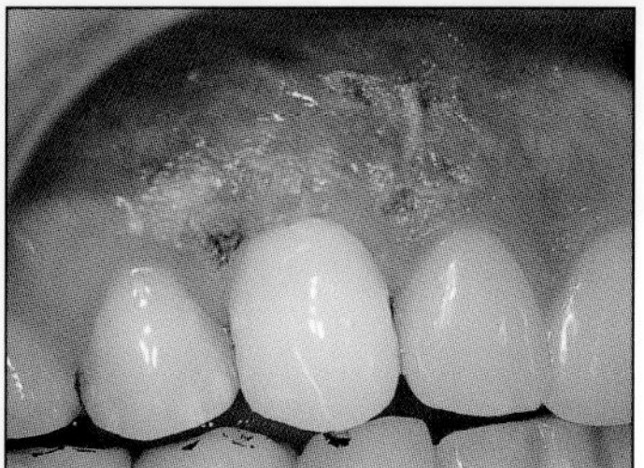

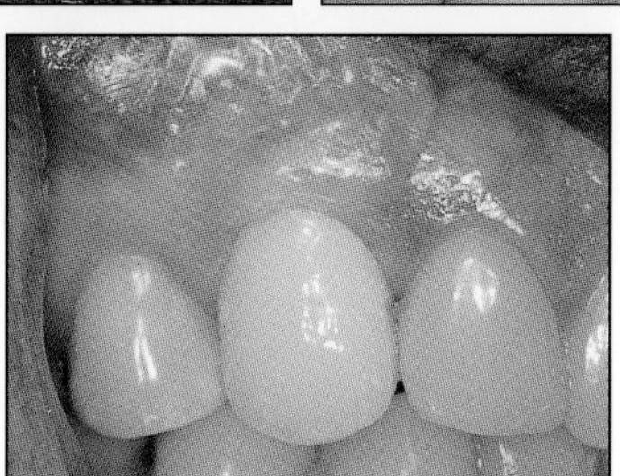

A custom ceramic abutment and provisional restoration were fabricated on the implant analog cast and delivered 2 months after implant placement and simultaneous soft tissue grafting. Laser soft tissue resurfacing was performed to blend the appearance of the soft tissues with the adjacent areas.

Final result — Total: 4 months

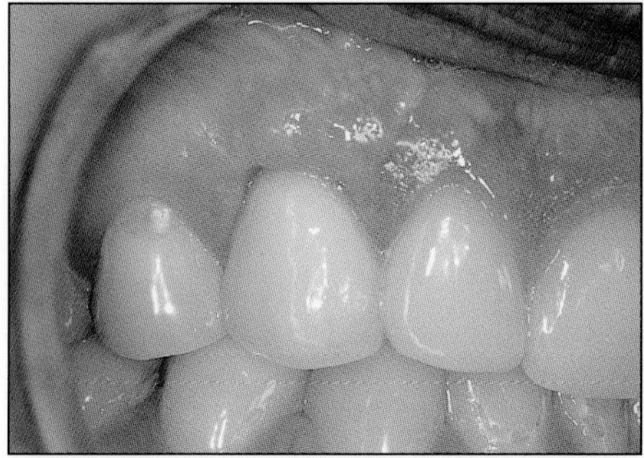

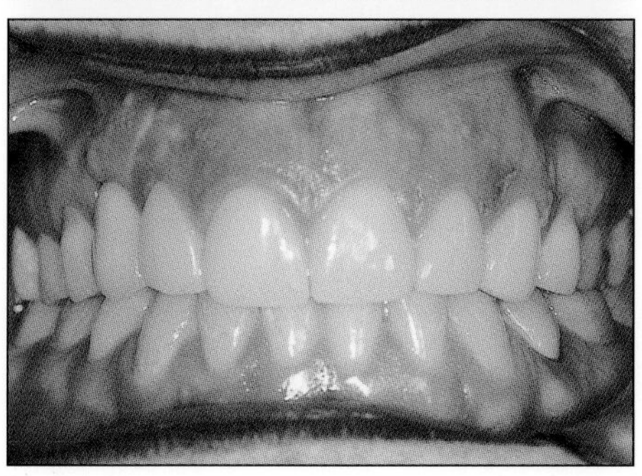

Correction of this small-volume esthetic ridge defect simultaneous with nonsubmerged implant placement with custom tooth-form healing abutment limited the site development to one surgical procedure and one minor laser soft tissue refinement procedure. In light of the previously failed implant, the patient greatly appreciated the reduced total treatment time of 4 months, made possible by simultaneous soft tissue grafting with nonsubmerged implant placment. This result was technically possible because of the abundant vestibular depth in the area, which facilitated coronal advancement of the cover flap and thereby enhanced the predictability of the soft tissue graft. The final result was inconspicuous and duplicated the esthetics that the patient had prior to fracture and loss of her maxillary canine. (Restoration by Dr Manuel Seage, Coral Gables, FL.)

Appendix: Treatment Algorithms for Esthetic Implant Therapy

Esthetic implant therapy can be as simple as removing a failed tooth with immediate replacement and site preservation with the Bio-Col alveolar ridge preservation technique, or as complex as a multidisciplinary approach involving multiple therapeutic modalities, as demonstrated in chapter 7. Although an algorithm for such complex therapy could never include every possible clinical scenario, the series of algorithms presented in this Appendix will lead the implant surgeon to appropriate treatment options for the vast majority of case types encountered in esthetic implant therapy.

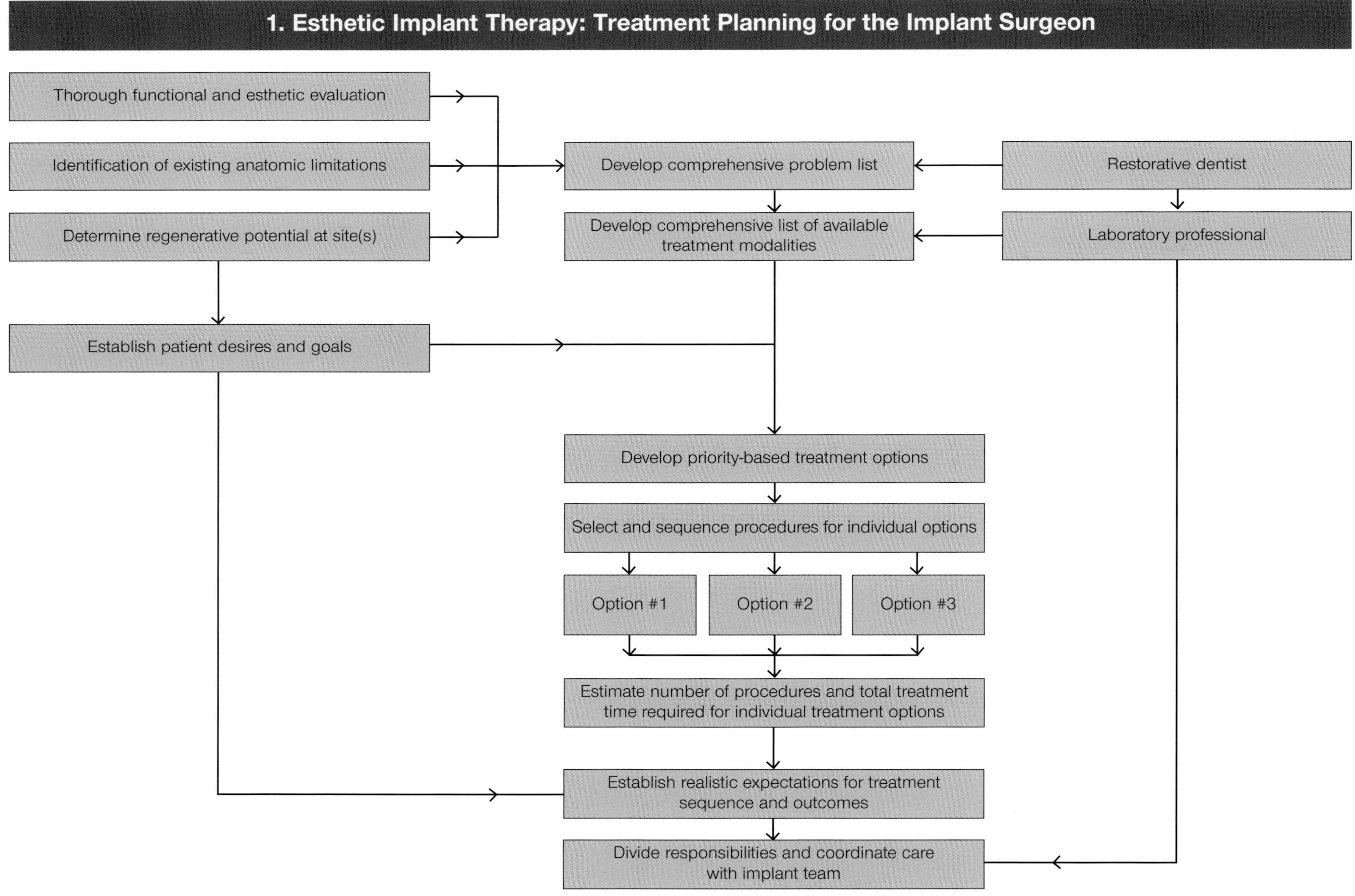
1. Esthetic Implant Therapy: Treatment Planning for the Implant Surgeon
Thorough functional and esthetic evaluation
Identification of existing anatomic limitations
Determine regenerative potential at site(s)
Establish patient desires and goals
Develop comprehensive problem list
Develop comprehensive list of available treatment modalities
Restorative dentist
Laboratory professional
Develop priority-based treatment options
Select and sequence procedures for individual options
Option #1
Option #2
Option #3
Estimate number of procedures and total treatment time required for individual treatment options
Establish realistic expectations for treatment sequence and outcomes
Divide responsibilities and coordinate care with implant team

2. Esthetic Implant Therapy: Special Treatment-Planning Considerations

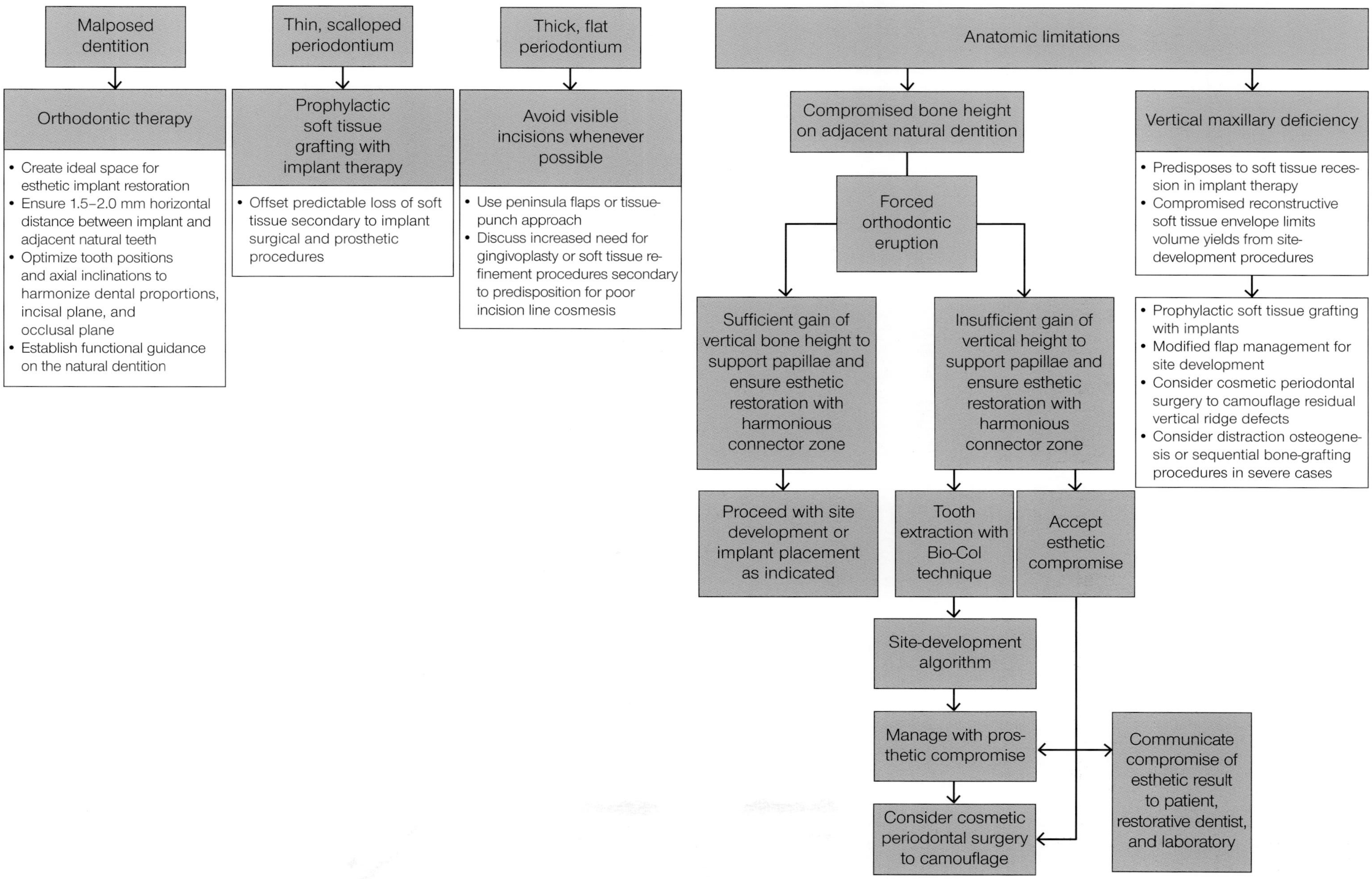

Malposed dentition
→ **Orthodontic therapy**
- Create ideal space for esthetic implant restoration
- Ensure 1.5–2.0 mm horizontal distance between implant and adjacent natural teeth
- Optimize tooth positions and axial inclinations to harmonize dental proportions, incisal plane, and occlusal plane
- Establish functional guidance on the natural dentition

Thin, scalloped periodontium
→ **Prophylactic soft tissue grafting with implant therapy**
- Offset predictable loss of soft tissue secondary to implant surgical and prosthetic procedures

Thick, flat periodontium
→ **Avoid visible incisions whenever possible**
- Use peninsula flaps or tissue-punch approach
- Discuss increased need for gingivoplasty or soft tissue refinement procedures secondary to predisposition for poor incision line cosmesis

Anatomic limitations
→ **Compromised bone height on adjacent natural dentition**
→ **Forced orthodontic eruption**
- → Sufficient gain of vertical bone height to support papillae and ensure esthetic restoration with harmonious connector zone
  - → Proceed with site development or implant placement as indicated
- → Insufficient gain of vertical height to support papillae and ensure esthetic restoration with harmonious connector zone
  - → Tooth extraction with Bio-Col technique → Site-development algorithm → Manage with prosthetic compromise → Consider cosmetic periodontal surgery to camouflage
  - → Accept esthetic compromise → Manage with prosthetic compromise ↔ Communicate compromise of esthetic result to patient, restorative dentist, and laboratory; → Consider cosmetic periodontal surgery to camouflage

→ **Vertical maxillary deficiency**
- Predisposes to soft tissue recession in implant therapy
- Compromised reconstructive soft tissue envelope limits volume yields from site-development procedures

→
- Prophylactic soft tissue grafting with implants
- Modified flap management for site development
- Consider cosmetic periodontal surgery to camouflage residual vertical ridge defects
- Consider distraction osteogenesis or sequential bone-grafting procedures in severe cases

3. Esthetic Implant Therapy: Site Preservation

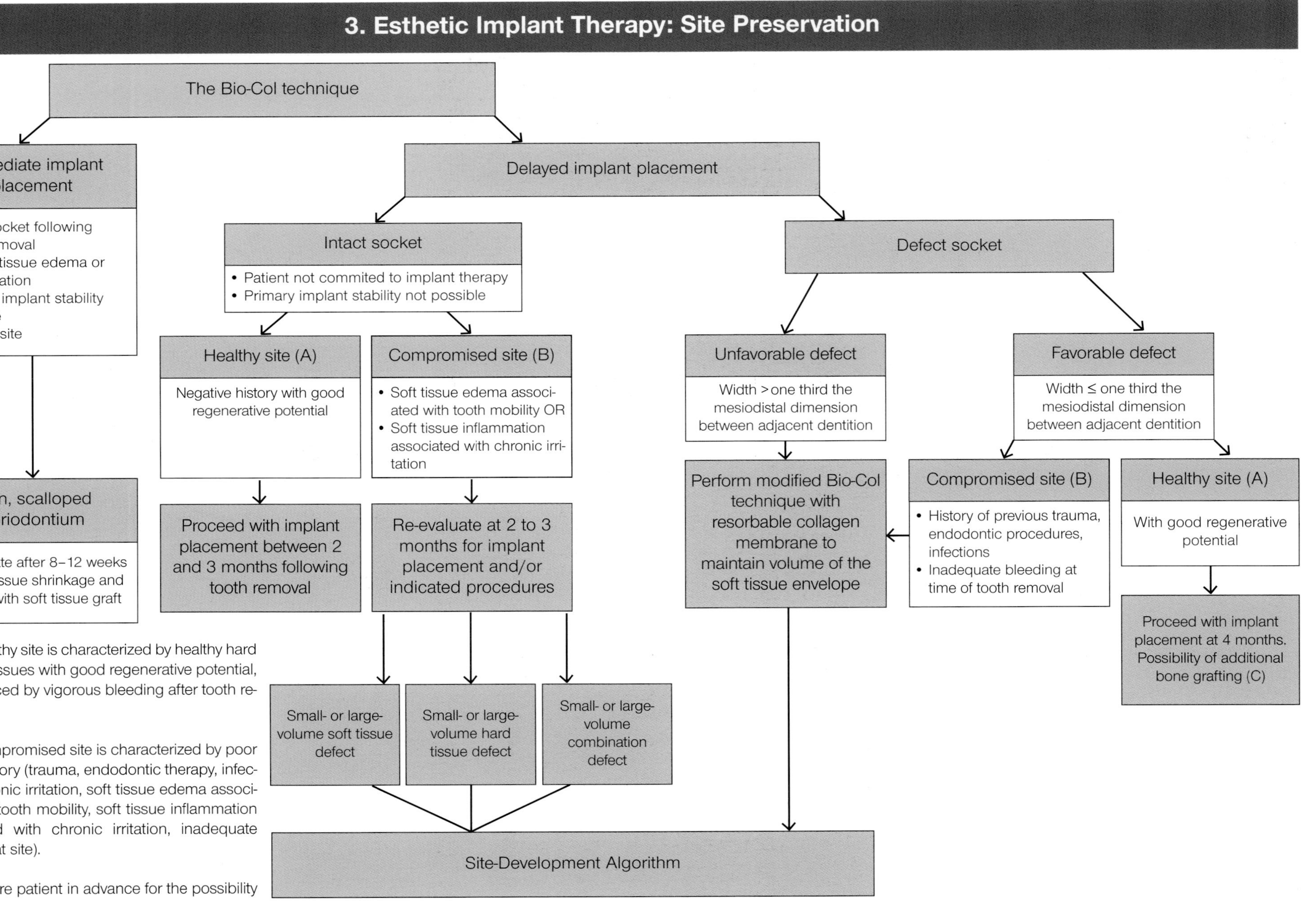

(A) A healthy site is characterized by healthy hard and soft tissues with good regenerative potential, as evidenced by vigorous bleeding after tooth removal.

(B) A compromised site is characterized by poor dental history (trauma, endodontic therapy, infections, chronic irritation, soft tissue edema associated with tooth mobility, soft tissue inflammation associated with chronic irritation, inadequate bleeding at site).

(C) Prepare patient in advance for the possibility that additional bone grafting may be needed if inadequate bone regeneration is discovered upon entry for implant placement.

4. Small-Volume Hard Tissue Ridge Defect

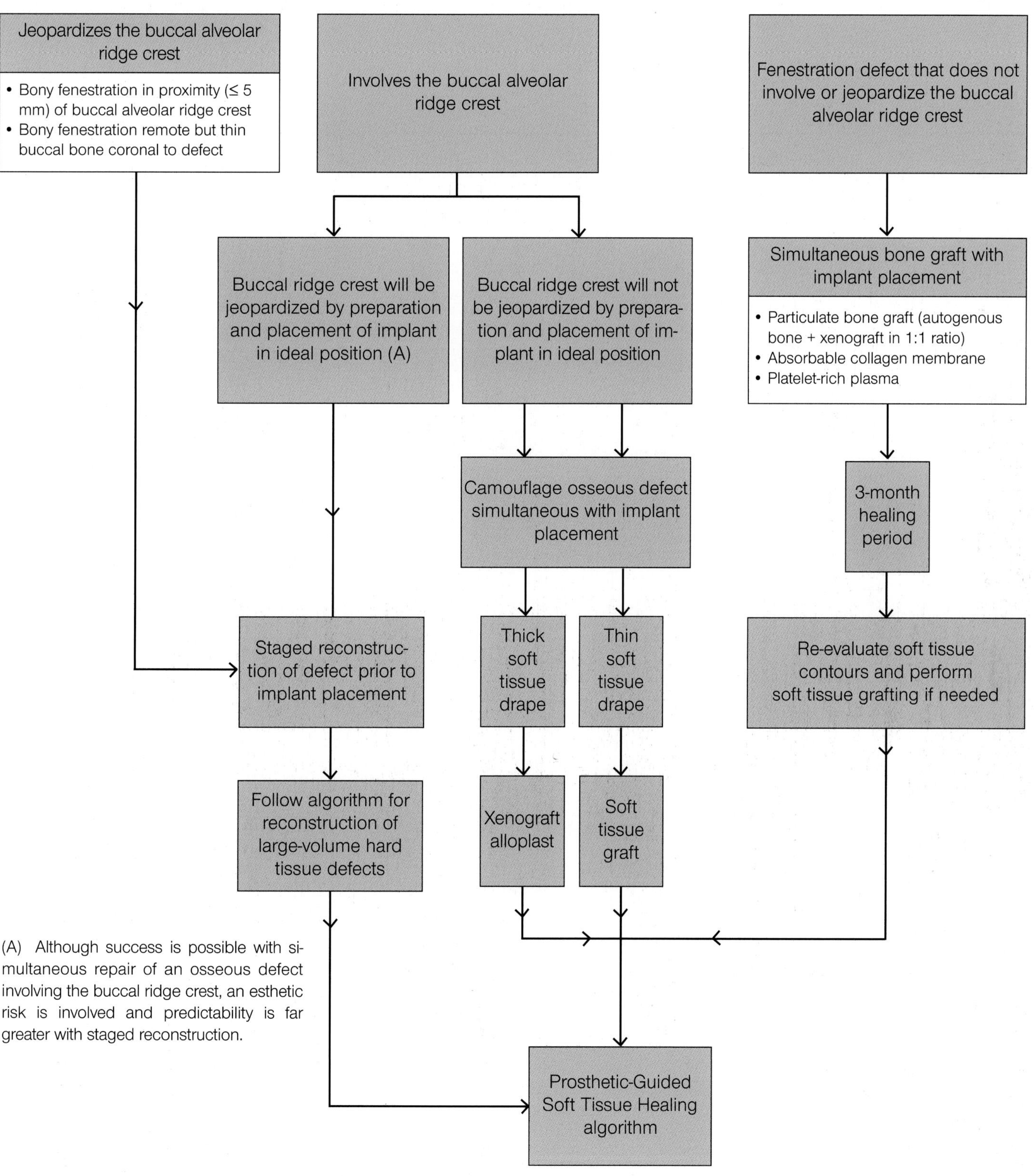

(A) Although success is possible with simultaneous repair of an osseous defect involving the buccal ridge crest, an esthetic risk is involved and predictability is far greater with staged reconstruction.

5. Large-Volume Hard Tissue Esthetic Alveolar Ridge Defect

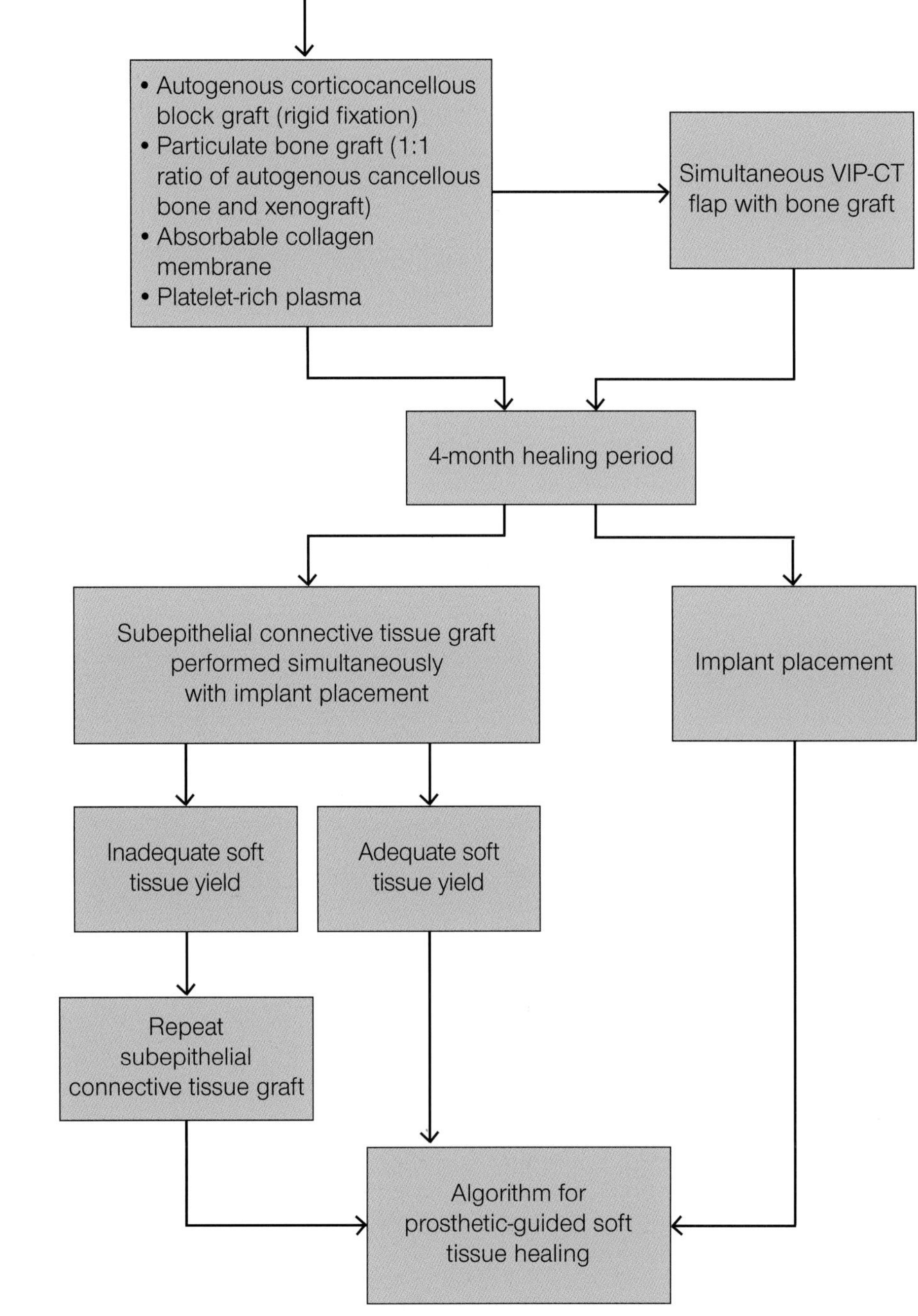

6. Small-Volume Soft Tissue Esthetic Alveolar Ridge Defect

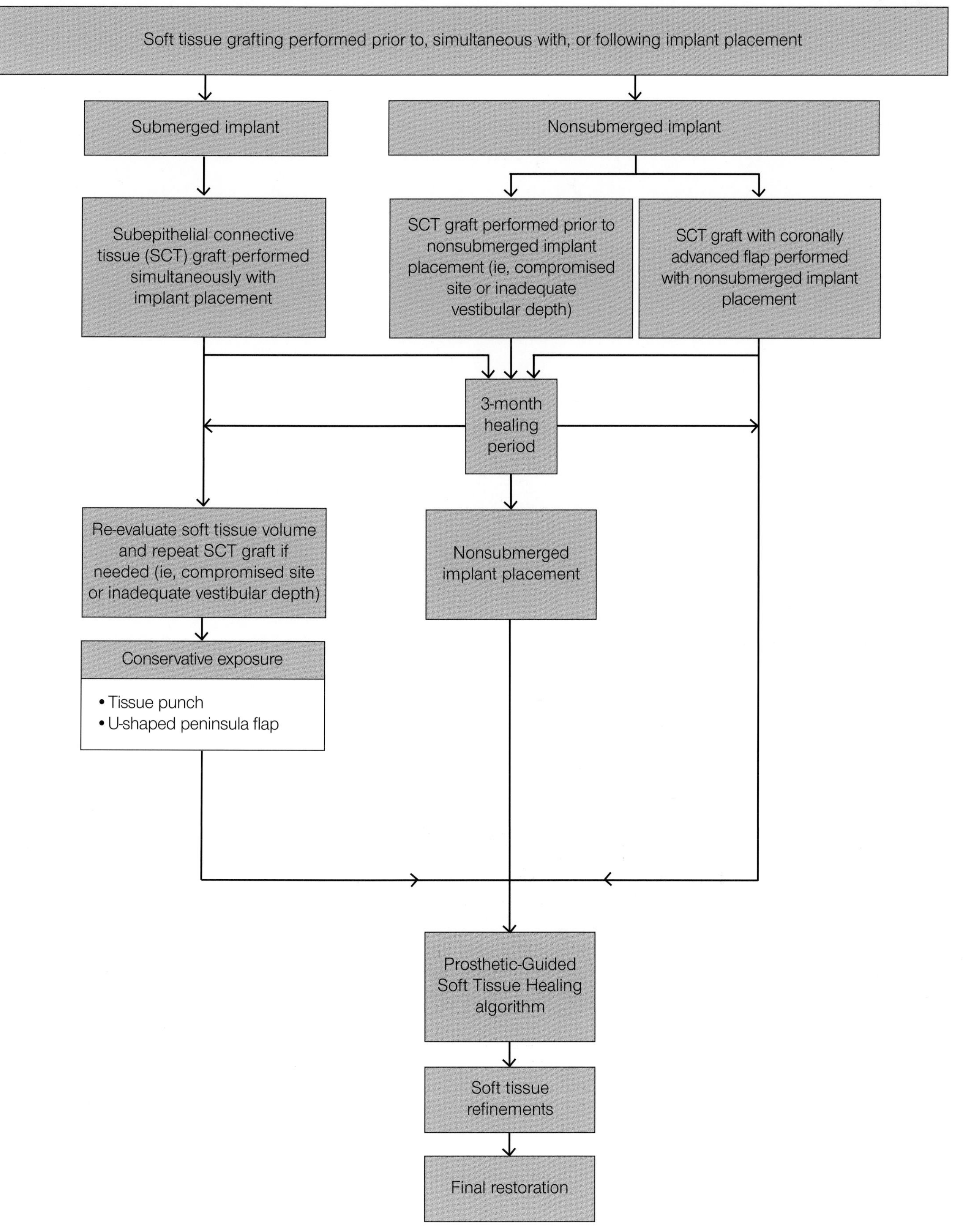

7. Large-Volume Soft Tissue Esthetic Alveolar Ridge Defect

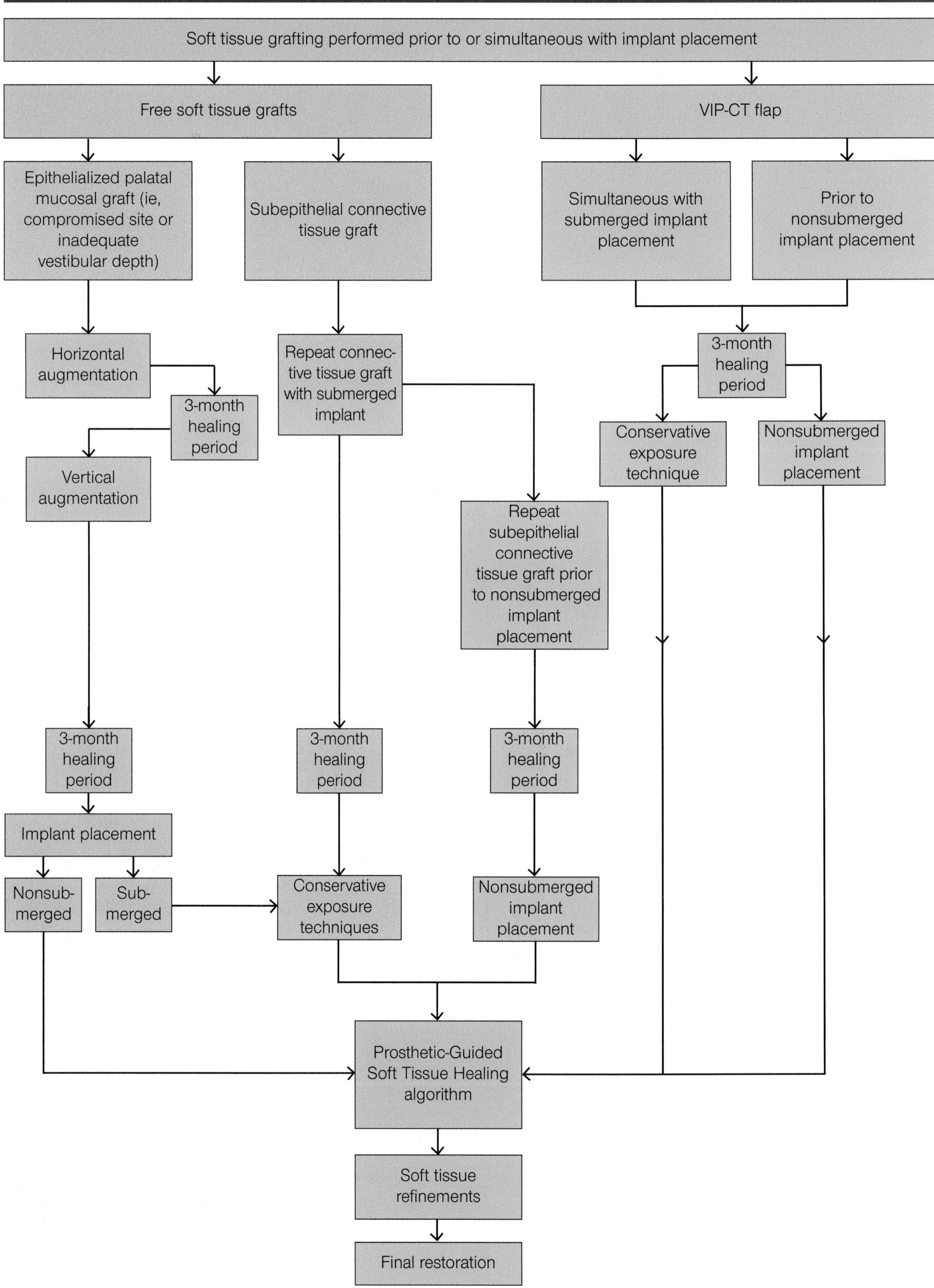

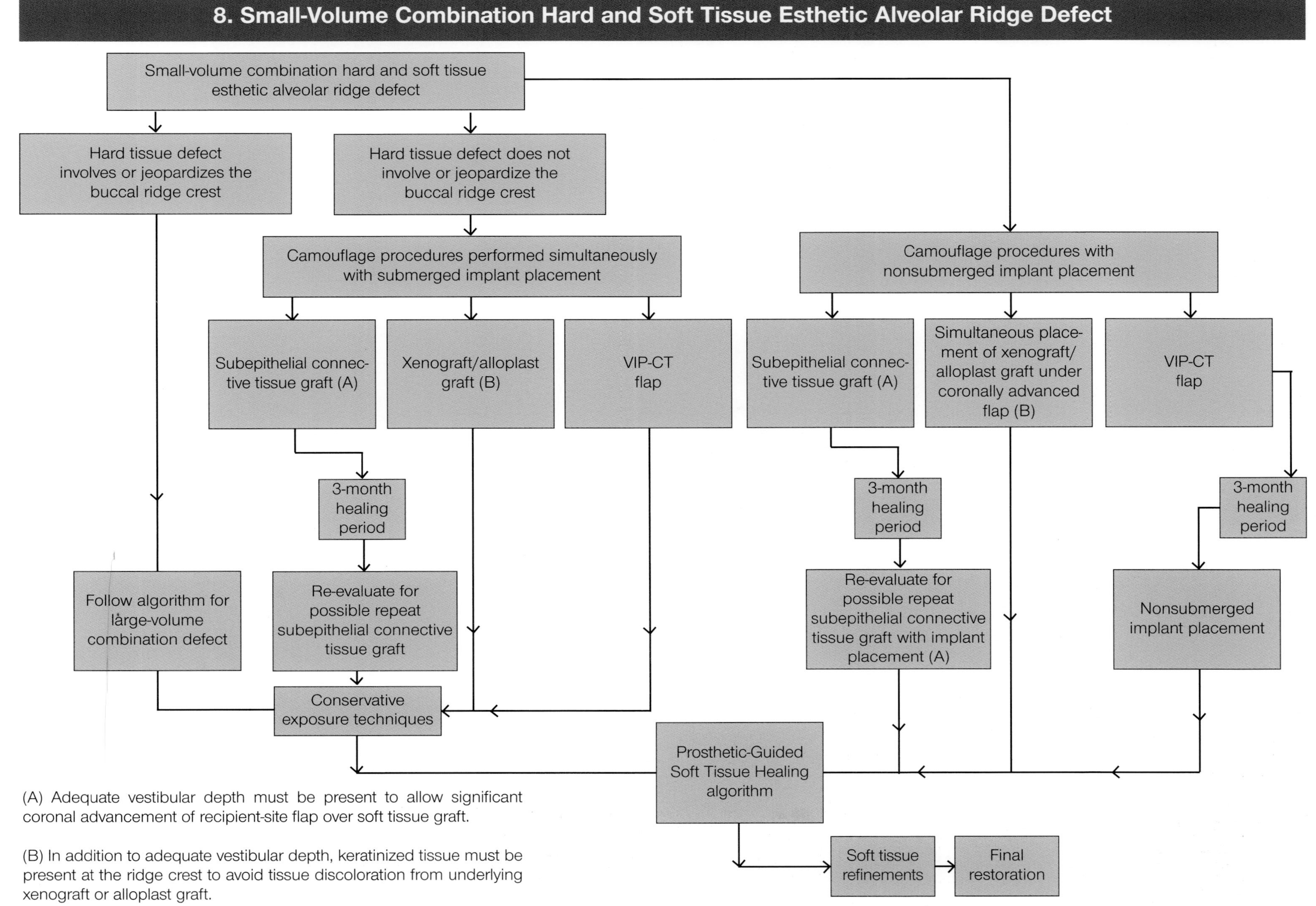

(A) Adequate vestibular depth must be present to allow significant coronal advancement of recipient-site flap over soft tissue graft.

(B) In addition to adequate vestibular depth, keratinized tissue must be present at the ridge crest to avoid tissue discoloration from underlying xenograft or alloplast graft.

9. Large-Volume Combination Hard and Soft Tissue Esthetic Alveolar Ridge Defect

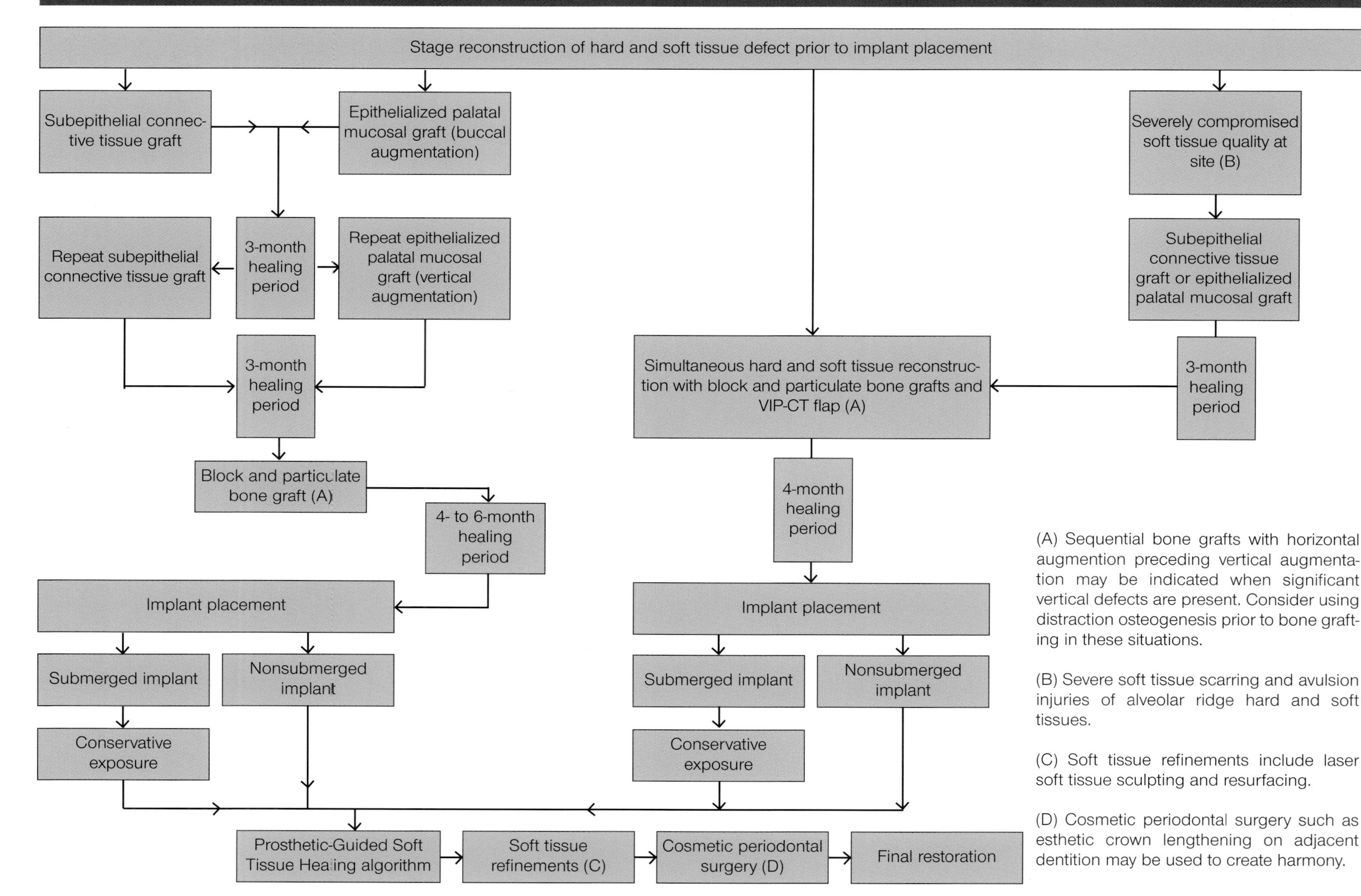

(A) Sequential bone grafts with horizontal augmention preceding vertical augmentation may be indicated when significant vertical defects are present. Consider using distraction osteogenesis prior to bone grafting in these situations.

(B) Severe soft tissue scarring and avulsion injuries of alveolar ridge hard and soft tissues.

(C) Soft tissue refinements include laser soft tissue sculpting and resurfacing.

(D) Cosmetic periodontal surgery such as esthetic crown lengthening on adjacent dentition may be used to create harmony.

10. Prosthetic-Guided Soft Tissue Healing

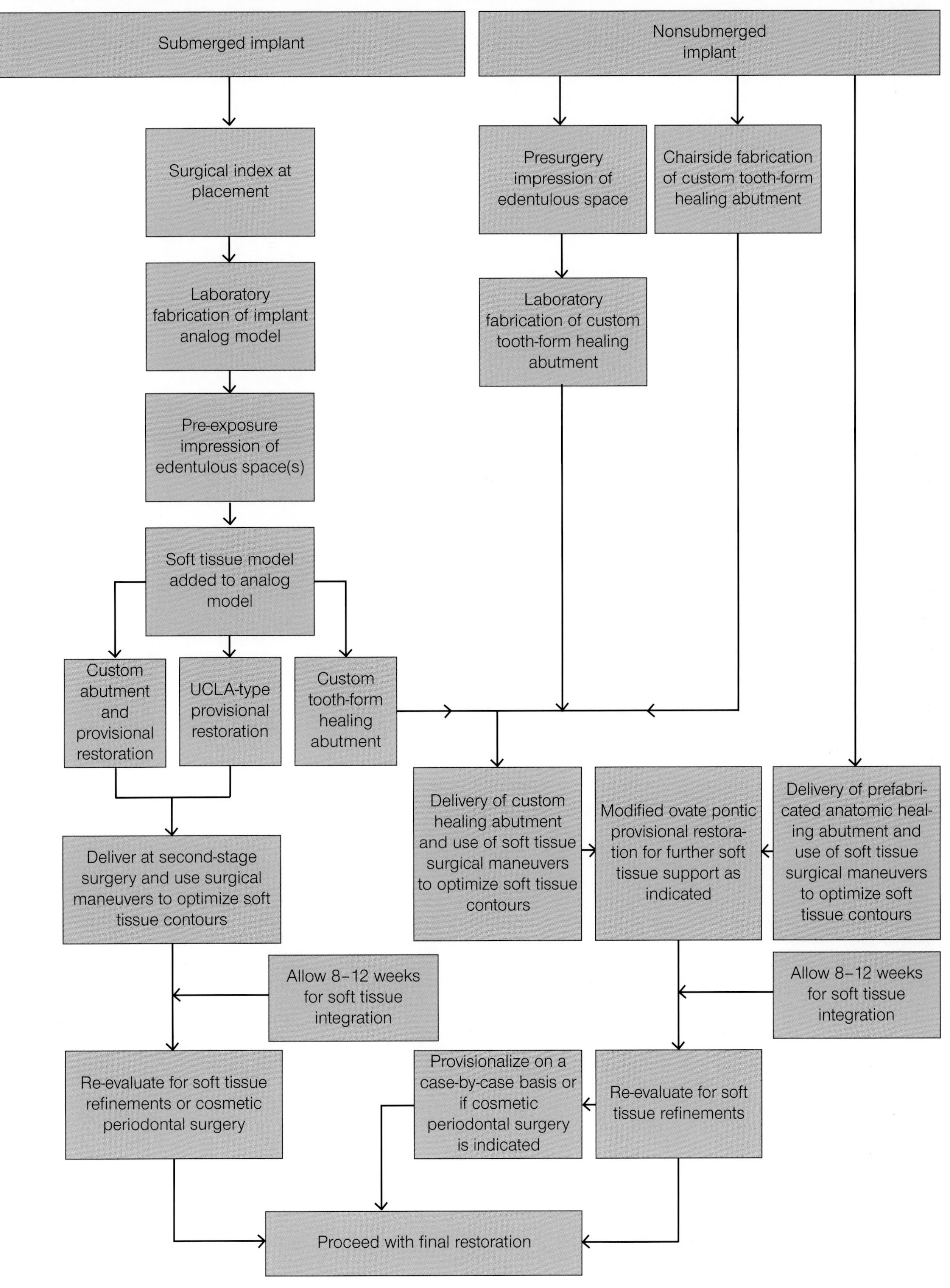

References

Chapter 1

1. Schroeder A, van der Zypen E, Stich H, Sutter F. The reaction of bone, connective tissue, and epithelium to endosteal implants with titanium-sprayed surfaces. J Maxillofac Surg 1981;9:15–25.
2. James RA, Kelln E. A histopathological report on the nature of the epithelium and underlying connective tissue which surround oral implants. J Biomed Mater Res 1974; 8:373–382.
3. Berglundh T, Lindhe J, Ericsson I, Marinello CP, Liljenberg B, Thomsen P. The soft tissue barrier at implants and teeth. Clin Oral Implants Res 1991;2:81–90.
4. Buser D, Weber HP, Donath K, Fiorellini JP, Paquette DW, Williams RC. Soft tissue reactions to non-submerged unloaded titanium implants in beagle dogs. J Periodontol 1992;63:225–235.
5. Berglundh T, Lindhe J, Jonsson K, Ericsson I. The topography of the vascular systems in the periodontal and peri-implant tissues dog. J Clin Periodontol 1994;21:189–193.
6. Berglundh T, Lindhe J. Dimension of the periimplant mucosa. Biological width revisited. J Clin Periodontol 1996; 23:971–973.
7. Abrahamsson I, Berglundh T, Wennström J, Lindhe J. The peri-implant hard and soft tissue characteristics at different implant systems. A comparative study in dogs. Clin Oral Implants Res 1996;7:212–220.
8. Ainamo J, Löe H. Anatomical characteristics of gingiva. A clinical and microscopic study of free and attached gingiva. J Periodontol 1966;37:5–13.
9. Carranza FA Jr, Itoiz ME, Cabrini RL, Dotto CA. A study of periodontal vascularization in different laboratory animals. J Periodontal Res 1966;1:120–128.
10. Kindlova M. The blood supply of the marginal periodontium in Macassus Rhesus. Arch Oral Biol 1965;10:869.
11. Karring T, Löe H. Blood supply of the periodontium. J Periodontal Res 1967;2:74.
12. Hansson BO, Lindhe J, Brånemark PI. Microvascualr topography and function in clinically healthy and chronically inflamed dentogingival tissues—A vital microscopic study in dogs. Periodontics 1968;6:264–271.
13. Carranza FA Jr (ed). Glickman's Clinical Periodontology, ed 5. Philadelphia: Saunders, 1979.
14. Kaplan GB, Pameijer CH, Ruben MP. Scanning electron microscopy of sulcular and junctional epithelia correlated with histology (Part 1). J Periodontol 1977;48:446–451.
15. Kobayashi K, Rose G, Mahan CJ. Ultrastructual histochemistry of the dentoepithelial junction. I. Phosphotungstic acid periodic acid–silver methenamine and periodic acid–thiosemicarbazide–silver proteinate. J Periodontal Res 1977;12:351–367.
16. Lindhe J, Karring T. Anatomy of the periodontium. In: Lindhe J, Karring T, Lang NR (eds). Clinical Periodontology and Implant Dentistry, ed 3. Copenhagen: Munksgaard, 1998.
17. Bauman GR, Rapley JW, Hallmon WW, Mills M. The peri-implant sulcus. Int J Oral Maxillofac Implants 1993;8: 273–280.
18. Meffert R. The soft tissue interface in the dental implantology. Implantologist 1986;5:55.
19. Zarb G, Schmill A. The longitudinal clinical effectiveness of osseointegrated dental implants: The Toronto study. Part 3: Problems and complications encountered. J Prosthet Dent 1990;64:185–194.
20. Mericske-Stern R. Clinical evaluation of overdenture restorations supported by osseointegrated titanium implants: A retrospective study. Int J Oral Maxillofac Implants 1990;5: 375–383.
21. Wennstrom J, Bengazi F, Lekholm U. The influence of the masticatory mucosa on the peri-implant soft tissue condition. Clin Oral Implants Res 1994;5:1–8.
22. Silverstein LH, Lefkove MD, Garnick JJ. The use of free gingival soft tissue to improve the implant/soft tissue interface. J Oral Implantol 1994;20:36–40.
23. Silverstein LH, Lefkove MD. The use of the subepithelial connective tissue graft to enhance both the aesthetics and periodontal contours surrounding dental implants. J Oral Implantol 1994;20:135–138.
24. Alpert A. A rationale for attached tissue at the soft tissue/ implant interface: Esthetic and functional dictates. Compend Contin Educ Dent 1994:15:356–366.

25. Artzi Z, Tal H, Moses O, Kozlovsky A. Muscosal considerations for osseointegrated implants. J Prosthet Dent 1993; 70:427–432.
26. Sclar AG. Use of the epithelialized palatal graft with dental implants in soft tissue esthetic procedures for teeth and implants. Oral Maxillofac Surg Clin North Am 1999;7:79–94.
27. Orban B, Kohler J. The physiologic gingival sulcus. Z Stomatol 1924;2:353.
28. Gottlieb B. Der Epithelansatz am Zahne. Dtsch Monatsschr Zahnhk 1921;39:142.
29. Waerhaug J. The gingival pocket. Odontol Tidskr 1952;60 (Suppl 1).
30. Orban B, et al. The epithelial attachment (the attached epithelial cuff). J Periodontol 1956;27:167.
31. Sicher H. Changing concepts of the supporting dental structure. Oral Surg Oral Med Oral Pathol 1959;12:31–35.
32. Stallard RE, Diab MA, Zandewr HA. The attaching substance between enamel and epithelium—A product of the epithelial cells. J Periodontol 1965;36:40.
33. Ussing MJ. The development of the epithelial attachment. Acta Odontol Scand 1956;13:123.
34. Waerhaug J. Current views on the epithelial cuff. Periodontics 1966;4:278.
35. Gargiulo AW, Wentz FM, Orban B. Dimensions and relations of the dentogingival junction in humans. J Periodontol 1961; 32:261.
36. Vacek JS, Gher ME, Assas DA, Richardson AC, Giambiaressi LI. The dimensions of the human dentogingival junction. Int J Periodontics Restorative Dent 1994;14:155–165.
37. Ingber JS, Rose LF, Coslet JG. The "biologic width"—A concept in periodontics and restorative dentistry. Alpha Omegan 1977;10:62–65.
38. Block PL. Restorative margins and periodontal health: A new look at an old perspective. J Prosthet Dent 1987;57:683–689.
39. Nevins M, Skurow HM. The intracrevicular restorative margin, the biologic width, and the maintenance of the gingival margin. Int J Periodontics Restorative Dent 1984;4:30–49.
40. Maynard JG, Wilson RD. Physiological dimensions of the periodontium significant to the restorative dentist. J Periodontol 1979;50:170–174.
41. Fugazzotto PA. Periodontal restorative interrelationships: The isolated restoration. J Am Dent Assoc 1985;110:915–917.
42. Sivers JE, Johnson GK. Periodontal and restorative considerations for crown lengthening. Quintessence Int 1985;16: 833–836.
43. Berglundh T, Lindhe J, Ericsson I, Marinello CP, Liljenberg B. Experimental breakdown of the peri-implant and periodontal tissues. A study in the beagle dog. Clin Oral Implants Res 1992;3:9–16.
44. Weber HP, Buser D, Donath K, et al. Comparison of healed tissues adjacent to submerged and non-submerged unloaded titanium dental implants. A histometric study in beagle dogs. Clin Oral Implants Res 1996;7:11–19.
45. Hürzeler MB, Quiñones CR, Schüpbach P, Vlassis JM, Strub JR, Caffesse RG. Influence of the superstructure of the peri-implant tissues in beagle dogs. Clin Oral Implants Res 1995; 6:139–148.
46. Chehroudi B, Gould TR, Brunette DM. The role of connective tissue in inhibiting epithelial downgrowth on titanium-coated percutaneous implants. J Biomed Mater Res 1992;26: 493–515.
47. Abrahamsson I, Berglundh T, Glantz PO, Lindhe J. The mucosal attachment at different abutments. An experimental study in dogs. J Clin Periodontol 1998;25:721–727.
48. Cochran DL, Hernman JS, Schenk RK, Higginbottom FL, Buder D. Biologic width around titanium implants. A histometric analysis of the implanto-gingival junction around unloaded and loaded non-submerged implants in the canine mandible. J Periodontol 1997;68:186–198.

Chapter 2

1. Chiche G, Pinault A. Artistic and scientific principles applied to esthetic dentistry. In: Chiche G, Pinault A (eds). Esthetics of Anterior Fixed Prosthodontics. Chicago: Quintessence, 1994:13–32.
2. Chiche G, Pinault A. Replacement of deficient crowns. In: Chiche G, Pinault A (eds). Esthetics of Anterior Fixed Prosthodontics. Chicago: Quintessence, 1994:53–74.
3. Levin EI. Dental esthetics and the golden proportion. J Prosthet Dent 1978;40:244–252.
4. Morley J. Smile design—Specific considerations. J Calif Dent Assoc 1997;25:633–637.
5. Olsson M, Lindhe J. Periodontal characteristics in individuals with varying form of the upper central incisors. J Clin Periodontol 1991;18:78–82.
6. Tarnow DP, Magner AW, Fletcher P. The effect of the distance from the contact point to the crest of bone on the presence or absence of the interproximal dental papilla. J Periodontol 1992;63:995–996.
7. Sullivan HC, Atkins JH. Free autogenous gingival grafts. III. Utilization of grafts in the treatment of gingival recession. Periodontics 1968;6:152–160.
8. Miller PD Jr. A classification of marginal tissue recession. Int J Periodontics Restorative Dent 1985;5(2):8–13.
9. Pasquinelli KL. The histology of new attachment utilizing a thick autogenous soft tissue graft in an area of deep recession: A case report. Int J Periodontics Restorative Dent 1995; 15:248–257.
10. Allen EP, Gainza CS, Farthing GC, Newbold DA. Improved technique for localized ridge augmentation: A report of 21 cases. J Periodontol 1985;56:195–199.

Chapter 3

1. Brånemark P-I, Zarb GA, Albrektsson T. Tissue-Integrated Prostheses: Osseintegration in Clinical Dentistry. Chicago: Quintessence, 1985:211–240.
2. Buser D, Dahlin C, Schenk RK. Guided-Bone Regeneration in Implant Dentistry. Chicago: Quintessence, 1984:207–233.
3. Palacci P, Ericsson I, Engstrand P, Rangert B. Optimal Implant Positioning & Soft Tissue Management for the Brånemark System. Chicago: Quintessence, 1995:59–70.

Chapter 4

1. Lekovic V, Kenney EB, Weinlaender M, et al. A bone regeneration approach to alveolar ridge maintenance following tooth extraction: Report of 10 cases. J Periodontol 1997;68:563–570.
2. Lang N, Becker W, Karring T. Alveolar bone formation. In: Lindhe J (ed). Textbook of Clinical Periodontology and Implant Dentistry, ed 3. Copenhagen: Munksgaard, 1998:906–932.

3. Clokie C. Material presented at the scientific sessions of the Canadian Association of Oral and Maxillofacial Surgery, Vancouver, 16 July 1998.
4. Lekovic V, Camargo PM, Klokkevold PR, et al. Preservation of alveolar bone in extraction sockets using bioabsorbable membranes. J Periodontol 1998;69:1044–1049.
5. Warrer K, Gotfredsen K, Hjorting-Hansen E, Karring T. Guided tissue regeneration ensures osseointegration of dental implants placed into extraction sockets. An experimental study in monkeys. Clin Oral Implants Res 1991;2:166–171.
6. Becker W, Becker B, Handelsman M, Oshsenbein C, Albrektsson T. Guided tissue regeneration for implants placed into extraction sockets: A study in dogs. J Periodontol 1991;62:703–709.
7. Klinge B, Alberius P, Isaksson S, et al. Osseous response to implanted natural bone mineral and synthetic hydroxylapatite ceramic in the repair of experimental skull bone defects. J Oral Maxillofac Surg 1992;50:241–249.
8. Wetzel AC, Stich H, Caffese RG. Bone apposition onto oral implants in the sinus area filled with different grafting materials: A histological study in beagle dogs. Clin Oral Implants Res 1995;6:155–163.
9. Valentini P, Abensur D. Maxillary sinus floor elevation for implant placement with demineralized freeze-dried bone and bovine bone (Bio-Oss): A clinical study of 20 patients. Int J Periodontics Restorative Dent 1997;17:232–241.
10. Valentini P, Abensur D, Densari D, et al. Histological evaluation of Bio-Oss in a 2-stage sinus floor elevation and implantation procedure: A human case report. Clin Oral Implants Res 1998;9:59–64.
11. Haas R, Mailath G, Dortbudak O, Watzek G. Bovine hydroxyapatite for maxillary sinus augmentation: Analysis of interfacial bond strength of dental implants using pull-out tests. Clin Oral Implants Res 1998;9:117–122.
12. Berglundh T, Lindhe J. Healing around implants placed in bone defects treated with Bio-Oss: An experimental study in the dog. Clin Oral Implants Res 1997;8:117–124.
13. Boyne PA. The use of particulate bone grafts as barriers, eliminating the use of membranes in guided tissue regeneration. Atlas Oral Maxillofac Surg Clin North Am 2001:9;485–491.

Chapter 5

1. Friedman N. Mucogingival surgery. Tex Dent J 1959;75: 358–362.
2. Miller PD Jr. Regenerative and reconstructive periodontal plastic surgery. Mucogingival surgery. Dent Clin North Am 1988;32:287–306.
3. Wennström JL. Mucogingival surgery. In: Lang NP, Karring T (eds). Proceedings of the 1st European Workshop on Periodontology. London: Quintessence, 1994:193–209.
4. Maynard JG Jr, Wilson RD. Physiologic dimensions of the periodontium significant to the restorative dentist. J Periodontol 1979;50:170–174.
5. Bauman GR, Rapley JW, Hallmon WW, et al. The peri-implant sulcus. Int J Oral Maxillofac Implants 1993;8: 273–280.
6. Meffert R. The soft tissue interface in dental implantology. Implantologist 1986;5:55–58.
7. Lang NP, Löe H. The relationship between the width of keratinized gingiva and gingival health. J Periodontol 1972;43: 623–627.
8. Karring T, Ostergaard E, Löe H. Conservation of tissue specificity after heterotopic transplantation of gingiva and alveolar mucosa. J Periodontal Res 1971;6:282–293.
9. Abrams L. Augmentation of the deformed residual edentulous ridge for fixed prosthesis. Compend Contin Educ Dent 1980;1:205–214.
10. Scharf DR, Tarnow DP. Modified roll technique for localized alveolar ridge augmentation. Int J Periodontics Restorative Dent 1992;12:415–425.
11. Reikie DF. Restoring gingival harmony around single tooth implants. J Prosthet Dent 1995;74:47–50.
12. Sullivan HC, Atkins JH. Free autogenous gingival grafts, I. Principles of successful grafting. Periodontics 1968;6(3): 121–129.
13. Gordon HP, Sullivan HC, Atkins JH. Free autogenous gingival grafts, II. Supplemental findings—histology of the graft site. Periodontics 1968;6(3):130–133.
14. Sullivan HC, Atkins JH. Free autogenous gingival grafts, III. Utilization of grafts in the treatment of gingival recession. Periodontics 1968;6(4):152–160.
15. Langer B, Calagna L. The subepithelial connective tissue graft: A new approach to the enhancement of anterior cosmetics. Int J Periodontics Restorative Dent 1982;2(2):23–34.
16. Reiser C, Bruno JF, Mahan PE, Larkin LH. The subepithelial connective tissue graft palatal donor site: Anatomic considerations for surgeons. Int J Periodontics Restorative Dent 1996;16:131–137.

Chapter 6

1. Axhausen W. The osteogenic phases of regeneration of bone. A historical and experiemental study. J Bone Joint Surg Am 1956;38:593.

Index

Page numbers followed by "f" denote figures; those followed by "t" denote tables